Handbook of AI-Based Models in Healthcare and Medicine

This handbook provides thorough, in-depth, and well-focused developments of artificial intelligence (AI), machine learning (ML), deep learning (DL), natural language processing (NLP), cryptography, and blockchain approaches, along with their applications focused on healthcare systems.

Handbook of AI-Based Models in Healthcare and Medicine: Approaches, Theories, and Applications highlights different approaches, theories, and applications of intelligent systems from a practical as well as a theoretical view of the healthcare domain. It uses a medically oriented approach in its discussions of human biology, healthcare, and medicine and presents NLP-based medical reports and medicine enhancements. The handbook includes advanced models of ML and DL for the management of healthcare systems and also discusses blockchain-based healthcare management. In addition, the handbook offers use cases where AI, ML, and DL can help solve healthcare complications.

Undergraduate and postgraduate students, academicians, researchers, and industry professionals who have an interest in understanding the applications of ML/DL in the healthcare setting will want this reference on their bookshelf.

Artificial Intelligence in Smart Healthcare Systems

Series Editors: Vishal Jain and Jyotir Moy Chatterjee

The progress of the healthcare sector is incremental as it learns from associations between data over time through the application of suitable big data and IoT frameworks and patterns. Many healthcare service providers are employing IoT-enabled devices for monitoring patient healthcare, but their diagnosis and prescriptions are instance-specific only. However, these IoT-enabled healthcare devices are generating volumes of data (Big-IoT Data), that can be analyzed for more accurate diagnosis and prescriptions. A major challenge in the above realm is the effective and accurate learning of unstructured clinical data through the application of precise algorithms. Incorrect input data leading to erroneous outputs with false positives shall be intolerable in healthcare as patient's lives are at stake. This new book series addresses various aspects of how smart healthcare can be used to detect and analyze diseases, the underlying methodologies, and related security concerns. Healthcare is a multidisciplinary field that involves a range of factors like the financial system, social factors, health technologies, and organizational structures that affect the healthcare provided to individuals, families, institutions, organizations, and populations. The goals of healthcare services include patient safety, timeliness, effectiveness, efficiency, and equity. Smart healthcare consists of m-health, e-health, electronic resource management, smart and intelligent home services, and medical devices. The Internet of Things (IoT) is a system comprising real-world things that interact and communicate with each other via networking technologies. The wide range of potential applications of IoT includes healthcare services. IoT-enabled healthcare technologies are suitable for remote health monitoring, including rehabilitation, assisted ambient living, etc. In turn, healthcare analytics can be applied to the data gathered from different areas to improve healthcare at a minimum expense.

This new book series is designed to be a first choice reference at university libraries, academic institutions, research and development centres, information technology centres, and any institutions interested in using, design, modelling, and analysing intelligent healthcare services. Successful application of deep learning frameworks to enable meaningful, cost-effective personalized healthcare services is the primary aim of the healthcare industry in the present scenario. However, realizing this goal requires effective understanding, application, and amalgamation of IoT, Big Data and several other computing technologies to deploy such systems in an effective manner. This series shall help clarify the understanding of certain key mechanisms and technologies helpful in realizing such systems.

Designing Intelligent Healthcare Systems, Products, and Services Using Disruptive Technologies and Health Informatics
Teena Bagga, Kamal Upreti, Nishant Kumar, Amirul Hasan Ansari, and Danish Nadeem

Next Generation Healthcare Systems Using Soft Computing Techniques
D.Rekh Ram Janghel, Rohit Raja, and Korhan Cengiz

Immersive Virtual and Augmented Reality in Healthcare: An IoT and Blockchain Perspective
Rajendra Kumar, Vishal Jain, Garry Han, and Abderezak Touzene

Handbook on Augmenting Telehealth Services: Using Artificial Intelligence
Edited by Sonali Vyas, Sunil Gupta, Monit Kapoor, and Samiya Khan

Machine Learning in Healthcare and Security: Advances, Obstacles, and Solutions
Edited by Prashant Pranav, Archana Patel, and Sarika Jain

Handbook of AI-Based Models in Healthcare and Medicine

Approaches, Theories, and Applications

Edited by
Bhanu Chander, Koppala Guravaiah,
B. Anoop, and G. Kumaravelan

CRC Press
Taylor & Francis Group
Boca Raton London New York

CRC Press is an imprint of the
Taylor & Francis Group, an **informa** business

First edition published 2024
by CRC Press
2385 NW Executive Center Drive, Suite 320, Boca Raton FL 33431

and by CRC Press
4 Park Square, Milton Park, Abingdon, Oxon, OX14 4RN

CRC Press is an imprint of Taylor & Francis Group, LLC

ISBN: 978-1-032-41915-2 (hbk)
ISBN: 978-1-032-42588-7 (pbk)
ISBN: 978-1-003-36336-1 (ebk)

DOI: 10.1201/9781003363361

Typeset in Times
by Deanta Global Publishing Services, Chennai, India

Contents

Preface

Artificial intelligence (AI), machine learning (ML), and deep learning (DL) have boosted the healthcare sector with their pioneering systematic approaches, which are accurate and relevant to the collection of tasks. The situation transformed even further with the recent COVID-19 pandemic. During the pandemic disaster, we saw a tremendous digital transformation, with the acceptance of disruptive machinery across different fields, with healthcare being one of them. Thus, people now make the highest priority of health, regardless of cost, making the health industry more prominent. Hence, the attention of the healthcare sector is on improving the health of people, lowering the price of health tests and care, and improving the patient experience.

In this context, AI progressively assists in noticing hidden insights into clinical decision-making, linking individuals with intelligent devices for self-management, extracting meaning from distant and unstructured data assets, remotely treating patients, and into drug discovery. ML is highly employed in the medical imaging field and facilitates several services like computer-aided analysis, X-rays, computerized tomography (CT) scans, magnetic resonance imaging (MRIs), and other image-guided therapy. DL builds on mathematical models that allow the healthcare sector to analyze data at exceptional speeds with high accuracy. It continues to make inroads into the industry. These technologies are connected, providing something different to the industry and changing how medical professionals manage their roles and patient care.

This book delivers a high-level understanding of healthcare and medicine applications for emerging technologies such as AI, ML, and DL, by covering innovative advances, concepts, and persistent challenges. In addition, the book also offers potential use cases where AI, ML, and DL can help solve malicious healthcare complications.

Chapter 1 explores the use of edge computing in healthcare. The chapter explores how to use edge computing technology to process the large amount of data generated by medical devices, electronic health records, and other sources locally, at or near the point of care, to reduce the latency associated with transmitting data to remote servers or data centres.

Chapter 2 examines the landscape of artificial intelligence within the current medical curriculum and makes an effort to understand how it can affect both current healthcare and the practice of medicine in the future.

Chapter 3 provides a deeper view of the current trends in AI-driven drug discovery, and how explainable AI is reinforcing the results from such machine intelligence concepts. The possible challenges that are perceived and how they need to be handled while introducing AI to the drug discovery practice are also included.

Chapter 4 performs a detailed study of a cirrhosis dataset. The outliers and missing values are detected through visualization, and they are handled through statistical imputation. In addition, unsupervised feature selection algorithms extra trees classifier and recursive feature elimination, and machine learning models logistic regression, decision tree, multilayer perceptron, AdaBoost, random forest, and XGBoost are used.

Chapter 5 aims to focus on the imaging techniques and principles of computed tomography, their main drawbacks, and the motivation behind deep learning-based 3D reconstruction. Details on the three techniques of volumetric reconstruction from two-dimensional X-ray images are covered and followed by a conclusion.

Chapter 6 discusses how X-ray imaging is one of the most popular diagnostic imaging techniques that plays a critical role in the diagnosis and treatment process. Proposed GAN-MLC, a CNN-LSTM description generator model for multi-label classification of X-ray images. In addition the proposed GAN-MLC will improve the feature learning for capturing disease-specific findings.

Chapter 7 and Chapter 10 present a curated selection of various machine learning and deep learning-based diabetic retinopathy (DR) detection models. The Chapter 7 review includes models for binary and multistage DR classification as well as detection and segmentation of four main lesions – namely microaneurysms, hemorrhages, cotton wool spots, and hard exudates. These DR-CAD systems can allow automatic detection of DR at an early stage, which allows the control of progressive damage to the retina. On the other hand, Chapter 10 provides an innovative and effective deep learning architecture for segmentation that makes use of U-Net as its major module and proposes RetinalAlexU-Net.

Chapter 8 illustrates deep learning methods to identify and categorize breast cancer from multi-modality images, namely mammogram, histopathology, magnetic resonance imaging, and ultrasound. An ensemble model comprising three different deep learning networks, namely VGG-16, ResNet-50, and Inception V3, was trained and tested, and their performance was studied. Further, the developed and trained ensemble model is accelerated using PYNQ hardware accelerators for optimal diagnostic performance.

Chapter 9 discusses how Alzheimer's disease (AD) is the most pervasive and incurable neurodegenerative ailment that wreaks havoc on the mind's memory. With an increasing number of persons suffering from AD, relying on traditional conceptions to identify the illness may be economically unsustainable. Hence, computer-aided approaches are being developed to mitigate these issues.

Chapter 10 discusses how the recent escalation in deep learning underpins a swarm of algorithms with an incredible potential to decipher the information contained within images. Among these algorithms, convolutional neural networks (CNNs) and vision transformers (ViTs) have evolved as contemporary architectures for capturing local and global image features, respectively.

Chapter 11 begins with extracting features from electroencephalography (EEG) signals and then generating images from those features using proposed generative adversarial networks. This work focuses on digits and character datasets.

Chapter 12 presents and analyzes the EEG brainwaves with their domain analysis, pre-processing, classification accuracy, and the cause-and-effect of various mental health disorders. Additionally, it examines the machine learning model for EEG analysis and classification techniques for better accuracy.

Chapter 13 covers the various levels of ML-based detection methods that have been utilized to interpret the electrocardiogram (ECG) signal. This chapter also covers an ML-based method for predicting abnormalities in ECGs based on low-amplitude fluctuations known as ventricular late potentials (VLPs). These ML-based algorithms have been demonstrated to provide significantly more satisfactory discoveries and early predictions when compared to manual detection approaches.

Chapter 14 discusses heart disease, the major cause of severity of cardiovascular disease (CVD), and the increase in death rate due to heart disease. A novel approach, "Heartcare Assistance System", is proposed, using a Random Forest classifier to predict heart risk and Kommunicate, an intelligent chatbot system, to help patients to look out for remedial measures for various heart-related queries.

Chapter 15 aims to record multiple sets of real-time nerve signals from given subjects by dint of a designed neurostimulator in the laboratory environment and its processing and extraction of diagnostic markers. Subsequently, a microcontroller-based decision-making platform is developed by analyzing the recorded signals.

Chapter 16 analyzes various working apps, such as Mayo Clinic Symptom Checker, WebMD Symptom Checker, Symptomate, Your.MD, Ada etc. These apps use text-based input from the user and predict the probable diagnosis based on a questionnaire. This chapter discusses working algorithms and diagnostic criteria. Patient profiles based on the most prevalent medical conditions were created and the workflows of the different apps have been comparatively analyzed. Furthermore, the challenges and issues related to the usage of such apps in the healthcare industry are elucidated.

Chapter 17 proposes reinforcement learning-based optimal treatment of acute inflammatory response with drug-dosage regulation, where the mathematical model of inflammation response is a well-known universal model. In the treatments, external disturbance and ineffective dosage cases have been considered to strengthen the immune system to prevent possible damage by considering the septic and aseptic dynamics of the inflammation response.

Chapter 18 presents the branch of science called histopathology, which is used for the identification of the signature of disease in cells of diseased tissue.

Chapter 19 emphasizes the need for the development of remedies and precautionary measures to protect the general populace from the widespread pathogenicity of infectious diseases. The highly mutable nature of the pathogens and their impact make it necessary to provide remedies as quickly as possible. This chapter predominantly focuses on how these epitopes elicit a reaction in the bodies, and how that knowledge can be harnessed to select the best possible combination of epitopes and vaccine formula. The selection of the most suitable antigens, linkers, and adjuvants is an important part of the process.

Chapter 20 presents a deep learning technique for drug target interaction (DTI) that has recently emerged as an innovative field of research. Deep learning algorithms are applied in this process to produce novel drug candidates that have the potential to be effective at searching through a wide range of molecules. In this chapter, a two-step approach is proposed for identifying potential drug molecules to combat COVID-19 and its variants: initially to induce generative adversarial networks (GAN) using reinforcement techniques to generate novel molecules; then, to determine the binding affinity between potential compounds and the target protease sequence, a deep learning-based unique drug target interaction (DTI) model is suggested. Finally, the binding affinity of the generated molecules is predicted against the 3CLPro main protease by using the proposed DTI model

Chapter 21 explains the importance of chatbots in healthcare. The chapter discusses the role of various deep learning algorithms to train and test models of X-ray and scan reports and integrate with medical chatbots to provide resourceful answers with appropriate remedial care and accurate diagnosis of reports to prescribe drugs or precautions as a response to queries of patients. It also deliberates on future challenges, limitations, regulatory standard issues, ethical problems, security glitches, and the scope of research in the field of deep learning chatbots.

Finally, Chapter 22 provides an overview of the types and efficacy of AI-assisted tools created by machine learning models and deep learning models used to solve learning issues in children with a variety of NDDs. The chapter summarizes the research, showing how AI tools can enhance social connection and supportive teaching.

We are sincerely thankful to the authors for their contributions. Our gratitude is also extended to the many anonymous referees involved in the revision and acceptance process of the submitted manuscripts. It would not have been possible to reach this publication quality without the contributions of the referees. The editors are sincerely thankful to the series editors Prof. Vishal Jain and Prof. Jyotir Chatterjee for providing constructive input and allowing an opportunity to edit this important book. As the editors, we hope this book will stimulate further research in medical image processing, theories, and applications, to utilize in real-world clinical settings. Special thanks go to our publisher, CRC Press/Taylor & Francis Group. We hope that this book will present promising ideas and outstanding research results.

Bhanu Chander
Dept. of CSE, IIIT Kottayam, Kerala, India
Koppala Guravaiah
Dept. of CSE, IIIT Kottayam, Kerala, India
Kumarvelan Gopalakrishnan
Dept. of CSE, Pondicherry University, Pondicherry, India
B. Anoop
Post Doc University of Texas Health Science Centre at San Antonio, TX, USA

About the Editors

Dr. Bhanu Chander, working as Assistant Professor at Indian Institute of Information Technology (IIIT-K), Pala, Kerala, India, graduated from Acharya Nagarjuna University, Andhra Pradesh, India, and received a postgraduate degree from the Central University of Rajasthan, India. Dr. Bhanu earned a Ph.D. in Machine Learning in Wireless Sensor Networks for Sensor Data Classification from Pondicherry University, India, in 2022. Dr. Bhanu's primary research interests are in the areas of wireless sensor networks, machine learning, and IoT security. As we know, computer science as a field has largely focused on problems relevant to the developed world. The internet and the world wide web have remained largely urban phenomena, which means that a significant fraction of the developing world, especially in rural and underdeveloped regions, remains disconnected from the rest of the world. Dr. Bhanu is an academic reviewer recognized by IEEE, ACM, and Springer, and has served for 16 various scientific journals and conferences in the review process of more than 50 articles. He contributed as a track chair and session chair for numerous international conferences and workshops, and performed as a technical program committee (TPC) member for several international conferences organized by IEEE, Springer, and ACM.

He is interested in machine learning techniques for energy-efficient 6G networks, blockchain technology for the security of the Internet of Things and wireless communications, analysis and verification of cryptographic protocols, and identification of novel features or misclassified features in satellite image analysis. He published eight articles in peer-reviewed journals, five international conferences, and eight book chapters (Elsevier, Wiley, CRC, and Springer). Presently, his main areas of interest include wireless sensor networks (WSN), IoT and healthcare, cryptography, machine learning, and deep learning.

Dr. Anoop, working as Postdoctoral Research Fellow at Glenn Biggs Institute for Alzheimer's and Neurodegenerative Diseases, University of Texas Health Science Centre, US, received a Ph.D. degree in the Development of Automated Methods for Retinal Optical Coherence Tomography Image Analysis from the National Institute of Technology, Surathkal, India, in 2021 and M.Tech on Signal Processing from National Institute of Technology, Calicut, India, 2013. He received the Best Paper award at the ninth International Conference on Pattern Recognition and Machine Intelligence, PReMI 2021 for the work entitled "Attention-Assisted Patchwise CNN for the Segmentation of Fluids from the Retinal Optical Coherence Tomography Images" Organized by Machine Intelligence Unit, Indian Statistical Institute (ISI), Kolkata, India, in December 2021. He attended the 43rd-annual International Conference of the IEEE Engineering in Medicine and Biology Society (EMBC21). Research fellow on a project entitled "Retinal Cysts Identification and Quantification from Low-SNR Optical Coherence Tomography Scans Using Image Processing Techniques" (funding agency: DST-SERB) from May 2017 to March 2020. He has membership in the professional bodies IEEE, IEEE Signal Processing, Engineering in Medicine and Biology Society, and Internet Society.

He published six articles in peer-reviewed journals and two book chapters. Presently, his main areas of interest include medical image processing, deep learning, GANs and auto-encoders.

Dr. Koppala Guravaiah, working as Assistant Professor at Indian Institute of Information Technology (IIIT-K), Pala, Kerala, India, completed a Ph.D. on the topic of Performance of Routing Protocols in Wireless Sensor Networks using River Formation Dynamics from National Institute of Technology Tiruchirappalli, India. His research interests include the Internet of Things (IoT), wireless sensor networks, MANETs, applications and security aspects in IoT, WSN, and MANETs, and natural language processing. He is an active speaker at various international and national conferences. He contributed as a track chair and session chair for numerous international conferences and workshops and pe0rformed as a technical program committee member for several international conferences. He has published in five journals, eight conferences, and contributed two book chapters in the areas mentioned above. He is a member of various professional research bodies, such as IEEE and ACM.

Dr. G. Kumaravelan currently serves as Associate Professor at Department of Computer Science, School of Engineering and Technology, Pondicherry University, Karaikal Campus, Karaikal, India. He received his M.Tech in Advanced Information Technology and his Ph.D. in Computer Science from Bharathidasan University, Trichy, India, in 2009 and 2013, respectively. He has published more than 25 research papers in reputed international journals indexed in Scopus and SCI and conferences including IEEE, SPRINGER, and ACM. He received two best paper awards in the international conferences organized by the IITs. He has received "Best Teacher Award" from Pondicherry University, based on students' evaluation, for the past six years (2013–14, 2014–15, 2015–16, 2016–17, 2017–18, and 2018–19). He has gained 17 years of rich teaching and research experience. He is an active reviewer in various international conferences and peer-reviewed journals, and has reviewed more than 200 papers. He has acted as a resource person in various FDPs, conferences, and seminars in higher educational institutions. He contributed as a track chair and session chair for numerous international conferences and workshops and performed as a TPC member for several international conferences. His research interests include the Internet of Things, cloud computing, big data analytics, wireless communications, and networking.

Contributors

A. Sathya Vani
Computer Science and Engineering,
    VIT-AP University,
Andhra Pradesh, India

Navya Aggarwal
Centre for Computational Biology and
    Bioinformatics, Amity Institute of
    Biotechnology, Amity University,
Noida, India

Santhosh Amilpur
Indian Institute of Information
    Technology Sri City,
Chittoor, AP

R. Babu
Department of Computational
    Intelligence, SRM Institute of
    Science and Technology,
Chennai, India

Hina Bansal
Centre for Computational Biology and
    Bioinformatics, Amity Institute of
    Biotechnology, Amity University,
Uttar Pradesh, India

Bibal Benifa
Department of Computer Science and
    Engineering, Indian Institute of
    Information Technology Kottayam,
Kerala, India

Selami Beyhan
Department of Electrical-Electronics
    Engineering, Izmir Democracy
    University,
Izmir, Turkey

Manabendra Bhuyan
Department of Electronics and
    Communication Engineering, Tezpur
    University,
Assam, India

E. Chandra Blessie
Coimbatore Institute of Technology,
Coimbatore, Tamil Nadu

C. Manjunath
School of Mechanical Engineering,
    REVA University,
Bengaluru, India

Meriç Çetin
Department of Computer Engineering,
    Pamukkale University,
Denizli, Turkey

Kunal Chaudhari
Department of Computer Engineering
    and IT, COEP Technological
    University (COEP Tech),
Pune, India

D. Sumathi
Department of Computer Science and
    Engineering, VIT-AP University,
Andhra Pradesh, India

Dipali Dakhole
Computer Science and Engineering
    Department, Presidency University,
Bengaluru, India

Chandra Mohan Dasari
Assistant Professor, Indian Institute of
    Information Technology Sri City,
AP, India

Nitu Dogra
Research Boulevard Technologies,
Uttar Pradesh, India

Lachit Dutta
Department of Electronics and
   Communication Engineering,
   Guwahati University,
Assam, India

A. Kannammal
Coimbatore Institute of Technology,
Tamil Nadu, India

Poonguzhali Elangovan
National Institute of Technology
   Puducherry,
Karaikal, India

Geostat
INRIA Bordeaux Sud-Ouest, Rue de la
   Vieille Tour,
Talence Cedex, France

Qazi Amanur Rahman Hashmi
Centre for Computational Biology and
   Bioinformatics, Amity Institute of
   Biotechnology, Amity University,
Noida, India

Anil Hazarika
Department of Physics, Cotton University,
Assam, India

Ketaki Jadhav
Department of Computer Engineering
   and IT, COEP Technological
   University (COEP Tech),
Pune, India

K. Jayashree
Department of Artificial Intelligence
   and Machine Learning, Panimalar
   Engineering College,
Chennai, India

Chinju John
Department of Computer Science and
   Engineering, Indian Institute of
   Information Technology Kottayam,
Kerala, India

Amit Joshi
Department of Computer Engineering
   and IT, COEP Technological
   University (COEP Tech),
Pune, India

A. Maria Jossy
SRM IST,
Tamil Nadu, India

K. Karthik
School of Computer Science and
   Engineering, Vellore Institute of
   Technology (VIT)
Vellore, India

Deepshikha Pande Katare
Proteomics and Translational
   Research Lab, Centre for Medical
   Biotechnology, Amity Institute of
   Biotechnology, Amity University,
Noida, India

R. Kayalvizhi
SRM IST,
Tamil Nadu, India

Manish Kumar
Department of Computer Science and
   Engineering, IIT Patna,
Bihar, India

Rahul Kumar
Healthcare Analytics and Language
   Engineering (HALE) Lab,
   Department of Information
   Technology, National Institute of
   Technology,
Karnataka, India

R. Mahalakshmi
Bio-intelligence Lab, Department of
   Computer Science and Engineering,
   Presidency University,
Bengaluru, India

Suman Kumar Maji
Department of Computer Science and
   Engineering, IIT Patna
Bihar, India

S. Malarvizhi
SRM IST,
Tamil Nadu, India

Meenakshi Malhotra
Dayananda Sagar University,
Bengaluru, India

Ruchi Jakhmola Mani
Proteomics and Translational
   Research Lab, Centre for Medical
   Biotechnology, Amity Institute of
   Biotechnology, Amity University,
Noida. India

H. Heartlin Maria
SRM IST,
Tamil Nadu, India

Tauheed Khan Mohd
Augustana College, Rock Island,
Illinois, USA

K.N. Praveena
Department of Computer Science and
   Engineering. Presidency University,
Bengaluru, India

Ritik Naik
Department of Computer Engineering
   and IT, COEP Technological
   University (COEP Tech),
Pune, India

Akarsh K. Nair
Department of Computer Science and
   Engineering, Indian Institute of
   Information Technology,
Kerala, India

Malaya Kumar Nath
National Institute of Technology
   Puducherry,
Karaikal, India

P. Kanishk
Coimbatore Institute of Technology,
Tamil Nadu, India

Shatanu Patil
SRM IST,
Tamil Nadu, India

Anabel Pineda-Briseno
National Technology of Mexico,
   Mexico

Angamba Meetei Potshangbam
Manipur University, Department of
   Biotechnology,
Imphal, India

R. Jayaparvathy
Sri Sivasubramaniya Nadar College of
   Engineering,
Chennai, India

Shalini Ramanathan
National Institute of Technology
   Tiruchirappalli,
Tamil Nadu, India

Mohan Ramasundaram
National Institute of Technology
   Tiruchirappalli,
Tamil Nadu, India

S. Barath Vignesh
Coimbatore Institute of Technology,
Tamil Nadu, India

S. Daphin Lilda
Sri Sivasubramaniya Nadar College of
    Engineering,
Chennai, India

S. Sowmya Kamath
Healthcare Analytics and Language
    Engineering (HALE) Lab, Department
    of Information Technology, National
    Institute of Technology,
Karnataka, India

Jayakrushna Sahoo
Department of Computer Science and
    Engineering, Indian Institute of
    Information Technology,
Kerala, India

Poonam Saini
Department of Computer Science and
    Engineering, Punjab Engineering
    College,
Chandigarh, India

Akshita Sakshia
Heritage Institute of Technology,
Kolkata, India

Nitigya Sambyal
Department of Computer Science and
    Engineering, Thapar Institute of
    Engineering and Technology,
Patiala, India

Ankur Saxena
Centre for Computational Biology and
    Bioinformatics, Amity Institute of
    Biotechnology, Amity University,
Noida, India

P. Antony Seba
Kumaraguru College of Technology,
Coimbatore, India

Amarprit Singh
Department of Electronics and
    Communication Engineering, Tezpur
    University,
Assam, India

Rishita Singh
Centre for Computational Biology and
    Bioinformatics, Amity Institute of
    Biotechnology, Amity University,
Noida, India

Tumul Vikram Singh
Centre for Computational Biology and
    Bioinformatics, Amity Institute of
    Biotechnology, Amity University,
Noida, India

Rupali Syal
Department of Computer Science and
    Engineering, Punjab Engineering
    College,
Chandigarh, India

Champak Talukdar
Department of Electronics and
    -Communication Engineering,
    Tezpur University,
Assam, India

Revathi Venkatraman
SRM IST,
Tamil Nadu, India

Priya Vijay
Department of Information Technology,
    Rajalakshmi Engineering College,
Chennai, India

K. Vijay
Department of Computer
  Science, Rajalakshmi Engineering
  College,
Chennai, India

Kiran Waghmare
Center for Development of Advanced
  Computing,
Mumbai, India

Ravina Yadav
Proteomics and Translational
  Research Lab, Centre for Medical
  Biotechnology, Amity Institute of
  Biotechnology, Amity University,
Noida, India

Hussain Yahia
Geostat, INRIA Bordeaux Sud-Ouest,
Cedex, France

About the Book

The edited book *Handbook of AI-Based Models in Healthcare and Medicine: Approaches, Theories, and Applications* is intended to discuss the evolution of future generation technologies for healthcare applications through the Internet of Things (IoT), artificial intelligence (AI), machine learning (ML), and deep learning (DL). The main focus of this volume is on all the related technologies, such as IoT, AI, ML, and DL, applied to healthcare to solve health-related issues easily with a single platform, so that undergraduate and postgraduate students, researchers, academicians, and industry people can easily understand the AI, machine learning, deep learning algorithms, and learning analytics in IoT-enabled technologies for healthcare applications.

AI and ML are highly employed in medical imaging and facilitate services like computer-aided analysis, X-rays, CT scans, MRIs, and other image-guided therapy. DL builds on mathematical models that allow the healthcare sector to analyze data at exceptional speeds with high accuracy. It continues to make inroads into the industry. These technologies are connected, providing something different to the industry and changing how medical professionals manage their roles and patient care. This book delivers a high-level understanding of healthcare and medicine applications with emerging technologies such as AI, ML, and DL by discovering innovative advances, concepts, and persistent challenges. In addition, the book also offers potential use cases where AI, ML, and DL can help solve malicious healthcare complications.

This book will help researchers and practitioners to understand the design architecture of different problems of healthcare with AI, ML, and DL algorithms through IoT.

1 Edge Computing in Healthcare
Concepts, Tools, Techniques, and Use Cases

Shalini Ramanathan, Anabel Pineda-Briseno, Tauheed Khan Mohd, and Mohan Ramasundaram

1.1 OVERVIEW

Edge computing is a method of computing that brings data storage and computation closer to the point where it's used to improve the speed of response and reduce bandwidth consumption. Figure 1.1 shows the basic architecture of edge computing. Healthcare providers can use edge computing and analytics to transform data into novel findings that can help improve patient outcomes while providing commercial and functional value. In healthcare, edge computing refers to the processing and analysis of data at the network's edge, which is closer to the origin of the data rather than at a centralized place. This approach involves deploying computing resources, such as servers and storing devices, at the centre of the network, such as in hospitals, clinics, and medical devices [1]. Edge computing in healthcare has the potential to revolutionize patient care by enabling real-time monitoring, faster and more accurate medical imaging, and personalized medicine. It can also support telemedicine, remote patient monitoring, and electronic health records (EHRs) by providing low-latency and high-bandwidth connectivity for remote consultations and faster and more efficient data processing at the point of care.

Edge computing in healthcare has the potential to enhance outcomes for patients, save money, and improve the effectiveness and safety of medical facilities. For example, edge computing can enable real-time patient monitoring, allowing healthcare providers to respond to emergencies quickly and efficiently. It can also reduce the latency associated with sending large image files to a centralized server, enabling faster and more accurate medical imaging. Edge computing is used with Internet of Things (IoT) devices, self-driving cars, and medical monitoring tools [2]. Utilizing edge computing in the healthcare sector provides a lot of benefits, like mobility, rural region accessibility, and workforce reduction. There have been several recent advancements in healthcare across a range of areas, including medical devices,

DOI: 10.1201/9781003363361-1

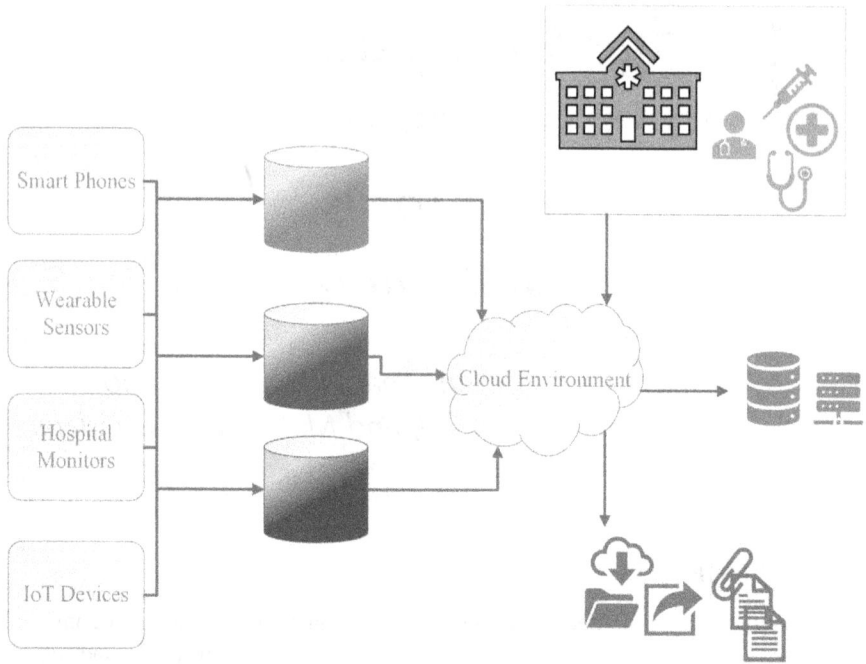

FIGURE 1.1   Basic architecture of edge computing

pharmaceuticals, digital health, and genomics. In medical devices, artificial intelligence- (AI-) powered medical devices are being developed that can improve diagnostic accuracy and enable personalized treatment plans [3]. Wearable gadgets like fitness trackers and smartwatches are being used for remote monitoring and early detection of health issues. 3D printing technology is being used to create customized medical implants and prosthetics, reducing the risk of rejection and improving patient outcomes. In pharmaceuticals, gene therapies are being developed that can cure genetic diseases by replacing or repairing defective genes. Immunotherapy drugs are being used to treat cancer by strengthening the immune system to fight cancer cells. Personalized medicine is becoming more common, using genetic testing to tailor treatment plans to a patient's unique genetic profile. In digital health, telemedicine and remote patient monitoring technologies are enabling virtual care and remote consultations between patients and healthcare professionals. EHR systems are being adopted widely to increase the precision and efficiency of healthcare services. Big data are being used to identify patterns and trends in patient data, improving diagnosis accuracy and treatment outcomes. In genomics, the cost of genetic sequencing is decreasing rapidly, making it more accessible and affordable for patients and healthcare providers. Advances in genetic factor editing knowledge, such as Clustered Regularly Interspaced Short Palindromic Repeats (CRISPR), are enabling precise modifications to genetic material, offering new possibilities for disease treatment and prevention. Genetic counselling and testing are becoming more common, allowing patients to make informed decisions about their health and treatment options based on their genetic information. These are a few examples of recent advancements in healthcare. The healthcare industry is continuously evolving with novel technologies and treatments, which are developed regularly. These advancements are improving patient outcomes, increasing access to healthcare, and enhancing the efficiency and effectiveness of healthcare delivery.

Advantages of using edge computing in the healthcare sector:

- Real-time processing: Edge computing enables instantaneous data analysis and processing, allowing healthcare professionals to make faster and better-informed decisions about patient care.
- Improved patient outcomes: Edge computing can improve patient outcomes by enabling real-time monitoring, personalized medicine, and faster and more accurate medical imaging.
- Reduced latency: Edge computing reduces the latency associated with sending data to a centralized server, enabling quicker and more competent data processing at the point of care.
- Enhanced security: Edge computing can enhance the security of patient data by processing and storing data locally, reducing the risk of data breaches and cyberattacks.
- Cost-effective: Edge computing can be more profitable than out-of-date computing models, as it reduces the need for expensive hardware and infrastructure.

Disadvantages of using edge computing in the healthcare sector:

- Limited processing power: Edge computing devices typically have limited processing power and storage capacity compared to centralized servers, which may limit their ability to process and analyze large amounts of data.
- Maintenance and management: Edge computing devices require regular maintenance and management, which can be challenging for healthcare organizations with limited resources.
- Data integration challenges: Integrating data from multiple sources can be challenging in an edge computing environment, which may lead to data silos and fragmented data.
- Dependence on network connectivity: Edge computing devices rely on network connectivity to communicate with other devices and systems, which may be unreliable in some settings.
- Data privacy concerns: Edge computing devices may store sensitive patient data locally, which may raise concerns about data privacy and security.

In summary, edge computing in healthcare is a promising approach to transform the healthcare industry by providing faster, more efficient, and more secure data processing at the point of care, ultimately improving patient outcomes and enhancing the quality of care [4]. Edge computing offers several benefits for the healthcare sector, but it also presents some challenges that need to be addressed to ensure successful implementation and adoption. Healthcare organizations should carefully consider the advantages and disadvantages of using edge computing and evaluate their specific needs and requirements before implementing this technology.

1.2   EDGE COMPUTING INTELLIGENCE

AI is playing an increasingly important role in edge computing [5]. It involves local data processing, somewhat quicker to the basis of the data than distributing it to a centralized information centre or cloud for dispensation. It allows for faster data processing, reduced latency, and improved efficiency. AI is being used in edge computing to enable intelligent decision-making. Considering autonomous vehicles, AI algorithms are used to examine IoT device information in real time, permitting vehicles to make immediate decisions without consuming the data at the centralized server for processing. Similarly, in industrial automation and robotics, AI algorithms are used to analyze sensor data to make decisions and perform actions in real time. AI uses edge computing to advance the proficiency of data processing. By using AI algorithms to analyze data at the edge, only relevant details are sent to the server to be examined further, limiting the quantity of information that needs to be analyzed, and thus minimizing the bandwidth requirements and storage costs. Furthermore, AI is being used in edge computing to improve security [6]. AI algorithms can detect anomalies in data at the edge, allowing for immediate responses to potential security threats before they become more serious. Overall, AI plays a critical role in edge computing by enabling real-time decision-making, improving efficiency, and enhancing security. Figure 1.2 summarises the various edge computing intelligence.

Machine learning (ML) is a subdivision of AI that encompasses training procedures to learn patterns and make calculations based on data [7]. It has an important role to play in edge computing, where data handling and investigation are performed at the edge of the computing network, nearer to the foundation of the data. Here are some examples of ML used with edge computing:

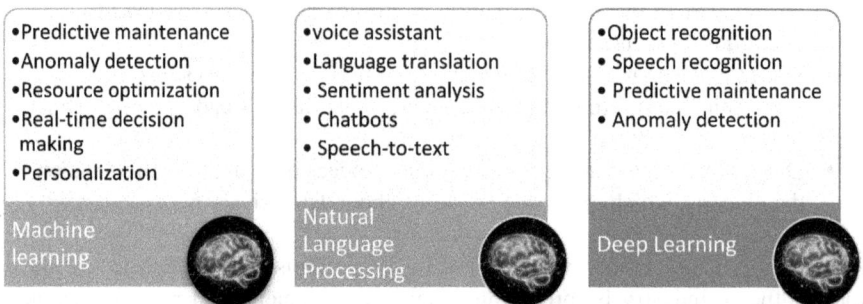

•Predictive maintenance •Anomaly detection •Resource optimization •Real-time decision making •Personalization	•voice assistant •Language translation • Sentiment analysis • Chatbots • Speech-to-text	•Object recognition • Speech recognition • Predictive maintenance • Anomaly detection
Machine learning	Natural Language Processing	Deep Learning

FIGURE 1.2   Various intelligence of edge computing

Predictive conservation: In numerous industries, ML is used to forecast when the apparatus is likely to nose-dive, allowing for proactive upkeep to be completed before the equipment breaks down. By processing sensor information at the edge of the computing network, ML algorithms can make predictions in real time, reducing downtime and maintenance costs.

Anomaly detection: ML algorithms can be used to detect anomalous behaviour in sensor data, such as sudden spikes or drops in temperature or pressure. These anomalies could indicate a potential problem, allowing for immediate action to be taken to prevent damage or failure.

Resource optimization: In edge computing environments, resources such as storage and processing power are limited. ML algorithms can be used to optimize resource usage by predicting when certain resources will be needed and when they can be freed up.

Real-time decision-making: ML algorithms can be used to scrutinize sensor data in real time and make decisions based on that data. For example, in autonomous vehicles, ML algorithms can analyze sensor data to make decisions about steering, braking, and acceleration without the need for human intervention.

Personalization: ML algorithms can be used to personalize experiences for users by analyzing data about their behaviour and preferences. In edge computing environments, this analysis can be performed in real time, allowing for personalized experiences to be delivered immediately.

Natural language processing (NLP) is a defined subclass of AI that involves the communication between individuals and supercomputers using natural language. NLP has a significant role to play in edge computing, where statistics processing and study are done at the place of the system, nearer to the source of the information. Some examples are voice assistants, language translation, sentiment analysis, chatbots, and speech-to-text. Voice aides like Siri, Alexa, and Google Assistant are becoming increasingly popular in edge computing environments [8]. NLP algorithms are used to interpret the user's voice commands and provide responses in real time. Language translation services in edge computing environments need to communicate with each other across language barriers, and NLP algorithms can be used to translate between languages in real time. Sentiment analysis and NLP algorithms benefit from the analysis of social media data in real time to determine the sentiment of content being shared. This information can be used to inform real-time decision-making or to identify potential issues that require immediate attention. Chatbots are becoming increasingly popular in edge computing environments where human interaction is required. NLP algorithms are used to interpret the user's messages and provide appropriate responses in real time. Speech-to-text with edge computing services is a need to convert speech to text in real time, and NLP algorithms can be used to transcribe the speech in real time, enabling faster and more accurate communication.

Deep learning is the process used to train artificial neural networks to recognize patterns among data [9]. It also plays a crucial role in processing and analyzing data to the advantage of the network system. Here are some of the key roles of deep learning in edge computing:

Object recognition: Deep learning procedures are used to identify objects in images or video feeds in real time. This is particularly useful in applications such as surveillance, robotics, and autonomous vehicles.

Speech recognition: Deep learning algorithms can be used to recognize and transcribe speech in real time, enabling more natural and efficient communication between humans and machines.

Predictive maintenance: In edge computing environments where equipment is monitored using sensors, deep learning algorithms can be used to predict when maintenance is required before equipment failure occurs.

Anomaly detection: Deep learning algorithms can be used to detect anomalous behaviour in sensor data, such as sudden spikes or drops in temperature or pressure. These anomalies could indicate a potential problem, allowing for immediate action to be taken to prevent damage or failure.

NLP has a critical role to play in edge computing by enabling voice assistants, language translation, sentiment analysis, chatbots, and speech-to-text capabilities, all of which contribute to more efficient and effective communication in edge computing environments. ML has enabled predictive maintenance, anomaly detection, resource optimization, real-time decision-making, and personalization [10]. By computing the data, deep learning algorithms enable more efficient and effective decision-making, leading to improved performance, reduced downtime, and enhanced user experiences.

1.3 AI-POWERED HEALTHCARE-BASED EDGE COMPUTING

Edge computing has the potential to transform healthcare by providing faster, better organized, and more secure information handling at the point of care [11]. Here are some applications of edge computing in healthcare:

- **Real-time patient monitoring:** It will enable real-time patient monitoring, allowing healthcare providers to monitor patients continuously and respond to emergencies quickly.
- **Telemedicine:** Edge computing can support telemedicine by providing low-latency and high-bandwidth connectivity for remote consultations, enabling healthcare professionals to provide real-time virtual care to patients in remote locations.
- **Wearable devices**: Wearable devices such as fitness trackers and smartwatches create significant data that will be processed at the edge.
- Edge computing can provide real-time insights into patient health, enabling healthcare providers to make more informed decisions about patient care.
- **Medical imaging:** Edge computing can enable faster and more accurate medical imaging by processing data locally, reducing the latency associated with sending large image files to a centralized server.

- **Medical attentive systems:** These provide a way for patients to call for help in an emergency, such as a fall or sudden illness.
- **Medical billing application:** This is used to manage the financial aspects of healthcare, such as billing patients, managing insurance claims, and processing payments.
- **Clinical verdict provision systems:** These provide healthcare professionals and real-time clinical information to aid in decision-making, such as prescribing medication or ordering tests.
- **Personalized medicine:** Edge computing can enable personalized medicine by processing patient data locally and providing real-time insights into patient health, allowing healthcare providers to customize treatment plans based on individual patient needs.
- **EHRs:** Edge computing can support EHRs by enabling faster data handling at the point of care, improving the standard of treatment, and reducing the risk of medical errors.
- **Medical imaging gears:** This includes X-ray machines, magnetic resonance imaging (MRI) scanners, computed tomography (CT) scanners, and ultrasound machines used to produce images of the inside of the human body.
- **Health information exchange platforms:** These enable the sharing of patient information between healthcare organizations, allowing for coordinated care and improved patient outcomes.

1.4 LEARNING SYSTEM OF EDGE COMPUTING

It is a disseminated computing standard to carry calculation and storage nearer to the place it is required, rather than relying on centralized cloud computing resources. In edge computing, computation is performed on devices that are closer to the data source, such as sensors, mobile devices, and IoT devices. The awareness behind edge-based computing will reduce the latency and bandwidth constraints associated with transmitting data to centralized computing resources, along with the potential safety with privacy concerns that arise when sensitive data is transmitted over the network. By performing computation at the computing edge of the structure, it can improve system performance, reduce network congestion, and enhance data confidentiality and refuge. Edge computing involves the deployment of computing infrastructure, such as servers, storage devices, and system equipment. These devices can be placed in a wide range of locations, from industrial sites and manufacturing facilities to remote locations and smart city environments. The edge computing ecosystem includes a wide range of devices, such as smartphones, tablets, wearables, and IoT devices, as well as edge servers and other network infrastructure. In addition, edge computing involves the use of forward-thinking knowledge, such as AI, ML, and natural language processing, to enable immediate processing and analysis of data at the computing of the edge network. It represents a new paradigm in disseminated computing which conveys computation and data storage faster to the site where it is wanted, enabling more efficient computing solutions for an extensive variety of claims, from smart cities to industrial automation and beyond. It relies on a wide range of technologies to enable the immediate processing of information in the computing part of the network. Some of the main technologies used in edge computing are listed below. IoT devices, such as sensors and connected devices, are a crucial element of edge-based computing. These devices generate large amounts of data that can be processed and analyzed with the computing edge-based network. Microservices construction is used to develop and model deployment of edge network applications [12]. This approach involves breaking down tasks into minor, self-governing components that can be arranged and installed separately. Containers are used to package and deploy edge computing applications. Containers provide a volatile and transportable way to deploy applications across different environments. Virtualization is used to create virtual machines that can be used to run edge computing applications. This approach provides a flexible and scalable way to deploy applications across different environments [13]. AI and ML technologies are used to enable real-time processing and analysis of data with the computing edge-based network. These technologies will perform everyday jobs, such as image reconstruction, NLP, image segmentation, object identification, and predictive measures. 5G and edge computing networks are being used to enable faster and more reliable connectivity between edge computing devices. This technology provides the low-latency and high-bandwidth needs for computing devices.

1.5   IMPACT ON HEALTHCARE

Edge-based computing systems have momentous problems in transforming healthcare by allowing current-time processing of healthcare data with edge computing systems. Here are some of the ways in which edge computing can have a significant impact on healthcare:

Real-time monitoring: It is used to monitor patients in real time, using wearable devices and other connected devices. This can help healthcare professionals to detect health problems early and provide timely intervention.

Faster diagnosis: Edge computing can enable faster and more accurate diagnosis of health problems by processing and analyzing medical images and other diagnostic data in real time at the point of care [14].

Remote patient monitoring: Edge computing can enable remote patient monitoring, allowing healthcare professionals to monitor patients in real time from remote locations. This can be particularly useful for patients with chronic conditions who require regular monitoring and intervention.

Predictive analytics: Edge computing can be used to perform predictive analytics on healthcare data, helping healthcare professionals to identify patterns and trends that may indicate potential health problems. This can enable proactive intervention and better healthcare outcomes.

Data privacy and security: Edge computing can help to address privacy and security concerns associated with healthcare data by processing and storing data locally, instead of transmitting it to unified cloud computing resources [15].

By leveraging edge computing, healthcare professionals can provide more efficient, effective, and personalized healthcare services, improving patient outcomes and reducing healthcare costs. It has significant potential to transform healthcare by enabling current-time processing and investigation of healthcare information. Several driving factors are fuelling the adoption of edge computing in healthcare. Here are some of the key factors: (i) Increase in healthcare data: With the growing use of connected devices, wearables, and other medical technologies, there is an important maximization in the quantity of healthcare material being generated. Edge structures can enable actual-time processing of data over improving healthcare outcomes. (ii) Need for instantaneous monitoring: Real-time intensive care of patients is vital in many healthcare settings, such as emergency rooms and critical care units. Edge computing can enable real-time monitoring of patients using connected devices, helping healthcare professionals detect health problems early and provide timely intervention. (iii) Remote patient monitoring: Remote patient monitoring is becoming increasingly important in healthcare, particularly for patients with chronic conditions who require regular monitoring and intervention. Edge computing can enable remote patient monitoring, allowing healthcare professionals to monitor patients in real time from remote locations. (iv) Need for faster diagnosis: Faster and more accurate diagnosis of health problems is critical in healthcare. Analysis of medical images with their diagnostic data at the point of care, help healthcare professionals to make faster and more accurate diagnoses.

Improving patient outcomes: Ultimately, the goal of healthcare is to improve patient outcomes. Edge computing can help to achieve this goal by enabling more efficient, effective, and personalized healthcare services, improving patient outcomes, and reducing healthcare costs. Therefore, the need for real-time monitoring, faster diagnosis, and improved patient outcomes is driving the adoption of edge computing in healthcare. By leveraging edge computing, healthcare professionals can provide more efficient and cost-effective healthcare services. Real-time cloud computing with edge computing performance can provide significant benefits in terms of speed and efficiency, compared to traditional cloud computing architectures [16]. Cloud computing resources are used to process and analyze data in real time, whereas edge computing is used to conduct local monitoring and examination of data at the network's edge, closer to the source of the data [17].

By combining these two technologies, real-time cloud computing with edge computing can provide several performance advantages, as shown in Figure 1.3.

By performing local monitoring and examination of data with the computing edge-based network, edge computing can significantly reduce latency, or the delay between the time when data is generated and when it is processed. This can enable real-time response to critical events, such as emergency medical situations, improving outcomes for patients. Edge computing can reduce the amount of data that needs to be transmitted over the network by performing local processing and analysis of

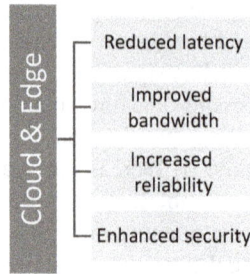

FIGURE 1.3 Advantages of combining cloud and edge computing

data. This can help to reduce network congestion and improve bandwidth, enabling faster and more efficient data transmission. Edge computing can provide increased reliability and resiliency, as data monitoring and examination can continue even if network connectivity is lost. This can be particularly important in healthcare, where real-time monitoring and intervention can be critical. Edge computing can provide enhanced security and privacy for healthcare data by processing and storing data locally with the computing edge-based network, rather than transmitting it to centralized cloud computing resources [18].

5G promises to reduce latency to less than one millisecond, which is critical for applications that require real-time processing and decision-making [19]. By processing data with the computing edge-based network, edge computing can further reduce latency, enabling new use cases such as autonomous vehicles, augmented reality, and remote surgery. 5G offers higher bandwidth compared to previous cellular network technologies, which is essential for transmitting large amounts of data quickly. It may process and monitor these data with the computing edge-based network, reducing the need to transmit large amounts of data to a centralized cloud. It can reduce the load on the central cloud, improving scalability and reducing costs. Edge computing can improve security by processing sensitive data locally, rather than transmitting it over the network to a central cloud. This reduces the risk of data breaches and improves data privacy. Edge computing can be deployed in various locations, such as at the network edge, in a device, or in a data centre. This flexibility enables organizations to deploy edge computing where it makes the most sense, based on their specific use cases and requirements.

Edge computing can be used in vehicular networks to process data generated by vehicles and other connected devices in real time, providing immediate feedback to improve safety, efficiency, and user experience. Virtual reality (VR) is a technology that immerses users in a simulated environment, while edge computing is a model of computing that brings processing and data storage toward the data source. Together, these technologies have the potential to transform healthcare by improving patient outcomes, reducing costs, and enhancing the patient experience. Here are some key features and benefits of VR and edge computing in healthcare: By processing data with the computing edge-based network, edge computing can reduce latency and provide real-time feedback to VR applications. This is critical for healthcare applications where real-time monitoring and feedback are essential, such as surgical procedures and physical therapy. VR and edge computing can improve patient outcomes by providing immersive and personalized experiences for patients. For example, VR can be used to provide virtual environments for patients undergoing painful procedures, such as chemotherapy or dental work, to distract them from pain and discomfort. Edge computing can reduce the need for expensive central cloud infrastructure, reducing costs and improving scalability. This can make VR applications more affordable and accessible for healthcare providers and patients. VR can be used for medical training and education, allowing healthcare professionals to practice procedures and techniques in a safe and controlled environment. Edge computing can provide real-time feedback and analysis, improving the effectiveness of training and education. Edge computing can improve data privacy and security by processing sensitive data locally, rather than transmitting it over the network to a central cloud. This reduces the risk of data breaches and improves data privacy. Therefore, the combination of VR and edge computing can improve patient outcomes. By processing data with the computing edge-based network, edge computing can reduce latency and improve real-time processing, making VR applications more effective and accessible for healthcare providers and patients.

1.6 COMBINING TECHNOLOGIES FOR INTELLIGENT COMPUTING

Cloud with edge computing balances two technologies that can work together to deliver a more efficient computing environment [20]. The task of a cloud environment in conjunction with an edge-based computing system is to provide a scalable, secure, and efficient computing environment that leverages the strengths of both technologies. By working together, cloud computing and edge computing can provide more effective solutions to an extensive variety of tasks, from smart cities to industrial automation. Here are some of the tasks, such as information processing and packing, scalability, security, and loading. Edge computing can be used to pre-process data locally before distributing it to the cloud environment for additional processing. This may help decrease the large amount of data required to be sent to the cloud, reducing expectancy and improving overall system performance. Edge computing devices can store frequently accessed data locally, reducing the need to access data from the cloud. This can help reduce network congestion and improve overall system performance. Cloud computing can provide scalable computing resources to support edge computing devices. For example, when edge devices experience a spike in demand, additional computing resources can be provisioned from the cloud to support the increased workload. Cloud computing can provide security services, such as identity and access management, data encryption, and threat detection, to protect edge computing devices from security threats [21]. Cloud computing can provide advanced analytics capabilities to process data collected from edge computing devices. This can help identify patterns, trends, and anomalies, enabling more effective decision-making.

1.7   EDGE COMPUTING-BASED USE CASES

There are many edge computing-based use cases in various industries, including healthcare, manufacturing, transportation, retail, and more. Here are some examples:

- **Healthcare**: Edge computing can enable real-time monitoring of patients using connected devices, enabling healthcare professionals to detect health problems early and provide timely intervention. Edge computing can also enable remote patient monitoring, allowing healthcare professionals to monitor patients in real time from remote locations. IoT devices such as wearable sensors and medical monitors can be used to collect real-time data about patients' vital signs and transmit them to cloud computing services for analysis. This can help healthcare providers monitor patients remotely and detect potential health issues before they become serious. Robotics is used in healthcare to perform tasks such as surgery and patient monitoring. Edge computing can be used to monitor the performance of these robots in real time, providing immediate feedback to improve their performance and reduce the risk of errors.
- **Transportation**: Edge computing can enable real-time monitoring of vehicles, drivers, and passengers, providing insights into safety, performance, and route optimization. This can help to reduce accidents, improve efficiency, and increase overall passenger knowledge [22].
- **Retail**: Edge computing can be used to personalize the shopping experience for customers by analyzing their behaviour and preferences in real time. This may assist in improving client satisfaction and increasing sales. Some IoT sensors may be utilized to collect data about consumer behaviour. They can process huge amounts of data with the computing edge-based network, providing immediate feedback to retailers to optimize their inventory management and improve customer experiences.
- **Smart cities**: Edge computing may be used to screen and scrutinize data from IoT sensors deployed throughout a city, providing insights into traffic flow, air quality, and supplementary important factors. These data can be transmitted to cloud computing services for analysis, enabling city planners to make data-driven decisions about infrastructure, transportation, and public safety. This can help to improve safety, efficiency, and quality of life for city residents.
- **Smart homes**: IoT-enabled devices such as thermostats, security cameras, and smart speakers can be connected to cloud computing services, which can store and analyze the data generated by these devices. This can enable homeowners to control their devices remotely and automate routine tasks, such as turning on the lights or adjusting the temperature.
- **Industrial automation**: IoT-enabled sensors can be used to monitor and control industrial processes, such as manufacturing and logistics. By connecting these sensors to cloud computing services, manufacturers can

optimize their operations, reduce downtime, and improve overall efficiency. Robotics is used in logistics to automate tasks such as picking, packing, and shipping. Edge computing can be used to monitor the performance of these robots in real time, identifying any issues or faults that may arise. The data can then be analyzed at the network's periphery, providing instant feedback that can be used to improve the robot's operation and minimize disruption [23].

- **Agriculture**: IoT sensors can track soil moisture, temperature, and various other environmental variables that influence crop growth. These data can be transmitted to cloud computing services for analysis, enabling farmers to make data-driven decisions about irrigation, fertilization, and other aspects of crop management. Robotics is increasingly used in agriculture to automate tasks such as planting, harvesting, and crop monitoring. Edge-based computing structures can be used to process data from robotics sensors in real time, providing immediate feedback on mud moisture, crop healthiness, and ecological issues that distress yield growth. These data can be used to optimize the use of resources and increase crop yields [24].

- **Smart manufacturing**: Edge computing can be used to monitor and analyze data from sensors and devices on factory floors, enabling real-time quality control and predictive maintenance. This may be utilized to reduce downtime and improve efficiency. IoT sensors may be utilized to monitor and control the production process in real time. Edge computing can process and analyze data with the computing edge-based network, providing immediate feedback to machines and devices to optimize their performance and reduce downtime. Robots are commonly used in manufacturing processes to perform repetitive tasks. Edge computing can be used to monitor the performance of these robots in real time, identifying any issues or faults that may arise. The data can then be analyzed with the computing edge-based network, providing immediate feedback to optimize the performance of the robots and reduce downtime.

- **Energy management**: IoT sensors can be used to collect data about energy usage and production. Edge-based computing systems would process these data, providing immediate feedback to energy managers to optimize energy usage and reduce costs.

These use cases for edge computing provide considerable advantages in terms of efficiency, efficiency, and reliability for a wide range of industries and applications. Processing the detailed local data with the edge computing of the network will help to make decisions that will improve outcomes for businesses and their customers.

1.8 SOFTWARE AND HARDWARE COMPANIES DEVELOPING HEALTHCARE TECHNOLOGIES

Figure 1.4 illustrates some edge computing tools used in healthcare and medicine:

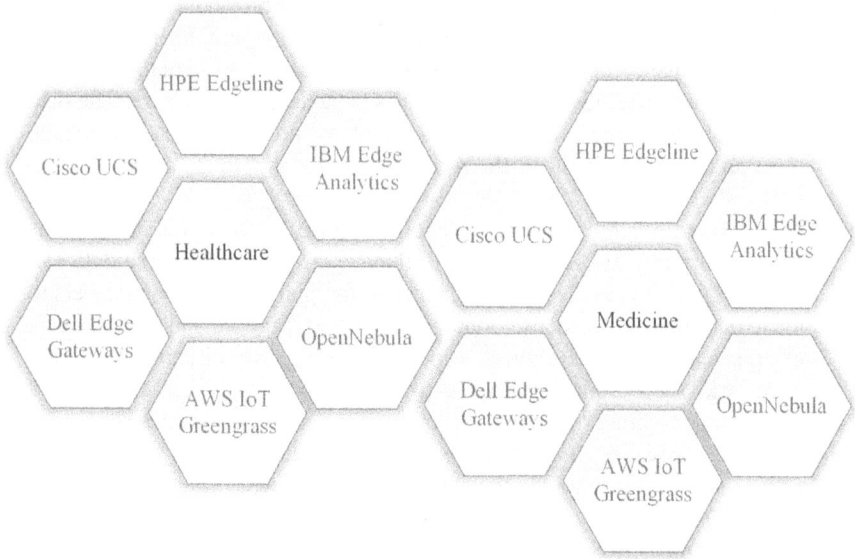

FIGURE 1.4   Edge computing tools used in healthcare and medicine

1. HPE Edgeline is a family of edge computing systems designed for health-care applications. These systems are intended to be installed with the computing edge-based network, allowing for real-time processing and analysis of healthcare data.
2. Cisco UCS is a platform designed for edge computing applications, including healthcare. It allows current-time processing of healthcare data and supports a wide variety of healthcare tenders, counting patient monitoring and predictive maintenance.
3. Dell Edge Gateways are edge computing devices designed for a range of applications, including healthcare. These devices enable real-time processing and analysis of healthcare data and can be used to support applications such as medical imaging and patient monitoring.
4. Amazon Web Services (AWS) IoT Greengrass is an edge computing platform that enables real-time processing and analysis of healthcare data. It supports various healthcare devices with remote patient monitoring and predictive maintenance.
5. IBM Edge Analytics is a platform designed for edge computing applications, including healthcare. It utilizes various healthcare data with medical appliances such as medical imaging and patient monitoring.
6. OpenNebula is an open-source cloud computing platform that can be used for edge computing applications in healthcare.
7. NVIDIA Clara AGX is an AI-based edge computing platform designed for healthcare. It enables real-time processing of medical imaging data and

supports a range of medical applications, including radiology, pathology, and medical research.

8. Developer Kit – Edge AI from Intel is a platform designed for developing and deploying AI models at the edge. It is particularly useful in medical imaging applications, allowing for real-time analysis and processing of large datasets.

9. Azure IoT Edge from Microsoft is a cloud-based edge computing platform that enables real-time processing of medical data. It supports a range of medical applications, including remote patient monitoring, predictive maintenance, and drug discovery.

10. IoT Edge with Google Cloud is a cloud-based edge computing platform that enables real-time processing of medical data. It helps with a range of medical instruments, counting disease diagnosis, drug discovery, and personalized medicine.

11. OpenVINO is an edge computing toolkit from Intel that enables developers to optimize AI models for edge devices. It utilizes a range of medical applications, together with medical imaging, disease diagnosis, and drug discovery.

12. Arm Cortex-M series is an array of microcontrollers designed for edge computing applications. They are particularly useful in medical applications that require low-power and low-cost solutions, such as medical sensors and wearable devices.

These technologies are used to enable real-time processing with the analysis of medical data.

1.9 HEALTHCARE IMPLEMENTATION TOOLS

EdgeCloudSim is a simulator that allows the simulation, modelling, and evaluation of edge computing structures. It is an extension of the CloudSim simulator, which is widely used for demonstrating and simulating cloud computing settings. EdgeCloudSim provides a flexible simulation system that enables researchers and practitioners to study various aspects of edge computing, such as workload allocation, resource management, and energy efficiency. **EmuFog** is an open-source simulation framework for fog computing environments. It is designed to simulate the behaviour of a large-scale fog computing network and provides a comprehensive set of tools for modelling, simulating, and analyzing fog computing systems. EmuFog allows researchers and practitioners to study various aspects of fog computing, such as resource management, workload allocation, and energy efficiency. **EmStar** is a distributed, open-source simulation framework used to investigate the efficiency and performance of edge computing systems. It is designed to simulate large-scale edge computing networks and provides a comprehensive set of tools for modelling, simulating, and analyzing edge computing systems. EmStar allows researchers and practitioners to study various aspects of edge computing, such as resource management, workload allocation, and energy efficiency. EmStar is a valuable tool for researchers and practitioners who are interested in studying and optimizing edge computing systems. It provides a flexible and extensible simulation framework that allows for the exploration of various scenarios and configurations, helping to advance the performance, energy productivity, and cost-efficacy of edge computing-based systems. **FogTorchII** is an open-source simulation framework designed to evaluate the performance of resource allocation policies in fog computing environments. It allows researchers and practitioners to model the behaviour of a large-scale fog computing network and simulate various scenarios to assess the effectiveness of different resource allocation strategies. It provides a detailed model of fog nodes, including their computational capabilities, memory, storage, and energy consumption. **IOTSim** is an open-source simulator designed to simulate the behaviour of large-scale IoT systems. It is a flexible and extensible simulation framework that allows researchers and practitioners to model, simulate, and analyze the performance of IoT systems under various conditions. This enables researchers to study the performance and energy efficiency of fog nodes under various workloads and resource allocation schemes. **PureEdgeSim** provides a model of the workload generated by edge devices, including the type of computation, data size, and arrival rate. This enables researchers to study the impact of workload characteristics on the performance of edge computing.

REFERENCES

1. Kauffmann, Jacob, Malte Esders, Lukas Ruff, Grégoire Montavon, Wojciech Samek, and Klaus-Robert Müller. "From clustering to cluster explanations via neural networks." *IEEE Transactions on Neural Networks and Learning Systems* (2022).
2. Patil, Shishir G., Paras Jain, Prabal Dutta, Ion Stoica, and Joseph Gonzalez. "POET: Training neural networks on tiny devices with integrated rematerialization and paging." *International Conference on Machine Learning* 162 (2022): 17573–17583. PMLR.
3. Ismail, Leila, and Rajkumar Buyya. "Artificial intelligence applications and self-learning 6G networks for smart cities digital ecosystems: Taxonomy, challenges, and future directions." *Sensors* 22, no. 15 (2022): 5750.
4. Gupta, Ishu, Ashutosh Kumar Singh, Chung-Nan Lee, and Rajkumar Buyya. "Secure data storage and sharing techniques for data protection in cloud environments: A systematic review, analysis, and future directions." *IEEE Access* 10 (2022): 71247–71277.
5. Zhu, Shiqiang, Yu Ting, Tao Xu, Hongyang Chen, Schahram Dustdar, Sylvain Gigan, Deniz Gunduz et al. "Intelligent computing: The latest advances, challenges, and future" *Intelligent Computing* 2 (2023): 0006.
6. Chang, Michael Alan, Aurojit Panda, Hantao Wang, Yuancheng Tsai, Rahul Balakrishnan, and Scott Shenker. "AutoTune: Improving end-to-end performance and resource efficiency for microservice applications." *arXiv Preprint ArXiv:2106.10334* (2021).
7. Zhong, Zhiheng, Minxian Xu, Maria Alejandra Rodriguez, Chengzhong Xu, and Rajkumar Buyya. "Machine learning-based orchestration of containers: A taxonomy and future directions." *ACM Computing Surveys (CSUR)* 54, no. 10s (2022): 1–35.
8. Wang, Xiaojie, Jiameng Li, Zhaolong Ning, Qingyang Song, Lei Guo, Song Guo, and Mohammad S. Obaidat. "Wireless powered mobile edge computing networks: A survey." *ACM Computing Surveys* 55 (2023): 1–37.

9. Hénaff, Olivier J., Skanda Koppula, Evan Shelhamer, Zoran Daniel, Andrew Jaegle, Andrew Zisserman, João Carreira, and Relja Arandjelović. "Object discovery and representation networks." In *Computer Vision–ECCV 2022: 17th European Conference, Tel Aviv, Israel, October 23–27, 2022, Proceedings, Part XXVII*, pp. 123–143. Springer Nature Switzerland, 2022.

10. Sudharsan, Bharath, John G. Breslin, Mehreen Tahir, Muhammad Intizar Ali, Omer Rana, Schahram Dustdar, and Rajiv Ranjan. "Ota-tinyml: over the air deployment of tinyml models and execution on iot devices." *IEEE Internet Computing* 26, no. 3 (2022): 69–78.

11. Goudarzi, Mohammad, Huaming Wu, Marimuthu Palaniswami, and Rajkumar Buyya. "An application placement technique for concurrent IoT applications in edge and fog computing environments." *IEEE Transactions on Mobile Computing* 20, no. 4 (2020): 1298–1311.

12. Deb, Debayan, Xiaoming Liu, and Anil K. Jain. "Faceguard: A self-supervised defense against adversarial face images." In *2023 IEEE 17th International Conference on Automatic Face and Gesture Recognition (FG)*, pp. 1–8. IEEE, 2023.

13. Gunasekaran, Hemalatha, K. Ramalakshmi, Shalini Ramanathan, and R. Venkatesan. "A deep learning CNN model for genome sequence classification." *Intelligent Computing Applications for COVID-19* (2021): 169–185. https://www.taylorfrancis.com/chapters/edit/10.1201/9781003141105-9/deep-learning-cnn-model-genome-sequence-classification-hemalatha-gunasekaran-ramalakshmi-shalini-ramanathan-venkatesan

14. Ramanathan, Shalini, and Mohan Ramasundaram. "Alzheimer's disease shape detection model in brain magnetic resonance images via whale optimization with kernel support vector machine." *Journal of Electrical Engineering and Technology* 18 (2022): 1–10.

15. Ramanathan, Shalini, Savita Goel, and Subramanian Alagumalai. "Comparison of cloud database: Amazon's SimpleDB and Google's Bigtable." In *2011 International Conference on Recent Trends in Information Systems*, pp. 165–168. IEEE, 2011.

16. Ghosh, Shreya, Anwesha Mukherjee, Soumya K. Ghosh, and Rajkumar Buyya. "STOPPAGE: Spatio-temporal data driven cloud-fog-edge computing framework for pandemic monitoring and management." *Software: Practice and Experience* 52, no. 12 (2022): 2700–2726.

17. Calheiros, Rodrigo N., Rajiv Ranjan, Anton Beloglazov, César A.F. De Rose, and Rajkumar Buyya. "CloudSim: A toolkit for modeling and simulation of cloud computing environments and evaluation of resource provisioning algorithms." *Software. Software: Practice and Experience* 41, no. 1 (2011): 23–50.

18. Goudarzi, Mohammad, Marimuthu Palaniswami, and Rajkumar Buyya. "Scheduling IoT applications in edge and fog computing environments: A taxonomy and future directions." *ACM Computing Surveys* 55, no. 7 (2022): 1–41.

19. Wang, Zhiyu, Mohammad Goudarzi, Jagannath Aryal, and Rajkumar Buyya. "Container orchestration in edge and fog computing environments for real-time iot applications." *Computational Intelligence and Data Analytics: Proceedings of ICCIDA 2022* (2022): 1–21.

20. Barbuto, Vincenzo, Claudio Savaglio, Min Chen, and Giancarlo Fortino. "Disclosing edge intelligence: A systematic meta-survey." *Big Data and Cognitive Computing* 7, no. 1 (2023): 44.

21. Pham, Truong An, Junjue Wang, Roger Iyengar, Yu Xiao, Padmanabhan Pillai, Roberta Klatzky, and Mahadev Satyanarayanan. "Ajalon: Simplifying the authoring of wearable cognitive assistants." *Software: Practice and Experience* 51, no. 8 (2021): 1773–1797.

22. Tong, Alexander, Nikolay Malkin, Guillaume Huguet, Yanlei Zhang, Jarrid Rector-Brooks, Kilian Fatras, Guy Wolf, and Yoshua Bengio. "Conditional flow matching: Simulation-free dynamic optimal transport." *arXiv preprint arXiv:2302.00482* (2023).

23. Abirami, S., and Shalini Ramanathan. "Linear scheduling strategy for resource allocation in cloud environment." *International Journal on Cloud Computing: Services and Architecture (IJCCSA)* 2, no. 1 (2012): 9–17.

24. Iftikhar, Sundas, Sukhpal Singh Gill, Chenghao Song, Minxian Xu, Mohammad Sadegh Aslanpour, Adel N. Toosi, Junhui Du et al. "AI-based fog and edge computing: A systematic review, taxonomy and future directions" *Internet of Things* 21 (2022): 100674.

2 History and Role of AI in Healthcare and Medicine

Dipali Dakhole and K.N. Praveena

2.1 INTRODUCTION

Artificial intelligence (AI) is a field of computer science that rose with the invention of robots. Author Karel Capek, in his play "Study of Healthcare" from 1921, first used the term "robot". Robots have replaced human work in factories since their invention. By using leather, wood, and artificial organs, Yan Shi, a Chinese mechanical engineer, created the first human-shaped construct. Leonardo da Vinci created a knight robot during the Renaissance. His meticulous sketches were used to create this robot. It could stand up, move around, and wave its hands. His inspirational work influenced the medical industry as well, and an American business created the da Vinci surgical system, which was eventually renamed the "Intuitive Surgical" system. Complex surgical operations like heart valve replacement, prostatectomies, and gynaecologic surgeries can be handled using da Vinci surgical equipment [1]. William Grey Water created the Machina Speculatrix, the first electronic autonomous robot, in 1948, to illustrate how the brain works. John McCarthy invented the term "artificial intelligence" in 1955 and described it as "the science and engineering of making intelligent machines" [2]. At the conference, he discussed the topic that gave rise to the interdisciplinary field of "artificial intelligence". It offered a theoretical foundation for applications that could include computer science [3]. Today, computers are capable of solving any complicated mathematical problems, which assists in the large-scale resolution of medical-related applications, and AI is formally a subfield of computer engineering because it employs fresh ideas and creative approaches to solve challenging computing issues. Modern cybernetics has made significant contributions to the growth of AI. Cybernetics uses technology to regulate, structure, and constrain any system.

The future of healthcare and medical systems will be enhanced and transformed by AI, which includes tasks carried out by computers that mimic human intellect. AI initially consisted of a straightforward set of "if, then" principles, but over time it has developed to be able to handle problems that are often only solved by human brains. AI has several subdomains, including the fields of machine learning (ML), deep learning (DL), and computer vision. The goal of ML is to utilize an algorithm or model to find hidden patterns in data that can be used to assess problems and find solutions. Instead of tackling such issues with static solutions, ML algorithms

DOI: 10.1201/9781003363361-2

or models are used in various clinical decision-making scenarios to individualize patient treatment. Many ML and robotics-based applications in healthcare have highlighted the potential of AI. Now, it is referred to as DL, which is widely used. In DL, the machine may decide for itself by using algorithms to build an artificial neural network (ANN) that functions similarly to the human brain. In computer vision, a computer learns from a collection of still photos or moving pictures. There is a demand for more precise image-based diagnosis and problem interpretation in medical fields like radiology. A crucial part of medical education is learning how to interpret radiological images. These clinical procedures and services are being addressed by AI technology. Additionally, it is assisting in the transformation of radiology education and image-based learning for the future [4]. In recent years, AI has been employed to enhance ways of gathering sensory input and turning it into useful models that perform even better than human brain functions. For instance, research is currently being done on the diagnosis of breast cancer during mammography screening, the effectiveness of robotic surgery, and emerging procedures using autonomous robotic systems.

The technical development of AI systems is crucial, but for its responsible and effective adoption, ethical and legal concerns must also be addressed. The components of systems that have a patient-physician interaction for all diagnostic procedures and treatments include ethical considerations and human consent. Real-world issues with new, promising technology will only be resolved if the public is involved. Furthermore, a group with tribal inequalities does not have any statistically notable relationship, indicating that tribal disparities are not just the depiction of certain patient groups in the training data. In similar research, a number of researchers claimed that AI systems could recognize numerous patient demographic characteristics. One study demonstrated that, from chest X-rays, it is possible to differentiate between patients and find out the sex of a person using AI. Meanwhile, other investigations discovered that the AI model could accurately predict the chronological age of patients by conducting tests with various medical images. Retinal scans have been utilized in ophthalmology to forecast gender, age, and cardiac indicators with the use of hypertension and smoking status. These findings confirm what has been known for more than a century about the importance of variables and possible confounding from clinical and epidemiological studies. They show that racial identity, age, and other demographic characteristics that are highly correlated with disease outcomes are also highly correlated with elements of medical imaging and may lead to bias in model results.

Practically, many published AI models are upfront but with bivariate evaluations of attributes and have a tendency to forecast medical results. Despite advanced AI models beginning to take other hazard aspects into account, that theoretically brings models with multiple features. The clinical and epidemiological research largely omits important demographic multiple features (such as age, gender, and tribal individuality). The idea that tribal pinpointing in DL models may be confused suggests one potential mechanism for tribal inequities brought on by AI models: the capacity of AI models to quickly determine a patient's race from X-rays. This hypothesis has not received as much attention as other demographic factors such as age and sex,

TABLE 2.1

Various Subdomains in Medical Science and their Applications

AI Application Area in Medical Science	Description of Application
Risk prediction and intervention	Based on EHR data, AI can calculate health risks to patients.
Population health management	AI-based semi-automated systems can reach out to patients to identify and close the care gap.
Medical advice and triage	AI can triage patient complaints and free up primary care access for more appropriate care.
Risk-adjusted panelling and resourcing	AI ensures clinicians have adequate time to address the queries of each patient by adjusting panel sizes based on complexity.
Remote patient monitoring	AI organizes huge amounts of data collected from smart devices to provide actionable clinical insights.
Digital health coaching	AI provides patients with self-management tools for chronic diseases.
Diagnostics	AI-powered PCP services can help regions with a lack of specialty care.
Clinical decision-making	AI built-in HER platform gives physicians evidence-based clinical suggestions.
Practice management	AI can automate repetitive administrative tasks.

and radiologists generally hold the tacit belief that it is nearly impossible to find out the race of a patient using medical image data and that most imaging works are fundamentally race-neutral, considering that the task is unaffected by the race of patient [5].

There are many more applications in the medical domain, as listed in Table 2.1. These applications have transformed the healthcare system using AI [6]. All of these are sorted into two categories: the virtual branch of AI and the physical branch of AI, as explained in the next sections.

2.1.1 THE VIRTUAL BRANCH OF ARTIFICIAL INTELLIGENCE

The virtual branch of AI in medicine has two primary subfields: ML and DL, as shown in Figure 2.1. The mathematical techniques that use DL to enhance learning through experience serve as the virtual component. ML algorithms can be classified into three categories: (1) unsupervised (ability to detect patterns), (2) supervised (algorithms for categorization and prediction based on prior data), and (3) reinforcement learning (using a specific problem space as the basis for a method that uses a series of incentives and penalties). First, AI has expedited and continues to speed up genetic and molecular medical discoveries by offering ML algorithms and knowledge management. An example of medical advances AI has resulted in is the discovery of new therapeutic targets because of unsupervised protein-protein interaction

```
                                    ┌── Unsupervised Learning
                        Machine     │
                    ┌── Learning  ──┼── Supervised Learning
                    │   (ML)        │
         Virtual    │               └── Reinforcement Learning
         Branch   ──┤               ┌── Unsupervised Learning
         of AI      │   Deep        │
                    └── Learning  ──┼── Hybrid
                        (DL)        │
                                    └── Supervised Learning
```

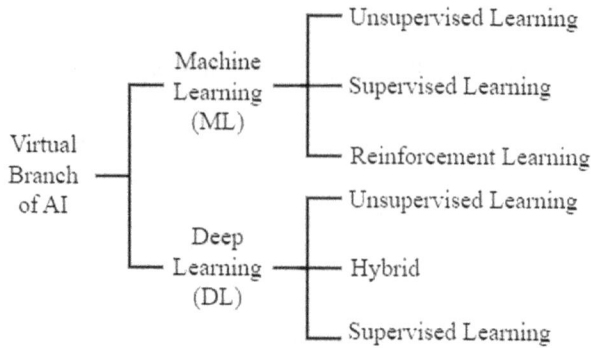

FIGURE 2.1　Types of virtual branch AI in medicine

algorithms. The strategy of evolutionary enhanced Markova clustering brought together flexible revolutionary algorithms and futuristic clustering methods, which are more authentic with reduced overfitting problems. They have been developed to discover DNA adaptation and RNA adaptation to predict hereditary diseases or behaviours [7]. Over 5,000 protein complexes could be predicted, and of them, no less than one gene ontology function item enriched more than 70% of the dataset. Overfitting problems arise if a model has more parameters than observations. Along with genetic applications, it is widely used in other healthcare systems.

Today, healthcare systems include larger-scale organizations in addition to the customary contacts between patients and doctors. The healthcare system must also always endeavour to improve itself by learning from its mistakes and implementing new procedures. A group of agents located in a shared environment interacts with one another in a multi-agent system (MAS). This procedure entails creating or joining an organization that makes substantial advancements with AI. For example, the creation of needlessly complicated ecosystems for the treatment of chronic mental illness in place of concentrating on medical expenses in public systems. In medical organizations, the MAS technique suggests studying patients' behaviour with medication consequences in a large ecosystem. A global healthcare platform enables practice mapping, streamlined standards, and better decision support through a proven rise in medication reaction, reduction in expenditures, and more effective treatments. Managers of health systems have been able to implement it; it is possible to examine the changes in the components of the social, medical, and criminal justice systems, as well as the dynamics of system performance. Electronic medical records that use certain algorithms to recognize people with genetic disorders or at a higher threat of developing a lingering ailment are among the virtual uses of AI. Allows employees to gather, and share their understanding to make ideal decisions in extent time. To reach the desired quality, the administration of healthcare processes and electronic medical records is crucial. Information from the inconsistently maintained patient records currently in use must be digitized and made available for epidemiological planning and research as both individual data and aggregated formats. To attain targeted efficacy and reduce costs, academics and the information technology sector must make significant efforts. For the healthcare system and knowledge acquisition, the majority of medical records currently exist as inaccessible silos that contain meaningless information. Collaboration between labs and clinics is necessary to speed up the use of electronic health records. Organizations should assist in the development of systems that can make sense of the data and encourage the collection of real-time data. Doctors and scientists must be allowed free access to aggregated data, and it must be made readily available at the point of service. New trends in discoveries in medical sciences must be disseminated via free sources. Each finding must be examined for its clinical application, as well as the dataset's simplicity, readability, and clinical utility. To upscale their medical value and lower healthcare costs, medical instruments or records are crucial parameters for individualized medication, early identification, and focused prevention.

2.1.2 THE PHYSICAL BRANCH OF ARTIFICIAL INTELLIGENCE

The second use of medical AI encompasses devices, medical machinery, and robots that are involved in the caretaking business and are referred to as "carebots". It involves the deployment of robot-assistants, for example, robot caretakers for elders who have cognitive impairment or restricted mobility. Carebots, a Japanese invention, are the supreme cutting-edge examples of this machinery. In surgery, robots can assist human doctors or even operate alone. One of the most stunning demonstrations of robot utility is their capacity to interact with and instruct autistic youngsters. Important ethical questions must be answered before AI robots may be used consistently in the current medical context, as well as in many other circumstances that could benefit from robotic assistance [8]. A fundamental difficulty in this emerging area of healthcare is the procedure requirements of varying psychological and physical conditions, their allocated results, along with ethical problems. In addition to the virtual and physical branches of AI, there are other applications too, which are used for finding the efficiency of treatments used in medical applications.

2.2 THE APPLICATION OF ROBOTS TO THE OBSERVATION OF THERAPY EFFICIENCY

In situations like rehabilitation, robots can also be useful in determining how human performance has evolved. AI may also be used to keep track of how drugs are administered specifically to particular malignancies, tissues, or organs. For instance, it is interesting to read about the recent advancement of nanorobots modified to address conveyance issues due to the challenges of therapeutic agent diffusion into interest areas. This issue arises when the psychotherapist tries to focus on the tumour's core, which is typically less vascularized and anoxic, but active. Authors have tried to use a natural substance in place of "intelligent" nanoparticles, in-order to get around the limits of mechanical-radioactive robotics [9]. They are researching a particular form of marine bacteria called *Magnetococcus marinas* for this purpose since it naturally moves to low-oxygen environments. An external magnetic source provides initial guidance, which is followed by the nanorobots' innate abilities. Covalent bonds between these nanorobots and nanoliposomes with therapeutic characteristics are possible. According to preliminary data, the gradient of the required medicine into the hypoxic zones has significantly increased. More study is required for the majority of these potential uses of AI in medicine, notably in the field of human-computer interactions. Moshimo Mori coined the term "uncanny valley" in 1970, with a primary emphasis on the human-robot interaction (HRI) discipline. This study evaluated humanoid robots for their supernatural and unpredictable nature as factors determining whether people view robots as being feared or accepted.

In a variety of clinical tasks, self-reported race is used to stratify AI performance in numerous healthcare applications, such as melanoma detection, mortality prediction, and algorithms that help forecast healthcare use. Furthermore, group affiliation and racial disparities do not have a substantial correlation. This shows that racial inequalities are not solely the result of these patients' training data. In similar research, a number of researchers claimed that AI systems could recognize numerous patient demographic characteristics. From chest X-rays, the investigations indicated that the AI model could reasonably predict the chronological age of patients, as well as forecast sex and differentiate between adult and paediatric patients. Retinal scans have been utilized in ophthalmology to forecast gender, age, and cardiac status. The results support which has been known from medical and epidemiological examination. They show that demographic variables that are highly correlated with disease outcomes, like age, sex, and race, are also highly interrelated with medical imaging and may cause bias in model results. Conceptually, many published AI models are just simple two-variable analysis (either potential of visual characteristics to forecast clinical outcomes). Most deep learning research in medicine has mainly ignored the important demographic factors, including age, sex, and racial identity. The conceptual underpinning of clinical and epidemiological research is multivariate modelling, despite more modern AI models beginning to incorporate additional risk factors. Findings highlighting the possibility of tribal identity confounding DL models point to one potential mechanism for tribal disparities brought on by AI models, which are openly capable of identifying a patient's history from medical photos. All radiographers believe that medical image processing is essentially race-neutral [10]. This is in contrast to other demographic information (like gender), where it is possible to determine a patient's race from medical images. Understanding how race affects medical imaging models is extremely important because the US Food and Drug Administration and other regulatory agencies are approving many AI-based models, which have medical images as a primary input. This understanding is important because there is a risk of bias loss in the medical system at a crucial part which is assumed to be race-neutral. In this work, we looked into how self-reported racial groups affect how accurately AI systems can identify a patient's race in medical imaging. To test whether AI models can accurately predict a person's race across a variety of imaging modalities, datasets, and clinical activities, we sought to analyze sizable publicly and privately available medical imaging datasets.

DL models are able to predict with accuracy, using both private and public data-sets, that it is possible to employ the patient's data with various clinical settings, formatting medical images, and population, irrespective of the patient's region [11]. This conclusion is startling because it is typically believed that only highly skilled humans can complete this activity. The careful elimination of features that encode parameters to render AI models "colour-blind" is one technique that is frequently suggested to reduce the known disparity in AI model performance. The study implies that this technique might be unachievable in medical image processing since tribal identification data looks to be exceedingly uneasy to segregate, despite the fact that this strategy has already been criticized as being ineffectual or even harmful in some situations. Any logical loss in resolution, the inclusion of noise, frequency distribution, or patch-based masking did not lessen the capacity to identify race. Even if we set aside the question of whether these strategies were helpful, it seems conceivable that it is improbable that these technical solutions will be successful and that methods for detecting racial bias, combined with models that are specifically designed to balance racial outcomes, should be thought of as the default strategy to maximize the security of AI in this situation. Even though it is changing, the regula-tory environment has not yet developed robust procedures to prevent unanticipated racial detection, either to recognize these talents in the models or to lessen the effects that may occur.

Furthermore, the constraints for investigations are the tribal identity label and the insignificant patient associates from various categories. Additionally, due to differences in how this group was documented across datasets, Hispanic patient populations were also omitted. Furthermore, there was no way to determine whether there was any remaining bone tissue on the photos because our studies to eliminate bone density only evaluated average body tissue pixels and brightness clipping at a 60% level. Future research might examine signal isolation prior to image reconstruction.

Finally, we should mention that the study did not uncover any brand-new racial differences in AI model performance. Instead, research that had already been pub-lished and that had revealed differences in some of the tasks we looked into served as the basis for the study. The outcomes of the study and the reported inequalities together imply that patient harm may result from the models' robust ability to iden-tify race in medical imagery. In other words, AI models appear to leverage their ability to anticipate the race of patients from their medical photos in order to provide varied health outcomes for those belonging to different racial groupings.

The study concluded by demonstrating how difficult it is to isolate the ability of medical AI systems to recognize self-reported racial identification from medi-cal imagery. We found that patient racial identity could be easily inferred from just medical picture data and that it would be applied to outside contexts and different imaging modalities. We strongly advise that everyone involved in the development, regulation, and use of DL models for medical image analysis exercise great caution, because such data may be abused to maintain or exacerbate the well-reported tribal inequities in medical science. This research suggests explicit model performance audits based on racial identity, sex, and age should be emphasized in future AI medical image processing, and that medical datasets should possibly include the self-documented race of patients.

AI is broadly defined as the use of computers to carry out operations that often require human intelligence, and has quickly emerged as a key component of medical research. According to the zeitgeist, a complete overhaul of the medical sector, including patient management, diagnosis, and treatment, is about to take place. Medical processes and decision-making are expected to change as a result of AI-based innovations, which also promise to bring about direct-to-consumer medical services and even robot-assisted healthcare [11–14]. However, there are many challenges in the AI framework. It is observed by many medical professionals that this is why it is evolving so slowly. Scepticism at this point is understandable. Currently, very few, if any, programmers actively serve as doctors. Despite being written more than 30 years ago, these remarks are still topical and relevant. While the AI revolution is being discussed, hospitals mostly carry on with "business as usual". Computers have undoubtedly revolutionized the healthcare industry, but most often they have replaced paper rather than human knowledge and skill. Patients are still virtually always evaluated, diagnosed, and treated with assistance from AI when they attend a medical facility.

Will AI in medicine live up to its promise? Maybe, but maybe not, if the current research priorities remain unchanged. Early medical AI was developed with the use of domain expertise, while modern machine learning algorithms frequently don't even need that. The new models are effective but frequently have inherent opaqueness; they fall short of the transparency standards set by their physicians and patient end-users. Clinicians and patients are left uninformed regarding how the model functions due to the inherent opacity, which is ascribed to a discrepancy between processing and the expectations of human interpretation and thinking. Lack of transparency makes doctors or patients unable to understand an algorithm because of proprietary secrets.

2.3   THE EFFECT OF BLACK-BOX AI

Black-box AI models lack a quality guarantee, don't inspire trust in organizations, and limit communication between doctors and patients. To improve the dependability of medical AI, healthcare should require clearness in facets of framework-building and evaluation.

2.3.1   THE GHOST OF AI PAST

Hypothesized artificial neuron systems with statistical skills gave rise to the area of AI in 1943. This discipline evolved alongside computers for a number of years, as new programmers that proved geometric theorems or resolved algebraic narrative problems using formal logic emerged. The first AI boom began in the 1960s when the standard switched from deduction through logic to knowledge-based systems.

Knowledge-based systems create a kind of customized "cookbook" by using domain expert knowledge through a ladder of "if, then" statements. AI started to tackle "real issues" for the first time, and the inclusion of reasoning gave the model some clearness by showing a trail of the inferences, which led to a lot of buzz, particularly in the healthcare industry. In a 1960 letter to the JAMA editors, the MYCIN system was the first significant attempt to imitate medical logistics, developed in the early 1970s. Knowledge-based systems, however, quickly showed their limitations in the face of sufficiently difficult issues. AI hype unexpectedly ended when James Lighthill published a paid report accusing researchers of exaggerating the capabilities of AI, leading to a significant decrease in funding. Thus, the AI boom came to a disappointing conclusion, and the "first AI winter" was born. When domain knowledge made significant economic advantages for the Digital Equipment Corporation in the 1980s and by 1986 had saved the company an estimated $40 million annually, a second AI boom had begun. With the help of additional businesses with significant financial incentives, the expert system market increased from a few million dollars to two billion dollars in less than ten years. The INTERNIST-1 system, which was first developed concurrently with MYCIN, had matured around this period. Through a diagnosis-ranking algorithm, this system aimed to develop and assess medical theories, but it was also inapplicable in real-world settings. Early on, there was scepticism regarding AI in medicine, but it soon spread to other sectors as well. The expert system market started to collapse in the late 1980s, as new research stopped finding its way into business. Once more, the AI trend ended in disappointment, and this sparked what was called the "second AI winter". Since then, machine learning, a new approach to AI, has largely replaced knowledge-based systems. It aims to link factors to respond using complex nonlinear functions immediately trained from the existing data without expert suggestions. As deep artificial neural networks (ANN) gained prominence throughout the 1990s and 2000s, machine learning research continued to advance. Although several early ANN decision support systems were made in the early 1990s, but with less accuracy than conventional regression models. We are currently experiencing a third wave of AI boom, driven by technological advancements, which allows us to recognize signals across space and time. It requires superfast computers and huge data to train deep neural networks, continuing the research in medicine.

2.3.2 THE GHOST OF AI PRESENT

By resolving numerous challenging issues, particularly in the areas of language and image processing, deep learning has renewed interest in AI. However, there are a number of ways that AI can fall short of being useful in the healthcare industry. A perfect model might not be used due to extrinsic issues like legal liability and data shortages. Furthermore, a lack of clearness in AI may be a fundamental issue that, if left unattended, could lead to an alternative AI winter in the field of healthcare. A large portion of contemporary machine learning was built for applications like internet promotion, where model efficiency is more crucial than its complexity. Even though DL models are effective, they are frequently deficient in clarity, making it difficult to know and understand why a model predicts something well. This is partially attributable to the extraordinarily complex "neural" connections and mathematical abstractions that these connections produce (such as the representation of pixel combinations in an image). It results in techniques like deep neural networks, where internal workings are hidden from the observer, like in "black boxes" [12]. Their utility in high-stakes decision-making is constrained by their lack of transparency and comprehensibility. Notably, black-box approaches (1) lack quality assurance, (2) do not foster trust, and (3) limit communication between clinicians and patients.

Some have claimed that there is no difference between a pharmacological intervention with a black-box ML model and an unidentified mechanism of action. After all, each of them may be thoroughly examined, trialled, and researched for their effects. The two technologies behave very differently within the context of the healthcare ecosystem, though. First, a note on quality control: AI in medical systems, even hidden AI (referred to as black-box AI), may have damaging preferences built into the model. A drug's mechanism is a natural phenomenon and cannot be regarded as innately biased. Second, if medical AI is not sufficiently transparent, patients might not trust it. In other words, even if they do not want explanations about, say, pharmacological processes, patients may nevertheless expect explanations from black-box models. Although factors other than a lack of openness can cause confidence to decline, this does not mean that it cannot as well. A patient's lack of confidence in a black-box model might undermine their faith in the model, even if their lack of confidence is factually incorrect because trust is dependent on subjective elements as well as objective ones. Contrarily, patients may not be interested in learning how a drug works; in this situation, keeping this information secret does not damage patients' confidence in the treatment. Obviously, as AI grows more pervasive, this could change. However, the patient's belief in medical AI will be contingent on a degree of clarity in the present, particularly in a context where AI-related disputes and catastrophes across multiple fields are being exposed. Third, in terms of the patient-physician conversation, black-box algorithms that can effectually make treatment value judgments may trump patient autonomy. Different from actually taking aspirin is being advised to do so. While there is typically just one correct diagnosis, there may be a wide range of viable therapies. The requirements and free will of each patient determine the "correct" course of action. Even if patients do not understand how a treatment works, they often need an explanation of why it is an acceptable alternative (based on efficacy, side effects, etc.) in order to choose the best course of action. The patient-physician relationship may suffer if such explanations are not given because it would be disrespectful to the patients' autonomy. Fourth, when it comes to validation, multiphase clinical trials are used to clinically validate medicinal therapies. The trials are open and tightly controlled. They also span a long period, requiring years of testing before being authorised for usage by people. Deep models frequently lack sufficient validation and have not yet been validated over long periods.

AI is an increasingly potent instrument that might "revolutionize" the healthcare industry. However, neglecting to acknowledge, and subsequently address, black-box AI's inherent limitations could result in the execution of a nascent technology that lacks quality of services, does not inspire reliability, and limits clinician-patient communication. As a substitute, we advocate for greater transparency in the medical arena to guarantee that AI in medicine is secure, efficient, and truly accepted by patients and healthcare experts. If not, trust might deteriorate, we might see another medical AI winter, and we would miss the true advantages that ML has the potential to offer.

2.4 CHATBOTS IN AI

Chatbots are developed for teaching and learning based on AI concepts. The findings demonstrate that a substantial amount of on-task activity was identified by the fundamental analysis of chat logs. Additionally, the research results point to chatbot technology as a potentially useful teaching and learning resource for distance learning and online instruction [13]. In a science lecture class, the usage of chatbots is also contrasted with the use of humanoid robots, and it was found that the visualisation provided by chatbots helped the students comprehend the lecture material more easily. However, research on chatbot use and development to enhance language learning is rather difficult to find. It might be challenging to locate studies on the usage and development of chatbots to improve language acquisition.

In order to offer a different viewpoint on how healthcare management systems are currently conducted, the health bot has been developed. Patient interaction with the platform is made simple by the health bot's user-friendly online and mobile app interfaces. As a result, the procedure is more interactive and user-friendly for patients, who can converse with the platform using human language. A strong NLP model processes free text classification with the help of free dialogs. It can be accessed via application programming interfaces (APIs) to provide services to third-party platforms [14].

2.5 CONCLUSION

In recent days, applications of AI are giving much more to human beings than our genetics. Therefore, it is widely used in medical sciences and healthcare systems. In healthcare, the goal of AI is to provide all kinds of services and practices, which are going to help the medical system to make accurate decisions and solutions.

AI is making evolutionary changes in the medical system by utilizing the huge amount of medical data available. This medical data must be utilized for developing patient-care applications as well as for advancing medical instruments' design and development. This article has explored both the physical and virtual aspects of AI. We examined the landscape of AI within the current medical student curricula and made an effort to understand how it can affect both current healthcare and the practice of medicine in the future.

REFERENCE LIST

1. Hamet, P, J Tremblay, Artificial intelligence in medicine. *Metabolism: Clinical and Experimental*, 69S, 2017 Apr, S36–S40.https://doi.org/10.1016/j.metabol.2017.01.011. Epub 2017 Jan 11. PMID: 28126242.

2. Kaul, V, S Enslin, SA Gross, History of artificial intelligence in medicine. *Gastrointestinal Endoscopy*, 92(4), 2020 Oct, 807–812. https://doi.org/10.1016/j.gie .2020.06.040. Epub 2020 Jun 18. PMID: 32565184.

3. Kulikowski, CA, An opening chapter of the first generation of artificial intelligence in medicine: The first Rutgers AIM workshop, June 1975. *Yearbook of Medical Informatics*, 10(1), 2015 Aug, 227–233. https://doi.org/10.15265/IY-2015-016. Epub 2015 Jun 30. PMID: 26123911. PMCID: PMC4587035.

4. Quinn, Thomas P, Stephan Jacobs, Manisha Senadeera, Vuong Le, Simon Coghlan, The three ghosts of medical AI: Can the black-box present deliver? *Artificial Intelligence in Medicine*, 124, 2022, 102158, ISSN 0933-3657. https://doi.org/10.1016/j.artmed.2021 .102158.

5. Gichoya, Judy Wawira, Imon Banerjee, Ananth Reddy Bhimireddy, John L Burns, Leo Anthony Celi, Li-Ching Chen, Ramon Correa, Natalie Dullerud, Marzyeh Ghassemi, Shih-Cheng Huang, Po-Chih Kuo, Matthew P Lungren, Lyle J Palmer, Brandon J Price, Saptarshi Purkayastha, Ayis T Pyrros, Lauren Oakden-Rayner, Chima Okechukwu, Laleh Seyyed-Kalantari, Hari Trivedi, Ryan Wang, Zachary Zaiman, Haoran Zhang, AI recognition of patient race in medical imaging: A modelling study. *Digital Health*, 4(Jun), 2022.

6. Lin, S, A clinician's guide to Artificial Intelligence (AI): Why and how primary care should lead the health care AI revolution. *Journal of the American Board of Family Medicine*, 35(1), 2022 Jan–Feb, 175–184. https://doi.org/10.3122/jabfm.2022.01.210226. PMID: 35039425.

7. Bakkar, N, T Kovalik, I Lorenzini et al, Artificial intelligence in neurodegenerative disease research: Use of IBM Watson to identify additional RNA-binding proteins altered in amyotrophic lateral sclerosis. *Acta Neuropathology*, 135(2), 2018, 227–247. https://doi.org/10.1007/s00401-017-1785-8.

8. Chakraborty, Chinmay, MM Kamruzzaman, Ibrahim Alrashdi, Ali Alqazzaz, New opportunities, challenges, and applications of edge-AI for connected healthcare in Internet of medical things for smart cities. *Journal of Healthcare Engineering*, 2022, 2040–2295. https://doi.org/10.1155/2022/2950699.

9. Yakar, Derya, Yfke P Ongena, Thomas C Kwee, Marieke Haan, Do people favor artificial intelligence over physicians? A survey among the general population and their view on artificial intelligence in medicine. *Value in Health*, 25(3), 2022, 374–381, ISSN 1098-3015. https://doi.org/10.1016/j.jval.2021.09.004.

10. Fischetti, Chanel, Param Bhatter, Emily Frisch, Amreet Sidhu, Mohammad Helmy, Matt Lungren, Erik Duhaime, The evolving importance of artificial intelligence and radiology in medical trainee education. *Acad Radiol.*, 29(Suppl 5), 2022, S70–S75. doi: 10.1016/j.acra.2021.03.023. PMID: 34020872.

11. Kulikowski, Casimir A, Beginnings of artificial intelligence in medicine (AIM): Computational artifice assisting scientific inquiry and clinical art – With reflections on present AIM challenges. *Yearbook of Medical Informatics*, 13, 2019, 68–84.

12. Yang, Guang, Ye Qinghao, Jun Xia, Unbox the black-box for the medical explainable AI via multi-modal and multi-centre data fusion: A mini-review, two showcases and beyond, two showcases and beyond. *Information Fusion*, 77, 2022, 29–52. ISSN 1566-2535. https://doi.org/10.1016/j.inffus.2021.07.016.

13. Haristiani, Nuria, Artificial intelligence (AI) chatbot as language learning medium: An inquiry. *Journal of Physics: Conference Series*, IOP Publishing, 2019. https://doi.org/10.1088/1742-6596/1387/1/012020.
14. Neelakandan, S, Maria V Vasileiou, Ilias G Maglogiannis, The health ChatBots in telemedicine: Intelligent dialog system for remote support. *Journal of Healthcare Engineering*, Hindawi. https://doi.org/10.1155/2022/4876512.

3 Drug Discovery Using Explainable AI Approaches
The Current Scenario

Chinju John, Akarsh K. Nair, and Jayakrushna Sahoo

3.1 INTRODUCTION

Drug discovery is composed of many processes, starting from disease recognition, cause identification, lead molecule creation and its improvisation, testing of the proposed drug, and finally its disposal to the target entities, with post-release effect studies by reputed administrative bodies. As the entire lifespan of these steps could take up to 15 to 20 years in the conventional pipeline, accelerating the entire course of actions without compromising on efficiency will be a great boon to the era, especially when viruses are mutating in a bewildering manner. Recent interventions by artificial intelligence (AI) in the drug discovery arena have helped to achieve reduced timelines to reach the final goal or "the cure".

There are well-performing and highly accurate AI-based models in machine learning (ML) and deep learning (DL), which have laid milestones in the drug discovery paradigm but are unable to explain the results they achieve or the approach they have followed to reach the results [1]. Since the conventional wet lab or *in silico* approaches are human-interfered procedures, the outcomes of such experiments tend to be more reliable, at least to the same extent as clinical testing. The trustworthiness of DL-guided models needs to be justified, as the succeeding phases of the outputs could put human lives at stake. Owing to this fact, the scientific community is working now on explainable AI models with high accuracy and reliability. The big data analysis from pharmaceutical research can be carried out with modern deep learning technologies and dig more into the toxicity prediction and omics of genomes and proteins [2].

The term "explainable AI" (XAI) deals with how an AI-based model can explain its decisions as per the end-users' questions. These explanations can be classified as "local" or "global" explanations, depending on their dimensional depth. It is considered to be an inevitable part of "third-wave AI systems". Interactive machine

DOI: 10.1201/9781003363361-3

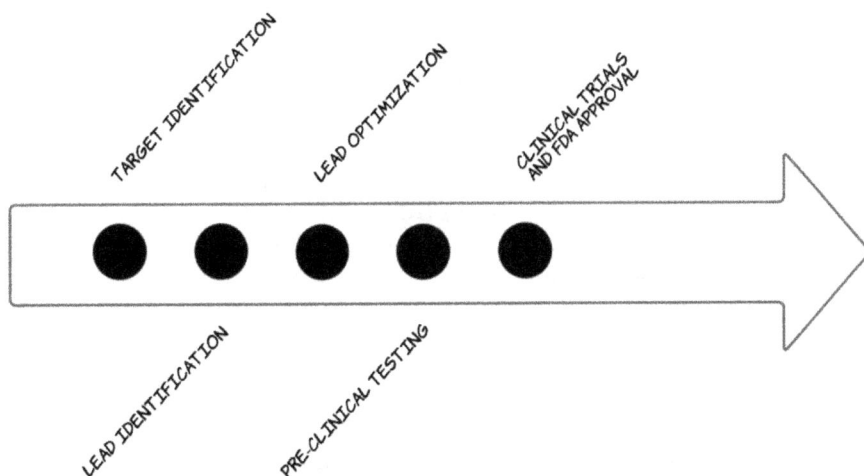

FIGURE 3.1 Drug discovery and development process

learning models (iMLs) are a variant of this, composed of algorithms that convey the procedure to the user and correct it if any changes are required [3]. Explainability of DL models associated with drug discovery is not a "cakewalk", as the AI models involved here determine the content, characteristics, and chemical feature explanations (for example, pharmacophores, functional groups, and physicochemical entities) [2] preserved from the drug candidates.

3.1.1 DRUG DISCOVERY PHASES

The entire drug discovery process (Figure 3.1) can be divided into two phases, comprising the drug discovery, its testing, and approval. Computer-aided drug discovery (CADD) methods have paved a pathway through milestones like protein or ligand structure-based methods and molecular docking studies to pick out lead compounds with the capability to be novel drugs. The past years have contributed significant innovations to these fields the changes from conventional to modern aspects which are detailed and discussed.

The subsequent sections of this chapter will focus on how XAI-influenced approaches are providing facelifts to the drug discovery phases, and what recent trends are reviving these phases.

3.2 DRUG TARGET IDENTIFICATION

A drug target, as defined by the *Oxford Dictionary of Biochemistry*, is "a biological entity that interacts with, and whose activity is modulated by a particular compound". Drugs are specific to their targets, which are classified as receptors, ion channels, enzymes, and carrier molecules. Identifying a putative therapeutic target that can be manipulated by a drug can be carried out with DL and ML approaches, which are versatile enough to use the information derived from biological, chemical, and topological properties of compounds to filter out the target from large-scale libraries [4]. Creating a causal connection between the target and the disease is the starting point of target identification. Gene expression is one of the most employed approaches to identifying the genes responsible for a disease. With the help of microarray and ribo nucleic acid-sequencing (RNA-Seq) technologies, a tremendous volume of sequence data is available these days, stored in publicly accessible databases such as the National Center for Biotechnology Information's (NCBI's) Gene Expression Omnibus (GEO), ArrayExpress, the Cancer Genome Atlas (TCGA), the Gene Expression Database (GXD). Predicting the differential expression of genes using the DL model called DEcode has opened new insights into differential expression of genes between tissues, differential transcript usage, and genome-wide gene expression [5].

Supervised machine learning models such as ElasticNet, k-nearest neighbours, Random Forest, and feed-forward neural networks are preferred for identifying tissue-specific drug targets [6]. A deep neural network (DNN) was employed to study the genotype-tissue expression (GTEx) data to reveal the differential expressions associated with soft tissue sarcomas and to differentiate the subtypes, a Random Forest ML model was used as the DNN model could not perform the same [7].

For the identification of anti-cancer drug targets, network-based and ML algorithms which take network features as input-based research are used these days. Decision trees are significant contributors in cancer target studies, but overfitting can limit their performance, and to overcome this, dimension-reduction and pruning strategies are employed [8]. DL models used for cancer drug target identifications and other disease targets are listed in Table 3.1. Once the drug target, which is usually a protein, is identified, it's necessary to identify the druggability characteristics. It is a postulation that considers the possibility of a drug adhering to a protein to change its functional role. The action of a drug and its target is like a lock-and-key mechanism, and the drug acts on protein pockets like a key in a keyhole. Hence, studying the physicochemical properties of the protein pockets can reveal the druggability of proteins.

Certain protein/target structures may not be available at publicly accessible data resources such as the Protein Data Bank (https://www.rcsb.org/), due to difficulties in crystallizing the molecule, or because the molecule is still under research. In such cases, DL methods are available these days as an alternative to traditional homology modelling techniques. In homology modelling, the FASTA format sequence of an unknown protein will be given along with the 3D structure of a known protein having a sequence identity of more than 30% for predicting the 3D structure of the unknown protein. Even if the template protein structure is not available, DL algorithms like CNN, RNN, variational autoencoders (VAEs), and generative adversarial networks (GAN) are capable of predicting promising target structures [14].

The Critical Assessment of Structure Prediction (CASP) evaluates predicted structures using a global distance test (GDT), and AlphaFold2 by DeepMind Technologies, based on DNN, scored a value of 92.4 for its predicted structures [15]. The predicted

TABLE 3.1

Deep Learning Models for Drug Target Identification

DL Algorithm Used	Input Data Used	Targeted Disease Type	Limitations	Reference
Deep neural networks	mRNA expression profile datasets from GEO	Lung adenocarcinoma	• The heterogeneity of data can cause biases in the yield • Limited data availability	[9]
DeepWalk graph-embedding algorithm	miRNA profiles associated with cancer types	Breast cancer, lung cancer, prostate cancer	• Experimental validation of the results is required	[10]
Convolutional neural networks, recurrent neural networks	Curated druggable proteins from the DrugBank and Therapeutic Target Database	General	• The non-availability of large-scale training and validation. • Extended efforts to fine-tune the model parameters are required to overcome limitations	[11]
XGBoost	Cancer-related lncRNAs	Cancer	• Imbalanced data and additional measures should be considered while dealing with such data.	[12]
Deep belief networks	Long noncoding RNAs	Cancer	• The dataset used has less-conserved biological properties. • Features are extracted by the network itself.	[13]

protein structure by AlphaFold2 has been shared via the European Molecular Biology Laboratory's European Bioinformatics Institute (EMBL-EBI), and it includes almost 98.5% of the human proteome (https://alphafold.ebi.ac.uk/). While the system has limitations, the CASP results ensure the capability of AlphaFold2 to unravel the 3D protein structure and thereby lift up biological research.

Our literature resources are rich in information related to diseases and associated proteins or other biomolecules; hence, they are the primary reference for such studies. There are natural language processing (NLP) AI models created to extract the associations between diseases and their responsible biomolecules, such as proteins or genes, from associated journal publications. BeFree is a supervised NLP kernel-based method that depends on the European Union's database of adverse drug reactions which is annotated by scientists [16], and DigSee collects text from PubMed abstracts to identify the genes and associated malfunctions leading to diseases from the sentences, calculating the ranking of the sentences using the Bayesian model [17]. A tool called TargetDB can aggregate the universally available information about a given target – such as paths to diseases, safety, 3D structures, ligandability, etc. – and represent it as an output for the user's best understanding [18]. A profuse database of genes and associated disease variants can be found in DisGeNET (https://www.disgenet.org/), which works on text-mining principles [19].

3.3 LEAD IDENTIFICATION

The National Cancer Institute (NCI) defines a lead compound as "a chemical compound which exhibits the potential to act against a disease target and to be developed as a new drug." Identifying a lead compound is as difficult as finding a needle in a haystack. The conventional computer-aided strategies for lead identification include virtual screening (target structure-based and ligand structure-based), *de novo* drug design (DNDD), and molecular docking studies. Structure-based virtual screening makes use of protein structures which are promising targets, the binding cavity identification of these proteins can help to choose the ligand molecules . If the ligands or drugs for a particular disease are already known, then ligand-based virtual screening is possible. Pharmacophores, which are the blueprints of a drug, can identify molecules with similar physicochemical properties. Quantitative structure–activity relationship (QSAR) studies are a subcategory of ligand-based drug design, where the relationship between biological activity and physicochemical properties of drug-like molecules can be determined. All these approaches can be used to identify potential lead molecules and to virtually screen large libraries of potential compounds [20]. A detailed representation is given in Figure 3.2.

Virtual screening filters databases with millions of chemical compounds that have drug-like characteristics. The alternative approach of DNDD is capable of designing completely new compounds using components from successful drug discoveries. AI has started to play a pivotal role in DNDD. MolAICal (https://molaical.github .io/), designed and implemented by Bai et al., is capable of designing new drugs in 3D formats scaffolded from protein pockets represented in 3D [21]. This tool has two components that make it function; the primary component uses DL and genetic

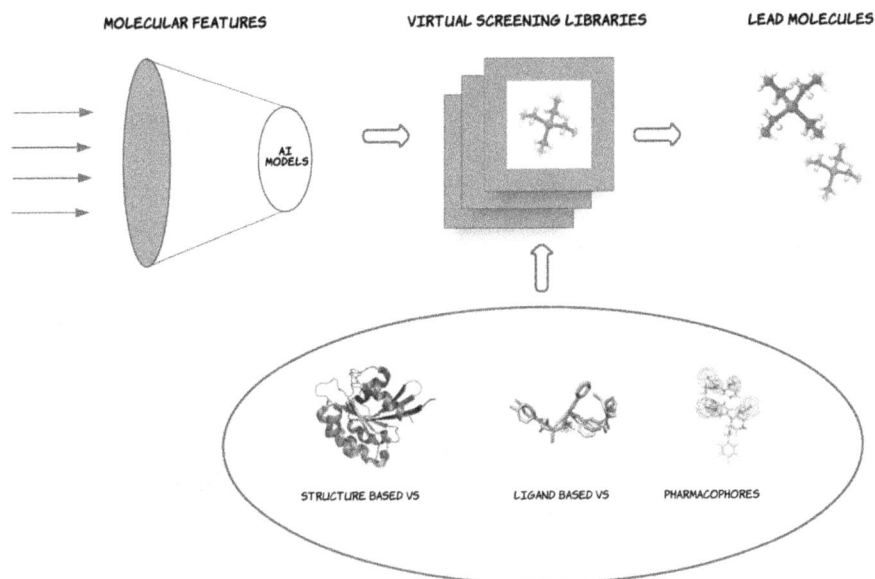

MOLECULAR FEATURES   VIRTUAL SCREENING LIBRARIES   LEAD MOLECULES

AI MODELS

STRUCTURE BASED VS   LIGAND BASED VS   PHARMACOPHORES

FIGURE 3.2 Outline of how AI-based models are used for lead identification

algorithm-employed modules, trained on drugs approved by the US Food and Drug Administration (FDA), and the second component makes use of the molecular docking technique along with a DL model trained on the ZINC database (https://zinc .docking.org/). Deep reinforcement learning (DRL) algorithm-based ReLeaSE combines two DNNs for the generative and predictive parts associated with DNDD [22]. The generative part controlled by one of the DNN modules is responsible for the production of novel compounds and the predictive part implemented by the second DNN performs the feature prediction of the generated compound.

A deep neural network model was designed and developed by Stokes et al. to replace the virtual screening of huge chemical libraries, which is expensive, time-consuming, and can fail to span the large chemical space [23]. They have considered the molecular representation of the property, which is to suppress the growth of *E. coli*. The model was trained with inhibitor molecules and then applied to multiple chemical libraries to identify potential lead compounds.

Therapeutic peptides, which can be used against the SARS-CoV-2 virus, were identified using DNNs, and the physicochemical properties of these peptides were calculated to characterize the inputs given and to guide the neural network to identify promising antiviral peptides [23].

To interpret the significance of identified peptides, they performed a composition analysis of the amino acids, which revealed the affinity measures towards the target proteins. Chemical sequences known as simplified molecular-input line-entry system (SMILES) strings are ubiquitous entities in drug repurposing [24]. SMILES can be coupled with amino acid (AA) sequences, 3D structures of promising molecules, and targeted proteins, to fetch promising features for the DL model's decision. Recent studies yielded DL models used to fight the SARS-CoV-2 virus by discovering therapeutic antibodies.

Designing lead molecules with desired features can be done through ML models, and various algorithms like variational auto encoders (VAE) and recurrent neural network (RNN) variants have shown impressive results. These models take SMILES strings as inputs and the grammar of these inputs is considered in generating new molecules. Generative models also incorporate different predictive models to calculate various absorption, distribution, metabolism, excretion, and toxicity (ADMET) features, while designing future possible drugs. Molecular graphs are an alternative to this problem; however, handling them on a computer is comparatively difficult. A DL model called MERMAID [25], based on RNN and Monte Carlo tree search (MCTS), can take a specific molecule as the beginning point for optimization. The authors of MERMAID have proposed single and multi-models focussed on optimizing the Quantitative Estimate of Drug-likeness (QED) score, they claim that molecules generated by the model are unique and state-of-the-art, and are high in number and similar in molecular weight.

Molecular dynamic simulations (MDS) can reveal the behaviour of molecules at atomistic levels. Protein–ligand interactions and binding stabilities can be measured using MD simulations, but these simulations have limitations, as they are time-consuming and very arduous. AI can bring these simulations to the next level by overcoming their limitations. A combination of 3D CNN and spatial-graph CNN was trained on free energies calculated from 15,000 small molecules, generated while they were transferred from cyclohexane to water. Other atomistic features were also considered for the purpose of the training, and the results were promising, with similar free-energy prediction accuracy scores similar to those of MD simulations [26].

3.4   LEAD OPTIMIZATION

The lead molecules are raw-form drugs, which need to be fine-tuned to become effective real drugs. These molecules are used as the starting point for detailed chemical modifications to further improve their target specificity, selectivity, pharmacokinetic activities, and safety profiles while maintaining the favourable properties of the lead compounds. Lead optimization involves recursions of the design–make–test–analyze (DMTA) steps. If the target structure is available, by performing drug-target interaction (DTI) studies, we can rationalize the drug design process.

The available computational methods for DTI studies can be classified as:

a) **Ligand-based methods**

Here, similar target proteins based on structure or sequence identity are exploited to predict the interactions with drug chemical structures, with QSAR support. The quality of a built QSAR model is not appreciable if the number of available active molecules of a target is low. QSAR models are limited in performance, as they consider only one target to predict the associated activity.

b) **Docking-based methods**

If the 3D structure of the target protein is known, studies of the molecular docking between the protein and lead molecules can unravel the interactions, and moleculardynamic simulations can measure the durability and stability of such interactions by mimicking the cellular environment. The limitation of this approach is that it is bound to protein structure availability, and wet lab procedures involved in depicting these structures are cumbersome.

c) **Chemogenomic methods**

Here, the dataset has binary classes labelled as positive and negative, consisting of the chemical structure and the drug target's biological sequences. This is used to train the model classifier (algorithm) and afterwards to detect unknown interactions [27].

Conventional approaches are being replaced with AI models; graph-based neural networks can learn the drug structure and drug-target interaction information, rather than taking them as strings, as strings may not be able to store structural information [28]. For graph-based DL model, the input is the drug-target pair and the output is a numerical value corresponding to the affinity of that pair. In the graphical representation, each node is a multi-dimensional binary feature vector, holding on the atom symbol information such as the count of adjacent atoms, the atom's implicit value, the number of adjacent hydrogens, and the aromatic features of the atom. DeepPurpose was introduced for customized DTI predictions [29]. It proposes separate encoders for compounds and protein molecules. The encoder-generated embeddings will be fed to a neural network decoder for generating predictions. The library is capable of providing continuous binding scores, such as inhibitory concentration (IC50) and binary outputs representing whether a protein interacts with a compound. Other DL models involved in DTI studies are listed in Table 3.2.

Software called DeepFrag was developed to improve the binding affinity of a lead molecule and can predict optimization factors [30]. DeepFrag was trained using crystal structures of proteins, after removing the co-crystallized ligands. The fingerprints predicted by the model were closely matched to the removed ligand fragments. This Python-based software is available as a browser app (http://durrantlab.com/deepfrag). Predictions made by DeepFrag were validated with experimentally identified ligands, and the suggestions recommended were implemented to check whether they provided optimization of the molecules [31].

A molecule can be modified through methods like adding atoms and by removing or adding bonds. A deep reinforcement learning (DRL) model can modify a molecule using a Markov decision-making process through the aforementioned steps. The proposed model MolDQN was compared with state-of-the-art models: junction tree variational autoencoder (JT-VAE), which is a deep generative model, and objective-reinforced generative adversarial networks (ORGAN), a molecule-generation algorithm that uses SMILES and follows DRL.

The drug candidates should possess the optimal pharmacokinetic and pharmacodynamic activity, to cure the disease without harming the healthy tissues of the

TABLE 3.2
DL Models for Drug-Target Interaction Studies

DL Algorithm Used	Input Data Used	Reference
Deep belief networks	Molecular descriptors (MDs) and molecular fingerprints (MFs), experimental drug–target pairs (EDTPs) for validation	[32]
Stacked autoencoder	Protein sequences such as position-specific scoring matrix (PSSM), along with drug molecules in the form of molecular fingerprints	[33]
Convolutional neural network-based model with two separate CNN blocks with three consecutive 1D convolution layers	Drug-target compound SMILES from PubChem	[34]
Convolutional neural networks with architecture similar to LeNet5	The chemical descriptors for chemical molecules were calculated by the PaDEL-Descriptor tool. For proteins, each feature was represented using a vector of 13-dimensional size.	[35]
Customized convolutional neural networks with drop-out layers and adaptive estimation	The protein's FASTA sequence and features were generated using the PROFIT web server and SMILES of drugs collected from Drug Bank.	[27]

target organism. To prevent the attrition of potential drug molecules during the clinical phases, several preventive measures were introduced, such as Lipinski's Rule of Five and ADMET assays for evaluating efficacy. The *in silico* ADMET screening software can design and identify novel or existing drug candidates, with promising performance during clinical testing, and can limit the count of compounds that need to be synthesized and profiled. There are ML-based predictive models which employ Bayesian neural networks (BNNs), Random Forest algorithms, and support vector machines (SVMs) [36]. A DL-based approach, with a hybrid architecture of DNN, gradient-boosting machine (GBM), and Gaussian process (GP) regression methods, could predict 18 different ADMET endpoints from the dataset provided by Merck [37]. The Tox21 challenge, which is designed to help scientists understand the potential of the chemicals and compounds under investigation, showcased DL-based methods excelling over shallow ML-based methods [38].

An XAI-based approach using integrated gradients of GNN models developed for predicting plasma protein binding, hERG channel inhibition, and cytochrome P450 inhibition can be referred in [39]. This approach revealed the molecular features and structural elements associated with the known pharmacophore motifs. Along with that, it revealed hidden ligand-target interactions.

3.5 PRECLINICAL TESTING

Preclinical studies in drug discovery are responsible for evaluating whether the drug is prepared for clinical trials by gauging its efficacy at a preliminary level, as well as pharmacokinetic activity, toxicity values, and safety-related information. During this phase, wide doses of drugs are tested using wet-lab-based *in vitro* (test tube or cell culture) and *in vivo* (animal experiments) models. The drug-target interactions are also studied through *in silico* (computer-generated) models.

Clinical phase attrition is caused by the compromised clinical performance of the identified compounds. The preclinical phase involves exclusive evaluations of the drug molecules identified from preceding phases. Cell- and animal-based models are used to study potential therapeutic interventions. Many drug-developing labs have started to use AI's benefits to perform these cumbersome and time-consuming tasks. Lundbeck pharmaceutical company is using AI solutions for the neuroscientific histopathological analysis of alpha-synuclein, associated with Parkinson's disease. With AI-powered image analysis, the risk of detecting vague and unclear targets and intra-observer variations can be minimized. The reproducibility of results is another advantage offered by the AI models.

The preclinical screening of drugs deals with the classification and precise sorting of cells; with an image analysis-based AI algorithm this can be made swift. The initial step in training the AI models is to preprocess the image data to contrast the target cells so that the model can interpret and learn the features for classification. The images that have features like wavelet-based texture or Tamura texture will be extracted, and dimension reduction of these features can be performed through principal component analysis (PCA). The machine should be fast enough to sort out the target cells from the given sample.

Drug administration and dosage determination is another area where AI models can be utilized. Ascertaining the optimum dose of the drug to be administered, to minimize its toxic effects, is always a crucial parameter to calculate. The neural network-based AI model AI-PRS (Artificial Intelligence – Parabolic Response Surface) can identify the drug and dose inputs that lead to the reduction of viral load [40]. The authors claim that this approach can guide the determination of the optimized population-wide and personalized dosing. The clinical studies conducted to test the efficiency of AI-PRS revealed that, compared to standard regimens, the tenofovir dosage suggested by AI-PRS (200 mg) can keep HIV infection to below 40 copies/mL with no relapse, and they have observed patients for a time period of 144 weeks.

A patient who was suffering from a threatening variant of prostate cancer was injected with a bromodomain inhibitor (ZEN-3694) and enzalutamide to reduce prostate-specific antigen levels, and the dose of the administered drug was guided by the AI platform CURATE.AI [41]. The dose adjustments made by the AI-based platform helped to improve the treatment efficacy and tolerance. It utilized a mathematical quadratic expression with variables of drug/dose and toxicity/efficacy plotted. A smooth curve in the plot indicated the success of crucial decisions of CURATE. AI. This platform has the potential to identify the optimal drug dosage for a patient

TABLE 3.3

AI-Based Models for Drug Dosage Determination in Clinical Studies

AI Platform	Purpose	Reference
comboFM (https://github.com/aalto-ics-kepaco/comboFM)	Drug combinations and dose determination on lymphoma cell lines during preclinical testing	[42]
ML-based relevance vector machines	Determination of warfarin dosage (for preventing blood clots)	[43]
Deep reinforcement learning model	For finding the ideal dose of anticoagulant Heparin	[44]
• ANN • Bayesian additive regression trees • Multivariate adaptive regression splines	Optimum dose determination of the drug Tacrolimus, which is an immunosuppressor	[45]
• Classification and regression trees • Multilayer perceptron network	Calculation of safe value for the initial dose of the cardiac drug digoxin	[46]

during treatment. More ML- and DL-based models for drug dosage identification are discussed in Table 3.3.

3.6 CLINICAL TESTING

When the preclinical studies are done, the winning drug candidates are used in clinical trials with real human beings. Clinical testing has three phases:

- **Phase One:** Safety testing of the proposed drug on a small population. These tests are designed to determine the safety and tolerability of a drug; if possible, pharmacokinetics and pharmacodynamics are also evaluated.
- **Phase Two:** Here, drugs are tested on a small group of human subjects suffering from a specific disease. Phase Two clinical studies correlate therapeutic doses for more-populated Phase Three studies. It usually lasts for 12 to 16 weeks.
- **Phase Three:** In this phase, studies are done on a larger number of patients. Phase Three trials investigate a new drug for a duration of six to 12 months or longer in a large patient population (100 patients or more) by providing a clinical environment living and assessing the efficacy and safety of the drug on a daily basis.

The clinical trials are followed by FDA reviews for the approval and commercialization of the drug. Figure 3.3 depicts how the compounds are filtered over time to get that single drug and reach FDA approval. The clinical trials may not always bring the best results, due to potential pitfalls such as choice of cohort (people groups) and

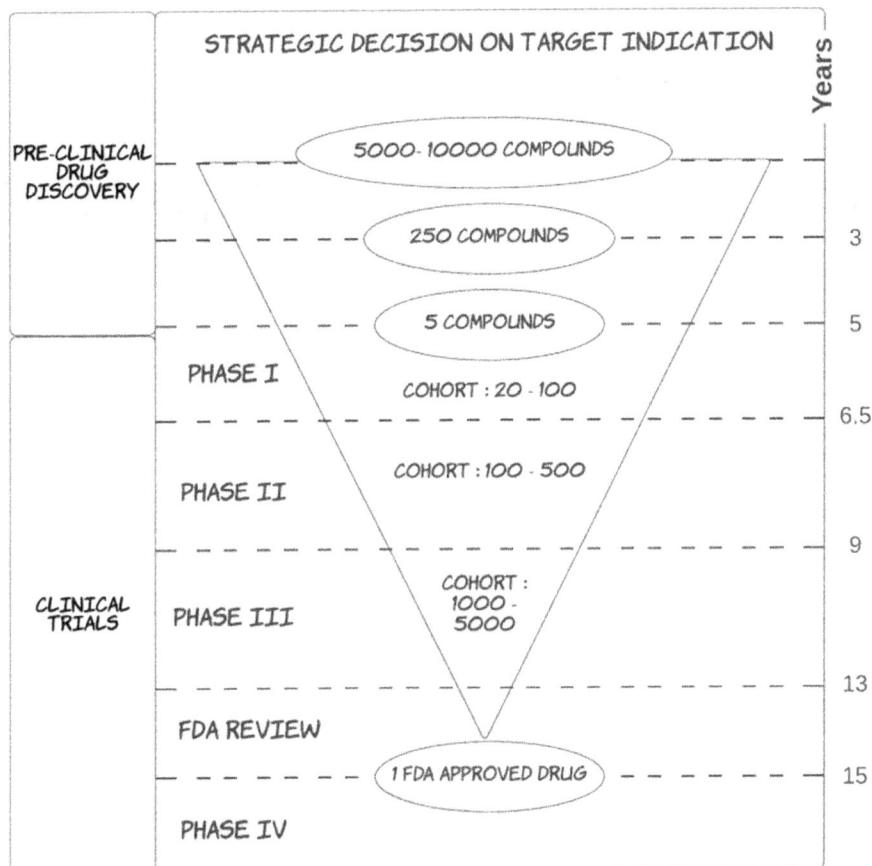

STRATEGIC DECISION ON TARGET INDICATION

Years

PRE-CLINICAL DRUG DISCOVERY

5000-10000 COMPOUNDS

250 COMPOUNDS — 3

5 COMPOUNDS — 5

PHASE I

COHORT : 20 - 100 — 6.5

PHASE II

COHORT : 100 - 500

— 9

CLINICAL TRIALS

PHASE III

COHORT : 1000 - 5000

— 13

FDA REVIEW

1 FDA APPROVED DRUG — 15

PHASE IV

FIGURE 3.3 The journey to the final approved drug from millions of compounds

the lack of technical infrastructure and intellectual support. Trustable and methodical adherence control, patient tracking, and clinical endpoint sensing systems play pivotal roles in clinical trials [47].

In the old days, identifying the eligible population for clinical trials was a challenging task. AI-assisted data analysis of the candidates' social media content has created a smoother data-mining platform. AI can be used to mine through online forums where patients discuss information about their medical conditions. NLP-based models can search hospital databases to identify potential candidates based on eligibility criteria.

The patients recruited as cohorts should adhere to the protocols of clinical trials, and data points will be collected to monitor the impact of the administered drug throughout the procedure. AI and ML models with wearable devices can be used for reliable and efficient patient monitoring. The disease diaries generated by such models – especially DL models, which are versatile enough to update measurement throughout recurrent training – can provide a detailed analysis of disease expression in a patient-specific way [48].

The results from succeeding phases may diverge at times if the drug benefits seen in short-duration testing fail to translate to the long-term endpoint. Some drugs could pass Phase Two with consistent endpoints but fail in Phase Three. DL models were used to predict the results of Phase Three from the features extracted from Phase Two-aggregated individual treatment effects [49]. Two DL models are used here: the first is an individual trough pharmacokinetic concentration (Ctrough) model which can predict the concentration of the drug used in Phase Three; the second model was built to detect the relationship between patient characteristics, Ctrough, and the test phase outputs. This approach provides a post-hoc prediction of results and can save the clinical trial coordinators from adverse outcomes in Phase Three. The applications for AI models are represented in Figure 3.4.

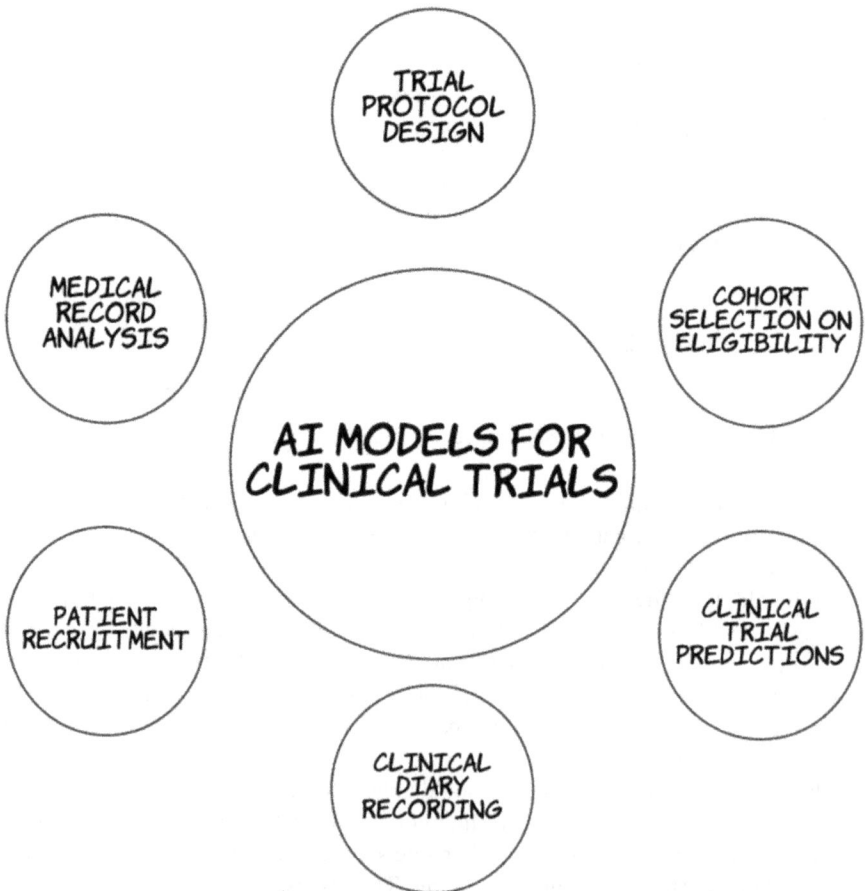

FIGURE 3.4 Applications of AI in clinical trials

The approved drugs which are available in the market and used by the population worldwide are monitored for side effects by the competent authorities in Phase Four clinical trials. These trials look for side effects that did not appear in earlier trials and may also study the effects of a new treatment for a prolonged period. It is also known as the post-marketing surveillance trial [50]. Advancements in the Internet of Things (IoT), AI, and AI's partnership with the healthcare sector are emerging trends these days; wearable devices and the retrieval and storage of the associated data in real time are promising for post-surveillance studies.

When AI components are used for evaluation in clinical trials, certain guidelines need to be followed, which were recommended by the Consolidated Standards of Reporting Trials-Artificial Intelligence (CONSORT-AI) in 2020. According to the proposal, investigators are obliged to submit clear descriptions of how the AI will be employed for input and output handling, what instructions and skills are required for controlling the AI components, and how AI will interact with humans for the analysis, especially while dealing with scenarios where errors occur [51].

3.7 DRUG REPURPOSING USING EXPLAINABLE AI MODELS

Drug repurposing or drug repositioning is the method of reusing the available approved drugs for common or rare diseases. This could solve the long wait for novel drugs by skipping preclinical discovery phases in drug development. Drug repositioning methods have had many success stories since multiple diseases are tagged to multiple targets [52]. Drug repurposing methods can be drug-centric, disease-centric, or combinations of these categories.

- **Disease-centric repositioning**: Here, the drugs developed for one disease are recommended for another drug based on the phenotypical similarity of the disease and its molecular signatures.
- **Drug-centric repositioning**: Here, the drugs are studied to compare the similarities in their molecular activity, and if the properties are similar and efficacy is good, those drugs will be recommended for clinical trials and market release.

When the COVID-19 pandemic was demanding fast cures, AI-based drug repurposing came to the rescue: 16 potential anti-HCoV repurposable drugs were identified using a network-based approach [53], and a multimodal DL approach revealed 12 promising drug targets [54]. An explainable computational data analysis approach for drug repositioning discovery was developed and implemented by Taie et al. for precision medicine through a novel patient group stratification method [55]. They used patient data collected on phenotypic and genotypic characteristics; the subpopulation was decided using heterogenous networks and then, for each subgroup, a drug-likeness score was calculated and assigned a rank for recommendation of repositioning. This method can be employed in clinical trials, as it can correlate the molecular profile of the drug and the subgroup population, thereby conducting a precise trial.

3.8 CHALLENGES AND LIMITATIONS OF EXPLAINABLE MODELS IN DRUG DISCOVERY

When it comes to biomedical application scenarios, one of the major challenges when integrating AI models is the explainability of the problem-solving mechanisms. Not just in the medical domain, but in any given application, an AI system should not only ensure good system performance with high levels of accuracy, but it should also provide high levels of interpretability and explainability to the end-user as well. It means that the end-user should be able to interpret the rationale behind choosing a particular approach for generating a solution over others. Even though the interpretability of AI models has been a long-existing problem in healthcare scenarios, considerable progress has not been made yet in generating a solid solution.

In certain healthcare scenarios associated with bioinformatics such as gene markers, the applicability of AI models and diagnostic applications still fails to provide a viable explanation. When we dive deep into the tasks associated with drug development and associated domains, several datasets are being employed to identify elements, patterns, and other markers. In such instances, the application of different approaches may produce entirely different results, even for identical datasets. Even though certain researchers claim that the complexity of certain tasks and the non-linear property of omics data are the primary reasons behind the issues, another major reason is that the non-interpretability of the AI model being deployed for the task makes the whole system highly opaque as a big, black box. Thus, there is a great need to develop explainable AI models that ensure high levels of functional transparency for both the users and the practitioners. Such models should give a clear understanding of not only why the system works, but also how it works.

Compared to other domains, the standards of interpretability and transparency required by biomedical applications are manifold, simply due to their special subjects and complex application scenarios. Blindly believing results generated by a non-interpretable AI model in drug development and related scenarios can lead to dangerous outcomes, due to the unpredictable nature of the results caused by the opaqueness of the system. The introduction of explainable AI into such systems has gradually reduced the barriers to understanding the functioning of such systems from an end-user's perspective. Even though XAI has introduced a certain level of explainability into such systems, it surely has many limitations as well. Certain challenges need to be tackled before successfully implementing explainable AI in biomedical applications. In this section, we will be discussing the limitations of XAI, especially in the context of drug development. Some of the major issues associated with XAI include the customization of AI models, the nonlinearity of training data, the complexity of the problem to be solved, biased perspectives in learning, and so on.

- Primarily, most of the state-of-the-art learning techniques were not devised specifically for biomedical applications. They were initially developed for other applications related to image processing, computer vision, or NLP-based tasks, and, over time, they were adopted for biomedical use cases, such as drug development, drug-to-drug interactions, and so on. When migrating such currently existing approaches to biomedical applications, achieving explainability is a highly tedious task. Hence, AI techniques should be customized initially, or else new ones should be developed for individual use cases and datasets, keeping better system performance and explainability as prime criteria. However, achieving such levels of model customization is a cumbersome task and needs a considerable amount of time to be developed, as AI modes are devoid of theoretical backing and guidance for executing such procedures. Additionally, the level of explainability required for individual systems and use cases may vary widely.

- Secondarily, the types of data involved in drug development and related tasks vary extremely. They are usually highly complex in nature, with huge volumes, varying from sequential data to complex omics data to normal text data or even spatiotemporal and image-based data. Thus, the volume, nonlinearity, and complexity of the data, along with the complexity of application domains, force AI models to compromise between achieving high performance and achieving interpretability. Usually, it is difficult to achieve high performance for any biomedical task. Considering the sensitivity of tasks when working with applications related to drug development, the system priority automatically gets aligned with attaining better performance rather than explainability. Even though there are certain AI models which offer high levels of explainability and average system performance, they would not be ideal choices for biomedical applications, due to the system performance failing to surpass a particular threshold.

- All these models rely upon the data on which they are trained and tested, and these data are collected from real-world patients' records and medical investigation reports, which contain highly sensitive and private information. The utmost care is required while dealing with such data, and unnormalized distribution should be prevented to avoid causing biased decisions.

- Learning biases generated by training models are also a major hurdle in biomedical applications, as these biases prevent the systems from delivering viable interpretations. The term bias refers to an AI system being biased towards a particular outcome or generating a wrong outcome [56]. Such learning bias can be caused by various issues, such as mismatched interactions between the methods employed and the data type being used, initialization of wrong parameters or faulty parameter tuning, imbalance in the training datasets, and so on. Such issues are highly complex and make it difficult for biomedical scientists to understand and debug the issues. The issues associated with learning bias are also referred to as learning security problems and lead to unjustifiable results because of the issues in the models.

- New, explainable AI approaches are usually generated on the assumption that the system exits in an idealistic condition, meaning that such techniques have the capability to generate complete high-performance results and are not prone to any sort of security issues. However, several widely employed

AI methods, such as kernel-based learning, ensemble learning, deep learning, and even federated learning, have a tendency or a possible tendency to showcase learning bias concerning the training data being used. For certain applications associated with drug development, fixing these security issues is more important than attaining explainability for the system, simply due to the sensitivity of the use cases [57].

In the current scenario, explainable AI has been under extensive research and various approaches, such as rule-based learning, process visualization, knowledge representation, human-centred computing, and so on, have been integrated into the systems to attain explainability [58]. Even though integrating such techniques has proven to be useful in generating explainable AI systems, especially in biomedical applications, overcoming certain challenges associated with novel explainable algorithm development requires far more effort than just such attempts at integration. It is totally possible that explainable AI approaches can enhance system efficiency and bring a certain degree of security and trust to traditional AI approaches, but such explainability should only be introduced into systems that have met the primary considerations associated with performance efficiency and systems security. It is necessary to carry out clinical trials as per the recommended guide lines and to adhere to ethical standards, especially when AI models are utilized [59].

Additionally, different matrices should also be used to achieve explainability in AI models, in order to satisfy the requirements of biomedical use cases. Explainable AI should make a system capable of delivering high performance along with unbiased results in an interpretable manner to upgrade system transparency and trustworthiness. As with conventional learning approaches, security issues can only be tackled efficiently once the models perform well enough and generate good system performance. Similarly, when it comes to explainability, we can expect the technology to be considered mature only once it can tackle such issues on its own and find stable applicability even in highly complex domains such as drug development and other biomedical applications.

3.9 CONCLUSION

The COVID-19 pandemic confronted the limitations and restrictions of traditional drug discovery concepts and accelerated the development of novel AI-involved approaches to fighting the virus. The leap from using only wet lab-accompanied procedures to using machine intelligence to make drug discoveries is phenomenal, but whether AI is capable of convincing human intelligence persists as a matter of discussion. The ubiquitous role of AI in our lives is inevitable, and with the advanced version of XAI, the explanations generated should be non-trivial, non-artificial, and the knowledge should be sharable for the respective scientific communities. For resolving drug discovery associated with XAI, collaborative efforts from deep learning experts, cheminformaticians, chemists, biologists, and experts from the field are required.

REFERENCES

1. E. B. Lenselink *et al.*, "Beyond the hype: Deep neural networks outperform established methods using a ChEMBL bioactivity benchmark set," *J. Cheminform.*, vol. 9, no. 1, pp. 1–14, 2017, doi: 10.1186/s13321-017-0232-0.
2. E. Gawehn, J. A. Hiss, and G. Schneider, "Deep learning in drug discovery," *Mol. Inform.*, vol. 35, no. 1, pp. 3–14, 2016, doi: 10.1002/minf.201501008.
3. A. Holzinger *et al.*, "Interactive machine learning: Experimental evidence for the human in the algorithmic loop: A case study on Ant Colony Optimization," *Appl. Intell.*, vol. 49, no. 7, pp. 2401–2414, 2019, doi: 10.1007/s10489-018-1361-5.
4. J. Vamathevan *et al.*, "Applications of machine learning in drug discovery and development," *Nat. Rev. Drug Discov.*, vol. 18, no. 6, pp. 463–477, 2019, doi:10.1038/s41573-019-0024-5.
5. S. Tasaki, C. Gaiteri, S. Mostafavi, and Y. Wang, "Differential gene expression," *Nat. Mach. Intell.*, doi: 10.1038/s42256-020-0201-6.
6. P. Mamoshina, M. Volosnikova, I. V. Ozerov, and E. Putin, "Machine learning on human muscle transcriptomic data for biomarker discovery and tissue-specific drug target identification," vol. 9, no. July, pp. 1–10, 2018, doi: 10.3389/fgene.2018.00242.
7. D. G. P. van IJzendoorn, K. Szuhai, I. H. Briaire-de Bruijn, M. Kostine, M. L. Kuijjer, J. V. M. G. Bovée, "Machine learning analysis of gene expression data reveals novel diagnostic and prognostic biomarkers and identifies therapeutic targets for soft tissue sarcomas," *PLoS Comput. Biol.*, vol. 15, no. 2, pp. 1–19, 2019, doi:10.1371/journal.pcbi.1006826.
8. Y. You *et al.*, "Artificial intelligence in cancer target identification and drug discovery," *Signal Transduct. Target. Ther.*, vol. 7, no. 1, pp. 1–24, 2022, doi: 10.1038/s41392-022-00994-0.
9. G. Selvaraj *et al.*, "Identification of target gene and prognostic evaluation for lung adenocarcinoma using gene expression meta-analysis, network analysis and neural network algorithms," *J. Biomed. Inform.*, vol. 86, no. May, pp. 120–134, 2018, doi: 10.1016/j.jbi.2018.09.004.
10. G. Li, J. Luo, Q. Xiao, C. Liang, P. Ding, and B. Cao, "Predicting microRNA-disease associations using network topological similarity based on DeepWalk," *IEEE Access*, vol. 5, pp. 24032–24039, 2017, doi: 10.1109/ACCESS.2017.2766758.
11. L. Yu, L. Xue, F. Liu, Y. Li, R. Jing, and J. Luo, "The applications of deep learning algorithms on in silico druggable proteins identification," *J. Adv. Res.*, vol. 41, pp. 219–231, 2022, doi: 10.1016/j.jare.2022.01.009.
12. X. Zhang, T. Li, J. Wang, J. Li, L. Chen, and C. Liu, "Identification of cancer-related long non-coding RNAs using XGboost with high accuracy," *Front. Genet.*, vol. 10, no. July, pp. 1–14, 2019, doi: 10.3389/fgene.2019.00735.
13. M. Madhavan and G. Gopakumar, "DBNLDA: Deep Belief Network based representation learning for lncRNA-disease association prediction," *Appl. Intell.*, vol. 52, no. 5, pp. 5342–5352, 2022, doi: 10.1007/s10489-021-02675-x.
14. B. Kuhlman and P. Bradley, "Advances in protein structure prediction and design," *Nat. Rev. Mol. Cell Biol.*, doi: 10.1038/s41580-019-0163-x.
15. O. Ronneberger *et al.*, "Highly accurate protein structure prediction with AlphaFold," *Nature*, vol. 596, no. August, 2021, doi: 10.1038/s41586-021-03819-2.
16. À. Bravo, J. Piñero, N. Queralt-Rosinach, M. Rautschka, and L. I. Furlong, "Extraction of relations between genes and diseases from text and large-scale data analysis: Implications for translational research," *BMC Bioinformatics*, vol. 16, no. 1, pp. 1–17, 2015, doi: 10.1186/s12859-015-0472-9.

17. J. Kim, J. J. Kim, and H. Lee, "An analysis of disease-gene relationship from Medline abstracts by DigSee," *Sci. Rep.*, vol. 7, no. January, pp. 1–12, 2017, doi: 10.1038/srep40154.
18. S. de Cesco, J. B. Davis, and P. E. Brennan, "TargetDB: A target information aggregation tool and tractability predictor," *PLOS ONE*, vol. 15, no. 9 September, pp. 1–12, 2020, doi: 10.1371/journal.pone.0232644.
19. J. Piñero, À. Bravo, N. Queralt-Rosinach, A. Gutiérrez-Sacristán, J. Deu-Pons, E. Centeno, J. García-García, F. Sanz, L. I. Furlong, "DisGeNET : a comprehensive platform integrating information on human disease-associated genes and variants," *Nucleic Acids Res.* vol. 45, no. October 2016, pp. 833–839, 2017, doi: 10.1093/nar/gkw943.
20. A. Talevi, "Computer-aided drug design: An overview," *Methods Mol. Biol.*, vol. 1762, no. 5, pp. 1–19, 2018, doi: 10.1007/978-1-4939-7756-7_1.
21. Q. Bai, S. Tan, T. Xu, H. Liu, "MolAICal : A soft tool for 3D drug design of protein targets by artificial intelligence and classical algorithm," vol. 22, no. April 2020, pp. 1–12, 2021, doi: 10.1093/bib/bbaa161.
22. M. Popova, O. Isayev, and A. Tropsha, "Deep reinforcement learning for de novo drug design," *Sci. Adv.*, vol. 4, no. 7, pp. 1–15, 2018, doi:10.1126/sciadv.aap7885.
23. J. M. Stokes *et al.*, "Article a deep learning approach," *Cell*, vol. 180, no. 4, pp. 688-702. e13, 2020, doi: 10.1016/j.cell.2020.01.021.
24. Y. Zhang, T. Ye, H. Xi, M. Juhas, and J. Li, "Deep learning driven drug discovery: Tackling severe acute respiratory syndrome coronavirus 2," vol. 12, no. October, pp. 1–8, 2021, doi: 10.3389/fmicb.2021.739684.
25. D. Erikawa, N. Yasuo, and M. Sekijima, "MERMAID: An open source automated hit-to-lead method based on deep reinforcement learning," *J. Cheminform.*, vol. 13, no. 1, pp. 1–10, 2021, doi: 10.1186/s13321-021-00572-6.
26. W. F. D. Bennett *et al.*, "Predicting small molecule transfer free energies by combining molecular dynamics simulations and deep learning," 2020, doi: 10.1021/acs.jcim .0c00318.
27. S. M. Hasan Mahmud, W. Chen, H. Jahan, B. Dai, S. U. Din, and A. M. Dzisoo, "DeepACTION: A deep learning-based method for predicting novel drug-target interactions," *Anal. Biochem.*, vol. 610, no. September, p. 113978, 2020, doi: 10.1016/j. ab.2020.113978.
28. T. Nguyen, H. Le, T. P. Quinn, T. Nguyen, T. D. Le, and S. Venkatesh, "GraphDTA: Predicting drug target binding affinity with graph neural networks," *Bioinformatics*, vol. 37, no. 8, pp. 1140–1147, 2021, doi: 10.1093/bioinformatics/btaa921.
29. K. Huang, T. Fu, L. M. Glass, M. Zitnik, C. Xiao, and J. Sun, "DeepPurpose: A deep learning library for drug-target interaction prediction," *Bioinformatics*, vol. 36, no. 22–23, pp. 5545–5547, 2020, doi: 10.1093/bioinformatics/btaa1005.
30. H. Green and J. D. Durrant, "DeepFrag: An open-source browser app for deep-learning lead optimization," *J. Chem. Inf. Model.*, vol. 61, no. 6, pp. 2523–2529, 2021, doi: 10.1021/acs.jcim.1c00103.
31. Z. Zhou, S. Kearnes, L. Li, R. N. Zare, and P. Riley, "Optimization of molecules via deep reinforcement learning," *Sci. Rep.*, vol. 9, no. 1, pp. 1–10, 2019, doi: 10.1038/ s41598-019-47148-x.
32. M. Wen *et al.*, "Deep-learning-based drug-target interaction prediction," *J. Proteome Res.*, vol. 16, no. 4, pp. 1401–1409, 2017, doi: 10.1021/acs.jproteome.6b00618.
33. L. Wang *et al.*, "A computational-based method for predicting drug-target interactions by using stacked autoencoder deep neural network," *J. Comput. Biol.*, vol. 25, no. 3, pp. 361–373, 2018, doi: 10.1089/cmb.2017.0135.
34. H. Öztürk, A. Özgür, and E. Ozkirimli, "DeepDTA: Deep drug-target binding affinity prediction," *Bioinformatics*, vol. 34, no. 17, pp. i821–i829, 2018, doi: 10.1093/ bioinformatics/bty593.

35. S. Hu, D. Xia, B. Su, P. Chen, B. Wang, and J. Li, "A convolutional neural network system to discriminate drug-target interactions," *IEEE ACM Trans. Comput. Biol. Bioinforma.*, vol. 18, no. 4, pp. 1315–1324, 2019, doi: 10.1109/tcbb.2019.2940187.

36. J. A. Keith *et al.*, "Combining machine learning and computational chemistry for predictive insights into chemical systems," 2021, doi: 10.1021/acs.chemrev.1c00107.

37. J. Ma, R. P. Sheridan, A. Liaw, G. E. Dahl, and V. Svetnik, "Deep neural nets as a method for quantitative structure – activity relationships," 2015, doi: 10.1021/ci500747n.

38. G. B. Goh, "Deep learning for computational chemistry," pp. 1–17, 2017, doi: 10.1002/jcc.24764.

39. M. Skalic, N. Weskamp, and G. Schneider, "Coloring molecules with explainable artificial intelligence for preclinical relevance assessment," 2021, doi: 10.1021/acs.jcim.0c01344.

40. Y. Shen *et al.*, "Harnessing artificial intelligence to optimize long-term maintenance dosing for antiretroviral-naive adults with HIV-1 infection," *Adv. Ther.*, vol. 3, no. 4, p. 1900114, 2020, doi: 10.1002/adtp.201900114.

41. A. J. Pantuck *et al.*, "Modulating BET bromodomain inhibitor ZEN-3694 and enzalutamide combination dosing in a metastatic prostate cancer patient using CURATE.AI, an artificial intelligence platform," *Adv. Ther.*, vol. 1, no. 6, pp. 1–9, 2018, doi: 10.1002/adtp.201800104.

42. H. Julkunen *et al.*, "Leveraging multi-way interactions for systematic prediction of preclinical drug combination effects," *Nat. Commun.*, vol. 11, no. 1, 2020, doi: 10.1038/s41467-020-19950-z.

43. A. Sharabiani, A. Bress, E. Douzali, and H. Darabi, "Revisiting warfarin dosing using machine learning techniques," *Comput. Math. Methods Med.*, vol. 2015, 2015, doi: 10.1155/2015/560108.

44. S. Nemati, M. M. Ghassemi, and G. D. Clifford, "Optimal medication dosing from suboptimal clinical examples: A deep reinforcement learning approach," 2016 38th Annual International Conference of the IEEE Engineering in Medicine and Biology Society (EMBC), Orlando, FL, USA, 2016, pp. 2978–2981, 2016, doi: 10.1109/EMBC.2016.7591355.

45. Y. H. Hu, C. T. Tai, C. F. Tsai, and M. W. Huang, "Improvement of adequate digoxin dosage: An application of machine learning approach," *J. Healthc. Eng.*, vol. 2018, 2018, doi: 10.1155/2018/3948245.

46. S. Imai, Y. Takekuma, T. Miyai, and M. Sugawara, "A new algorithm optimized for initial dose settings of vancomycin using machine learning," *Biol. Pharm. Bull.*, vol. 43, no. 1, pp. 188–193, 2020, doi: 10.1248/bpb.b19-00729.

47. S. Harrer, P. Shah, B. Antony, and J. Hu, "Artificial intelligence for clinical trial design," *Trends Pharmacol. Sci.*, vol. 40, no. 8, pp. 577–591, 2019, doi: 10.1016/j.tips.2019.05.005.

48. V. T. Tran, C. Riveros, and P. Ravaud, "Patients' views of wearable devices and AI in healthcare: Findings from the compare e-cohort," *npj Digit. Med.*, vol. 2, no. 1, pp. 1–8, 2019, doi: 10.1038/s41746-019-0132-y.

49. Y. Qi and Q. Tang, "Predicting Phase 3 clinical trial results by modeling Phase 2 clinical trial subject level data using deep learning." *Proc. Mach. Learn. Res.*, vol. 106, pp. 288–303, 2019.

50. F. Cascini, F. Beccia, F. A. Causio, A. Melnyk, A. Zaino, and W. Ricciardi, "Scoping review of the current landscape of AI-based applications in clinical trials," *Front. Public Heal.*, vol. 10, 2022, doi: 10.3389/fpubh.2022.949377.

51. S. Francisco *et al.*, *HHS Public Access*, vol. 2, no. 10, pp. 1–25, 2021, doi: 10.1016/S2589-7500(20)30218-1.Corresponding.

52. R. Gupta, D. Srivastava, M. Sahu, S. Tiwari, R. K. Ambasta, and P. Kumar, *Artificial Intelligence to Deep Learning: Machine Intelligence Approach for Drug Discovery*, vol. 25, no. 3, Springer International Publishing, 2021.

53. Y. Zhou, Y. Hou, J. Shen, Y. Huang, W. Martin, and F. Cheng, "Network-based drug repurposing for novel coronavirus 2019-nCoV/SARS-CoV-2," *Cell Discov.*, vol. 6, no. 1, 2020, doi: 10.1038/s41421-020-0153-3.

54. S. A. Hooshmand, M. Zarei Ghobadi, S. E. Hooshmand, S. Azimzadeh Jamalkandi, S. M. Alavi, and A. Masoudi-Nejad, "A multimodal deep learning-based drug repurposing approach for treatment of COVID-19," *Mol. Divers.*, vol. 25, no. 3, pp. 1717–1730, 2021, doi: 10.1007/s11030-020-10144-9.

55. Z. Al-Taie *et al.*, "Explainable artificial intelligence in high-throughput drug repositioning for subgroup stratifications with interventionable potential," *J. Biomed. Inform.*, vol. 118, p. 103792, 2021, doi: 10.1016/j.jbi.2021.103792.

56. H. Han, "Diagnostic biases in translational bioinformatics," *BMC Med. Genomics*, vol. 8, no. 1, pp. 1–17, 2015, doi: 10.1186/s12920-015-0116-y.

57. H. Han and X. Jiang, "Overcome support vector machine diagnosis overfitting," *Cancer Inform.*, vol. 13, no. s1, p. CIN.S13875, 2014, doi: 10.4137/cin.s13875.

58. G. Vilone and L. Longo, "Explainable artificial intelligence: A systematic review," *Decis. Anal. J.*, vol. 7, p. 100230, 2020, doi:10.1016/j.dajour.2023.100230.

59. A. K. Nair, E. D. Raj, and J. Sahoo, "An overview of artificial intelligence for advanced healthcare systems," *Digit. Health Transform. Blockchain Artif. Intell.*, vol. 1, pp. 141–160, 2022.

4 Supervised Learning Models for Diagnosing Severity of Cirrhosis Disease

Akshita Sakshi, J.V. Bibal Benifa, and P. Antony Seba

4.1 INTRODUCTION

Many researchers and medical professionals have been using various AI techniques to help the healthcare industry. The liver is the second-largest and an important organ of the human body. One of the most fatal liver diseases is cirrhosis. Cirrhosis is a condition in which the liver gradually becomes scarred and cannot function properly. It is caused by long-term damage to the liver from alcohol abuse, viral hepatitis, fatty liver disease, or certain medications [1–4]. Cirrhosis can also be caused by other diseases that affect the bile ducts and lead to problems with bile production. It can cause permanent damage to the liver's ability to function and may eventually lead to death if not treated. Cirrhosis has caused more than 1.32 million deaths globally [5]. This research focuses on the prediction of cirrhosis disease by applying machine learning (ML) algorithms. Since this problem comes under supervised learning, this research work performs a detailed study on the cirrhosis dataset and makes use of the decision tree [6, 7], logistic regression, [8, 9] multilayer perceptron, random forest, AdaBoost [10], and XGBoost algorithms to predict the stages of cirrhosis.

The outliers are detected through visualization and the data instances of the outliers are dropped [11]. Missing values are imputed through a statistical approach, by considering the skewness of the variable. Appropriate feature encoding has been applied to qualitative variables and the dataset is split in a stratified manner, as training and testing datasets. Feature selection is an important aspect of building machine learning models [12–17]. The features in the dataset are checked for redundancy using Pearson correlation and the chi-squared test of independence [18, 19]. Supervised feature selection algorithms – Extra Trees classifier (ETC) and Recursive Feature Elimination (RFE) – are applied to identify the relevant attributes. Exploratory data analysis [20] is carried out in this work to prepare the data for model building and then to predict the stages of cirrhosis [21–27].

DOI: 10.1201/9781003363361-4

4.2 LITERATURE REVIEW

Data preprocessing and feature selection are important tasks which are to be done before building predictive models. Features present in a dataset may be relevant or redundant and feature selection methods may be parametric or non-parametric, but the features that best explain the outcome are identified to improve the performance of the model. Several research works have been done in liver disease prediction, and various learning algorithms are used to make predictions of the disease using different datasets.

For predicting patients' liver illness, Ketan et al. examined many ML models, including logistic regression, decision trees, the K-nearest neighbours algorithm, random forest, gradient boosting, and XGBoosting [22]. The Indian liver patient dataset (ILPD) from the University of California (UCI) Machine Learning Library, which included 583 Indian liver patients, was used, and the missing values were filled in with the median, duplicate values were removed, and resampling was used to enhance performance. Random forest was the feature selection technique employed, and it was found that random forest (63%), Light Gradient Boosting Machine (Light GBM) (63%), and AdaBoost (62%) provided superior accuracy compared to other algorithms. Hence, it was determined that Light Gradient Boosting Machine (Light GBM) was the most effective algorithm.

Rakshith et al. employed the UCI ILPD dataset, which includes the following ten variables: age, gender, total bilirubin, direct bilirubin, total proteins, albumin, albumin/globulin (A/G ratio), serum glutamate pyruvate transaminase (SGPT), serum glutamic oxaloacetic transaminase (SGOT), and alkaline phosphatase [23]. There were 167 people without liver disease among the 415 entries it included. The purpose of this research was to make it easier to forecast liver disease, decrease the number of fatalities caused by liver disease, and improve physician identification of liver illness. The dataset underwent data preprocessing, and the classification methods K-nearest neighbour (KNN), support vector machine (SVM), artificial neural networks (ANN), and Naive Bayes were used. It was found that SVM and ANN provided the maximum accuracy, with respective values of 100% and 99.9%.

Nazmun et al. employed the Indian Liver Patient Dataset (ILPD), which is accessible through the UCI Machine Learning Repository [24]. There are 583 records altogether in this collection, 416 of which are of individuals with liver disease and 167 without. Male records numbered 441 and female records numbered 142. This research was carried out using the open-source Weka toolset. The major emphasis was on ensemble learning techniques (bagging, boosting, and stacking), and boosting algorithms like AdaBoost and LogitBoost were employed. The LogitBoost algorithm had the greatest accuracy of all the methods, coming in at 71.53%.

Yang et al. compared the performance of classification models created using a deep learning-based algorithm to that of traditional non-deep learning-based algorithms ANN (artificial neural network), MLR (multinomial logistic regression), SVM (support vector machine), and RF (random forest). They focused on the performance of classification models created using a deep learning-based algorithm to score liver fibrosis (random forest). Automated feature categorization and fibrosis scoring were accomplished using deep learning networks based on transfer learning and the AlexNet convolutional network [25].

Shivala Vishnu Murty and Kiran Kumar used a liver dataset collected from the Amrutha Group of Hospitals located in Srikakulam, Andhra Pradesh, India [26]. The dataset contains 11 attributes, with the first 10 attributes being considered as input or independent attributes, and the 11th attribute being the target attribute, which represents the class of the patient as either 0 (non-diseased) or 1 (diseased). The dataset consisted of a total of 882 instances, out of which 403 were of class 0 and 479 were of class 1. The authors compared the performance of several models, including the multilayer feed forward deep neural network (MLFFDNN) with an accuracy of 98%, naive Bayes (NB) with an accuracy of 71%, C4.5 decision tree with an accuracy of 97%, alternative decision (AD) tree with an accuracy of 92%, random belief (RBF) network with an accuracy of 83%, support vector machine with an accuracy of 73%, and XGBoost with an accuracy of 99%. The primary focus of this research was on boosting techniques, in which the authors first tuned several hyperparameters such as L2 regularization, logistic loss function, learning rate, and number of estimators for the XGBoost model.

Bihter Das assessed the efficacy of several disease-detection techniques offered by the statistical analysis system (SAS) software package, including neural networks, auto-neural networks, high performance (HP), SVM, HP forests, HP trees (decision trees), and HP neural network nodes [27]. The assessment was done using the Indian Liver Patient Dataset (ILPD). It was found that in the training phase, HP Forest produced the maximum accuracy, while in the validation phase, the neural network produced the highest accuracy rate. The training was completed after the dataset was randomly divided into training (80%) and validation (20%) datasets using the HP variable selection node to identify less significant characteristics.

Saima et al. in their research work utilized a dataset from the UCI machine learning repository to predict liver disease [17]. Initially, the data was preprocessed to eliminate any noisy data, and the LASSO (least absolute shrinkage and selector operator) feature extraction method was used to select the most important features. Then, they implemented classification algorithms such as logistic regression, decision tree, random forest, AdaBoost, SVM, KNN, LDA, and gradient boosting to construct models. The models were evaluated using a tenfold cross-validation technique. It was found that the Decision Tree algorithm had the highest accuracy of 94.28%.

Muktevi et al. evaluated five classifiers for the identification of liver disease: naive Bayes, logistic regression, support vector machine, random forest, and k-nearest neighbour [28]. The objective of the investigation was to use several machine learning algorithms to identify liver infections. A Kaggle dataset of 583 examples was used to create the dataset. The results showed that logistic regression outperformed.

Despite tremendous research work [22–31] done in predicting liver disease and its stages, it has been felt that important clinical attributes which help in prediction can be identified to build predictive models. In this work, various feature selection methods are applied to identify the important features, and predictive models have been built to predict the stages of cirrhosis.

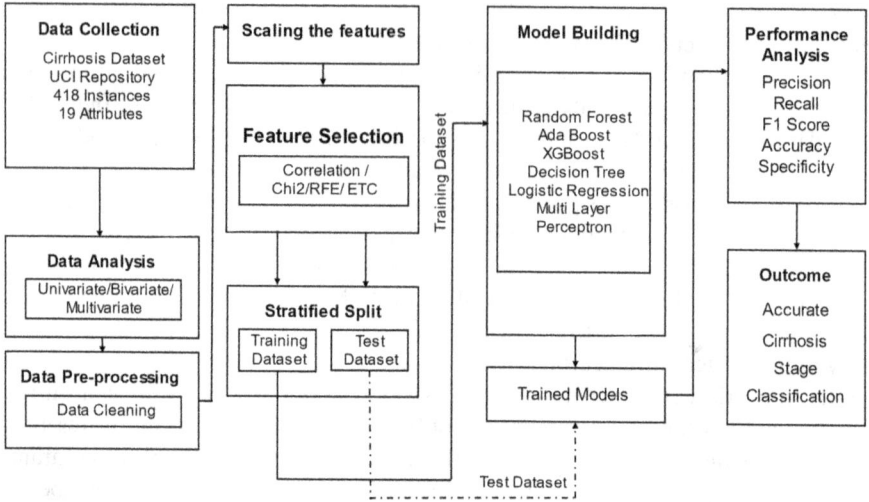

FIGURE 4.1   Cirrhosis severity classification architecture

4.3   METHODOLOGY

Exploratory data analysis is applied to the cirrhosis dataset to understand the characteristics of each variable in the dataset and handle missing values and outliers, and various feature selection methods are adapted to identify the relevant and redundant features. Each stage of the machine learning pipeline architecture is visualized to make observations and to get insights. Several machine learning models have been built and their performance has been evaluated. The complete machine learning pipeline architecture for cirrhosis severity classification is shown in Figure 4.1.

4.3.1   DATASET

The dataset was collected from Kaggle, a website for data scientists and machine learning enthusiasts [32]. The dataset has both quantitative and qualitative features. In total, it has 19 variables with 418 data instances. Its description and attributes are given in Table 4.1.

4.3.2   DATA PREPROCESSING

The distribution of the variables present in the dataset has been studied through data visualization [33] and the dataset has been subjected to machine learning pipeline architecture to analyze the data to make observations and to derive insights.

TABLE 4.1
Dataset Description

Sl. No.	Attributes	Description
1.	N_Days	Number of days between registration and the earlier of death transplantation, or date of the study analysis (July 1986)
2.	Status	Status of the patient (C is "censored", CL is "censored due to liver tx", D is "death")
3.	Drug	type of drug (D-penicillamine, placebo)
4.	Age	age in [days]
5.	Sex	M: "male", F: "female"
6.	Ascites	Presence of ascites (N: "No", Y: "Yes")
7.	Hepatomegaly	Presence of hepatomegaly (N: "No", Y: "Yes")
8.	Spiders	Presence of spiders (N: "No", Y: "Yes")
9.	Edema	Presence of edema (N: "no edema and no diuretic therapy for edema", S: "edema present without diuretics or edema resolved by diuretics", Y: "edema despite diuretic therapy")
10.	Bilirubin	Serum bilirubin (mg/dL)
11.	Cholesterol	Serum cholesterol (mg/dL)
12.	Albumin	Albumin (g/dL)
13.	Copper	Urine copper (µg/day)
14.	Alk-Phos	Alkaline phosphatase (U/liter)
15.	SGOT	SGOT (U/mL)
16.	Triglycerides	Triglycerides (mg/dL)
17.	Platelets	Platelets (mL/1000)
18.	Prothrombin	Prothrombin time in seconds (s)
19.	Stage	Histologic stage of disease (1, 2, 3, or 4)

4.3.3 OUTLIER DETECTION

Outliers are data values that are very different from the other values in the dataset. Outliers occur due to human errors and instrumental errors, which occur during data collection. Outliers in the data may affect the model fitting. Outliers can be detected through visualization using a box plot that considers the interquartile range to calculate the lower and upper fences that are 1.5 times away from the interquartile range (IQR), as shown in Equations 4.1 and 4.2.

$$\text{Lower Fence} = Q1 - (IQR \times 1.5) \tag{4.1}$$
$$\text{Upper Fence} = Q3 + (IQR \times 1.5) \tag{4.2}$$

Where Q1 is the 25th-quartile data and Q3 is the 75th-percentile data.

4.3.4 IMPUTATION

Missing values in the dataset lead to unreliable measures of the model's performance. Instances of data with missing values can be dropped or imputed. In this work, qualitative and quantitative attributes are imputed through statistical measures like mean, median, and mode.

4.3.5 FEATURE ENCODING

Feature encoding is an essential preprocessing step for the structured dataset in supervised learning. Since the machine learning algorithms cannot understand categorical attributes, it is essential to encode the attributes. Nominal attributes are those that do not follow any order, such as, for example, the gender of a person. Ordinal attributes are those where the order is essential, such as, for instance, a person's income or a student's grade. Almost every attribute is nominal and applied label encoding. Only one attribute was ordinal and applied ordinal encoding.

4.3.6 FEATURE SCALING

Feature scaling is the process of standardizing the attributes in a fixed range. Feature scaling is mainly done either by normalization or standardization. StandardScaler has been used here to standardize features. This transforms each attribute's value to a mean of zero and a standard deviation of one. StandardScaler has been used, since most of the attributes followed a normal distribution.

4.3.7 SPLITTING THE DATASET

The dataset is split into training (80%) and test (20%) datasets in a stratified manner for building and validating the model. The dataset is split in a stratified manner to overcome the data imbalance issue. The training dataset is used for model building, and the test dataset is used to validate the model.

4.3.8 FEATURE SELECTION

Feature selection helps to identify the important attributes for model building. The cirrhosis dataset consists of 19 independent variables. Relationships among the independent variables are checked using Pearson correlation (r), as given in Equation 4.3. The non-parametric statistical test is also used to identify attribute relationships.

$$r = \frac{\sum (x_i - \bar{x})(y_i - \bar{y})}{\sqrt{\sum (x_i - \bar{x})^2 \sum (y_i - \bar{y})^2}} \tag{4.3}$$

x_i and y_i are variable samples and r ranges from −1 to +1, where zero specifies that there is no relation between the two variables. If the value is greater than zero, it indicates a positive relationship between two variables; if the value is less than zero, it indicates a negative relationship between two variables. The chi-squared test for independence is done in this work to identify the relationship between categorical attributes using Equation 4.4. The test statistic score is compared to the critical value to accept or reject the null hypothesis.

$$X_C^2 = \frac{\Sigma(O_i - E_i)^2}{E_i} \tag{4.4}$$

Where c is the degree of freedom, O_i is the observed value, and E_i is the expected value. The Spearman correlation uses ranks to find the correlation values; therefore, this correlation is suited for ordinal data. The formula for the Spearman correlation is shown in Equation 4.5.

$$p = 1 - \frac{6\Sigma d_i^2}{n\left(n^2 - 1\right)} \tag{4.5}$$

The Spearman correlation coefficient, p, takes values between the range +1 and −1. A +1 indicates that there exists a perfect association of ranks, $p = 0$ indicates no association between ranks, and $p = -1$ indicates that there exists a perfect negative association of ranks. If p is closer to zero, then the associations are weaker. The correlation was performed with a p-value of 0.05. All ten features with p-values closer to zero were considered.

The extremely randomized trees classifier, or extra trees classifier (ETC), is an ensemble learning method used to select important features from the cirrhosis dataset. Random samples are used to build each decision and a k-feature from the feature set is given to each test node of each tree. Based on the Gini index, each decision tree chooses the optimum feature to split the data. In order to accomplish feature selection, each feature is ranked by its Gini importance in descending order, and the top k-features are considered the optimum features.

Recursive feature elimination (RFE) is used for feature elimination by fitting a model. Once the relevant features are determined, it then removes the irrelevant features one at a time in each iteration. It takes two arguments: the first is the algorithm and the second is the number of features. For example, if a decision tree is selected as an algorithm, RFE will apply a decision tree to the data and determine the essential features. The crucial features will vary from model to model; the second argument takes the number of significant features needed. The main drawback of RFE is that the number of features has to be selected in advance to avoid using recursive feature elimination cross-validation (RFECV). RFECV will perform cross-validation on the data and predict the n essential features of the dataset. In this work, RFECV has been used for the feature selection.

4.3.9 MODEL BUILDING

Machine learning models based on entropy, ensemble, and perceptron techniques have been built to classify the severity of cirrhosis disease. The ensemble techniques are preferred, since the size of the dataset used in this work is small.

4.3.9.1   Logistic Regression

Logistic regression is a supervised algorithm used for classification. First, the weighted sum of the independent features is calculated by Equation 4.6, then the result is passed through the sigmoid function in Equation 4.7, which will give us a value between zero and one. The lower the value is to one, the higher the probability of a "Yes" result (i.e., the person has cirrhosis).

$$y' = w^T x + b \tag{4.6}$$

Where b is the bias and w^T is the weight.

$$\sigma(z) = \frac{1}{1 + e^{-z}} \tag{4.7}$$

4.3.9.2   Decision Tree

The decision tree is a common algorithm used in supervised learning. It is a tree model with three nodes: decision, root, and leaf nodes. First, the best attribute must be chosen before the splitting can start. For that, the information gain and the entropy of each attribute have to be calculated by Equation 4.8. The attribute having the highest attribute will be the decision node. Entropy is the uncertainty of data, so the attributes having lower entropy should be considered first. Information gain is the difference in the values before and after the split of an attribute, calculated by Equation 4.9. This calculation is then done in a recursive process until it reaches the max_depth specified by the user.

$$E = -\sum_{i=1}^{N} p_i log_2 p_i \tag{4.8}$$

Where p_i is the probability of randomly selecting an input in class i.

$$information\ gain = 1 - entropy \tag{4.9}$$

4.3.9.3   Random Forest

The random forest classifier uses ensemble learning techniques to build classification and regression models. The main disadvantage of the decision tree is overfitting; the random forest classifier solves this problem, i.e., it minimizes the high variance of the data using the bagging technique. Since it is a classification problem, the bagging technique resamples the training data and makes a prediction for each subset. The majority prediction is then taken as the final prediction of this model.

4.3.9.4   AdaBoost

AdaBoost is a type of boosting algorithm. It is a sequential learning process, i.e., if multiple models are implemented, then each model will depend on the others. First, it assigns weights to every record, where weight = 1 / (number of records), then a stump is created, which is a tree-like structure that has a root node and leaf node with a depth of one; for each independent feature, a stump is created sequentially. After the entropy of every stump is calculated, the one having the lowest entropy is selected as the first base model. Then, the prediction takes place after the total error – which is the summation of all sample weights of misclassified data points – is calculated. After that, the performance of the stump is calculated using Equation 4.10. If misclassification happens, then the weight of those records is increased, while the weight of other records is decreased. Weights of the incorrectly and correctly classified records (W_{ic} and W_c, respectively) are updated using Equations 4.11 and 4.12. Next, AdaBoost calculates the normalized weight by dividing the updated weight by the total summation of the updated weights. After this, a new dataset using the normalized weights is created again. The decision tree made in each iteration will have a prediction, and the prediction with the majority vote is considered the final prediction.

$$performance\ of\ stump = \frac{1}{2}\log_e\left(\frac{1-TE}{TE}\right) \quad where\ TE = Total\ Error \quad (4.10)$$

$$W_{ic} = old\ Weight * e^{Performance\ of\ the\ stump} \quad (4.11)$$

$$W_c = old\ Weight * e^{-Performance\ of\ the\ stump} \quad (4.12)$$

4.3.9.5 XGBoost

Ensemble learning typically has two types of algorithms: bagging and boosting. XGBoost, also known as extreme gradient boost, is one of the boosting algorithms. In this work, XGBoost has been used to classify the severity of cirrhosis disease. XGBoost gives very high speeds since it gives parallelization and cache optimization; it is superior in terms of performance as well, as it provides auto-pruning and regularization, which helps make the model robust and prevents model overfitting. Scalability, treatment of missing values, and nonlinearity are further benefits of XGBoost. Residuals are calculated, which is the output score minus probability score probability, and then a tree is constructed for classification. The similarity score of the left, right, and root nodes is computed by Equation 4.13. In order to decide the order of attributes, the information gain of the tree is calculated, which is given by equation 4.14. The attribute having the highest gain will be considered first for splitting.

$$similarity\ score = \frac{\Sigma(residuals)^2}{\Sigma\left(probability\left(1-probability\right)+\lambda\right)} \quad (4.13)$$

Where λ is the regularization parameter.

$$Information\ gain = 1 - entropy \quad (4.14)$$

4.3.9.6 Multilayer Perceptron

Multilayer perceptron (MLP) is a type of feedforward artificial neural network. It is composed of the input layer, output layer, and hidden layers. The first process in MLP is forward propagation, and the data is propagated from the input layer to the output layer. The first step is to calculate the product of input and weights, as shown in Equation 4.15, and then the product Z1 is passed to the activation function.

$$Z1 = x_1 * w_1 + x_2 * w_2 + b \qquad (4.15)$$

In this cirrhosis severity prediction, the ReLU activation function is used for regularization. The main advantage of ReLU is that it solves the vanishing gradient descent problem. The range of the ReLU activation function is from zero to infinity. The value obtained after applying the activation function is then passed to hidden layers and then to the output layer. Likewise, the target variable, $Y1$, is also calculated using Equation 4.16.

$$Y1 = Z_1 * w_1 + Z_2 * w_2 + b \qquad (4.16)$$

After forward propagation, the backpropagation process takes place in this process. We first try to minimize the error by using a loss function, then update the weight and bias. The new weight and bias are given by Equations 4.17 and 4.18.

$$W_{new} = W_{old} - \eta \frac{\partial L}{\partial W_{old}} \qquad (4.17)$$

$$B_{new} = B_{old} - \eta \frac{\partial L}{\partial B_{old}} \qquad (4.18)$$

Where η= learning rate and $\eta \frac{\partial L}{\partial W_{old}}$, $\eta \frac{\partial L}{\partial B_{old}}$ can be calculated using the chain rule of partial differentiation.

4.4 RESULTS AND DISCUSSION

Univariate analysis is done on all attributes, and it has been identified that the features *Triglycerides, Copper, Cholesterol,* and *Bilirubin* have a lot of outliers, but they are not removed since it can lead to information loss; hence, those outliers' values are imputed with either the mean or median of each particular feature. The boxplot visualization of the variables is shown in Figure 4.2.

The numerical features (*Cholesterol, Copper, Alk-Phos, SGOT, Triglycerides, Platelets,* and *Prothrombin*) have missing values and are handled by imputing the mean of each feature. Categorical features like *Status, Drug, Ascites, Hepatomegaly,* and *Spiders* have missing values and are handled by imputing the mode of each particular feature. Label encoding is applied to categorical features (*Sex, Ascites, Spiders, Hepatomegaly, Drug*). In the *Sex* feature, female is encoded as 1 and male

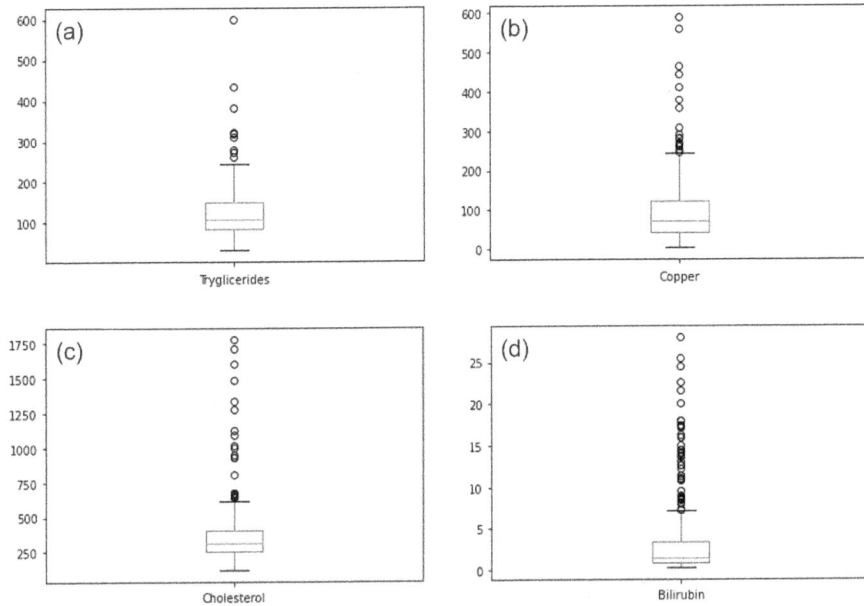

FIGURE 4.2   a. Triglycerides. b. Copper. c. Cholesterol. d. Bilirubin

is encoded as 0, in *Ascites, Hepatomegaly,* and *Spiders*, yes is encoded as 1 and no is encoded as 0, in *Drug*, D-penicillamine is encoded as 0 and placebo as 1, and ordinal encoding is applied on *Edema*. Status is shown by mapping Y as 0, N as 1, and S as 2, where Y means edema is present despite diuretic therapy, N means there is no edema and no diuretic therapy for edema, and S means edema is present without diuretics, or else edema was resolved by diuretics. For the attribute *Status*, D (death) is encoded as 0, C (censored) as 1, and CL (censored due to liver transplant) as 2. The bivariate analysis of the attributes, which explains the pairwise relationship between attributes, is shown in Figure 4.3.

It has been observed from the pair plot that there is no linear relationship between the variables. The attributes are scaled further using StandardScaler and then feature selection is performed. Different feature selection methods are applied and in each method, the ten best essential features are selected. First, the Pearson correlation is applied to the cirrhosis dataset and is visualized using a heatmap, as shown in Figure 4.4.

It has been identified that there are no highly correlated features. Spearman correlation analysis is done and the features with their corresponding p-values are given in Table 4.2.

The chi-squared test is applied and the ten best features (*Sex, Drug, Alk-Phos, SGOT, Albumin, Prothrombin, Triglycerides, Bilirubin, Copper, Hepatomegaly*) are selected. A supervised feature selection algorithm, extra trees classifier with ten estimators, and criterion entropy are applied, and the selected features are: *Age, Bilirubin, Albumin, Cholesterol, Triglycerides, SGOT, Platelets, Prothrombin,*

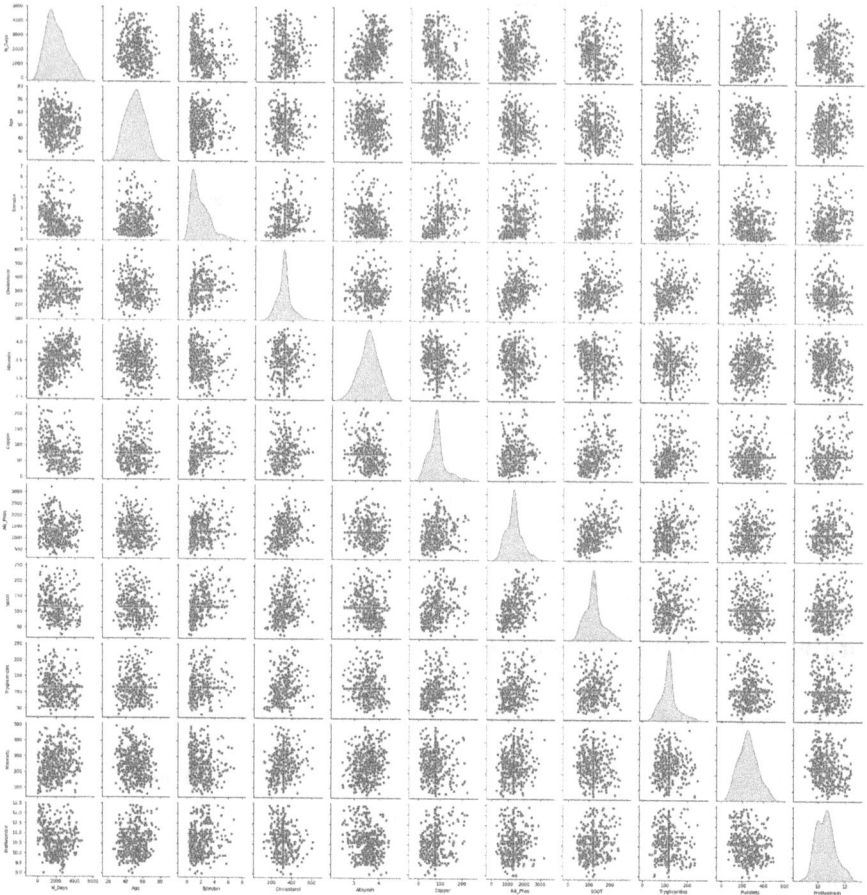

FIGURE 4.3 Pairwise relationship of attributes

Edema, SGOT, and *Copper.* A recursive feature elimination learning algorithm with a gradient boosting classifier as an estimator is used to identify the features which best explain the target *(Age, Hepatomegaly, Bilirubin, Cholesterol, Albumin, Copper, Alk-Phos, SGOT, Triglycerides, Platelets, Prothrombin).* With each feature set selected, machine learning models were built and the performance of the models was estimated. In this work, six models were built: XGBoost, AdaBoost, decision tree, random Forest, logistic regression, and multilayer perceptron. Starting with XGBoost, the max_depth parameter is 20 and the min_child_weight is five. For the model built using AdaBoost, the n_estimators parameter is 25 and learning_rate is fixed as one. For the random forest classifier model, the n_estimators parameter is set as 100 and the criterion used to find the best attribute is entropy. For the decision tree classifier, the max_depth parameter is set as 20. The performance metrics of the various models built are shown in Table 4.3.

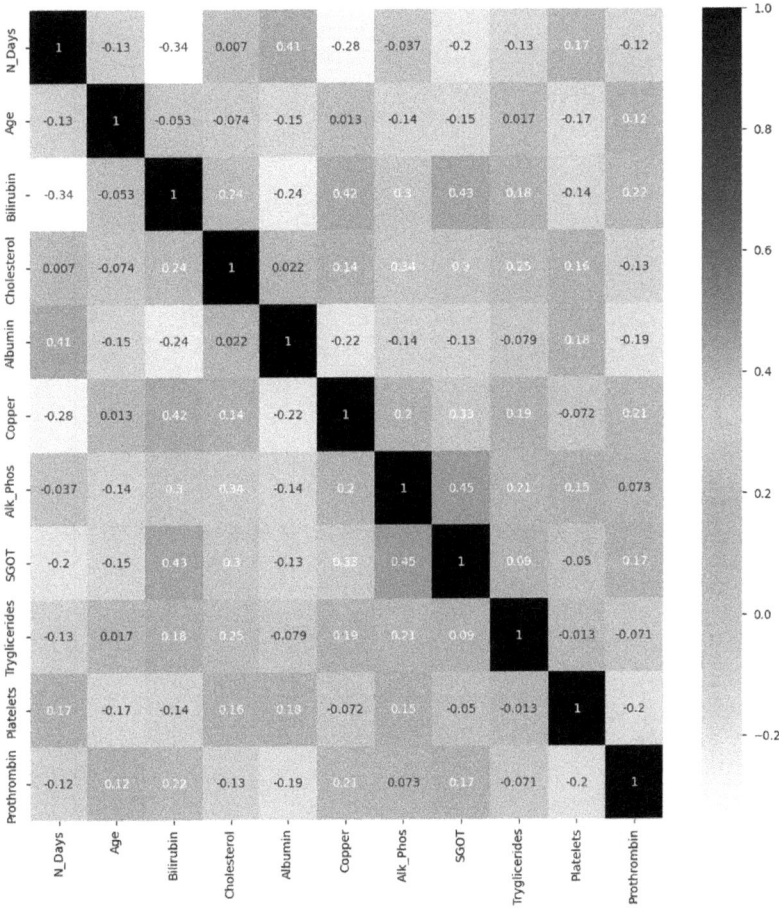

FIGURE 4.4 Heatmap of cirrhosis dataset

TABLE 4.2
Spearman Correlation (P) Values

P-Value	Feature
0.000001	Edema
0.000022	Ascites
0.000116	Bilirubin
0.000414	Platelets
0.000519	Copper
0.020488	Spiders
0.021125	SGOT
0021886	Hepatomegaly
0.026497	Cholesterol
0.0266	Albumin
0.048024	Sex

TABLE 4.3
Performance Metrics

Metrics	Feature Selection Method	XGBoost	AdaBoost	Random Forest	Decision Tree	Logistic Regression	Multilayer Perceptron
Accuracy	Chi-Squared	43.19	53.17	46.59	40.47	38.09	23.00
	ETC	42.83	49.20	44.13	39.68	40.47	39.70
	Spearman Correlation	44.55	42.85	39.00	38.88	43.65	43.70
	RFE	44.55	46.82	46.89	39.68	38.09	27.80
Precision	Chi-Squared	45	48	38	40	35	19
	ETC	48	50	41	40	39	42
	Spearman Correlation	44	39	38	38	41	41
	RFE	46	45	43	40	36	53
Recall	Chi-Squared	46	53	42	40	38	23
	ETC	48	49	44	40	40	40
	Spearman Correlation	46	43	40	39	44	44
	RFE	47	47	48	40	38	28
F1 Score	Chi-Squared	44	50	43	40	33	13
	ETC	47	48	44	40	40	40
	Spearman Correlation	45	40	39	38	41	41
	RFE	46	46	45	40	37	23
Specificity	Chi-Squared	61	57	60	50	44	72
	ETC	57	61	62	48	56	62
	Spearman Correlation	56	53	55	49	59	60
	RFE	57	49	61	49	59	56

The models built using the features selected by ETC yields better performance when compared to the feature sets identified as best by other feature selection methods. Chi-squared yields the maximum accuracy for the model built using AdaBoost in classifying the stages of cirrhosis.

4.5. CONCLUSION

Predictive analytics models have shown promise in predicting the risk of cirrhosis, a chronic liver disease. These models use statistical and machine learning techniques to analyze large datasets of patient information and identify patterns and predictors of disease progression. Several studies have demonstrated the efficacy of predictive analytics models in predicting the risk of cirrhosis and identifying high-risk patients who may benefit from early intervention. These models can be used to inform clinical decision-making and prioritize resources for preventative measures, such as lifestyle modifications, medication therapy, and liver transplantation. However, it is important to note that predictive analytics models are not foolproof and may have limitations. These models rely heavily on the quality and completeness of the data used to train them and may not account for certain factors that could influence disease progression. In addition, the interpretation and implementation of these models in clinical practice require careful consideration of ethical, legal, and social implications.

Univariate, bivariate, and multivariate analysis is done to study the variables and the data instances. Feature importance in predicting the stages of cirrhosis is considered in this work to identify the relevant features for model building. The selected features are used to build state-of-the-art machine learning models and are estimated using accuracy as the performance metric. The AdaBoost model outperforms the others, with the features selected using chi-squared methodology and the model yielding 53.17% accuracy.

REFERENCES

1. Ashley Spann, Angeline Yasodhara, Justin Kang, Kymberly Watt, Bo Wang, Anna Goldenberg, Mamatha Bhat, "Applying Machine Learning in Liver Disease and Transplantation: A Comprehensive Review," *Hepatology*, Vol. 71, No. 3, pp. 1093–1105, DOI: 10.1002/hep.31103, March 2020.
2. Tsehay Admassu Assegie, Rajkumar Subhashni, Napa Komal Kumar, Jijendira Prasath Manivannan, Pradeep Duraisamy, Minychil Fentahun Engidaye, "Random Forest and Support Vector Machine Based Hybrid Liver Disease Detection," *Bulletin of Electrical Engineering and Informatics*, Vol. 11, No. 3, pp. 1650–1656, DOI: 10.11591/eei.v11i3.3787, June 2022.
3. Xieyi Pei, Qingqing Deng, Zhuo Liu, Xiang Yan, Weiping Sun, "Machine Learning Algorithms for Predicting Fatty Liver Disease," *Annals of Nutrition and Metabolism*, Vol. 77, No. 1, pp. 38–45, DOI: 10.1159/000513654, June 2021.
4. Hye Won Lee, Joseph J. Y. Sung, Sang Hoon Ahn, "Artificial Intelligence in Liver Disease," *Journal of Gastroenterology and Hepatology*, Vol. 36, No. 3, pp. 539–542, DOI: 10.1111/jgh.15409, March 2021.
5. https://www.ncbi.nlm.nih.gov/pmc/articles/PMC8177826/.

6. Harsh H. Patel, Purvi Prajapati, "Study and Analysis of Decision Tree Based Classification Algorithms," *International Journal of Computer Sciences and Engineering*, Vol. 6, No. 10, pp. 74–78, DOI: 10.26438/ijcse/v6i10.7478, October 2018.

7. Nazmun Nahar, Ferdous Ara, "Liver Disease Prediction by Using Different Decision Tree Techniques," *International Journal of Data Mining & Knowledge Management Process*, Vol. 8, No. 2, pp. 01–09, DOI: 10.5121/ijdkp.2018.8201, March 2018.

8. Maher Maalouf, "Logistic Regression in Data Analysis: An Overview," *International Journal of Data Analysis Techniques and Strategies*, Vol. 3, No. 3, p. 281, DOI: 10.1504/ijdats.2011.041335, July 2011.

9. Ahmad Shaker Abdalrada, Omar Hashim Yahya, Abdul Hadi M. Alaidi, Nasser Ali Hussein, Haider T. H. Alrikabi, Tahsien Al-Quraishi Al-Quraishi, "A Predictive Model for Liver Disease Progression Based on Logistic Regression Algorithm," *Periodicals of Engineering and Natural Sciences (Pen)*, Vol. 7, No. 3, p. 1255, DOI: 10.21533/pen.v7i3.667, September 2019.

10. Anjna Jayant Deen, Manasi Gyanchandani, "Improved Machine Learning Using Adaptive Boosting Algorithm in Membrane Protein Prediction," *International Journal of Innovative Technology and Exploring Engineering*, Vol. 8, No. 12, pp. 3131–3137, DOI: 10.35940/ijitee.k2207.1081219, October 2019.

11. Egawati Panjei, Le Gruenwald, Eleazar Leal, Christopher Nguyen, Shejuti Silvia, "A Survey on Outlier Explanations," *The VLDB Journal*, Vol. 31, No. 5, pp. 977–1008, DOI: 10.1007/s00778-021-00721-1, September 2022.

12. Mehmet Akif Hasiloglu, Ayse Kunduraci, "A Research Study on Identifying the Correlation between Fourth Graders' Attitudes and Behaviors toward the Environment," *International Education Studies*, Vol. 11, No. 6, p. 60, DOI: 10.5539/ies.v11n6p60, May 2018.

13. Dr K. Vaneja, Ramesh Kumar, "Analysis of Feature Selection Algorithms on Classification: A Survey," *International Journal of Computer and Applications*, Vol. 96, No. 17, pp. 29–35, DOI: 10.5120/16888-6910, June 2014.

14. Pradnya Kumbhar, Manisha Pravin Mali, "A Survey on Feature Selection Techniques and Classification Algorithms for Efficient Text Classification," *International Journal of Science and Research (IJSR)*, Vol. 5, No. 5, pp. 1267–1275, DOI: 10.21275/v5i5.nov163675, May 2016.

15. Samreen Naeem, Aqib Ali, Salman Qadri, Wali Khan Mashwani, Nasser Tairan, Habib Shah, Muhammad Fayaz, Farrukh Jamal, Christophe Chesneau, Sania Anam, "Machine-Learning Based Hybrid-Feature Analysis for Liver Cancer Classification Using Fused (MR and CT) Images," *Applied Sciences*, Vol. 10, No. 9, p. 3134, DOI: 10.3390/app10093134, April 2020.

16. Abhishek Aravind, Avinash G. Bahirvani, Ronald Quiambao, Teresa Gonzalo, "Machine Learning Technology for Evaluation of Liver Fibrosis, Inflammation Activity and Steatosis (LIVERFASt™)," *Journal of Intelligent Learning Systems and Applications*, Vol. 12, No. 2, pp. 31–49, DOI: 10.4236/jilsa.2020.122003, May 2020.

17. Saima Afrin, F. M. Javed Mehedi Shamrat, Tafsirul Islam Nibir, Mst. Fahmida Muntasim, Md. Shakil Moharram, M. M. Imran, Md Abdulla, "Supervised Machine Learning Based Liver Disease Prediction Approach with LASSO Feature Selection," *Bulletin of Electrical Engineering and Informatics*, Vol. 10, No. 6, pp. 3369–3376, DOI: 10.11591/eei.v10i6.3242, December 2021.

18. Richa Singhal, Rakesh Rana, "Chi-Square Test and Its Application in Hypothesis Testing," *Journal of the Practice of Cardiovascular Sciences*, Vol. 1, No. 1, p. 69, DOI: 10.4103/2395-5414.157577, January 2015.

19. Sölpük Turhan Nihan, "Karl Pearsons Chi-Square Tests," *Educational Research and Reviews*, Vol. 15, No. 9, pp. 575–780, DOI: 10.5897/err2019.3817, May 2020.

20. Kabita Sahoo, Abhaya Kumar Samal, Jitendra Pramanik, Subhendu Kumar Pani, "Exploratory Data Analysis Using Python," *International Journal of Innovative Technology and Exploring Engineering*, Vol. 8, No. 12, pp. 4727–4735, DOI: 10.35940/ijitee.l3591.1081219, October 2019.

21. Ming Huang, Fuzhen Zhuang, Xiao Zhang, Xiang Ao, Zhengyu Niu, Min-Ling Zhang, Qing He, "Supervised Representation Learning for Multi-label Classification," *Machine Learning*, Vol. 108, No. 5, pp. 747–763, DOI: 10.1007/s10994-019-05783-5, May 2019.

22. Ketan Gupta, Nasmin Jiwani, Neda Afreen, Divyarani D, "Liver Disease Prediction Using Machine Learning Classification Techniques," in *2022 IEEE 11th International Conference on Communication Systems and Network Technologies (CSNT)*, pp. 221–226. IEEE, 2022.

23. D. B. Rakshith, Mrigank Srivastava, Ashwani Kumar, S. P. Gururaj, "Liver Disease Prediction System Using Machine Learning Techniques," *International Journal of Engineering Research and Technology (IJERT)*, Vol. 10, No. 6, pp. 949–951, 2021.

24. Nazmun Nahar, Vicky Barua, Ferdous Ara, Mohammad Shahadat Hossain, Md. Arif, Md. Arif Istiek Neloy, Karl Andersson. "A Comparative Analysis of the Ensemble Method for Liver Disease Prediction," DOI: 10.1109/ICIET48527.2019.9290507, 2019.

25. Yu Yang, Jiahao Wang, Chan Way Ng, Yukun Ma, Shupei Mo, Eliza Li Shan Fong, Jiangwa Xing, Ziwei Song, Yufei Xie, Ke Si, Aileen Wee, Roy E. Welsch, P. T. C. So, H. Yu, "Deep Learning Enables Automated Scoring of Liver Fibrosis Stages," *Sci Rep*, Vol. 8, p. 16016, DOI: 10.1038/s41598-018-34300-2, 2018.

26. Sivala Vishnu Murty, R. Kiran Kumar, "Accurate Liver Disease Prediction with Extreme Gradient Boosting," *International Journal of Engineering and Advanced Technology*, Vol. 8, No. 6, pp. 2288–2295, 2019.

27. Bihter Das, "A Comparative Study on the Performance of Classification Algorithms for Effective Diagnosis of Liver Diseases, Sakarya University," *Journal of Computer and Information Sciences*, Vol. 3, No. 3, pp. 366–375, 2020.

28. Muktevi Srivenkatesh, "Performance Evolution of Different Machine Learning Algorithms for Prediction of Liver Disease," *International Journal of Innovative Technology and Exploring Engineering*, Vol. 9, No. 2, pp. 1115–1122, 2019.

29. Moloud Abdar, Mariam Zomorodi-Moghadam, Resul Das, I-Hsien Ting, "Performance Analysis of Classification Algorithms on Early Detection of Liver Disease," *Expert Systems with Applications*, Vol. 67, pp. 239–251, DOI: 10.1016/j.eswa.2016.08.065, 2017.

30. Moloud Abdar, Neil Yuwen Yen, Hung Jason Chi-Shun, "Improving the Diagnosis of Liver Disease Using Multilayer Perceptron Neural Network and Boosted Decision Trees," *Journal of Medical and Biological Engineering*, Vol. 38, No. 6, pp. 953–965, DOI: 10.1007/s40846-017-0360-z, 2018.

31. Rong-HoLin, "An Intelligent Model for Liver Disease Diagnosis," *Artificial Intelligence in Medicine*, Vol. 47, No. 1, pp. 53–62, 2009.

32. https://www.kaggle.com/datasets/fedesoriano/cirrhosis-prediction-dataset (accessed on 16th June 2022).

33. P. Antony Seba, J. V. Bibal Benifa, "Perceptive Analysis of Chronic Kidney Disease Data Through Conceptual Visualization," in Das, A.K., Nayak, J., Naik, B., Vimal, S., Pelusi, D. (eds) *Computational Intelligence in Pattern Recognition. CIPR 2022. Lecture Notes in Networks and Systems*, Vol. 480. Springer, Singapore. https://doi.org/10.1007/978-981-19-3089-8_11.

5 3D Volumetric Computed Tomography from 2D X-Rays
A Deep Learning Perspective

Manish Kumar, Suman Kumar Maji, and Hussein Yahia

5.1 INTRODUCTION

Computed Tomography (CT) is an imaging technique used to capture detailed information about the human body . The word tomography comes from the Greek word *tomos*, which means "a slice or a section or a cut", and *graphein*, which means "to write or to record". Thus, computed tomography is a method that computes a record of slices. These slices are created by using a special device known as a scanner, or a CT scanner [1].

CT scanners are electronic machines used to scan a body part and create a picture or image of the scanned body part. The picture created by scanning the body part is also known as a "slice". A slice is a two-dimensional (2D) image. It captures the details of the scanned body part and presents it in two-dimensional form. After one slice of the image is created, the next slice is created by moving the scanner over the body. In this way, a CT scanner creates a number of slices of the scanned body part [1, 2]. Then, these slices are placed one on the other like a sliced loaf of bread to form a three-dimensional (3D) image, which is known as computed tomography or computerized tomography. Thus, the CT image is three-dimensional, created by two-dimensional slices of X-ray images imposed one on the other. Earlier CT scanners produced slices in a serial manner, one after another. But modern CT scanners produce continuous picture slices by moving the scanner in a helical or spiral manner. That is why these are known as helical or spiral CT scanners. These scanners are more advantageous than normal scanners because, for instance, these scanners are faster than normal CT scanners. These scanners also produce better-quality pictures and capture in-depth details of the scanned body part. Also, these scanners capture small abnormalities in the body better than earlier CT scanners [1, 3].

CT scanners are used in the medical field to diagnose cancer, circulatory system diseases like coronary artery disease, thrombosis, and vascular aneurysms, as well

DOI: 10.1201/9781003363361-5

TABLE 5.1
List of Abbreviations

Full Form	Abbreviation
Computed tomography	CT
Digitally reconstructed radiograph	DRR
Convolutional neural network	CNN
Generative adversarial network	GAN
Deep neural network	DNN

as spinal conditions, abscesses, kidney and gallbladder stones, inflammatory diseases like ulcerative colitis, head injuries, and injuries to the skeletal system and internal organs. CT scanners are also used to diagnose abnormalities in the brain and other cognitive impairment diseases like Alzheimer's [1].

Figure 5.1 shows a block diagram of a computed tomography machine. The main components of a CT machine are:

- **Detectors:** An ionization chamber filled with xenon gas, sealed at both ends, and flanked by two conductors that make up a capacitor make up the detector.
- **DC voltage supply:** A high-DC voltage supply is applied to an X-ray tube.
- **X-ray tube:** The X-ray tube emits X-rays allowed to pass through the patient.
- **Computer machine: This** captures the rays passed through the patient and applies some mathematical formulation to generate the image slices.

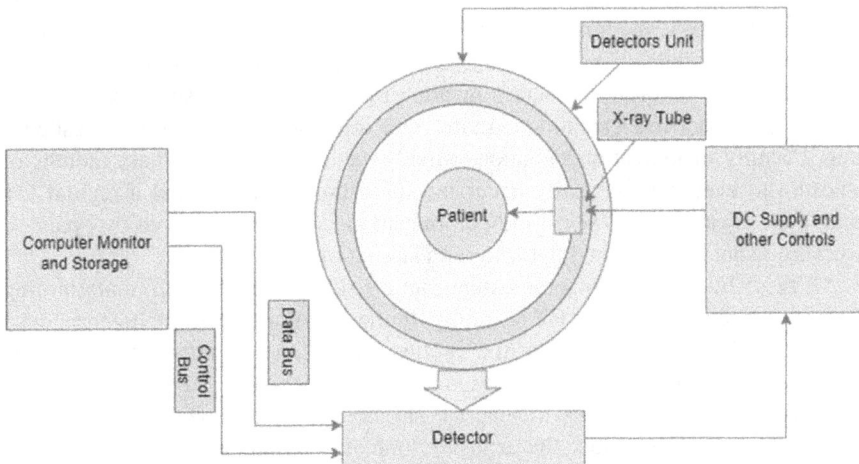

FIGURE 5.1   Block diagram of CT scan machine.

- **Control bus:** This controls the number of radiations to be passed through the patient and also controls the operations of the computer.
- **Data bus:** This carries data from the detectors to the computer system to process and generate the image [4].

5.2   IMAGE ACQUISITION USING CT SCANNERS

Conventional X-ray scanners contain a fixed X-ray tube, but CT scanners contain a motorized X-ray tube. The motorized X-ray tube revolves around the side of the circular opening known as the gantry, which has a donut-like structure. The patient is made to lie inside the gantry and the X-ray tube, which is rotating around the gantry, shoots a narrow X-ray beam through the body of the patient. The digital detectors, which are placed directly opposite the X-ray tube in the gantry, capture the rays passed through the patient's body, creating an image. The microcomputer controls the X-ray tube and detectors, and then passes the image to the computer machine to generate an image slice after applying some mathematical formulations. The thickness of this slice ranges between one and ten millimetres. After creating one slice, the motorized bed is moved inside the gantry to generate the next slice. The same procedure is followed again to generate another image slice, and this process is followed until the required number of slices is collected [4].

The slices generated are two-dimensional and can be stacked together by the computer to generate a three-dimensional CT image. The 3D CT image captures the details of the scanned body part in depth, which helps the physician check for abnormalities in the bones, skeleton, organs, and tissues [2].

5.3   DRAWBACKS OF CT SCANNERS

CT scanning helps capture the internal structure of the body in a convenient way. It helps diagnose the deadliest diseases, like cancer. But CT scans use X-rays, which are harmful to the body. It is important to note that the everyday exposure to ionization radiation to an average person in the US is about three millisieverts (mSv) per year, due to the naturally present ionization radiation in outer space or naturally occurring radioactive elements like radon. One low-dose CT scan of the chest contains 1.5 mSv of ionization radiation, which is about equivalent to six months of exposure to everyday, naturally occurring ionization radiation, and a regular CT scan of the chest contains seven mSv of ionization, equivalent to about two years of exposure to naturally occurring background radiation [2].

All these limitations, to some extent, put a risk to patient health, undermining the wide range of benefits of CT scanning. In the age of artificial intelligence, deep learning has been shown to perform exceptionally well in the area of 3D volumetric reconstruction of CT images from captured 2D slices. Also, deep learning-based methods have a proven ability to generate 2D slices from a single CT image. These factors have helped to reduce the exposure time of CT scanners, thereby mitigating their harmful effects. In this chapter, we will talk about these existing computational and deep learning-based methods [5].

5.4   3D CT RECONSTRUCTION: PROBLEM FORMULATION

Using two-dimensional X-ray image slices, 3D CT reconstruction generates three-dimensional CT images. The two-dimensional X-ray image cannot capture the behaviour of real-world objects in detail. So, it is necessary to reconstruct a three-dimensional CT scan, which can help us visualize volumetric objects. A vast amount of information about real-world objects that could be extremely helpful in the medical field is lost in X-ray imaging. The inner shape of the body is projected on a flat 2D image, which is inherently a lossy process, and to regenerate the original three-dimensional structure is a daunting process; therefore, there is a great necessity for a technique in which X-ray images can be used to generate three-dimensional objects [3, 5].

The problem of 3D CT reconstruction can be formulated as a series of 2D projections $X_1, X_2, ..., X_N$, where $X_i \in \mathbb{R}^{H_{2D} \times W_{2D}}$ and N is the number of projections, such that $1 < i < N$. The target is to generate 3D volume Y from these 2D projections. The predicted output is given by $Y_{pred} \in \mathbb{R}^{C_{3D} \times H_{3D} \times W_{3D}}$ and the ground truth value is $Y_{truth} \in \mathbb{R}^{C_{3D} \times H_{3D} \times W_{3D}}$, so that Y_{pred} and Y_{truth} are the same size. Each value in Y_{truth} and Y_{pred} is of voxel intensity. The problem is tackled by using a mapping function F, which maps the 2D projections onto 3D volumetric images. The input to this function F is $X_1, X_2, ..., X_N$, and Y_{pred}, which can be expressed in Equation 5.1, as the output,

$$F (X_1, X_2, ..., X_N) = Y_{pred} \tag{5.1}$$

The series of 2D projections $X_1, X_2, ..., X_N$ ($X_i \in \mathbb{R}^{H_{2D} \times W_{2D}}$) are stacked to form a 3D tensor $Z \in \mathbb{R}^{N \times H_{2D} \times W_{2D}}$, which is provided as an input to the function F [6].

5.5   MOTIVATION FOR 3D CT RECONSTRUCTION

Computational and deep learning techniques have found widespread utility in the medical domain, namely in MRIs [7, 8], microscopy [9, 10], ultrasounds, X-rays [11, 12], etc. There are multiple reasons to design computational and deep learning-based methods to generate 3D volumetric images from 2D slices. Firstly, X-ray images cannot capture all the details of the scanned body part. The X-ray images are two-dimensional in nature, which loses information when the body part is scanned, as the body part is 3D in nature. Therefore, three-dimensional reconstruction of two-dimensional X-ray images is necessary to regain all the lost information.

Secondly, the CT imaging process exposes patients to higher levels of ionization radiation, which is harmful to the body – especially for pregnant women and children – and can cause deadly diseases like cancer. Deep learning- and computational-based methods reduce the exposure time and limit ill effects.

Also, 3D CT scanners are costly and are not feasible everywhere. So, there is a great need to develop a computational solution which can effectively provide a 3D view of the body from two-dimensional X-ray images.

Furthermore, during CT scanning, patients have to lie down on the CT scan machine, which is not a good position to diagnose spine-related problems like lumbar disc herniation and cervical spondylosis. During spine-related diagnosis, the patient is required to be standing in a straight position during the scan.

5.6 TRADITIONAL COMPUTATIONAL TECHNIQUES FOR 3D CT RECONSTRUCTION

3D CT reconstruction is a mathematical technique in which CT images are generated by 2D X-ray images taken at different angles around the patient. Some of the methods for 3D CT reconstruction are listed below:

Analytical Methods: There are various types of analytical methods for 3D CT reconstruction. Of them, the most commonly used is the filtered backpropagation (FBP) type. In this technique, one-dimensional filters are used in the projection data and then the projection data is projected in the image space. This method is computationally efficient and stable. FBP methods have been used since the 1970s [6, 11, 13]. Until 1980, two-dimensional parallel and fan-beams were popular. Then, multi-slice and helical with narrow detectors came in the late-1980s [14]. During the 2000s, multi-slice and helical with wide-range detectors that range up to 320 detectors 16 centimeters wide became popular [15, 16]. Three-dimensional filtered backpropagation methods are used in CT scanners that have more than 16 detectors. CT scanner users are not very aware of the internal functioning of the reconstruction methods; they are mainly confined to adjusting the parameters of the CT scanners to improve the image standard. The reconstruction gauze, also known as "kernel" or "procedure" by some users, is the principal condition that most helps to improve the image standard. There is a compromise between noise and spatial sharpness for each kernel. A smoother kernel helps reduce disturbance in the image, but reduces the spatial resolution of the image [8, 10]. On the other hand, a sharper kernel helps improve the spatial resolution but it leads to increased noise in the image. So, the selection of the kernel should be based on the application of the CT scanners [7, 9]. For example, scanners used for brain examination require low noise and low spatial resolution, whereas scanners used for bone examination require sharper kernels, compromising noise for high spatial resolution. Another important parameter is slice thickness, which is used to control the resolution in a longitudinal direction, affecting the tradeoff between noise, radiation dose, and spatial resolution [2].

Iterative Methods: In iterative methods, optimization consists of regularization and data precision. The optimization process consists of forward and backward iterations of projections between the image space and the projection space. Iterative methods are advantageous over analytical methods, because, as compared to the focal point of analytical methods, X-ray beam spectrum, detector geometry, photon scattering, and geometry can be easily incorporated in iterative methods, which leads to lower image noise and higher spectral resolution. It also reduces windmills, metal artefacts, and beam hardening in images [17]. The images of analytical and iterative methods are different because of the data handling methods. The spatial resolution in the IR method depends on the noise and contrast of the surrounding structure, because of factors like regularization during optimization [18, 19]. Experiments on different methods have shown the effect of noise dependency and contrast on spatial resolution. The amount of radiation dose in IR methods depends on the diagnostic task because of this dependency. A small radiation dose is allowed for low-contrast detection tasks. Proper clinical evaluation and parameter optimization are required before these methods can be used in routine practice [2].

The advent of neural networks (NNs) has greatly contributed to healthcare monitoring, and 3D CT reconstruction is one area that has greatly benefited. In the following section, we give a brief overview of neural networks.

5.7 DEEP NEURAL NETWORKS

Deep neural networks (DNNs) are a type of artificial neural network (ANN) with many more hidden layers than other ANNs. ANNs are shallow networks that are commonly used in machine learning tasks to solve simple tasks. However, a deep neural network contains thousands of hidden layers, which can solve more complex real-time problems. Deep neural networks consist of an input layer which receives the input for the network, a number of hidden layers containing neurons connected to each other, which process the input and extract the important information from it, and an output layer which gives the result after processing from the hidden layer. Figure 5.2 below shows a shallow neural network and a deep neural network (DNN). The data to the networks are A1, A2, and A3. Outputs from the networks are B1, B2, and B3. The number of hidden layers is different in each network [20]. Deep neural networks contain a greater number of hidden layers than shallow networks, which helps to extract more information from the input data and in turn helps to provide better results than shallow neural networks. Y1, Y2, Y3, and Y4 are the neurons in the hidden layer, which are connected to each other and help to extract meaningful information from the inputs. The weights and biases change as data values pass from one layer to another from input to output. This is known as a forward pass. After the forward pass, the output values at the output layer are equated with the ground truth values. Errors are propagated back to the input, which is known as a backward pass. The backward pass helps minimize errors and improves the accuracy of the model [5].

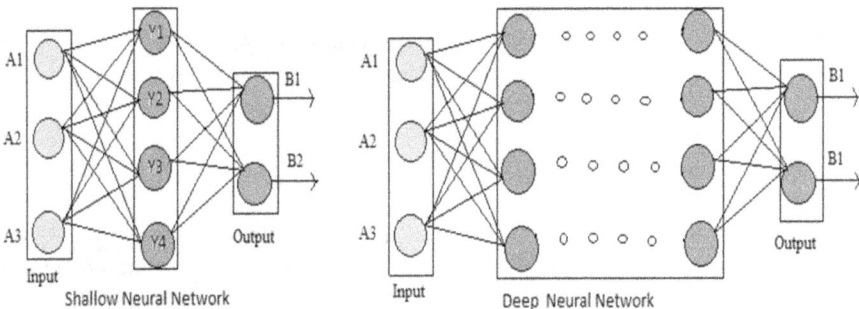

FIGURE 5.2   Deep neural network vs shallow neural network.

Due to the abundance of data readily available, deep learning is growing quickly in every sphere of life. It is replacing knowledge-based applications that have pre-defined knowledge. The use of a lot of data to train deep neural networks is producing cutting-edge results. Earlier, neural networks were not of much use because of the unavailability of large amounts of data and processing units like GPUs (graphics processing units) and TPUs (tensor processing units) [20].

Nowadays, deep learning is used in every domain to solve problems which were not feasible or require many resources, like data, processing units like GPUs, and time. They are called deep neural networks because they contain neural networks with millions of variables in them. The tuning of these variables is known as the learning of the network. This tuning is done by providing a large amount of data so that the network can learn the relationship between the ground truth and the input variables. At first, the model will give random results, but as training goes on, it gets better and gives good results. Training accuracy and training loss are used as measures to calculate the training performance of the neural network. Once training is done, the model is evaluated on an unseen dataset known as a test dataset [21]. This evaluation tells us the actual performance quality of the model. Deep learning models during training extract the important features present in the training images and then predict the output of unseen test images based on the features learned by the training. Therefore, the models require a lot of data so that they can learn all the important features present in the images. Overfitting occurs when the model memorizes the training data and fails to perform well on the unseen data when there is less data.

5.8 CONVOLUTIONAL NEURAL NETWORKS

A class of neural networks called convolutional neural networks – also known as ConvNets or CNNs – is used to process data like images, videos, and signals, among other things. A digital image consists of a series of pixel values stored in a grid-like structure. These pixel values denote the colour and the brightness of the image pixel.

Like the human brain, convolution neural networks help process data of an image for computers. The human brain processes information through large and complex structures consisting of neurons. Similarly, convolutional neural networks consist of deep hidden layers which can obtain simpler types of features like lines, edges, etc., and complex features like faces and objects from an input image. So, it is like an eye for the computer [3]. A CNN typically consists of three kinds of layers:

1. Convolution layer
2. Pooling layer
3. Fully connected layer

Convolution layer: This is the primary layer that is utilized in the process of obtaining various kinds of features from the input layer. The kernel also known as the filter is made to run over the input image and obtains the important attributes from the given image. Each time the kernel runs over the image, it performs the dot operation with the input image pixel values and gives a two-dimensional output known as an activation map [22]. The size of the sliding of the kernel is known as stride. Consider an image of size $W \times W \times D$ pixels, where D is the number of channels. When D_{out} number of kernels, each of size $F \times F$ with stride (S) and padding (P) are applied on the image, it gives $W_{out,}$ as in Equation 5.2 below:

$$W_{out} = (W - F + 2P)/S + 1 \qquad (5.2)$$

The size of the output volume is $W_{out} \times W_{out} \times D_{out}$.

Pooling layer: This layer reduces the computational cost and the dimensions of the attribute map by removing the most important features. There are various kinds of pooling layers. The most routinely used are max pooling and average pooling layers. In max pooling, the greatest pixel value is selected from the region of the image, and in standard pooling, all the pixel values over the region are averaged to give the output feature map [22]. Consider an activation map of $W \times W \times D$ pixels at a particular stage, where D is the number of channels, having filter size $F \times F$ and of stride (S) gives $W_{out,}$ as in Equation 5.3 below:

$$W_{out} = (W - F) / S + 1 \qquad (5.3)$$

The size of the output volume is $W_{out} \times W_{out} \times D$.

Fully connected layer: In a completely associated layer, neurons from one layer are associated with each neuron in the following layer. So, this forms a full connection between each layer and the following layer. The final layer is prior to the fully connected layers at the network's end [3].

Take the CIFAR-10 dataset as an example: here, there are 60,000 images across ten different classes in the dataset. The classes are truck, ship, horse, frog, airplane, automobile, cat, dog, bird, and deer, which are labelled from zero to nine, respectively. Out of 60,000 images, 50,000 images are pre-owned to train the CNN architecture and 10,000 pictures are used to test the trained network. Convolution, max pooling, and fully connected are the three layers that make up a straightforward CNN architecture. 50,000 images are used to train the network, which learns important features from the training images. The accuracy of the trained model is verified with testing data after the network has been trained [22].

Figure 5.3 shows the CNN architecture. It has two max pooling layers and two convolution layers. The network receives an input image sized $12 \times 12 \times 3$ pixels, having 3 channels and length and width of 12, and processes it through the Cov1 layer to generate an output image sized $32 \times 32 \times 32$ pixels, with 32 channels used. After that, it is sent to the max pooling layer, which extracts useful features to reduce the feature map. So, it reduces the size of the image to $16 \times 16 \times 32$ pixels. Now, this passed to the Cov2 layer and then the max pooling layer giving output image sized $8 \times 8 \times 64$ pixels, where the number of channels used is 64. Finally, the fully connected layer connects all the preceding and succeeding neurons and maps the features to the output labels [3].

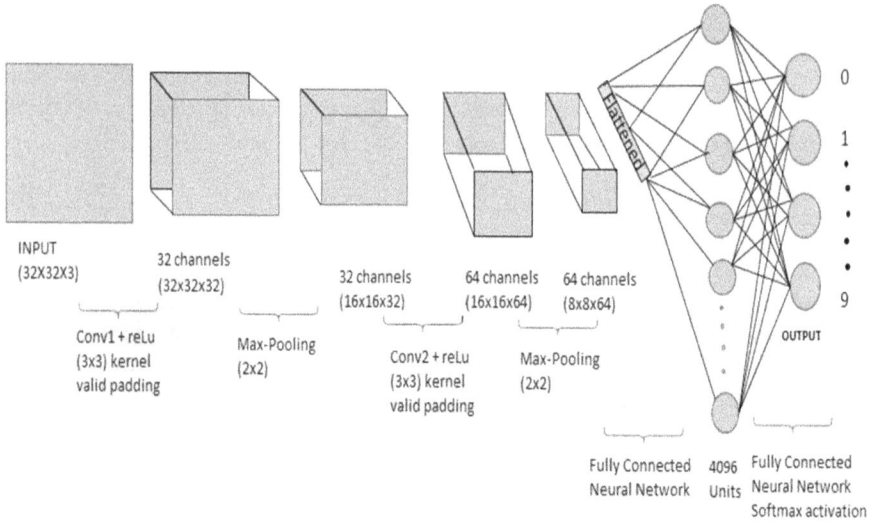

FIGURE 5.3   CNN architecture.

5.9   DEEP LEARNING TECHNIQUES FOR 3D CT RECONSTRUCTION

As deep learning has progressed, it has given state-of-the-art in every domain. In the medical field, deep learning is used in the classification of medical data, the segmentation of organs from medical images, 3D CT reconstruction, medical image denoising, and many other domains [17, 23]. It is used to classify whether a disease is present in images or not. Also, in segmentation like generating 3D images of organs from CT scan images. Denoising the background noise in X-ray and computed tomography pictures by deep convolutional networks helps to better understand the disease present in the body. There has been ongoing research in medical imaging using deep learning and it has helped a lot by providing state-of-the-art technologies. But there are some fields, like 3D CT reconstruction, in which much is needed to be explored [24].

Here, we will be focusing on deep neural network-based methods, which have manifested great results compared to traditional methods in 3D CT reconstruction. Deep learning-based methods have advanced significantly as a result of the abundance of available data. CNN-based methods, GAN (Generative Adversarial Network)-based methods like cyclic GAN, and a recent method based on transformers have shown better results than traditional statistical modelling-based methods. All these procedures have provided state-of-the-art three-dimensional reconstruction from two-dimensional X-ray images [20].

CT recreation from 2D X-beam pictures utilizing profound learning-based strategies can be sorted into three methods, as shown in Figure 5.4. In the first method, by using a single X-ray image, a deep learning model can estimate multiple CT images

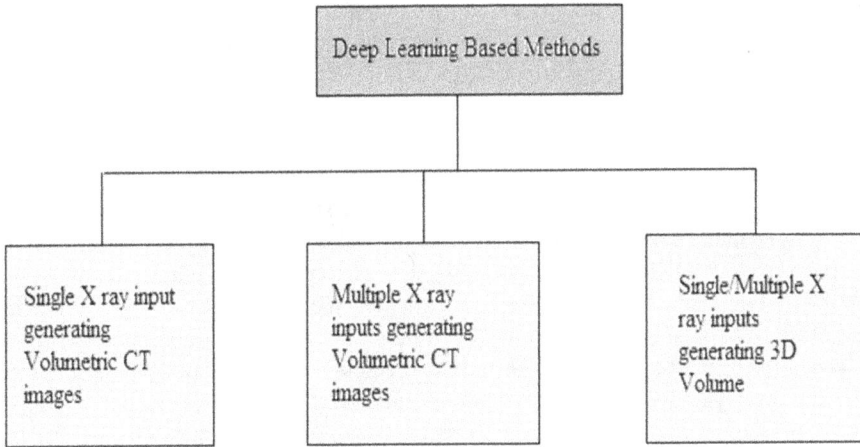

FIGURE 5.4   Deep learning-based procedures for 3D CT reconstruction.

of various depths, thereby giving a 3D understanding. Secondly, given multiple two-dimensional X-ray images as input, a deep learning model can generate a great number of CT images, thereby enabling further insight. Thirdly, by using a single X-ray image, a deep learning model can generate a 3D structure of the scanned body part [22]. We will talk about the various deep learning models under these three categories in the following subsections.

5.9.1   SINGLE X-RAY INPUT TO GENERATE VOLUMETRIC CT IMAGES

CT restoration from two-dimensional X-ray images has not been observed for long; only in recent years has it evolved. Shen et al. [6] developed a deep CNN-based encoder-decoder architecture comprising three modules – a representation network, a transformation network, and a generation network – to reconstruct volumetric CT images. The experiment is conducted with different input projections (one, two, five, and ten), which are stacked together. The experiment was carried out for three different cases: lung, upper abdomen, and head and neck. The experiment gives promising results. Zhiqiang Tan et al. [11] developed XctNet, which uses a single X-ray image to reconstruct three-dimensional CT images. It uses prior knowledge from X-ray images and helps in the reconstruction of CT images. The proposed method is based on U-Net and comprises a self-attention module and a multiscale feature fusion module. Almeida et al. [13] reconstructed three-dimensional CT images using a single X-ray image by a novel deep convolutional encoder-decoder-based architecture for lower limbs. The architecture gives promising results. Jiang et al. [15] developed a GAN-based architecture for CT restoration from a single X-ray image of the lung and upper abdomen. Peng et al. [16] developed a two-stage deep CNN-based network used to restore 3D CT volumes from a single 2D X-ray input. The images used to train the architecture were from LIDC/IDRI (Lung Image Database Consortium/

Image Database resource Initiative) collection, which is a publicly available dataset. From the 1018 chest CT volumes, the 780 best CT volumes were chosen. Out of these 70 were used for testing, 700 for training, and ten for validation of the model. This is the foremost effort in radiograph synthesis. Yu et al. [25] developed a deep neural network-based architecture using an algorithm called filtered backpropagation (FBP), which is used to restore 3D CT volumes from single-input two-dimensional X-ray images. It contains a projection generation stage, an FBP layer, and a CT fine-tuning stage. The network beats the ultra-modern technology. Estelle Loyen et al. [14] developed a deep CN-based network to restore 3D CT volumes from single 2D X-ray input images. The network is trained to locate the position of a tumor in the brain. The standardized root-mean-square error is used to compute the error between the ground truth CT image and the predicted volumetric images. Hisaichi et al. [26] developed a CNN-based network named X2CT-FLOW, which uses a single two-dimensional input X-ray image to reconstruct volumetric chest images. PSNR (peak signal to noise ratio) with SSIM (structural similarity index) value is used to calculate the standard of the predicted CT image and MAE (mean absolute error), RMSE (root mean square error) are used to compute the error between the ground truth reconstructed image and the output chest CT images. The summary of all the papers discussed here is listed in Table 5.2.

TABLE 5.2
Summary of Papers for Category One

Author	Contribution
Liyue Shen et al. [6]	Encoder-decoder-based model using single or multiple projection views to generate 3D volumetric images.
Zhiqiang Tan et al. [11]	A deep learning-based model similar to InceptionNet that was used to create 3D volumetric CT images from a solitary X-ray image.
Diogo F. Almeida et al. [13]	As a data augmentation technique, an encoder-decoder model with skip associations and a multi-dimensional Gaussian gauge is used to generate three-dimensional medical image volumes using a single X-ray image.
Ling Jiang et al. [15]	Developed a GAN-based architecture for lung and upper abdominal CT reconstruction using a solitary X-ray image.
Cheng Peng et al. [16]	Using a single 2D X-ray input, a two-stage deep CNN network can recreate 3D CT volumes. The model is trained using the publicly available LIDC/IDRI dataset.
Jianqiao Yu et al. [25]	An FBP- (filtered backpropagation-) based deep CNN network is used to recreate 3D CT volumes using a single-input 2D X-ray image. It has a stage for projection generation, an FBP layer, and a stage for CT fine-tuning.
Estelle Loyen et al. [14]	A CNN-based network for reconstructing a single two-dimensional X-ray input image into a 3D CT volume. The network has been trained to identify a brain tumour's location.
Hisaichi Shibata et al. [26]	Deep CNN-based network named X2CT-FLOW, which uses a single 2D input X-ray image to reconstruct volumetric chest images.

5.9.2 MULTIPLE X-RAY INPUT TO GENERATE VOLUMETRIC CT IMAGES

Ying et al. [18] proposed a GAN-based architecture for 3D CT reconstruction using two X-ray images. The architecture uses a separate encoder for each of the input X-ray images, which leads to a complex architecture and requires plenty of reckoning resources. Ratul et al. [19] developed a GAN- and deep CNN-based architecture to restore volumetric images from biplanar X-ray images and beat the state-of-the-art technology. Shen et al. [27] use geometric image priors for three-dimensional CT restoration from multiple two-dimensional X-ray images, which enhances the CT reconstruction process. Ge et al. [28] developed a deep learning-based novel architecture comprising two separate modules for 3D CT reconstruction and segmentation of the cervical vertebra. The architecture uses two projections anterior-posterior (AP) and lateral (LAT) as inputs and generates the 3D volume of the object. Afshar et al. [29] developed the framework known as CARISI, which makes use of the inter-slice interpolation method to restore three-dimensional CT volumes from multiple two-dimensional X-ray image slices. The encoder-decoder architecture that is utilized in the reconstruction of a brain tumour's shape is the foundation of the architecture. The model is evaluated on a real-time dataset consisting of 3064 segmented brain tumour images. Santarelli et al. [30] proposed a deep CNN-based inter-slice interpolation method to reconstruct 3D volumetric images from multiple X-ray images. The method enhances the image quality and speed of reconstruction by using geometric image priors and an inter-slice interpolation method. PSNR and SSIM values are used to compare the ground truth image with the reconstructed image. The MSE and RMSE values are used to compute the errors between the ground truth image and the reconstructed image. The above papers are summarized in Table 5.3 below.

5.9.3 SINGLE/MULTIPLE X-RAY INPUT TO GENERATE 3D VOLUME

Three-dimensional reconstruction from two-dimensional X-ray images results in CT volumetric images which can be estimated to get the volumetric view of the body part scanned. Henzler et al. [31] were, to the best of our knowledge, the first to restore three-dimensional cranial volumes using a single 2D X-ray image. They use deep CNN-based architecture that has skip connections with residual learning. The model is trained using two-dimensional X-ray images and the corresponding 3D CT images of 175 different mammalian classes. Shiode et al. [32] designed a GAN-rooted model to get volume out of two-dimensional X-ray images, using a statistical structure model (SSM) and CNN-based neural network to restore three-dimensional volume from two-dimensional X-ray images of bones. Bayat et al. [33] reconstruct spine posture from two orthogonal-view X-ray images. The architecture Transvert is based on an encoder-decoder deep CNN model consisting of three structures: a sagittal encoder, a coronal encoder, and a 3D decoder. These three structures are integrated by map and fuse block. Hangkee Kim et al. [34] developed a CNN model to restore leg bones from two-dimensional X-ray images, using bounding boxes to extract the features and a statistical shape model (SSM) parameter to fine-tune the

TABLE 5.3

Summary of Papers in Category Two

Author	Contribution
Xingde Ying et al. [18]	Reconstructed a 3D CT volume from two orthogonal X-rays using GAN.
Md Aminur et al. [19]	Proposed an architecture based on GAN and deep CNN to reassemble volumetric CT images using orthogonal X-ray images.
Liyue Shen et al. [27]	Used geometric image priors for three-dimensional CT restoration from multiple X-ray images, which enhances the CT reconstruction process.
Rongjun Ge et al. [28]	Proposed deep learning-based novel architecture comprising two separate modules for 3D CT reconstruction and segmentation of cervical vertebra. The architecture uses two projections AP and LA as inputs and generates the 3D volume of the object.
Parnian Afshar et al. [29]	Based on the inter-slice interpolation method, the framework known as CARISI can restore 3D CT volumes from multiple X-ray image slices. The encoder-decoder architecture that is utilized in the reconstruction of the brain tumor's shape is the foundation of the model.
Chiara Santarelli et al. [30]	The CNN-based inter-slice interpolation technique is used to reconstruct multiple X-ray images into 3D volumetric images. Using geometric image priors and the inter-slice interpolation method, the method improves image quality and speeds up reconstruction.

model. In cases where bounding boxes are not able to extract the features, feature ellipses and feature points are used. Jana Cavojska et al. [12] developed a deep neural network-based architecture to estimate the three-dimensional structure of bones using a pair of two-dimensional X-ray images. Transfer learning and the triplet loss function are used in combination with KNN (K-nearest neighbor) classifiers to differentiate between bones. The approach is compared with eight other approaches and shows that this method works better than others. Yifan Wang et al. [35] developed a deep neural network-based model called DeepOrganNet, which reconstructs multiple 3D meshes of the organ using a solitary X-ray projection view. The model extracts features using smooth deformation fields and leverages latent descriptors which are extracted from two-dimensional X-ray images. MobileNet is used to reconstruct multiple view meshes of the organ. Catherine Namayega et al. [36] used deep CNN-based network U-Net to reconstruct the 3D volume of the scapula bone using biplanar X-ray images. However, the model does not fit well to real-time datasets. Weinan Song et al. [37] developed a two-phase deep neural network-based model which uses a single panoramic X-ray image to reconstruct the 3D volume of the oral cavity. The first stage uses a GAN-based architecture to project two-dimensional features into three-dimensional space and the second stage reconstructs 3D volume from the 2D input image. The model is evaluated using a real-time dataset and gives amazing results. Yoni Kasten et al. [38] developed a GAN-based deep neural network to reconstruct 3D volume out of a single two-dimensional X-ray image of synovial joints. The papers discussed in this category are summarized in Table 5.4 below.

TABLE 5.4
Summary of Papers in Category Three

Author	Contribution
Philipp Henzler et al. [31]	A model rooted on encoder-decoder with skip connections and a fusion step makes a single X-ray image into a three-dimensional volume.
Ryoya Shiode et al. [32]	GAN-based model to get the volume out of two-dimensional X-beam pictures which utilizes factual shape model (SSM) and CNN-based brain organization to remake 3D volume from two-dimensional X-beam pictures of bones.
Amirhossein Bayat et al. [33]	Reconstructed spine posture from two orthogonal-view X-ray images. The proposed architecture "Transvert" is based on an encoder-decoder deep CNN model.
Hangkee Kim et al. [34]	CNN model that uses bounding boxes to extract features and statistical shape model (SSM) parameters to fine-tune the model to restore leg bones from two-dimensional X-ray images.
Jana Cavojska et al. [12]	Deep neural network-based architecture to estimate the 3D shape of bones using a pair of two-dimensional X-ray images. Transfer learning and triplet loss function are used in combination with kNN classifiers to differentiate between bones.
Yifan Wang et al. [35]	DeepOrganNet, which reconstructs multiple 3D meshes. The model extracts features using smooth deformation fields and leverages latent descriptors which are extracted from X-ray images. MobileNet is used to reconstruct multiple view meshes of the organ.
Catherine Namayega et al. [36]	Using biplanar X-ray images, a deep CNN-based network can reconstruct the 3D volume of the scapula bone. The model, on the other hand, is hard to apply to real-time datasets.
Weinan Song et al. [37]	Formulated a two-stage deep CNN-based model that reconstructs the oral cavity's volume using a single panoramic X-ray image. The first stage projects two-dimensional features into 3D space using a GAN-based model, and the second stage reconstructs 3D volume from the 3D input image.
Yoni Kasten et al. [38]	Crafted a deep convolutional neural network to restore 3D volume from two orthogonal planar X-ray input images of knee and hip bones.

5.10 RESULTS ANALYSIS

In this section, we review the performance and results of some prominent deep learning models belonging to the three different categories of 3D CT reconstruction.

5.10.1 CATEGORY ONE: SINGLE X-RAY INPUT TO GENERATE VOLUMETRIC CT IMAGES

This category uses single X-ray input to generate multiple CT volumetric images. A representative concept diagram for understanding the operation of CT slice generation using a single X-ray input image is shown in Figure 5.5. One of the prominent methods in this category was proposed by Liyue Shen et al. [6]. In this work, a

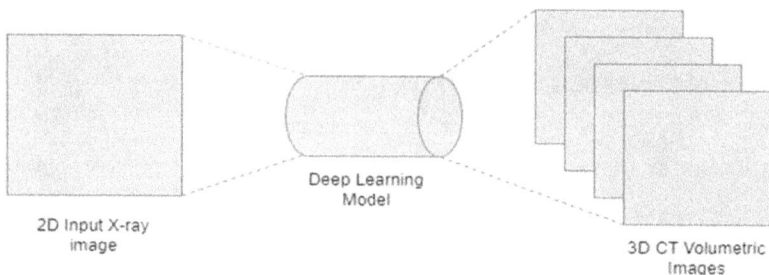

FIGURE 5.5 Concept diagram of single X-ray input to generate volumetric CT images.

hierarchical encoder-decoder-based network is used to create three-dimensional CT images using a solitary X-ray image [20]. There are three parts to the architecture: the generation network, transformation network, and representation network. The generation module generates the corresponding 3D CT images rooted in the features learned from the representation network, which extracts the important features from the given X-ray image. With convolution and deconvolution operations, the transformation network serves as a link between the generation network and the representation network, facilitating the mapping of two-dimensional features onto 3D features. The model is trained using a lung and abdominal dataset gathered from the patients of Stanford Hospital (not publicly available due to patient privacy). Due to the non-availability of CT and X-ray pairs for training the model, CT-DRR pairs are generated by the cone beam-based method [11]. Augmentation techniques like translation and rotation are applied to increase the dataset. The dataset contains 720 DRR for training and 120 DRR for validation. Six hundred unseen DRR are used for testing. Adam optimizer is used to adjust the network's parameters and minimize the loss function through backpropagation. Results of CT reconstruction for the lung with input two-dimensional X-ray and ground truth are shown in Figure 5.6. The predicted CT slice is nearly the same as the ground truth value and the difference between the ground truth and the prediction shows that predicted CT images are nearly the same as the ground truth CT image. Testing a single sample for 3D CT reconstruction took about 0.5 seconds.

Another prominent method in this category is by Zhiqiang Tan et al. [11], who developed a deep CNN-based architecture to reconstruct CT volumetric images using a solitary X-ray input image. An encoder-decoder framework serves as the foundation for the architecture, which includes a self-attention technique for adaptive optimization of features, a 3D branch generation module to generate the details of the features extracted, and multiscale feature fusion to enhance the precision of the CT reconstruction. The model is trained using the publicly available LIDC-IDRI dataset [6]. The LIDC-IDRI dataset contains 1024 chest CT images, which are processed to get two-dimensional X-ray-equivalent DRR images by digital reconstruction radiograph algorithm. The model is trained using the two-dimensional DRR images and 3D CT volumetric images. The trained model is evaluated on a testing dataset. The reconstructed volumetric image is very close to the ground truth image.

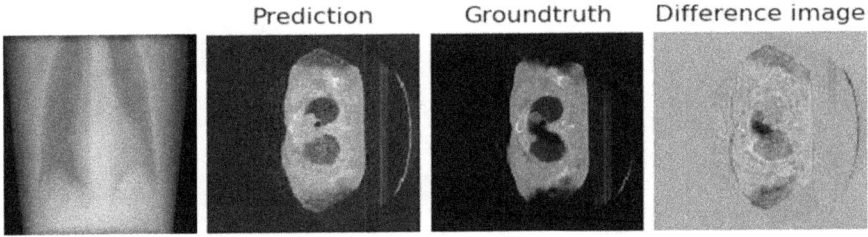

FIGURE 5.6   Shows (i) the input image, (ii) the predicted lung CT, (iii) ground truth CT, and (iv) the difference image.

The model is able to reconstruct the internal structure of the CT image clearly. The contours of the rib area are clearly visible and the internal organs in the middle are reconstructed well. The main reason for this is the adaptive learning rate and the self-attention mechanism which improved the overall reconstruction of the images. The augmentation techniques helped retain fine details from the reconstructed CT slices, like contours and edges.

Lastly, one more method proposed by Almeida et al. [13] is presented here. A solitary two-dimensional X-ray image is used as the input for a deep CNN-based encoder-decoder framework with skip connections for 3D CT reconstruction of the lower limbs. The network architecture is inspired by Henzler et al. The network converts two-dimensional features (128 × 128) gradually into a 3-dimensional (128 × 128 × 128) volume by using 3D convolution layers. The dataset consists of 344 lower limb CT scans. 230 CT scans were taken of male subjects, while 114 CT scans were taken of female subjects, with an average age of 65. On these CT scans, the digitally reconstructed radiograph (DRR) method is used to generate the corresponding two-dimensional X-rays [22]. The hold-out method is used to divide the dataset into 100 testing sets and 244 training sets. The Adam optimizer and a learning rate of 1e-4 are used to train the model for up to 1000 epochs.

The trained architecture is assessed on an unseen testing dataset. Reconstructed CT images of the hip crop are generated with the help of an actual CT image and a single-input image. The reconstructed CT image is nearly the same as the ground truth CT image. The contours of the reconstructed CT image are clearly visible and spacing between the bones is maintained properly. The soft tissues of the hip crop are estimated well, regardless of the fact that the dataset contains some CT images of older patients. But, the overall anatomical structure of the hip bone is reconstructed well.

5.10.2   CATEGORY TWO: MULTIPLE X-RAY INPUTS TO GENERATE VOLUMETRIC CT IMAGES

This category uses multiple input X-ray inputs to generate multiple CT volumetric images. A representative concept diagram for understanding the operation of CT slice generation using multiple X-ray input images is shown in Figure 5.7. In this

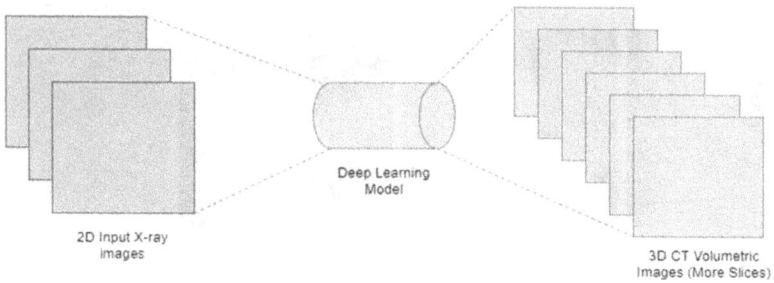

FIGURE 5.7 Concept diagram of multiple X-ray inputs to generate more volumetric CT images.

category, the first method we will discuss is proposed by Xingde Ying et al. [18]. The authors proposed a GAN framework that uses two orthogonal biplanar input images to reconstruct 3D CT volume [6, 11]. This was the first architecture which used two biplanar input images to reconstruct CT volumetric images. The architecture uses a generator consisting of three encoder-decoder modules. The two encoder-decoder modules, working in parallel, are used to process the two input images, i.e., anterior-posterior and lateral. The third encoder-decoder module is kept in between these two encoder-decoder frameworks to fuse the information from these two modules, which helps to reconstruct a better volumetric CT.

The network is trained using a standard procedure, in which discriminators and generators are trained separately. The network is learned using the Adam optimizer, with an initial learning rate of 2e-4 and a linear decrease in learning rate after 50 epochs. The network performs well after being trained to 100 epochs. The model was learned using the LIDC-IDRI dataset, which is accessible to the general public. 1018 chest CT scans are included in the dataset [6]. We use these CT scans and digitally reconstructed radiographs because the X-ray chest dataset with the corresponding CT volumes is unavailable. The network can be trained with these, and the CT volumes that correspond to them can be used as ground truth CT volumes. After preprocessing, 916 CT scans are chosen for the network's training and 102 CT scans can be used to test the network.

The results of the 3D CT reconstruction are generated with two orthogonal input X-ray images and the actual CT image. The results are nearly the same as the actual CT image. When using the method X2CT-GAN+B, where +B represents biplanar two-dimensional X-ray input images, results are good as compared to single X-ray input image method X2CT-GAN+S by four percents. This is due to the complementary features from the biplanar input image. The CT-reconstructed images produced by X2CT-GAN+B produce sharper boundaries covering finer details of the organ, as compared to the single-input X-ray model, which gives blurry outputs; images reconstructed from this method are not of good quality. The evaluation of the trained model is also done with real-world X-ray data. The results are significantly plausible.

The next method in this category is by Aminur et al. [19]. The author proposed a class-conditioned network that is used to restore CT volumes from two orthogonal

X-ray images. The author proposed three modules: deep feature transformation (DFT), which is used to modulate two-dimensional features spatially by affine transformation and heighten it along the third axis; adaptable feature fusion (AFF), which is used to remove the reconstruction problem from the unrestricted data; and depth aware connection (DAC), which is used to remove unnecessary features and bridges the 2D and 3D feature maps [13, 16]. The network is based on X2CT-GAN and contains two parallel encoder-decoder modules to process input biplanar X-ray images and a third module named fuse, which is in the middle of these two modules, to combine the information from both modules.

The network is trained on the publicly available LIDC-IDRI dataset. The LIDC-IDRI dataset contains 1024 chest CT images, which are processed to get two-dimensional X-ray-equivalent DRR images by digital reconstruction radiograph algorithm [6]. The model learns using the two-dimensional DRR images and 3D CT volumetric images. The model is trained with 916 images and remaining images are used for testing the model. The Adam optimizer is used to train the network for up to 100 epochs at a learning rate of 2e-3. The learning rate decreases by 30% after 50 epochs. The network is trained by using two different approaches: firstly, by incorporating pixel-wise and voxel-wise L1 loss known as CCX-rayNet, and, secondly based on a GAN known as CCX-rayGAN. The result of the proposed CCX-rayGAN+B, where B is used for biplanar input images, is compared with the state of the X2CTGAN+B, and from the results of the CCX-rayGAN+B we can conclude that the proposed results are far better than X2CTGAN+B, as the visual quality of the reconstructed CT images has improved dramatically.

5.10.3 CATEGORY THREE: SINGLE/MULTIPLE X-RAY INPUTS TO GENERATE 3D VOLUME

This category uses single/multiple X-ray inputs to generate CT volumes. A representative concept diagram for understanding the operation of 3D CT volume generation using a single/multiple X-ray input image is shown in Figure 5.8. In this category, the first method we will discuss is proposed by Philipp Henzler et al. [31]. The method known as single image tomography (SIT) is used to restore three-dimensional

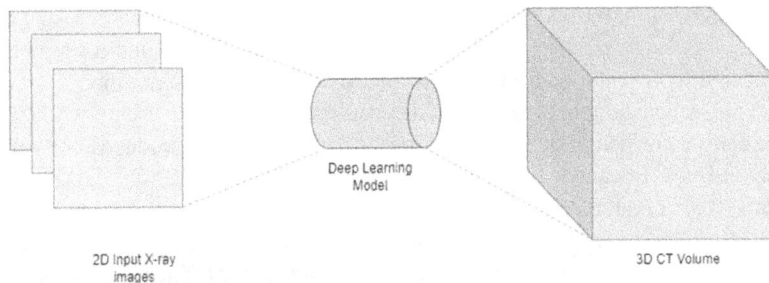

Deep Learning
Model

2D Input X-ray
images

3D CT Volume

FIGURE 5.8 Concept diagram of single/multiple X-ray inputs to generate CT volumes.

volumes from a solitary two-dimensional X-ray image. A deep CNN-based method for restoring three-dimensional CT volumes from a single X-ray image is described in this paper. The encoder-decoder framework is the foundation of the architecture. The data for the architecture is a single two-dimensional X-ray image with a size of 256×256 pixels and the output from the network is a three-dimensional volume comprising $128 \times 128 \times 128$ density volume of 3D CT scan. The encoder part extracts the feature information, reduces the resolution, and generates more complex features by decreasing the size vertically and increasing the channels, which leads to an increase in the size of the network horizontally. The decoder part (blue blocks) increases the resolution again without reducing the number of channels. This resolution is increased by using deconvolution or up-sampling. The skip interconnections are made from the encoder part of the network to the decoder part of the network which helps in passing fine details like edges from the two-dimensional image to the high-resolution 3D volume [20].

The training data for the network consists of half a million two-dimensional X-ray images of 175 distinct mammalian species. A great amount of two-dimensional X-ray images and their three-dimensional volumes are included in the dataset. The preparation of the organization is finished on four Nvidia Tesla K80 gas pedal cards, which decreases the preparation time to one day. As this is a regression problem, the loss function is L2-norm (Euclidean) loss [3, 24]. The evaluation of the network is done both on a validation dataset which comprises synthetic X-rays generated from 3D CT volumes and on real X-rays where ground truth images are not available. The outcome is obtained from a real X-ray image. From the outcomes, we can conclude that the model is able to restore the three-dimensional volume from the two-dimensional real unseen X-ray images effectively, although the ground truth CT volume is not available and the model is trained on artificial X-ray images. The output three-dimensional volume matches exactly with the actual volume and the model is able to generate the three-dimensional volume from the single two-dimensional X-ray input effectively.

The next method in this category is by Amirhossein Bayat et al. [33], who proposed a deep neural network-based architecture named Transvert, which reconstructs the 3D structure of spine posture by using two orthogonal input X-ray images. There are three blocks in the Transvert: a 3D decoder, a sagittal encoder, and a coronal encoder. A block called map&fuse brings these three blocks together. The map&fuse block is used to convert two-dimensional information from coronal and sagittal views into intermediate latent information in three dimensions. Using channel-wise consolidation, this latent information is then combined into a single three-dimensional representation and decoded into a 3D voxel representation.

Two publicly available lung nodule datasets are used to train the network: a lung nodule dataset consisting of 800 CT images that are utilized to produce DRR images, as well as 154 CT scans in a company dataset. The training dataset and the validation dataset are created by dividing the total dataset in half at a five-to-one ratio. The Hausdorff distance and Dice coefficient between the predicted and actual vertebral CT masks are used to evaluate the model's performance [25]. The proposed architecture for three-dimensional reconstructed shapes contains an encoder's self-attention layer and adversarial training-enhanced performance, emanating in a Dice value of 95.52% and a Hausdorff distance of less than 5.11 mm. By putting together the predicted three-dimensional vertebrae at their respective centroid locations, the spine's 3D volume can be restored.

Another method in this category is by Yoni Kasten et al. [38]. The authors proposed an end-to-end deep CNN-based method for reconstructing three-dimensional volumes of knee bones from two orthogonal two-dimensional X-ray images presented in this paper. The architecture is based on V-Net containing 3D convolution layers of filter size $(3 \times 3 \times 3)$ and encoding and decoding layers having skip connections between them. The last $(1 \times 1 \times 1)$ convolution layer outputs five channels representing five classes and a SoftMax layer after it. The classes zero to four represent the knee bones' anatomical partitioning. The network is trained with synthetic X-ray images generated from CT scans by using DRR technology and on both unsupervised and supervised losses. Adam enhancer with initial learning rate of 10^{-2} is used to train the network which is reduced after every 10th epoch by a factor of ten. The training and testing datasets consist of 18,810 and 20 scans respectively, generated by using augmentation by rotation [14].

The trained network is evaluated on 20 test images by Dice and Chamfer metrics. The Marching Cube algorithm is used to reconstruct 3D meshes from the predicted labels. The greater the value of Dice and the lower the merit of Chamfer, the better the results [39].

5.11 CONCLUSION

CT scanning uses X-rays, which are harmful to the body – especially for children and pregnant women – and exposure to these harmful rays can lead to deadly diseases like cancer [1]. Also, two-dimensional X-ray images cannot capture the volumetric view or detailed information of the body part scanned [2]. Earlier traditional and computational-based methods, like iterative and analytical methods, were used, but these approaches necessitate hundreds of projection views and a full rotational body scan, putting the patient at greater risk of radiation exposure. So, here, we have discussed deep learning-based methods which reconstruct CT volumetric images using single/multiple two-dimensional X-ray images and help diagnose the abnormalities present in the body using a volumetric view [1, 4, 6].

Starting with an introduction to CT scanning and an explanation of the block diagram of CT scanning, we then discussed the drawbacks of CT scanning and the motivation for this work. Traditional methods to reconstruct CT images are explained here briefly. But, due to the advancement in artificial intelligence, deep CNN-based methods are used nowadays to restore CT images from two-dimensional X-ray images [2, 4]. The deep learning methods are divided into three categories based on a survey of the literature. The experimentation work is performed using some papers from each of the three categories of deep learning-based procedures and the results of these methods show that deep learning-based procedures outperform traditional methods and give superior outcomes.

REFERENCE LIST

1. https://www.nibib.nih.gov/science-education/science-topics/computed-tomography-ct.
2. https://www.imagewisely.org/Imaging-Modalities/Computed-Tomography/Image-Reconstruction-Techniques.
3. https://medium.com/@draj0718/convolutional-neural-networks-cnn-architectures-explained-716fb197b243.
4. https://www.daenotes.com/electronics/industrial-electronics/ct-scanner.
5. https://www.tutorialspoint.com/python_deep_learning/python_deep_learning_deep_neural_networks.htm.
6. Shen, L., Zhao, W., & Xing, L. (2019). Patient-specific reconstruction of volumetric computed tomography images from a single projection view via deep learning. *Nature Biomedical Engineering*, 3(11), 880–888.
7. Aetesam, H., & Maji, S. K. (2021). Noise dependent training for deep parallel ensemble denoising in magnetic resonance images. *Biomedical Signal Processing and Control*, 66, 102405.
8. Aetesam, H., & Maji, S. K. (2022). Attention-based noise prior network for magnetic resonance image denoising. *IEEE International Symposium on Biomedical Imaging ISBI 2022*, Kolkata, India.
9. Maji, S. K., & Yahia, H. (2019). A feature based reconstruction model for fluorescence microscopy image denoising. *Scientific Reports*. Nature Publishing Group, 9(1), 7725.
10. Maji, S. K., & Boulanger, J. (2021). A variational model for Poisson Gaussian Joint denoising deconvolution. *IEEE International Symposium on Biomedical Imaging ISBI 2021*, Nice, France.
11. Tan, Z., Li, J., Tao, H., Li, S., & Hu, Y. (2022). XctNet: Reconstruction network of volumetric images from a single X-ray image. *Computerized Medical Imaging and Graphics*, 98, 102067.
12. Čavojská, J., Petrasch, J., Mattern, D., Lehmann, N. J., Voisard, A., & Böttcher, P. (2020). Estimating and abstracting the 3D structure of feline bones using neural networks on X-ray (2D) images. *Communications Biology*, 3(1), 1–13.
13. Almeida, D. F., Astudillo, P., & Vandermeulen, D. (2021). Three-dimensional image volumes from two-dimensional digitally reconstructed radiographs: A deep learning approach in lower limb CT scans. *Medical Physics*, 48(5), 2448–2457.
14. Loÿen, E., Dasnoy-Sumell, D., & Macq, B. (2022, October). 3DCT reconstruction from a single X-ray projection using convolutional neural network. In *2022 IEEE International Conference on Image Processing (ICIP)* (pp. 1111–1115). IEEE.
15. Jiang, L., Zhang, M., Wei, R., Liu, B., Bai, X., & Zhou, F. (2021, November). Reconstruction of 3D CT from A single X-ray projection view using CVAE-GAN. In *2021 IEEE International Conference on Medical Imaging Physics and Engineering (ICMIPE)* (pp. 1–6). IEEE.
16. Peng, C., Liao, H., Wong, G., Luo, J., Zhou, S. K., & Chellappa, R. (2021, May). Xraysyn: Realistic view synthesis from a single radiograph through CT priors. In *Proceedings of the AAAI Conference on Artificial Intelligence* (Vol. 35, No. 1, pp. 436–444).
17. Sidky, E. Y., & Pan, X. (2008). Image reconstruction in circular cone-beam computed tomography by constrained, total-variation minimization. *Physics in Medicine and Biology*, 53(17), 4777.
18. Ying, X., Guo, H., Ma, K., Wu, J., Weng, Z., & Zheng, Y. (2019). X2CT-GAN: Reconstructing CT from biplanar X-rays with generative adversarial networks. In: *Proceedings of the IEEE/CVF Conference on Computer Vision and Pattern Recognition* (pp. 10619–10628).

19. Ratul, M. A. R., Yuan, K., & Lee, W. (2021, April). CCX-rayNet: A class conditioned convolutional neural network for biplanar X-rays to CT volume. In: *2021 IEEE 18th International Symposium on Biomedical Imaging (ISBI)* (pp. 1655–1659). IEEE.

20. https://towardsdatascience.com/a-comprehensive-guide-to-convolutional-neural-networks-the-eli5-way-3bd2b1164a53.

21. Ge, R., He, Y., Xia, C., Xu, C., Sun, W., Yang, G., ... Zhu, Y. (2022). X-CTRSNet: 3D cervical vertebra CT reconstruction and segmentation directly from two-dimensional X-ray images. *Knowledge-Based Systems*, 236, 107680.

22. https://towardsdatascience.com/convolutional-neural-networks-explained-9cc5188c4939.

23. Shen, L., Zhao, W., Capaldi, D., Pauly, J., & Xing, L. (2022). A geometry-informed deep learning framework for ultra-sparse 3D tomographic image reconstruction. *Computers in Biology and Medicine*, 148, 105710.

24. ShamanthHampali. (2021). 3D shape reconstruction of knee bones from low radiation X-ray images using deep learning. UWSpace.

25. Yu, J., Liang, H., & Sun, Y. (2022, October). Deep learning single view computed tomography guided by FBP algorithm. In *2022 12th International Conference on Information Science and Technology (ICIST)* (pp. 237–247). IEEE.

26. Shibata, H., Hanaoka, S., Nomura, Y., Nakao, T., Takenaga, T., Hayashi, N., & Abe, O. (2021). X2CT-FLOW: Maximum a posteriori reconstruction using a progressive flow-based deep generative model for ultra-sparse-view computed tomography in ultra-low-dose protocols. arXiv Preprint ArXiv:2104.04179.

27. Shen, L., Zhao, W., Capaldi, D., Pauly, J., & Xing, L. (2022). A geometry-informed deep learning framework for ultra-sparse 3D tomographic image reconstruction. *Computers in Biology and Medicine*, 148, 105710.

28. Ge, R., He, Y., Xia, C., Xu, C., Sun, W., Yang, G., ... Zhu, Y. (2022). X-CTRSNet: 3D cervical vertebra CT reconstruction and segmentation directly from two-dimensional X-ray images. *Knowledge-Based Systems*, 236, 107680.

29. Afshar, P., Shahroudnejad, A., Mohammadi, A., & Plataniotis, K. N. (2018, October). CARISI: Convolutional autoencoder-based inter-slice interpolation of brain tumor volumetric images. In: *2018 25th IEEE International Conference on Image Processing (ICIP)* (pp. 1458–1462). IEEE.

30. Santarelli, C., Argenti, F., Uccheddu, F., Alparone, L., & Carfagni, M. (2020). Volumetric interpolation of tomographic sequences for accurate 3D reconstruction of anatomical parts. *Computer Methods and Programs in Biomedicine*, 194, 105525.

31. Henzler, P., Rasche, V., Ropinski, T., & Ritschel, T. (2018, May). Single-image tomography: 3D volumes from two-dimensionalcranial X-rays. In *Computer Graphics Forum* (Vol. 37, No. 2, pp. 377–388).

32. Shiode, R., Kabashima, M., Hiasa, Y., Oka, K., Murase, T., Sato, Y., & Otake, Y. (2021). 2D–3D reconstruction of distal forearm bone from actual X-ray images of the wrist using convolutional neural networks. *Scientific Reports*, 11(1), 1–12.

33. Bayat, A., Sekuboyina, A., Paetzold, J. C., Payer, C., Stern, D., Urschler, M., ... Menze, B. H. (2020, October). Inferring the 3D standing spine posture from two-dimensionalradiographs. In *International Conference on Medical Image Computing and Computer-Assisted Intervention* (pp. 775–784). Springer.

34. Wu, D., Kim, K., El Fakhri, G., & Li, Q. (2017). Iterative low-dose CT reconstruction with priors trained by artificial neural network. *IEEE Transactions on Medical Imaging*, 36(12), 2479–2486.

35. Wang, Y., Zhong, Z., & Hua, J. (2019). DeepOrganNet: On-the-fly reconstruction and visualization of 3D/4D lung models from single-view projections by deep deformation network. *IEEE Transactions on Visualization and Computer Graphics*, 26(1), 960–970.

36. Namayega, C., Malila, B., Douglas, T. S., & Mutsvangwa, T. E. (2020, October). Contour detection in synthetic bi-planar X-ray images of the scapula: Towards improved 3D reconstruction using deep learning. In *2020 20th International Conference on Bioinformatics and Bioengineering (BIBE)* (pp. 303–307). IEEE.

37. Song, W., Liang, Y., Yang, J., Wang, K., & He, L. (2021, May). Oral-3D: Reconstructing the 3D structure of oral cavity from panoramic X-ray. In *Proceedings of the AAAI Conference on Artificial Intelligence* (Vol. 35, No. 1, pp. 566–573).

38. Kasten, Y., Doktofsky, D., & Kovler, I. (2020). End-to-end convolutional neural network for 3D reconstruction of knee bones from bi-planar X-ray images. In *Machine Learning for Medical Image Reconstruction: Third International Workshop, MLMIR 2020, Held in Conjunction with MICCAI 2020, Lima, Peru, October 8, 2020, Proceedings 3* (pp. 123–133). Springer International Publishing.

39. Sohan, K., & Yousuf, M. A. (2020, November). 3D bone shape reconstruction from two-dimensional X-ray images using MED generative adversarial network. In *2020 2nd International Conference on Advanced Information and Communication Technology (ICAICT)* (pp. 53–58). IEEE.

6 GAN-Based Encoder-Decoder Model for Multi-Label Diagnostic Scan Classification and Automated Radiology Report Generation

Rahul Kumar, K. Karthik, and S. Sowmya Kamath

6.1 INTRODUCTION

Radiologists analyze diagnostic medical images of patients on a daily basis to arrive at a diagnosis. However, the process of such analysis, interpretation, and creation of textual diagnostic reports for each scan demands skills such as extensive knowledge of anatomy, visual symptoms that manifest the disease-specific interpretation, and knowledge of correlation with other diagnostic results like pathology, etc. Creation of diagnostic reports is a challenging process even for experienced radiologists, often exacerbated by the cognitive exhaustion introduced due to repetitive manual analysis of hundreds of different radiology images each day. It has been reported that the average diagnostic error is in the range of three to five percent, which translates to more than 40 million annual global instances that have a significant adverse impact on patient well-being [1]. Genuine factors that may cause such inevitable lapses typically include an acute shortage of trained radiology staff, a large volume of diagnostic scans performed on a daily basis in busy hospital scenarios, the need for fast analysis, cognitive biases, and human exhaustion, to name a few [2].

Making computers automatically understand the contextual content in an image and offer a reasonable description in natural language is now a task of critical importance, due to the enormous volume of the data available, further compounded by its streaming nature. In clinical practice, medical specialists and researchers usually write diagnosis reports to record microscopic findings from images, so automatic captioning on medical images will benefit healthcare providers with valuable insights and reduce their burden across the overall clinical workflow. The medical

DOI: 10.1201/9781003363361-6

image captioning challenge [3] aims to advance methodological development in mapping visual information from medical images to condensed textual descriptions. The captioning task can be seen as a part of the medical image classification task [4, 5], and can be a significant addition to healthcare information management systems (HIMS) software.

Image processing and computer vision- (CV-) based techniques have been applied to design applications for surgical and imaging interventions. Such systems extend clinical decision-making capabilities for healthcare professionals by automating certain tasks related to diagnosis, or by forecasting the severity of several abnormalities and radiology reports [6, 7]. Incorporating artificial intelligence (AI) in these systems to support learning behaviour is of critical importance so that systems can detect abnormalities at the earliest disease onset in a wide variety of diagnostic media, like radiology, computed tomography (CT) scans, magnetic resonance imaging (MRI), etc. The radiologist can utilize these insights to enable and optimize the quality of diagnosis.

Medical reporting procedures for radiology images include the radiologist scanning the target body part of the patient and noting various findings and observations evident through the scan. Sometimes, related or unrelated findings about other body parts can be observed in a single image. Those findings and other observations then lead to a further consolidated overall diagnostic report about the patient, which is known as the impression. The scan images are also assigned proper tags for future categorization and recording purposes. Automated multi-label scan classification is seen as a potential solution for managing diagnostic scans and addressing problems such as scan image analysis, disease detection, and more. Image captioning concepts can address the combined problem of identifying the primary content and objects of a given image and generating natural language descriptions based on the content and objects present, the relationship between objects, and the context of other secondary objects in the image. Hence, a text description (a caption for a given image) is required to qualify the syntactical and semantic requirements of the targeted language.

Learning image feature representations can provide a base for the description generation task, and can also be a bottleneck, due to the very limited availability of datasets in the case of medical images. A generative adversarial network (GAN) combines two networks training together in an adversarial setup, with complementary goals. The generator part of the GAN-multi label classification (MLC) model generates new images from noisy samples, trying to fool the discriminator, which is training to classify given images as real images from the dataset or fake images generated by the generator part of the same model. This adversarial training results in the discriminator learning better feature representation of given images, getting better at classifying real vs. fake images, while the generator gets closer to generating real-looking images which were never present in the dataset. In this work, we adapt GANs to enable better feature learning in an adversarial training setup, thus improving classification for various diseases and tag prediction for description generation for diagnostic scans.

The main contribution here is the introduction of GANs that are adapted to improve feature learning performance in an adversarial training setup, for the task of multi-disease classification. The image representation and encoding approaches are based on convolutional neural networks (CNN)-MLC and tag prediction for description generation, experimentally validated and benchmarked on a standard dataset. The suggested approach can be deployed as a support system for pathologists in a faster analysis of X-Ray images for efficient diagnosis. The rest of this chapter is organized as follows: Section 6.2 discusses existing works in the area of interest. In Section 6.3, we present the specifics of the proposed method for medical image description using GANs. The implementation details and experimental results are presented in Section 6.4, followed by a conclusion with a discussion of future work.

6.2 RELATED WORK

Recent works in the area of computer vision that explore novel approaches for modelling images have significantly contributed to advancements in the area of image classification. The success of long short-term memory (LSTMs) for the natural language translation task enables ways to improve CNN- and recurrent neural network (RNN)-based image captioning solutions. Transfer learning techniques enable models pre-trained on huge datasets to be leveraged and subsequently adapted for domain-specific tasks. Inspired by inter-language translation models, Vinyals et al. [8] proposed a show-and-tell image captioning model. The proposed approach is an encoder-decoder-based model with a CNN-based encoder and an RNN-based decoder, utilizing the CNN model's ability to represent features of an image in a fixed-length vector. Prior to this approach, many researchers addressed the image captioning problem by co-embedding images with text in the same vector space and ranking and retrieving the closest description to the query image [9–11]. Karpathy et al. [12] used neural networks to co-embed given images and descriptions in the same vector space. However, the limited quality of the generated natural language description remained unaddressed in these approaches.

Detecting abnormalities and visual symptoms of various diseases from diagnostic images is a well-researched problem typically viewed as a binary or multi-label classification problem. When addressed as a multi-class classification, different combinations of labels are taken as an individual class and X-rays are classified against a combination of tags occurring in the dataset. This approach, while it provides a robust solution for combinations occurring in the dataset, fails with unseen combinations, which often occur in the case of real-life applications. Moreover, classic training approaches suffer from limitations caused by the scarcity of datasets. Basic GANs are focused on generating new data and have been successfully extended to generate novel images of faces and style transfer techniques in many recent works [13, 14]. Yu et al. [13] proposed deep convolutional generative adversarial network (DCGAN) with many improvisation techniques for training GANs and learned feature representation in the discriminator part were further used for the classification task.

CatGAN [15] utilizes the available ground truth along with images in discriminator training as a K-class classifier, while ensuring an equal distribution across all

K-classes in generated images. Odena et al. [16] presented a K+1 class discriminator for training GANs for image generation as well as multi-class image classification. Salehinejad et al. [17] presented an approach to overcome an imbalanced dataset with an over-representation of common medical problems and a paucity of data from rare conditions using GANs to generate novel images, which were later used to improvise deep convolutional neural networks (DCNN)-based classifiers for five diseases.

Li et al. [18] proposed the Knowledge-driven Encode, Retrieve, Paraphrase (KERP) model for knowledge-based and information retrieval-oriented medical report generation. They used graph learning and natural language modelling to align visual observations with available medical domain knowledge. Yuan et al. [19] encoded multi-view visual features into sentence representations using sentence-level attention mechanisms to enable report generation for lung X-ray images. Chen et al. [20] devised a memory-driven transformer architecture to record crucial information related to the visual aspects of the image. Endo et al. [21] proposed an information retrieval-based language generation model to generate free text clinical reports, using self-supervised contrastive learning. They reported more accuracy in reports and better generalization with their model. A multi-task learning framework for the prediction of tags and the generation of reports was proposed by Jing et al. [22], who incorporated CNNs with LSTM. The model is capable of not only generating high-level impressions, but also generating detailed descriptive findings. Xue et al. [23] used a text-image embedding network integrated with multi-level attention models in an end-to-end CNN-RNN architecture for learning distinctive image and text representations [24]. These models have shown promising results so far. PadChest by [25] is an initiative that involved trained physicians manually annotating 27% of the Unified Medical Language System Concept Unique Identifiers (UMLS-CUI) dataset samples. They then used an RNN attention method to label the remaining images and proposed a hierarchical taxonomy to categorize radiographic findings.

Based on a detailed review of existing works, certain crucial observations were made. Most works used a pre-trained multi-class classifier as a feature extractor, where the neural network was not trained with a wide variety of images to learn the features. It was also observed that multi-class objective K+1 classes (K for real images, plus one for fake) were used for image generation, while the max pooling layer can cause spatial information loss. A separate classifier was used for each clinical task (such as multi-label classification and report generation), instead of designing an end-to-end framework. A summary of a few key existing works is tabulated in Table 6.1. Recent works in the area of computer vision that explore novel approaches for modelling images have significantly contributed to advancement in the area of image classification. The recent success of LSTMs for natural language translation tasks enables the exploration of novel ways to improve CNN-RNN-based image captioning tasks. Transfer learning techniques can be adopted to leverage models pre-trained over huge datasets, while generative adversarial networks are being explored for a variety of tasks such as dataset augmentation to improve neural model training performance.

TABLE 6.1
Summary of Key Existing Works

Authors	Method	Advantages	Limitations
Vinyals et al. [8]	Generating captions for images using LSTM and CNN	End-to-end trainable framework	Uses pre-trained multi-class classifier as feature extractor
Springenberg et al. [15]	Unsupervised and semi-supervised learning with GANs	Multi-class classifier as GAN-discriminator	Multi-class objective K-classes image generation oriented
Odena et al. [16]	Semi-supervised learning with GAN	Multi-class classifier as GAN -Discriminator	Multi-class objective K+1 classes (K real + 1 fake)
Yu et al. [13]	GAN using all deep convolution net without pooling	stable to train, discriminator can serve as classifier	Used for image generation
Salehinejad et al. [17]	Dataset enhancement using GANs to model new X-rays	New generated images improves classifier efficiency	Separate Classifier No end-to-end framework

6.3 PROPOSED APPROACH

The proposed approach is a GAN-based multi-label classifier (GAN-MLC), which is depicted in Figure 6.1. In GAN-MLC, the generator has the same goal as in a basic GAN, i.e., to learn to generate images that fool the discriminator into classifying an image as real, but for the discriminator, the objective to classify images as real or fake differs in terms of how real and fake are implicitly defined. In standard GANs, the discriminator is not restricted in how it learns to discriminate between real and fake. The discriminator is only required to detect features present in a real image but yet not modelled by the generator model, at least not correctly. In GAN-MLC, the overall loss is the summation of discriminator loss over real images and images generated by generator. In the case of the NIH Chest X-Ray Dataset [26], 14 distinct labels are provided. Images from the real dataset along with corresponding labels are used to train the network, whereas images generated by network G are supplied to discriminator D with labels showing no relation to classes from the dataset. Thus, class labels supplied with images are used to translate the "real" and "fake" information about the images. This translation removes the necessity to provide real/fake information separately and enables the discriminator to be trained to classify images against real and fake, and against underlying classes.

Algorithm 1 illustrates the training process of the GAN-MLC model. During the training process, both the discriminator and the generator are trained jointly in an

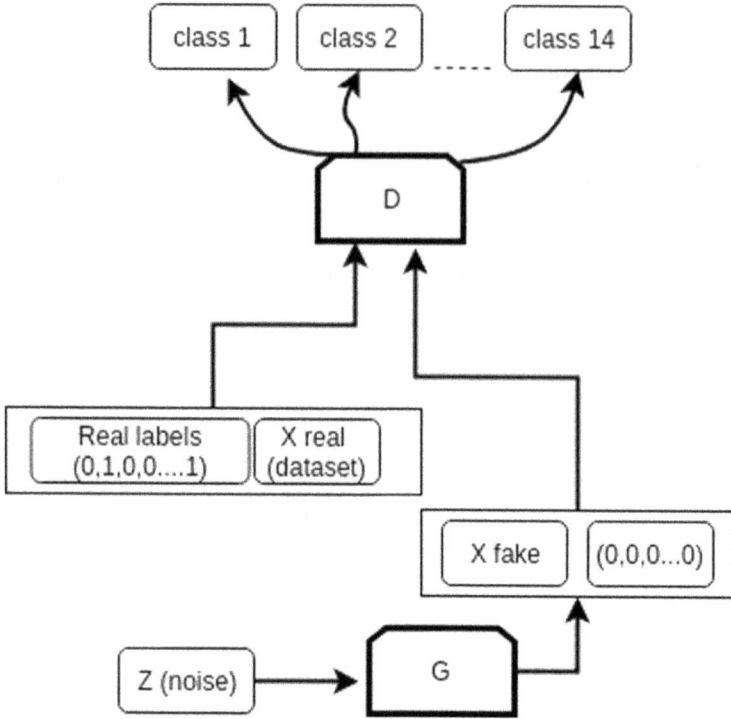

FIGURE 6.1 GAN-MLC framework

alternative manner using gradient descent. First, the generator generates a batch of images, then, the parameters of model G are fixed while a single iteration of gradient descent is performed on discriminator D and the gradient is propagated back through the discriminator. Next, model D's parameters are fixed, and the generator is trained for a single iteration of gradient descent. The generator begins with a noise input (z) with normal distribution and learns to map to G(z, θ_g) with objective function to achieve the highest D(G(z, θ_g)), given by Equation 6.1, where D learns to map input X to binary vector Y representing the label associated with the image, predicting the probability of given example X belonging to each of the classes with objective function. The overall objective function for GAN-MLC, also known as a min-max game with zero-sum, where the generator tries to minimize V and the discriminator tries to maximize it, is given as:

$$\min_{G} \max_{D} V(D,G) = E_{X \sim P_{data}(x)}\left[\log D(x)\right] + E_{z \sim P_Z}(z)\left[\log(1 - D(G(z)))\right]$$

(6.1)

$$\min_{G} V(G) = E_{z \sim P_Z(z)}\left[\log(1 - D(G(z)))\right].$$

(6.2)

$$\max_{D} V(D) = E_{X \sim P_{data}(x)} \left[\log D(x) \right] + E_{z \sim P_z}(z) \left[\log(1 - D(G(z))) \right] \quad (6.3)$$

To keep the GAN-MLC stable while training, many techniques are used, including replacing deterministic spatial pooling function layers and using strided convolution layers in the discriminator to make it learn the spatial downsampling function while training. Also in the generator, fractional-strided convolution layers are used to enable learning on the upsampling function. Batch normalization is used for the input to all intermediate layers to have zero means and unit variance, except for the last layer of the generator and the input layer of the discriminator.

ALGORITHM 1: GAN-MLC TRAINING PROCESS

1. for each iteration do
2. Generator draw M noise samples $\{(z^1, y_g), ..., (z^M, y_g)\}$ from noise prior $p_g(z)$, where

   $y_g = [0_1, ..., 0_{classes}]$;
3. Draw m examples $\{(x^1, y^1), ..., (x^m, y^m)\}$ from data generating distribution P_d (x);
4. Perform gradient descent on the parameters of D with regard to the negative likelihood of D on minibatch;
5. Generator draw M noise samples $\{(z^1, y_g), ..., (z^M, y_g)\}$ from noise prior $p_g(z)$, where

   $y_g = [0_1, ..., 0_{classes}]$;
6. Perform gradient descent on the parameters of G with regard to the negative likelihood of G on minibatch of noise sample;

6.3.1 Diagnostic Report Generation

The description generation model consists of a CNN followed by an RNN model, modelled as an encoder and decoder network. While training, the overall goal is to maximize the likelihood of labels provided with training-embedded images. LSTM layers further take a sequence of encoded inputs and learn to decode them to sequence one word after another. Figure 6.2 depicts the architecture designed for generating the descriptions for the X-ray images.

The overall objective for the description generator is given by Equation 6.4, to maximize the probability of correct description, where I is an encoded image and S is the target description sentence. Since S is a sentence, a sequence of maximum length N will be expanded to $S_0, S_1, ... S_{N-1}$, and the objective function is given, as shown in Equation 6.5.

$$\theta^* = \arg\max_{\theta} \sum \log p(S|I, \theta) \quad (6.4)$$

$$\log p(S \mid I, ,) = \sum_{T=0}^{N} \log p(S_T \mid I, S_0, S_1, ... S_T - 1) \quad (6.5)$$

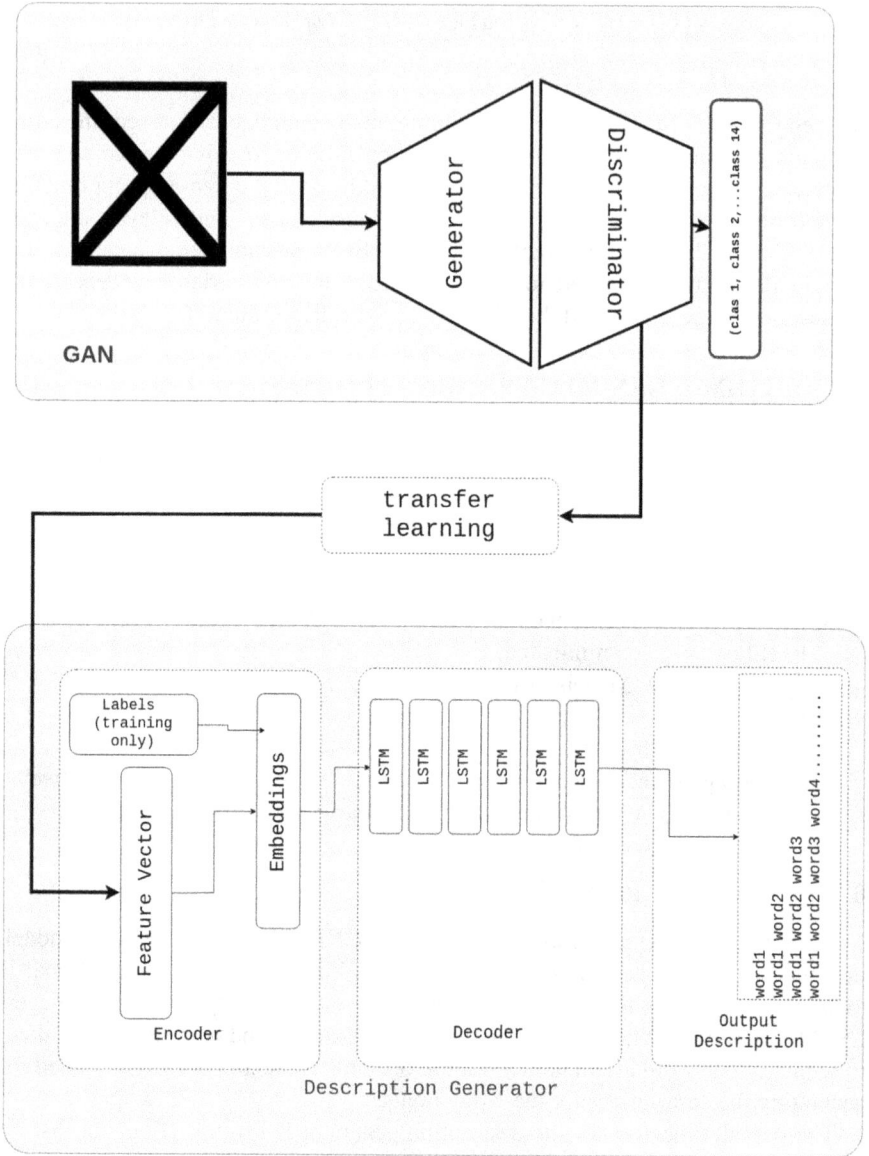

FIGURE 6.2 Description of generation architecture

In recurrent neural networks, variable length sequence is predicted until the previous state (T − 1) can be remembered by a fixed size cell state (h_{T-1}), which makes RNNs a natural choice for sequence modelling. In the description generation task, during training, the encoder network takes an input image, extracts features from the image, and combines them with the description encoded using word embedding learned over the whole vocabulary. Transfer learning is used to encode the given image in the feature vector, using the saved discriminator model form GAN-MLC after removing the classifier (fully connected) layers. The output of the last convolution layers in the GAN-MLC discriminator is a representation of the input image in a fixed-length vector. The description available for training images is processed into a vocabulary, a set of all unique tokens after removing stop words. As an input to the decoder, every token is represented by one hot encoding of the length of the vocabulary size. This can be further optimized by learning embedding for the given vocabulary and then using the embedding size vector to represent an input/output token. The decoder takes the output of the encoder and predicts the description for the given input image. For a given batch of images, features extracted by the encoder are combined with the sequence generated using the description for the batch. The decoder is an LSTM-based recurrent neural network, which takes image features and previously predicted words as inputs and predicts the next word for the sentence. Words in the ground truth description are encoded as an embedding of length 256, while the feature extractor output image is encoded as a vector of length 1024. Input at stage T, after already predicting T_1 words, is computed as per Equation 6.6, where I is the image encoded as a feature vector by the encoder.

$$X_T = (I \| X_1, X_2, \ldots X_{T-1}) \qquad (6.6)$$

Generator G is a seven-layer model with an input shape (batch size, 100), which is upsampled to an output shape (224, 224, 1) using transpose convolutions implemented using the Conv2DTranspose layer from Keras layers. The BatchNormalization layer is stacked after all Conv2DTranspose layers except the output layers of G, to ensure input to each layer has zero mean and unit variance, where the activation function used for generator G is rectified linear unit (ReLU). Reshape, BatchNormalization, and ReLU [27] are implemented using Keras layers as well. Figure 6.3 shows the layered architecture of the generator model. As shown in Figure 6.4, the discriminator model was implemented as six convolutional layers stacked with two fully connected layers. For spatial downsampling, strided convolution was used with a stride of two. Batch normalization is used for all convolution layers except the input layer, along with a dropout layer with a dropout of 0.3 on top of LeakyReLU as the activation function for all convolution layers with an alpha of 0.2. Filter size is 5×5 for all convolutional layer (CN) layers. The feature extractor part takes an input image of dimensions (224, 224, 1) and outputs a feature vector of dimension 1026. The classifier layers consist of two fully connected layers with a sigmoid activation function with 14 outputs for probabilities for different labels. LeakyReLU, Conc2D, BatchNormalization, Dropout, Flatten, and Dense classes from Keras were used to implement this model. The image encoder is implemented using a saved multi-label classifier taking an input image of dimension (224, 224, 1), while the output is collected from the last convolution layers and stacked with an embedding layer, giving an embedding vector of a length of 256, followed by a dropout layer. This input

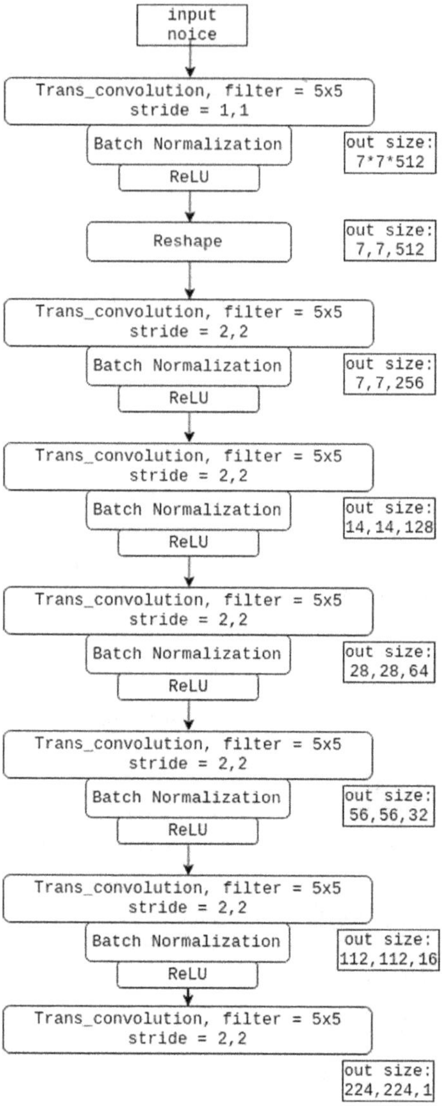

FIGURE 6.3 Generator model architecture

feature vector is then combined with word embedding and fed into two LSTM layers with 256 cells each. A CUDA deep neural network long short-term memory (CuDNNLSTM) layer was used to implement LSTM layers instead of standard LSTM layers because it takes less time when trained with Compute Unified Device Architecture (CUDA)-enabled GPU. The various experiments undertaken and the observed results are elaborated in Section 6.4.

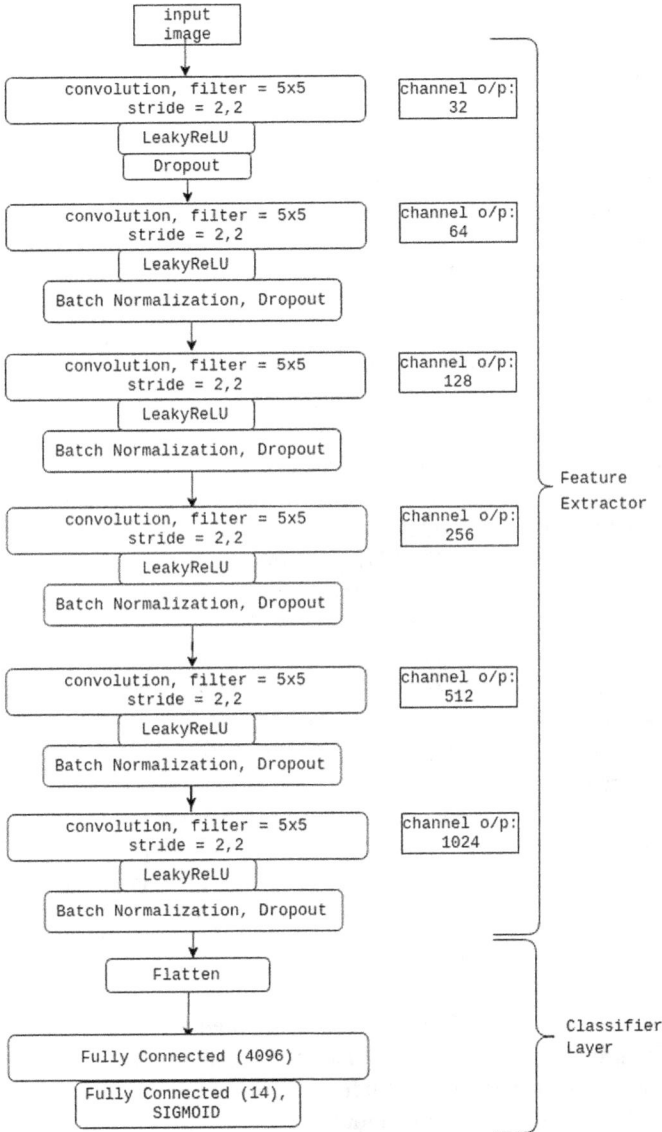

input
image

convolution, filter = 5x5
stride = 2,2

channel o/p:
32

LeakyReLU

Dropout

convolution, filter = 5x5
stride = 2,2

channel o/p:
64

LeakyReLU

Batch Normalization, Dropout

convolution, filter = 5x5
stride = 2,2

channel o/p:
128

LeakyReLU

Batch Normalization, Dropout

convolution, filter = 5x5
stride = 2,2

channel o/p:
256

LeakyReLU

Batch Normalization, Dropout

Feature
Extractor

convolution, filter = 5x5
stride = 2,2

channel o/p:
512

LeakyReLU

Batch Normalization, Dropout

convolution, filter = 5x5
stride = 2,2

channel o/p:
1024

LeakyReLU

Batch Normalization, Dropout

Flatten

Classifier
Layer

Fully Connected (4096)

Fully Connected (14),
SIGMOID

FIGURE 6.4 Discriminator model architecture

6.4 EXPERIMENTAL EVALUATION AND RESULTS

For experimental validation of the proposed model, we used two different datasets: the NIH Chest X-rays dataset and the IU X-rays dataset. The NIH Chest X-rays dataset contained 11,2000 images with a dimension of 1024 × 1024 pixels. For training GAN-MLC and CNN-MLC, 60,241 images tagged with the label "No Findings" were removed, and the resulting dataset was resized to 224 × 224 pixels, with only a single channel to reduce computation resource consumption without losing too much resolution. The training set contained 50,048 images, while the validation set contained 1711 images belonging to 14 classes. Input images were also normalized to have pixel values between negative one and one, before being fed to the GAN-MLC model. Both G and D were trained using the Adam optimizer with a learning rate of 1e-5 and a momentum term of 0.5 for 80 epochs. G was trained twice in an epoch. All the models were implemented in Keras using Tensorflow as a backend.

For the description generator, the IU X-ray dataset was used for 7470 images along with their descriptions. Images were resized to 224 × 224 pixels with a single channel. The MLC-GAN discriminator and CNN-MLC pre-trained on the NIH Chest X-rays dataset were used for feature extraction. To further save computational resources, features extracted once were saved and reused to compare models. Description data was pre-processed by converting all the tokens to lowercase and a vocabulary of 2057 unique words was created by removing non-alphanumeric characters. For the decoder network, the Adam optimizer was used with a learning rate of 0.000001 with a decay of 0.0000001. Standard evaluation metrics like Bilingual Evaluation Understudy Score (BLEU) [28] and Area Under Receiver Operating Characteristic Curve (AUC) were used for evaluating the performance. AUC is used to evaluate multi-label classification models by degree of separability. How well a classifier can differentiate between classes is measured on a scale of zero to one; in this work, the objective is to classify X-rays for the presence or absence of disease. BLEU is used to evaluate the generated description sentences by comparing them to the reference descriptions and to evaluate the multi-label classification model by degree of separability. BLEU checks the similarity between a candidate report and a set of reference reports and returns a score computed as per Equation 6.7, where C(i) is the number of tuples in the candidate report. In our work, if C equals "no acute cardiopulmonary abnormality", then C(1) = 4, C(2) = 3, ... and C(4) = 1.

$$BLEU-(i) = \frac{Matched(i)}{C(i)} \tag{6.7}$$

The GAN-MLC is trained on 51,750 images distributed in a batch size of 128 images per batch from the NIH Chest X-Rays dataset. Due to an imbalance in the number of images per class, images with no findings were removed to train the GAN-MLC. Further experimentation on resizing input X-ray images from a dimension of 128 × 128 to 224 × 224 resulted in generated improved images in less time on the above-mentioned architecture. The resulting images generated at different epochs to the final epoch are shown in Figures 6.5 and 6.6.

The summary of observed results obtained for different models experimented with for the task of multi-label disease classification is shown in Table 6.2. It is clear that the VGG-19 model pre-trained on ImageNet images achieved the best AUC values when compared to other models. For a textual description of the reports, the proposed GAN-MLC showed improvement over the standalone model trained on the same dataset, the results of which are shown in Table 6.3.

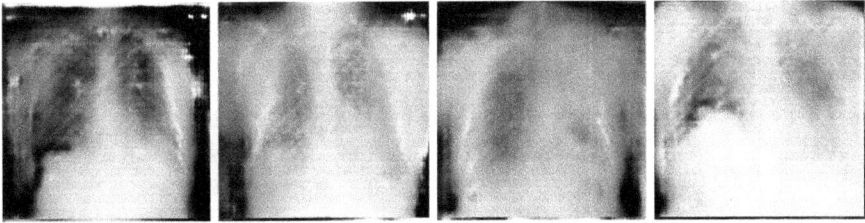

FIGURE 6.5 Generated images – sixth epoch, GAN-MLC, six-layer generator with an input image size of 128 × 128

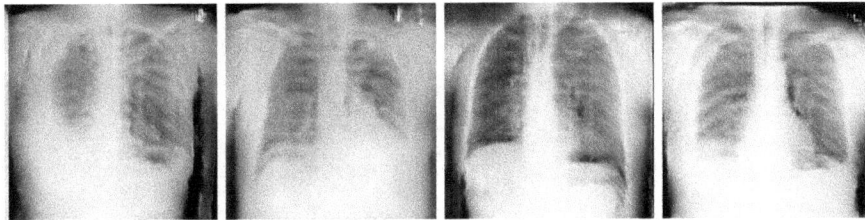

FIGURE 6.6 Generated images – 43rd epoch, GAN-MLC, six-layer generator with an input image size of 128 × 128

TABLE 6.2
Summary of Multi-label Classification Results

Methods	Architecture	AUC (in %)
Standalone CNNs model6l	6l-BN-relu, strided-conv	72
GAN-MLC-model6l as discriminator	6l-BN-relu, strided-conv	78
VGG-19, standalone	Pre-trained on Imagenet	83
GAN-MLC, VGG-19 as discriminator	6l-BN-relu, strided-conv	61 (unstable GAN)

To compute the BLEU score, each report in the training dataset is considered and the report given by the DL model for each image under test is taken as a source of perspective. The quantity of distinctly unique sentences produced for each of the test-set images is determined independently. References are then assessed on each of the different candidate sets. Finally, the model that achieved the highest BLEU-4 score is noted, and the results are tabulated in Table 6.3. Overall, when the training results were observed, the pre-trained VGG-19 model when trained in a GAN setup showed no improvement for convolution layers that were frozen to preserve learning. Also, VGG uses max pooling as a sub-sampling technique, which results in an unstable GAN while training.

TABLE 6.3

Summary of Description Generation Results

Encoder	BLEU1	BLEU2	BLEU3	BLEU4
CNN model standalone	0.126	0.0917	0.0803	0.056
VGG-19 standalone	0.202	0.134	0.097	0.079
GAN-MLC model	0.247	0.178	0.134	0.092

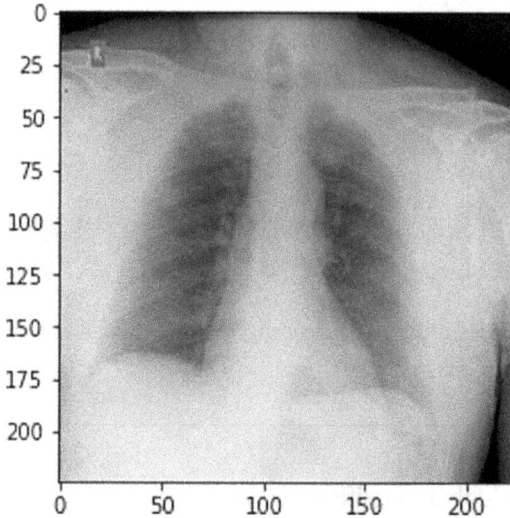

FIGURE 6.7 Test X-ray image for which the description generated is "no acute cardio-pulmonary abnormality the lungs are clear bilaterally specifically no evidence of focal consolidation pneumothorax or pleural effusion cardio mediastinal silhouette is unremarkable visualized osseous structures of the thorax are without acute abnormality"

6.5   CONCLUSION AND FUTURE WORK

In this chapter, an adversarial training approach is developed to train a multi-label classifier with generative networks in an adversarial manner. CNN models with multi-label classification as an objective are trained on the NIH Chest X-ray dataset with and without a generative network training in an adversarial setup trying to generate new X-rays. Both training approaches were further tested by using MLC as a feature extractor in a CNN-RNN description generator framework. In terms of multi-label classification (tag generation), CNN-based MLC when training with an adversarial G learns better with an AUC improvement of six percent compared to CNN-based MLC trained in a standard (standalone) manner. Furthermore, CNN-LSTM description generators also show improvement when GAN-MLC is used to encode images into a feature vector, as compared to a standard CNN-MLC as a feature extractor. A pre-trained VGG-16 model that uses max pooling as a spatial dimensional sub-sampling technique was employed, which results in an unstable GAN when using VGG-16 as a discriminator in GAN. Further optimization techniques are required to train a GAN with a pre-trained model as the discriminator. For description generation, an attention mechanism can be applied to further improve generated description relevance. A generative network training in adversarial setup along with a multi-label classifier improves classification accuracy as well as reduces chances of classifier overfitting while training on restricted datasets, by generating new images and directly tuning feature modelling while training. Another way to improve the framework is to use GANs with self-attention capabilities and transfer learning.

FUNDING DETAILS

This work was carried out with the authors' research interest and was not supported by any funding agency.

DISCLOSURE STATEMENT

The authors report there are no competing interests to declare.

DATA AVAILABILITY STATEMENT (DAS)

The datasets that were used and analyzed as part of the current study are openly and publicly available at the following: Indiana Dataset - https://www.kaggle.com/raddar/chest-xrays-indiana-university

REFERENCES

1. J. N. Itri, R. R. Tappouni, R. O. McEachern, A. J. Pesch, and S. H. Patel, "Fundamentals of diagnostic error in imaging," *Radiographics*, vol. 38, no. 6, 2018, pp. 1845–1865.
2. National Quality Forum, *Improving diagnostic quality and safety*. National Quality Forum, Washington, DC, 2017.
3. A. G. S. de Herrera, C. Eickhoff, V. Andrearczyk, and H. Muller, "Overview of the imageCLEF 2018 caption prediction tasks," *CLEF Working Notes, CEUR*, 2018.
4. M. Villegas, H. Muller, A. Gilbert, L. Piras, J. Wang, K. Mikolajczyk, A. G. Herrera, S. Bromuri, M. A. Amin, and M. K. Mohammed, "General overview of imageCLEF at the CLEF 2015 labs," in *International Conference of the Cross-Language Evaluation Forum for European Languages*. Springer, 2015, pp. 444–461.
5. G. Seco, A. de Herrera, R. Schaer, S. Bromuri, and H. Muller, "Overview of the imageCLEF 2016 medical task," *Working Notes of CLEF*, 2016.
6. K. Karthik and S. S. Kamath, "A hybrid feature modeling approach for content-based medical image retrieval," in *2018 IEEE 13th International Conference on Industrial and Information Systems (ICIIS)*. IEEE, 2018, pp. 7–12.

7. K. Karthik and S. S. Kamath, "Deep neural models for automated multi-task diagnostic scan management—Quality enhancement, view classification and report generation," *Biomedical Physics & Engineering Express*, vol. 8, no. 1, 2021, p. 015011.

8. O. Vinyals, A. Toshev, S. Bengio, and D. Erhan, "Show and tell: A neural image caption generator," in *Proceedings of the IEEE Conference on Computer Vision and Pattern Recognition*, 2015, pp. 3156–3164.

9. M. Hodosh, P. Young, and J. Hockenmaier, "Framing image description as a ranking task: Data, models and evaluation metrics," *Journal of Artificial Intelligence Research*, vol. 47, 2013, pp. 853–899.

10. Y. Gong, L. Wang, M. Hodosh, J. Hockenmaier, and S. Lazebnik, "Improving image-sentence embeddings using large weakly annotated photo collections," in *European Conference on Computer Vision*. Springer, 2014, pp. 529–545.

11. V. Ordonez, G. Kulkarni, and T. L. Berg, "Im2text: Describing images using 1 million captioned photographs," in *Advances in Neural Information Processing Systems*, 2011, pp. 1143–1151.

12. A. Karpathy, A. Joulin, and L. F. Fei-Fei, "Deep fragment embeddings for bidirectional image sentence mapping," in *Advances in Neural Information Processing Systems*, 2014, pp. 1889–1897.

13. Y. Yu, Z. Gong, P. Zhong, and J. Shan, "Unsupervised representation learning with deep convolutional neural network for remote sensing images," in *International Conference on Image and Graphics*. Springer, 2017, pp. 97–108.

14. J.-Y. Zhu, T. Park, P. Isola, and A. A. Efros, "Unpaired image-to-image translation using cycle-consistent adversarial networks," in *Proceedings of the IEEE International Conference on Computer Vision*, 2017, pp. 2223–2232.

15. J. T. Springenberg, "Unsupervised and semi-supervised learning with categorical generative adversarial networks," arXiv preprint arXiv:1511.06390, 2015.

16. A. Odena, "Semi-supervised learning with generative adversarial networks," arXiv preprint arXiv:1606.01583, 2016.

17. H. Salehinejad, S. Valaee, T. Dowdell, E. Colak, and J. Barfett, "Generalization of deep neural networks for chest pathology classification in x-rays using generative adversarial networks," in *2018 IEEE International Conference on Acoustics, Speech and Signal Processing (ICASSP)*. IEEE, 2018, pp. 990–994.

18. C. Y. Li, X. Liang, Z. Hu, and E. P. Xing, "Knowledge-driven encode, retrieve, paraphrase for medical image report generation," in *Proceedings of the AAAI Conference on Artificial Intelligence*, vol. 33, no. 1, 2019, pp. 6666–6673.

19. J. Yuan, H. Liao, R. Luo, and J. Luo, "Automatic radiology report generation based on multi-view image fusion and medical concept enrichment," in *International Conference on Medical Image Computing and Computer-Assisted Intervention*. Springer, 2019, pp. 721–729.

20. Z. Chen, Y. Song, T.-H. Chang, and X. Wan, "Generating radiology reports via memory-driven transformer," arXiv preprint arXiv:2010.16056, 2020.

21. M. Endo, R. Krishnan, V. Krishna, A. Y. Ng, and P. Rajpurkar, "Retrieval-based chest x-ray report generation using a pre-trained contrastive language-image model," in *Machine Learning for Health. PMLR*, 2021, pp. 209–219.

22. B. Jing, P. Xie, and E. Xing, "On the automatic generation of medical imaging reports," arXiv preprint arXiv:1711.08195, 2017.

23. Y. Xue, T. Xu, L. R. Long, Z. Xue, S. Antani, G. R. Thoma, and X. Huang, "Multimodal recurrent model with attention for automated radiology report generation," in *International Conference on Medical Image Computing and Computer-Assisted Intervention*. Springer, 2018, pp. 457–466.

24. X. Wang, Y. Peng, L. Lu, Z. Lu, and R. M. Summers, "Tienet: Text-image embedding network for common thorax disease classification and reporting in chest x-rays," in *Proceedings of the IEEE Conference on Computer Vision and Pattern Recognition*, 2018, pp. 9049–9058.
25. A. Bustos, A. Pertusa, J.-M. Salinas, and M. de la Iglesia-Vaya, "Padchest: A large chest x-ray image dataset with multi-label annotated reports," *Medical Image Analysis*, vol. 66, 2020, p. 101797.
26. X. Wang, Y. Peng, L. Lu, Z. Lu, M. Bagheri, and R. M. Summers, "Chestx-ray8: Hospital-scale chest x-ray database and benchmarks on weakly-supervised classification and localization of common thorax diseases," in *Proceedings of the IEEE Conference on Computer Vision and Pattern Recognition*, 2017, pp. 2097–2106.
27. V. Nair and G. E. Hinton, "Rectified linear units improve restricted Boltzmann machines," in *Proceedings of the 27th International Conference on Machine Learning (ICML-10)*, 2010, pp. 807–814.
28. K. Papineni, S. Roukos, T. Ward, and W.-J. Zhu, "Bleu: A method for automatic evaluation of machine translation," in *Proceedings of the 40th Annual Meeting on Association for Computational Linguistics*. Association for Computational Linguistics, 2002, pp. 311–318.

7 A Survey of Machine Learning- and Deep Learning-Based Techniques for Diabetic Retinopathy Screening

Nitigya Sambyal, Poonam Saini, and Rupali Syal

7.1 INTRODUCTION

Diabetic retinopathy (DR) is an ophthalmic condition associated with diabetes, which is also identified as a primary cause of visual impairment worldwide [1]. The World Health Organization (WHO) predicts that the total percentage of patients with DR is estimated to increase to 4.4% by 2030 [2]. According to a recent study, DR is also identified as the fifth-most common cause of moderately severe visual impairment (MSVI) [3]. Diabetic retinopathy (DR) is identified as progressive damage to the retina, which may cause blurred vision or even irreversible blindness in extreme cases [4]. The main risk factors for DR are high levels of glucose in the blood, the presence of high blood pressure, dependence on insulin, nutritional and genetic factors, etc.

7.1.1 RETINA

The retina is a thin (0.5 millimetre) tissue lining present at the back of the eye on the eye's interior. Any damage to the retina obstructs the receiving and processing of light, which further prevents the brain from receiving visual information, ultimately leading to blindness. Figure 7.1 shows a brief overview of the retina when viewed through an ophthalmoscope.

The main components of the retina are optic disc (nerve), blood vessels, fovea, and macula [5]. The optic disc (optic nerve head) is a circular or white area present in the centre of the retina and is used to transmit visual information from the retina to the brain. Blood vessels are the extensive vascular structure network that maintains the functionality of the retina. The central retinal artery (CRA) enters the eye at the optic disc, from where it divides into two major branches. These branches further

DOI: 10.1201/9781003363361-7

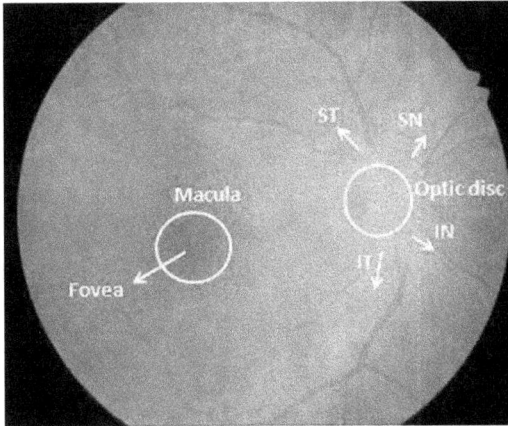

FIGURE 7.1   An overview of the retina. IT: Inferior temporal, ST: Superior temporal, IN: Inferior nasal, SN: Superior nasal

sub-divide into arterioles; namely the superior nasal, inferior temporal, superior temporal, and inferior nasal arterioles. The macula is the central part of the retina and measures five millimetres in diameter. The fovea is a blood vessel-free reddish spot present at the centre of the macula which provides sharp central vision.

7.1.2   DIABETIC RETINOPATHY

The severity and duration of hyperglycemia, genetic evolution, and metabolic control density are the prime factors leading to DR [6]. Traditionally, ophthalmologists have examined the fundus photographs of patients to determine the presence of cues associated with DR. The common DR-associated retinal lesions are hemorrhages, microaneurysms, soft exudates, and hard exudates [7, 8], as illustrated in Figure 7.2. Hemorrhages, also known as red lesions, are dot, blot and flame-shaped and may occur in deeper or more superficial layers of the retina [2]. Microaneurysms are circular in shape and have an approximate size of 100–120 micrometres [9]. Cotton wool spots are small, white, puffy patches with smooth edges [10]. Hard exudates are identified as bright yellow spots caused by the leakage of fats and proteins on the retina [11]. Based on the magnitude of DR severity, the fundus images can be classified into various stages, from healthy to mild to severe to most severe [12].

The fundus photography captures the rear of the eye, known as the fundus, using a specialized fundus camera with a microscope attached to it. The fundus images enable easy immediate review, image magnification, enhancement, and manipulation. This allows effortless monitoring and control of the progression of DR. The manual inspection of fundus images by ophthalmologists using a fundus camera is tedious, time-consuming, and subject to human error [13]. To overcome these limitations and to allow accurate mass screening, (need for) diabetic retinopathy computer-aided diagnosis (DR-CAD) system has become indispensable [14]. Such automated systems can aid in early diagnosis, which in turn can control vision

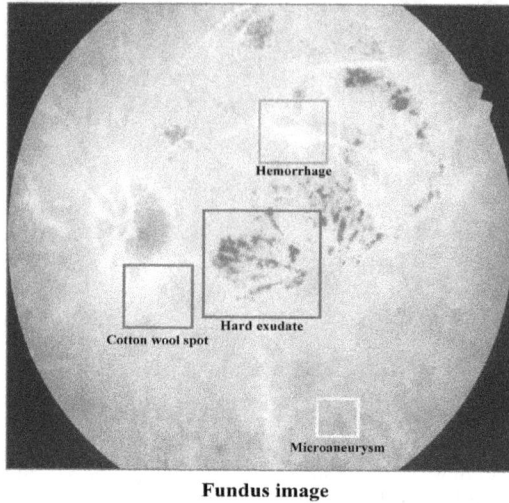

Fundus image

FIGURE 7.2 Retinal abnormalities associated with diabetic retinopathy

deterioration, thereby reducing and possibly preventing the risk of blindness among diabetic patients [15]. The CAD system developed using machine learning (ML) and deep learning (DL) algorithms can enable the speedy interpretation of medical image findings without the need of a skilled professional [16, 17]. The ML algorithms – namely artificial neural networks (ANN), decision trees, k-nearest neighbour (KNN), random forest, and support vector machines (SVM) – are based on expert knowledge and require manual feature extraction and a lot of time for tuning features. On the contrary, deep learning algorithms like convolutional neural networks (CNN), generative adversarial networks (GANs), recurrent neural networks (RNN), etc. are faster and more accurate, as they automatically extract desirable features from the image by learning through multiple levels of abstraction [18–20].

This chapter provides a critical review of various dot, blot DR-CAD systems consisting of DR classification and retinal lesion detection models that have been proposed to date.

This chapter is organized into seven sections. Section 7.2 focuses on the basic structure and components of a DR-CAD system. Section 7.3 provides an outline of the research papers reviewed. Section 7.4 presents an overview of the literature corresponding to the binary and multistage classification of DR. Section 7.5 presents a review of various models used in the detection and segmentation of retinal abnormalities in fundus images. In Section 7.6, a methodology has been proposed for automatic detection of DR. Section 7.7 presents the findings of the review along with a future scope.

7.2 DR-CAD SYSTEM

A complete DR-CAD system helps in the identification of DR, along with the detection and segmentation of retinal lesions, for better severity analysis. However, there may be some systems that focus on either the classification of DR or retinal lesion detection in fundus images. Figure 7.3 presents a complete structure of basic

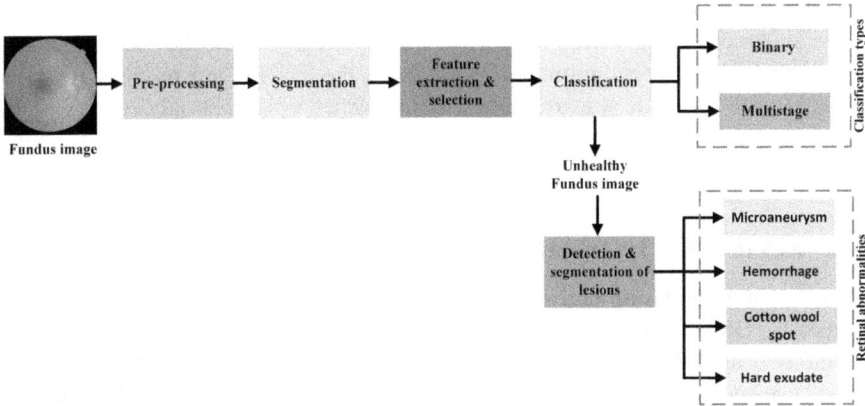

FIGURE 7.3 A DR-CAD system

DR-CAD systems consisting of five main components: preprocessing, segmentation of region of interest (ROI), feature extraction and selection, classification, and retinal lesion detection.

A DR-CAD system consists of five main phases:

1. **Preprocessing:** This phase focuses on the improvement of image quality by suppressing distortions or noise, image brightness normalization, and enhancement of significant features for better processing. In DR-CAD systems, it helps in the suppression of anatomical regions like blood vessels and optic disc to clearly visualize the retinal abnormalities.

2. **Segmentation:** In this phase, the anatomical structures are segmented so that the region of interest can be obtained for further processing. Segmentation of other anatomical structures like blood vessels and the optic discs is done from fundus images, to better visualize the candidate lesion regions.

3. **Feature extraction and selection:** This phase helps in the extraction of significant features from the segmented image. Initially, the pixel- or region-level features are extracted from the candidate retinal lesions. The best-performing features are selected to form a feature vector.

4. **Classification:** The features extracted in the above step are then used to categorize the retinal images into various classes. Based on the features extracted from the preprocessed, segmented fundus image, it is classified as either healthy or unhealthy. For multistage classification, the unhealthy fundus image can be further classified, depending on the severity of the disease.

5. **Detection and segmentation of retinal lesions:** To allow for better severity screening of DR, the retinal lesions from the unhealthy fundus images can also be detected and segmented. This helps in determining the number of lesions, their size, and their location, which can further allow physicians to better assess the disease severity.

Due to manual feature extraction process, traditional machine learning and image processing methods have been found to be inadequate in the detection and classification of diabetic retinopathy images. Due to this, the focus of our research has now shifted to the use of deep learning-based approaches which not only require minimal image processing but also ensure improved accuracy by automatically learning through multiple levels of abstraction [21].

7.3 REVIEW OF LITERATURE CLASSIFICATION

This section provides an outline of the literature reviewed, based on the task performed for DR screening. The entirety of the literature is initially categorized based on the two main tasks performed: classification and segmentation. Both of these tasks have been performed by machine learning and deep learning-based techniques [22]. An overview of the review structure followed in this paper is clearly illustrated in Figure 7.4.

Here, classification aims at the identification of the severity stage of DR by analysis of the fundus image. Some researchers have focused their work on the binary classification of fundus images, i.e., healthy vs. unhealthy. Meanwhile, others have performed multistage classification of detected unhealthy images. Detection and segmentation of lesions involve the identification and classification of various retinal lesions like hemorrhages, microaneurysms, cotton wool spots, and hard exudates in the fundus image. In recent years, both of these tasks have been effectively performed by machine learning and deep learning techniques [23, 24].

Machine learning techniques involve manually extracting and selecting features from fundus images, which are then employed in the classification of abnormalities

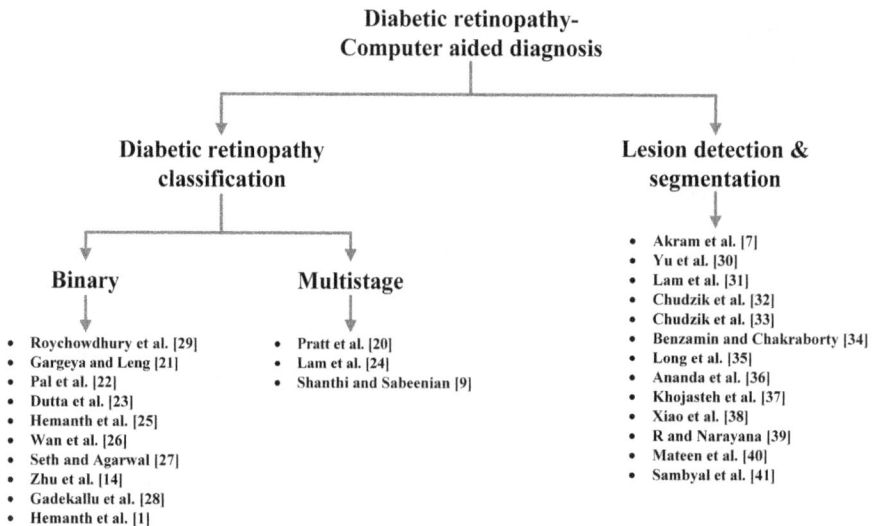

Diabetic retinopathy-Computer aided diagnosis

Diabetic retinopathy classification

Lesion detection & segmentation

- Akram et al. [7]
- Yu et al. [30]
- Lam et al. [31]
- Chudzik et al. [32]
- Chudzik et al. [33]
- Benzamin and Chakraborty [34]
- Long et al. [35]
- Ananda et al. [36]
- Khojasteh et al. [37]
- Xiao et al. [38]
- R and Narayana [39]
- Mateen et al. [40]
- Sambyal et al. [41]

Binary

- Roychowdhury et al. [29]
- Gargeya and Leng [21]
- Pal et al. [22]
- Dutta et al. [23]
- Hemanth et al. [25]
- Wan et al. [26]
- Seth and Agarwal [27]
- Zhu et al. [14]
- Gadekallu et al. [28]
- Hemanth et al. [1]

Multistage

- Pratt et al. [20]
- Lam et al. [24]
- Shanthi and Sabeenian [9]

FIGURE 7.4 An outline of the review of literature

using classifiers like ANN, SVM, KNN, etc. [25, 26]. On the other hand, deep learning models like DNN, CNN, autoencoders, etc. use automatic feature extraction and classification models for accurate disease prediction [18, 27, 28]. Both techniques help in the detection of DR, which leads to better disease management.

7.4 CLASSIFICATION

This section summarizes various ML- and DL-based techniques employed in the classification of DR. Roychowdhury et al. [29] in 2014 proposed a CAD system for generating DR severity grades by fundus image analysis. The authors used machine learning classifiers – SVM, gaussian mixture model (GMM), KNN, and AdaBoost to distinguish between lesion and non-lesion regions. The model was trained and tested on the DIARETDB1 and MESSIDOR datasets respectively . The background region consisting of the optic disc and vasculature was segmented from the fundus image using a minimum-intensity maximum-solidity algorithm. Thereafter, the AdaBoost algorithm was employed for the selection of the top 30 features for the classification of fundus images. The foreground region was classified as candidate bright lesions and red lesions. The hard exudates and cotton wool spots were identified as bright lesions, whereas hemorrhages and microaneurysms were categorized as red lesions. GMM obtained optimum results for bright lesion classification, whereas KNN was preferred for red lesion classification. Overall, the DREAM model achieved a sensitivity of 100%, with a specificity of 53.16% and area under the receiver operating characteristic curve (AUC) of 0.904.

Pratt et al. [30] performed five-stage DR classification using CNN with Gaussian initialization and categorical cross entropy loss function on a Kaggle fundus image set. The model was trained using stochastic gradient descent with Nestrov momentum and obtained a specificity of 95%, accuracy of 75%, and 30% sensitivity.

Gargeya and Leng [31] developed a robust DR screening model using CNN. The proposed model comprised five residual blocks with four, six, eight, ten, and six layers and a convolutional visualization layer with 1024 filters at the end. An average pooling followed by a softmax layer provided class probabilities for accurate binary classification. The model was trained on the EyePACS dataset and tested on the MESSIDOR-2 and e-Ophtha datasets. On the MESSIDOR-2 dataset, the model achieved 93% sensitivity, 87% specificity, and 0.94 AUC, whereas on the e-Ophtha dataset, 90% sensitivity, 94% specificity, and 0.95 AUC were obtained.

Pal et al. [32] examined the performance of various ML classifiers to determine signs of DR in fundus scans of the retinal images. The dataset understudy was taken from a University of California Irvine (UCI) machine learning repository consisting of 1151 instances with 19 numeric values, and the models were evaluated on both Python and Weka tools. The performance of SVM with linear kernel surpassed other classifiers by obtaining an accuracy of 74.65% on Python and 67.87% on Weka.

Dutta et al. [33] evaluated the performance of ANN, DNN, and CNN for DR classification, using a Kaggle fundus image set. After noise removal and segmentation of bright backgrounds, statistical features like standard deviation, average, median, etc. were extracted from the images. When trained on these statistical features, DNN outperformed NN, with a test accuracy of 82.3%. However, when trained on image data, CNN obtained the highest test accuracy of 78.3%.

To better assess the severity of the disease, the classification of the severity stage of DR was proposed by Lam et al. [34]. The authors used a pre-trained GoogLeNet model for DR detection after preprocessing the images using the contrast-limited adaptive histogram equalization (CLAHE) technique. The proposed GoogLeNet classification model achieved a validation accuracy of 74.5%, 68.8%, and 57.2% on 2-ary, 3-ary, and 4-ary, respectively, using the Kaggle and MESSIDOR-1 datasets.

A modified Hopfield neural network (MHNN) model for DR classification was proposed by Hemanth et al. [35] using fundus images collected from Lotus Eye Care Hospital in India. After image preprocessing, the MHNN was trained using six textural features extracted from the image set. The model delivered an accuracy of 99.25% for the detection of both healthy and DR images.

Wan et al. [36] compared the state-of-the-art ImageNet models – namely AlexNet, GoogLeNet, VGGNet, and ResNet – for the identification of healthy or unhealthy fundus images. The performance of these ImageNet models with hyperparameter tuning and transfer learning was analysed on the Kaggle fundus image set. The accuracy details of various models are shown in Figure 7.5. It was observed that the overall classification results improved after hyperparameter tuning, with VGGNet-s providing an excellent accuracy of 95.68%.

Seth and Agarwal [37] performed DR screening of fundus images using VGGNet asfeature extractor and SVM as classifier. The model hyperparameters were tuned using the grid search technique to obtain sensitivity and specificity of 0.93 and 0.83 respectively on the EyePACS dataset.

Shanthi and Sabeenian [12] also proposed multistage DR classification using modified AlexNet architecture. The model was validated on a MESSIDOR dataset

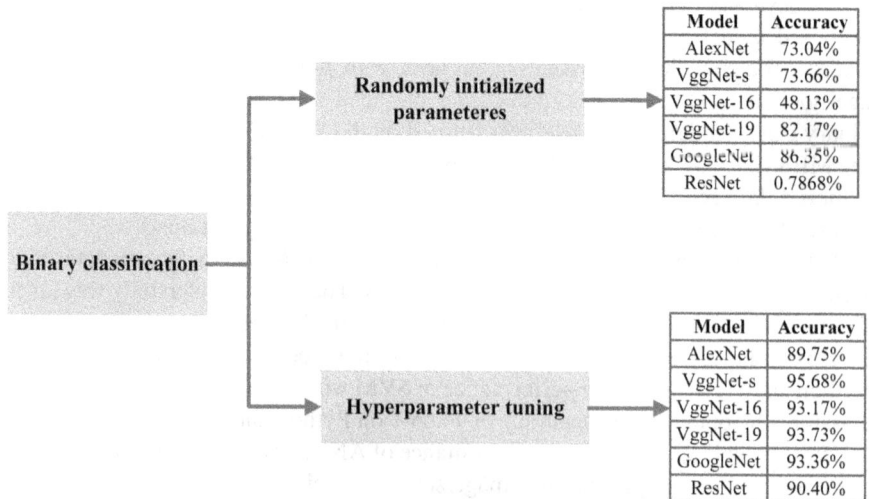

Model	Accuracy
AlexNet	73.04%
VggNet-s	73.66%
VggNet-16	48.13%
VggNet-19	82.17%
GoogleNet	86.35%
ResNet	0.7868%

Model	Accuracy
AlexNet	89.75%
VggNet-s	95.68%
VggNet-16	93.17%
VggNet-19	93.73%
GoogleNet	93.36%
ResNet	90.40%

FIGURE 7.5　Binary classification results by Wan et al. [36]

and obtained classification accuracies of 96.6% for healthy, 96.2% for DR stage 1 , 95.6% for DR stage 2 , and 96.6% for DR stage 3 .

Zhu et al. [25] combined the classifier for microaneurysm detection with the classifier for the classification of fundus images. The canny edge detection with a threshold value of 0.1 was used for the detection of the candidate microaneurysm region. Thereafter, naive Bayes employing colour and shape features was used to verify true microaneurysm regions. This was followed by a final DR prediction using six features, namely Mascount, Masmgray, Gmgray, Gstd, Ggrad, and Vdense. The proposed cascade framework obtained an AUC of 0.908 on the Lariboisière dataset and 0.832 on MESSIDOR datasets.

Gadekallu et al. [38] also conducted binary classification of fundus images with DNN using the Diabetic Retinopathy Debrecen dataset from the UCI machine learning repository. After the removal of outliers and normalization of the dataset, PCA was employed to retain only significant features. These selected features were used for the training of DNN with parameter tuning performed using Grey Wolf Optimization (GWO). This model showed exemplary performance compared to SVM, naive Bayes, decision tree, and XGBoost, with 97% accuracy, 91% sensitivity, and 97% specificity.

Hemanth et al. [1] designed a hybrid model by combining deep learning and image processing techniques for the classification of DR using the MESSIDOR fundus dataset. The authors applied CLAHE individually to the R, G, and B channels of the images and then concatenated these resulting channels to obtain an image with improved quality. This was followed by classification with a CNN model, which achieved an accuracy of 97%, sensitivity of 94%, and specificity of 98%.

Table 7.1 provides a summary of the various research studies discussed above for the classification of DR.

Discussion: The section discusses research work on binary and multistage classification of DR using machine learning and deep learning approaches. Various authors have employed machine learning-based techniques like KNN, SVM, decision trees, and ANN [25, 32, 37, 39]. To overcome the inherent limitation of machine learning models, deep learning models for DR classification have been explored in various studies [1, 12, 20, 34, 36, 38]. Deep learning models allow automatic extraction and selection of significant features, which help to classify fundus images more accurately. It has also been observed that deep learning models are more suitable for unstructured input data and achieve higher performance than traditional machine learning models.

7.5 SEGMENTATION

This section summarizes various AI-based techniques used in the detection and segmentation of retinal abnormalities associated with DR [40]. The four retinal lesions associated with DR are microaneurysms (MA), hemorrhages (HE), cotton wool spots (CWS) or soft exudates (SE), and hard exudates (EX). Akram et al. [10] suggested the detection of retinal lesions using a hybrid fuzzy classifier. After background subtraction and removal of noise, blood vessels and the optic disc were

TABLE 7.1

Method, Dataset, Classification, Classifier, Results, and Future Work of the Selected Studies for DR Classification

Method, Year	Dataset	Classification	Classifier	Results	Future work
Roychowdhury et al. [39], *2014*	DIARETDB1 and MESSIDOR	Binary	GMM + KNN + AdaBoost	• Sensitivity = 100%, Specificity = 53.16%, AUC = 0.904	• Effect of cost-sensitive SVM and AdaBoost for lesion classification can be analysed • Detection of neovascularization, vascular bleeding, and drusen can be undertaken
Pratt et al. [30], *2016*	Kaggle	Five-stage	CNN	• Sensitivity = 30%, Specificity = 95%, Accuracy = 75%	• Results must be validated on more datasets
Gargeya and Leng [31], 2017	EyePACS, MESSIDOR-2 and e-Ophtha	Binary	CNN	• On MESSIDOR-2: Sensitivity = 93%, Specificity = 87%, AUC = 0.94 • On e-Ophtha: Sensitivity = 90%, Specificity = 94% and AUC = 0.95	• Evaluation using geographic variation within training and test sets can be done • Patients' demographic information can be incorporated for improved performance
Pal et al. [32], 2017	UCI	Binary	SVM, naive Bayes, KNN and decision tree	• SVM with linear kernel achieved best classification accuracy • Python: Accuracy = 74.65% • Weka: Accuracy = 67.87%	• Deep neural networks can be explored for accuracy improvement

(Continued)

TABLE 7.1
(Continued)

Method, Year	Dataset	Classification	Classifier	Results	Future work
Dutta et al. [2018], 2018	Kaggle	Binary	NN, DNN, CNN (VGG-16)	• DNN obtained best accuracy of 82.3% when trained with statistical data • CNN obtained best accuracy of 78.3% when trained with image data	• Statistical and image data can be combined to develop a standalone application • The existing model can be extended to NPDR classification
Lam et al. [34], 2018	Kaggle and MESSIDOR-1	Multistage	GoogLeNet	• Binary classification accuracy = 74.5% • 3-ary classification accuracy = 68.8% • 4-ary classification accuracy = 57.2%	• 4-ary classification accuracy can be improved by exploring residual networks
Hemanth et al. [35], 2018	Fundus image set from Lotus Eye Care Hospital, India	Binary	MHNN	• Detection of healthy images: Sensitivity = 99%, Specificity = 99%, Accuracy = 99.25% • Detection of DR images: Sensitivity = 99%, Specificity = 99%, Accuracy = 99.25%	• Additional features and combination features can be studied for better classification • Models with less training time can be explored
Wan et al. [36], 2018	Kaggle	Binary	AlexNet, VGGNet, GoogLeNet and ResNet	• Best performance of VGGNet-s with hyperparameter tuning • Sensitivity = 86.47%, Specificity = 97.43%, Accuracy = 95.68%, AUC = 0.97	• Model should be modified to enable multistage classification of DR • More datasets should be considered to ensure generalizability
Seth and Agarwal [37], 2018	EyePACS	Binary	SVM with linear kernel	• Sensitivity= 93% and Specificity= 83%	• Model should be validated on more datasets

(Continued)

TABLE 7.1
(Continued)

Method, Year	Dataset	Classification	Classifier	Results	Future work
Shanthi and Sabeenian [12], 2019	MESSIDOR	Multistage	Modified AlexNet	• Healthy retina: Sensitivity = 95.3%, Specificity = 97.3%, • Accuracy = 96.6%, Precision=95.3% • DR stage 1: Sensitivity = 88%, Specificity = 98.3%, Accuracy = 96.2%, Precision = 93% • DR stage 2: Sensitivity = 90.1%, Specificity = 97.6%, Accuracy = 95.6%, Precision = 94% • DR stage 3: Sensitivity = 96%, Specificity = 96.6% Accuracy = 96.6%, Precision = 86%	• The algorithm should be tested on datasets with more instances
Zhu et al. [25], 2019	Lariboisière and MESSIDOR	Binary	SVM	• AUC = 0.908 on Lariboisière • AUC= 0.832 on MESSIDOR	• Improved models for precise segmentation of lesions should be proposed for accurate DR grading
Gadekallu et al. [38], 2020	Diabetic Retinopathy Debrecen dataset, UCI	Binary	DNN	• Sensitivity = 91%, Specificity = 97%, Accuracy = 97%, Precision = 96.5% Recall = 97%,	• The model can be validated on datasets with more instances and images with higher dimensions
Hemanth et al. [1], 2020	MESSIDOR	Binary	CNN	• Sensitivity = 98%, Specificity = 94%, Accuracy = 97%, Precision = 94% Recall = 94%, F-score = 94%, G-mean = 95.9%	• More datasets should be used for evaluating the model

segmented from input retinal images. Thereafter, a fuzzy neural network consisting of fuzzy self-organizing layers was used in the pre-classification task and bright and dark lesion detection was performed by a multilayer perceptron (MLP). The proposed model achieved a dark lesion (HE and MA) detection accuracy of 95.97% for DRIVE and STARE databases and an overall accuracy of 94.7% for bright lesions (EX and CWS).

Yu et al. [41] performed a CNN-based pixel-level detection of exudates using the e-Ophtha-EX dataset. After the removal of the optic disc and blood vessels from the fundus image, CNN was trained on image patches sized 64×64 using 150 epochs. The pixel-wise accuracy, sensitivity, and specificity as reported by the model were 91.92%, 88.85%, and 96% respectively on the test set.

Lam et al. [42] performed segmentation of retinal lesions using a GoogLeNet model. The model when trained for 600 epochs with a 0.001 learning rate and 0.5 dropout in the last fully connected layer to obtain a five-class classification accuracy of 95% and binary classification accuracy of 98% on randomly selected image patches from the Kaggle test set.

Chudzik et al. [43] proposed the detection of MA using CNN with a batch size of 128 and 0.0001 as the initial learning rate. After noise removal and image resizing, the dataset was augmented by artificial transformations like rotation horizontal and vertical reflections for better training of CNN. The model showed the highest average FROC score of 0.355 on the ROC dataset and 0.392 on the DIARETDB1 dataset.

Exudate segmentation using a fully convolutional neural network (FCNN) was also performed by Chudzik et al. [44] using e-Ophtha datasets. The performance of CNN was improved by employing an auxiliary codebook formed through the propagation of every training patch through FCNN, but collection of outputs was done only for the selected intermediate convolutional layer. The output of both models was merged to obtain the final segmented results. The model, having been trained on e-Ophtha-MA and tested on e-Ophtha-EX, obtained 99.98% specificity, 86.66% sensitivity, and 0.982 as AUC.

Benzamin and Chakraborty [45] performed the detection of exudate from fundus images using an eight-layer CNN trained on 32×32 image patches using the IDRiD dataset. This model underwent training for 1500 epochs and achieved 98.29% sensitivity, 41.35% specificity, and 96.6% accuracy.

Long et al. [46] proposed a method consisting of fuzzy c-means (FCM) clustering and SVM for the detection and classification of EX. After optic disc segmentation, FCM was used to obtain a local dynamic threshold of 30×40 image patches for segmentation of EX. Thereafter, eight features – namely mean green-channel intensity, grey intensity, mean hue, mean saturation, mean value of retinal image in HSV colour model, energy, standard deviation, and mean gradient magnitude were used to train SVM with radial basis function (RBF) kernel for EX classification. The model obtained a mean sensitivity of 76.5% on e-Ophtha and 97.5% on the DIARETDB1 dataset.

Ananda et al. [47] proposed a model i.e. modified U-Net for multiclass lesion segmentation. in the original U-Net model ReLU was replaced by leaky ReLU and a batch normalization layer was added before each pooling operation to obtain the modified U-Net model. The model used a binary cross entropy loss function and also calculated the Dice score. This model was trained using the IDRiD dataset and was tested on the MESSIDOR dataset, where it obtained better lesion segmentation results than the original U-Net and SegNet models. The model successfully obtained a Dice coefficient of 0.7082, 0.7125, 0.7793, and 0.6920 for EX, SE, HE, and MA respectively on the test set.

Khojasteh et al. [48] compared the performance of various classifiers: CNNs, ResNet-50 + SVM, ResNet-50 + Optimum path forest, ResNet-50 + KNN, and Discriminative Restricted Boltzmann Machines (DRBM) for EX detection. The models were trained using 25 × 25 exudate and non-exudate patches from the DIARETDB1 and e-Ophtha datasets. It was noted that ResNet-50 + SVM surpassed the rest of the classifiers under study, with accuracies of 98.2% and 97.6% respectively.

Xiao et al. [49] proposed pixel-level segmentation of retinal lesions from fundus images using a holisticallynested edge detection network (HEDNet) incorporated into conditional generative adversarial network (cGan) with a standard PatchGAN discriminator. HEDNet builds upon VGGNet and generates semantically meaningful edge maps to identify object contours. The cGan was used as the discriminator, as it learns the joint distribution of the input with a segmentation map conditioned on the output. The proposed model minimizes the segmentation loss and maximizes the discriminator classification loss, obtaining an average precision (AP) of 43.92%, 48.39%, 84.05%, and 48.12% for MA, SE, EX, and HE, respectively.

Deepa and Narayana [50] extracted the candidate MA regions using thresholding and morphological operations. Thereafter, the number of candidate regions and the mean intensity of the red and green planes were used as features to train a feed-forward neural network. The model obtained 100% sensitivity, 100% specificity, 98.89% accuracy, and 98.83% precision on the DIARETDB1 dataset.

Mateen et al. [51] performed EX detection by merging extracted features from Inception V3, ResNet-50, and VGGNet-19. Initially, GMM was used to localize the EX region in fundus images and, thereafter, features from various networks were joined into the fully connected layer for classification of non-exudate and exudate by softmax layer. The model delivered accuracy of 98.43% and 98.91% on the e-Ophtha and DIARETDB1 datasets, respectively.

Sambyal et al. [52] suggested a modified U-Net architecture for pixel-wise segmentation of MA and EX from retinal images (Figure 7.6). The architecture consisted of pre-trained ResNet-34 as the encoder, middle convolution layers, and U-Net blocks as the decoder and merge layer. The intermediate output from the encoder was also provided as the input to the corresponding U-Net block in the decoder for accurate lesion segmentation. On the IDRiD dataset, the model achieved 99.95% accuracy for both MA and EX semantic segmentation. This model when trained on e-Ophtha and tested on the IDRiD dataset, achieved 99.89% accuracy for both MA and EX.

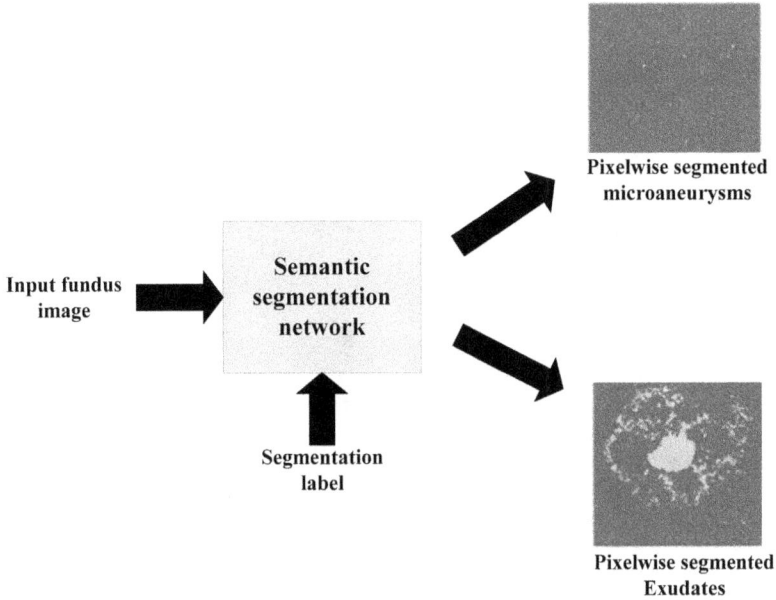

FIGURE 7.6   Pixel-wise segmentation of microaneurysms and exudates [52]

The details of the above-discussed research studies into the detection and segmentation of retinal lesions associated with DR have been compiled in Table 7.2.

Discussion: This section discusses research work done for the segmentation of various retinal lesions associated with DR. Most authors employ deep learning models as they are more suitable for accurate detection and classification of retinal lesions, which vary in size, shape, and colour. Authors reported Dice scores as high as 0.9999 for exudates and 0.99998 for MA using e-Ophtha as the training set and IDRiD as the test set [52]. Ananda et al. [47] reported the highest Dice score of 0.7125 for SE and 0.7793 for HE using IDRiD as the training set and MESSIDOR as the test set. In general, there is less research work focusing on the detection of hemorrhages and cotton wool spots. Further, ensemble models can be explored for improvement in existing methods for retinal lesion segmentation.

7.6   PROPOSED METHODOLOGY

Computer-aided diagnosis (CAD) is a computer-based system that assists doctors in faster evaluation and analysis of abnormalities, thereby enabling early and accurate detection of the disease. In this section, a hybrid deep learning model has been proposed for the detection of DR. The proposed DR-CAD solution performs automatic classification and segmentation of retinal lesions from unhealthy fundus images. Figure 7.7 shows the schematic of the proposed DR-CAD.

TABLE 7.2

Method, Dataset, Lesion, Model, Results, and Future Work of the Selected Studies for Detection and Segmentation of DR-Associated Retinal Lesions

Method, Year	Dataset	Lesion Detection	Classifier	Results	Future Work
Akram et al. [10], 2012	DRIVE, STARE, DIARETDB0, and DIARETDB1	MA, HE, CWS, and EX	Hybrid fuzzy classifier	• DRIVE: Accuracy = 96.14% for dark lesions and 96.23% for bright lesions • STARE: Accuracy = 95.98% for dark lesions and 95.71% for bright lesions • DIARETDB0: Accuracy = 91.26% for dark lesions and 93.89% for bright lesions • DIARETDB1: Accuracy = 91.60% for dark lesions and 93.10% for bright lesions	• DNN-based models can be explored for improved lesion detection accuracy
Yu et al. [41], 2017	e-Ophtha-EX	EX	CNN	• Sensitivity = 88.85%, Specificity = 96%, Accuracy = 91.92%, F-Score = 92.61%	• More benchmark datasets should be used for model validation
Lam et al. [42], 2018	e-Ophtha and Kaggle	MA, HE, EX, and CWS	GoogLeNet	• Five-class Accuracy = 95% • Binary Accuracy = 98%	• Model can be modified to detect neovascularization
Chudzik et al. [43], 2018	ROC and DIARETDB1	MA	CNN	• For ROC: FROC score = 0.355 • For DIARETDB1: FROC score = 0.392	• Forward propagation step can be parallelized across multiple devices to reduce time

(Continued)

TABLE 7.2
(Continued)

Method, Year	Dataset	Lesion Detection	Classifier	Results	Future Work
Chudzik et al. [44], 2018	e-Ophtha-MA and e-Ophtha-EX	EX	CNN	• Sensitivity = 86.66%, Specificity = 99.98%, AUC = 0.982	• Segmentation of red lesions can be performed by modifying the model
Benzamin and Chakraborty [45], 2018	IDRiD	EX	CNN	• Sensitivity = 98.29%, Specificity = 41.35%, Accuracy = 96.6%	• Effect of image patch size on detection of exudates can be studied • Results should be validated on more datasets
Long et al. [46], 2019	e-Ophtha-EX and DIARETDB1	EX	SVM with RBF kernel	• e-Ophtha-Ex: Sensitivity = 76.5%, PPV = 82.7%, F-Score = 76.7% • DIARETDB1: Sensitivity = 97.5%, Specificity = 97.8%, Accuracy =97.7%	• Detection of exudates suffers due to poor contrast between it and background • Overall accuracy relies significantly on optic and blood vessel detection results
Ananda et al. [47], 2019	IDRiD and MESSIDOR	EX, SE, HE, and MA	Modified U-Net	• Dice = 0.7082 for EX • Dice = 0.7125 for SE • Dice = 0.7793 for HE • Dice = 0.6920 for MA	• Ensemble models for improvement of Dice score can be investigated

(Continued)

TABLE 7.2 (Continued)

Method, Year	Dataset	Lesion Detection	Classifier	Results	Future Work
Khojasteh et al. [48], *2019*	DIARETDB1 and e-Ophtha	EX	CNNs, ResNet50 + SVM, ResNet50 + OPF, ResNet50 + KNN and DRBM	• ResNet50 + SVM provided best performance for EX detection • For DIARETDB1: Sensitivity = 99%, Specificity = 96%, Accuracy = 98.2% • For e-Ophtha: Sensitivity = 98%, Specificity = 95%, Accuracy = 97.6%	• Computationally efficient classifiers can be explored • Specificity of the detection model can be improved using approaches such as Twin SVM • DNN such as generative adversarial networks can be investigated for exudate detection
Xiao et al. [49], *2019*	IDRiD	MA, SE, EX, HE	HEDNet + cGAN	• Microaneurysm: AP = 43.92% and F-1 score = 42.98% • Soft exudate: AP = 48.39% and F-1 score = 43.98% • Hard exudate: AP = 84.05% and F-1 score = 69.08% • Hemorrhage: AP = 48.12% and F-1 score = 45.76%	• Combination of other models can be explored for improved lesion segmentation
Deepa and Narayana [50], *2020*	DIARETDB1	MA	Feed-forward NN	• Sensitivity = 100%, Specificity = 100%, Accuracy = 98.89%, Precision = 98.83%	• Classification can be done by taking more features
Mateen et al. [51], *2020*	e-Ophtha, DIARETDB1	EX	CNN	• On e-Ophtha: Accuracy = 98.43% • On DIARETDB1: Accuracy = 98.91%	• Model can be modified to include segmentation of HE and MA

(Continued)

TABLE 7.2
(Continued)

Method, Year	Dataset	Lesion Detection	Classifier	Results	Future Work
Sambyal et al. [52], 2020	e-Ophtha, IDRiD	MA, EX	Modified U-Net	• On IDRiD: Sensitivity = 99.85%, Specificity = 99.95%, Accuracy = 99.88%, Dice = 0.9998 for both MA and EX • Trained on e-Ophtha and tested on IDRiD: Sensitivity = 99.88%, Specificity = 99.89%, Accuracy = 99.98%, Dice = 0.9998 for MA • Trained on e-Ophtha and tested on IDRiD: Sensitivity = 99.88%, Specificity = 99.89%, Accuracy = 99.98%, Dice = 0.9999 for EX	• Model can be extended to detect HE and CWS • Model can be validated on clinically acquired datasets

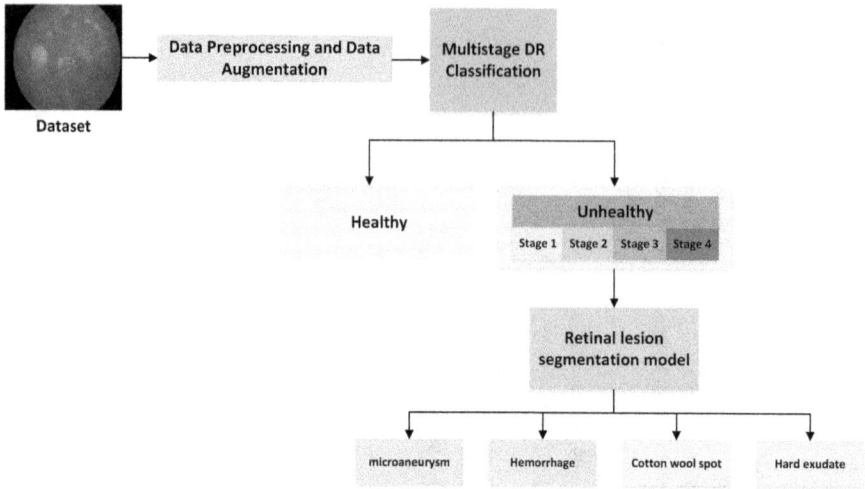

FIGURE 7.7 Proposed methodology

The methodology consists of the following steps:

1. The first step is to select an appropriate dataset for multistage DR classification and lesion segmentation. For classification, the severity grading of fundus images is required. For segmentation, pixel-wise labelling (i.e., healthy or unhealthy) is required for accurate detection of lesions.
2. The next step is to preprocess the data to enhance the quality of the fundus images. This includes the removal of noise, image resizing, and data augmentation like flipping, rotation, zooming, scaling, etc. Finally, the preprocessed fundus images are segmented into two sets for the training and testing of the model.
3. The third step is to classify the images on the basis of their severity stage, from the healthy to the most severe stage. For this purpose, various CNNs can be used, as discussed in Section 7.4.
4. The next step is to detect various retinal lesions from the unhealthy fundus images. For this purpose, various deep learning models can be used, as discussed in Section 7.5. It is observed that in comparison to other techniques, the U-Net-based deep learning model provides better results, in terms of accuracy and Dice score.
5. The last stage is to evaluate the model in terms of various performance parameters, by comparing the results with the ground truth. This helps to determine the reliability of the model in assessing the severity of the disease.

Hence, the proposed comprehensive DR-CAD system will enable better severity analysis of the disease.

7.7 CONCLUSION

This chapter details various AI-based models that have been used for the classification of DR and detection & segmentation of the retinal lesions associated with it. Screening of DR using CAD systems includes five major tasks: preprocessing, segmentation of anatomical structures, feature extraction & selection, detection, and segmentation of retinal lesions. The preprocessing phase enables enhancement of the quality of fundus images by contrast adjustment and noise removal. This is followed by segmentation phase, wherein less significant anatomical structures are discarded. The significant features are selected from the resultant fundus image and are then used to train the classification and lesion detection models. The machine learning models rely on handcrafted feature extraction and selection, whereas deep learning models automatically extract significant features over several hidden layers in the network. Various authors have proposed approaches for binary and multistage (from healthy stage to most severe stage) classification of fundus images using classifiers like SVM, CNN, DNN, etc. It has been observed that most of the recent literature to date focuses more on binary classification, i.e., the classification of fundus images as healthy or unhealthy. Thus, new techniques and models must be proposed to extend the existing research to the multistage classification of DR. The detection and segmentation of retinal lesions like microaneurysms, cotton wool spots, hard exudates, and hemorrhages help in determining the location and size of the problem regions. This in turn helps the physician in accurately assessing the severity of DR. A DR-CAD system can eliminate the probability of human error and allows speedy and accurate mass screening of fundus images. This will enable not only the early detection of DR but also the control of the associated irreversible vision loss. In the future, various deep learning-based hybridization techniques can be developed for more accurate DR detection. Also, advanced automatic hyperparameter tuning methods can be explored for faster and better network convergence. Further, an automated system may be developed with extended capabilities, like the detection of other retinal abnormalities such as glaucoma, macular edema, and abnormal blood vessel growth.

REFERENCES

1. Hemanth DJ, Deperlioglu O, Kose U. An enhanced diabetic retinopathy detection and classification approach using deep convolutional neural network. *Neural Comput Appl* 2020;32(3):707–21. https://doi.org/10.1007/s00521-018-03974-0.
2. Mumtaz R, Hussain M, Sarwar S, Khan K, Mumtaz S, Mumtaz M. Automatic detection of retinal hemorrhages by exploiting image processing techniques for screening retinal diseases in diabetic patients. *Int J Diabetes Dev Ctries* 2018;38(1):1–8. https://doi.org/10.1007/s13410-017-0561-6.
3. Thomas RL, Halim S, Gurudas S, Sivaprasad S, Owens DR. IDF Diabetes Atlas: A review of studies utilising retinal photography on the global prevalence of diabetes related retinopathy between 2015 and 2018. *Diabetes Res Clin Pract* 2019;157:1–13. https://doi.org/10.1016/j.diabres.2019.107840.

4. Huang X, Wang H, She C, Feng J, Liu X, Hu X, et al. Artificial intelligence promotes the diagnosis and screening of diabetic retinopathy. *Front Endocrinol (Lausanne)* 2022;13:1–12. https://doi.org/10.3389/fendo.2022.946915.

5. Kolb H. Simple anatomy of the retina. *Webvision Organ Retin Vis Syst* 1995: – .

6. Saleh E, Błaszczyński J, Moreno A, Valls A, Romero-Aroca P, de la Riva-Fernández S, Słowiński R. Learning ensemble classifiers for diabetic retinopathy assessment. *Artif Intell Med* 2018;85:50–63. https://doi.org/10.1016/j.artmed.2017.09.006.

7. Devaraj D, RS, Prasanna Kumar SC. A survey on segmentation of exudates and micro-aneurysms for early detection of diabetic retinopathy. *Mater Today Proc*, Elsevier Ltd; 2018, p. 10845–50. https://doi.org/10.1016/j.matpr.2017.12.372.

8. Kaur J, Mittal D. A generalized method for the segmentation of exudates from patho-logical retinal fundus images. *Biocybern Biomed Eng* 2018;38(1):27–53. https://doi.org/10.1016/j.bbe.2017.10.003.

9. Shankar K, Sait ARW, Gupta D, Lakshmanaprabu SK, Khanna A, Pandey HM. Automated detection and classification of fundus diabetic retinopathy images using synergic deep learning model. *Pattern Recognit Lett* 2020;133:210–6. https://doi.org/10.1016/j.patrec.2020.02.026.

10. Akram UM, Khan SA. Automated detection of dark and bright lesions in retinal images for early detection of diabetic retinopathy. *J Med Syst* 2012;36(5):3151–62. https://doi.org/10.1007/s10916-011-9802-2.

11. Imani E, Pourreza H. A novel method for retinal exudate segmentation using signal seperation algorithm. *Comput Methods Programs Biomed* 2016;133:195–205. https://doi.org/10.1016/j.cmpb.2016.05.016.

12. Shanthi T, Sabeenian RS. Modified alexnet architecture for classification of diabetic retinopathy images. *Comput Electr Eng* 2019;76:56–64. https://doi.org/10.1016/j.compeleceng.2019.03.004.

13. Szolovits P. Possibilities for healthcare computing. *J Comput Sci Technol* 2011;26(4):625–31. https://doi.org/10.1007/s11390-011-1162-3.

14. Anwar SM, Majid M, Qayyum A, Awais M, Alnowami M, Khan MK. Medical image analysis using convolutional neural networks: A review. *J Med Syst* 2018;42(11):1–13. https://doi.org/10.1007/s10916-018-1088-1.

15. Faust O, Acharya UR, Ng EYK, Ng KH, Suri JS. Algorithms for the automated detection of diabetic retinopathy using digital fundus images: A review. *J Med Syst* 2012;36:145–57. https://doi.org/10.1007/s10916-010-9454-7.

16. Shweta, EA, Saha S, Bhattacharyya P. Deep learning architecture for patient data de-identification in clinical records. *Proc Clin Nat Lang Process Work* 2016:32–41.

17. Santosh KC, Roy PP. Arrow detection in biomedical images using sequential classi-fier. *Int J Mach Learn Cybern* 2018;9(6):993–1006. https://doi.org/10.1007/s13042-016-0623-y.

18. Razzak MI, Naz S, Zaib A. Deep learning for medical image processing: Overview, challenges and future. *Classif BioApps* 2018:323–50. https://doi.org/10.1007/978-3-319-65981-7_12.

19. Kaushik P, Gupta A, Roy PP, Dogra DP. EEG-based age and gender prediction using deep BLSTM-LSTM network model. *IEEE Sens J* 2019;19(7):2634–41. https://doi.org/10.1109/JSEN.2018.2885582.

20. Lahmar C, Idri A. On the value of deep learning for diagnosing diabetic retinopathy. *Health Technol (Berl)* 2022;12(1):89–105. https://doi.org/10.1007/s12553-021-00606-x.

21. Srinivas M, Roy D, Mohan CK. Discriminative feature extraction from X-ray images using deep convolutional neural networks. *2016 IEEE International Conference on Acoustics, Speech, and Signal Processing (ICASSP)*, 2016:917–21.

22. Lahmar C, Idri A. Deep hybrid architectures for diabetic retinopathy classification. *Comput Methods Biomech Biomed Eng Imaging Vis* 2022:1–19. https://doi.org/10.1080/21681163.2022.2060864.

23. Deepa V, Kumar CS, Cherian T. Ensemble of multi-stage deep convolutional neural networks for automated grading of diabetic retinopathy using image patches. *J King Saud Univ Comput Inf Sci* 2021. https://doi.org/10.1016/j.jksuci.2021.05.009.

24. Ayala A, Ortiz Figueroa T, Fernandes B, Cruz F. Diabetic retinopathy improved detection using deep learning. *Appl Sci* 2021;11(24). https://doi.org/10.3390/app112411970.

25. Zhu CZ, Hu R, Zou BJ, Zhao RC, Chen CL, Xiao YL. Automatic diabetic retinopathy screening via cascaded framework based on image- and lesion-level features fusion. *J Comput Sci Technol* 2019;34(6):1307–18. https://doi.org/10.1007/s11390-019-1977-x.

26. Zhao JJ, Pan L, Zhao PF, Tang XX. Medical sign recognition of lung nodules based on image retrieval with semantic features and supervised hashing. *J Comput Sci Technol* 2017;32(3):457–69. https://doi.org/10.1007/s11390-017-1736-9.

27. Zhang W, Zhong J, Yang S, Gao Z, Hu J, Chen Y, Yi Z. Automated identification and grading system of diabetic retinopathy using deep neural networks. *Knowl Based Syst* 2019;175:12–25. https://doi.org/10.1016/j.knosys.2019.03.016.

28. Krizhevsky, Alex, Ilya Sutskever GEH. ImageNet classification with deep convolutional neural networks. *Adv Neural Inf Process Syst* 2012;2012:1097–105. https://doi.org/10.1201/9781420010749.

29. Roychowdhury S, Koozekanani DD, Parhi KK. DREAM: Diabetic retinopathy analysis using machine learning. *IEEE J Biomed Heal Inform* 2014;18(5):1717–28. https://doi.org/10.1109/JBHI.2013.2294635.

30. Pratt H, Coenen F, Broadbent DM, Harding SP, Zheng Y. Convolutional neural networks for diabetic retinopathy. *Procedia Comput Sci* 2016;90:200–5. https://doi.org/10.1016/j.procs.2016.07.014.

31. Gargeya R, Leng T. Automated identification of diabetic retinopathy using deep learning. *Am J Ophthalmol* 2017;124(7):962–9. https://doi.org/10.1016/j.ophtha.2017.02.008.

32. Pal R, Poray J, Sen M. Application of machine learning algorithms on diabetic retinopathy. *2017 2nd IEEE International Conference on Recent Trends in Electronics, Information & Communication Technology (RTEICT)*, 2017, pp. 2046–51.

33. Dutta S, Manideep BC, Basha SM, Caytiles RD, Iyengar NCSN. Classification of diabetic retinopathy images by using deep learning models. *Int J Grid Distrib Comput* 2018;11(1):99–106. https://doi.org/10.14257/ijgdc.2018.11.1.09.

34. Lam C, Yi D, Guo M, Lindsey T. Automated detection of diabetic retinopathy using deep learning. *AMIA Jt Summit Transl Sci Proceeding* 2018;124:147–55. https://doi.org/10.1016/j.ophtha.2017.02.008.

35. Hemanth DJ, Anitha J, Indumathy A. Diabetic retinopathy diagnosis in retinal images using hopfield neural network. *J Med Syst* 2018;62:893–900. https://doi.org/10.1080/03772063.2016.1221745.

36. Wan S, Liang Y, Zhang Y. Deep convolutional neural networks for diabetic retinopathy detection by image classification. *Comput Electr Eng* 2018;72:274–82. https://doi.org/10.1016/j.compeleceng.2018.07.042.

37. Seth S, Agarwal B. A hybrid deep learning model for detecting diabetic retinopathy. *J Stat Manag Syst* 2018;21(4):569–74. https://doi.org/10.1080/09720510.2018.1466965.

38. Gadekallu TR, Khare N, Bhattacharya S, Singh S, Maddikunta PKR, Srivastava G. Deep neural networks to predict diabetic retinopathy. *J Ambient Intell Humaniz Comput* 2020:1–14. https://doi.org/10.1007/s12652-020-01963-7.

39. Roychowdhury S, Koozekanani DD, Parhi KK. DREAM: Diabetic retinopathy analysis using machine learning. *IEEE J Biomed Heal Inform* 2014;18(5):1717–28. https://doi.org/10.1109/JBHI.2013.2294635.

40. Soni A, Rai A. A novel approach for the early recognition of diabetic retinopathy using machine learning. *2021 International Conference on Computer Communication and Informatics (ICCCI)*, 2021. https://doi.org/10.1109/ICCCI50826.2021.9402566.

41. Yu S, Xiao D, Kanagasingam Y. Exudate detection for diabetic retinopathy with convolutional neural networks. *39th Annual International Conference of the IEEE Engineering in Medicine and Biology Society*. IEEE, 2017, pp. 1744–7. https://doi.org/10.1109/EMBC.2017.8037180.

42. Lam C, Yu C, Huang L, Rubin D. Retinal lesion detection with deep learning using image patches. *Invest Ophthalmol Vis Sci* 2018;59(1):590–6.

43. Chudzik P, Majumdar S, Calivá F, Al-Diri B, Hunter A. Microaneurysm detection using fully convolutional neural networks. *Comput Methods Programs Biomed* 2018;158:185–92. https://doi.org/10.1016/j.cmpb.2018.02.016.

44. Chudzik P, Al-Diri B, Caliva F, Ometto G, Hunter A. Exudates segmentation using fully convolutional neural network and auxiliary codebook. *Annual International Conference of the IEEE Engineering in Medicine and Biology Society EMBS*, 2018, pp. 770–3. https://doi.org/10.1109/EMBC.2018.8512354.

45. Benzamin A, Chakraborty C. Detection of hard exudates in retinal fundus images using deep learning. *2nd International Conference on Imaging, Vision & Pattern Recognition*, 2018, pp. 465–9. https://doi.org/10.1109/ICSCAN.2018.8541246.

46. Long S, Huang X, Chen Z, Pardhan S, Zheng D. Automatic detection of hard exudates in color retinal images using dynamic threshold and SVM classification: Algorithm development and evaluation. *BioMed Res Int* 2019:1–13.

47. Ananda S, Kitahara D, Hirabayashi A, Udaya Kumar Reddy KR. Automatic fundus image segmentation for diabetic retinopathy diagnosis by multiple modified U-nets and segnets. *Asia-Pacific Signal and Information Processing Association Annual Summit and Conference APSIPA ASC*. IEEE, 2019, pp. 1582–8. https://doi.org/10.1109/APSIPAASC47483.2019.9023290.

48. Khojasteh P, Passos Júnior LA, Carvalho T, Rezende E, Aliahmad B, Papa JP, Kumar DK. Exudate detection in fundus images using deeply-learnable features. *Comput Biol Med* 2019;104:62–9. https://doi.org/10.1016/j.compbiomed.2018.10.031.

49. Xiao Q, Zou J, Yang M, Gaudio A, KItani K, Smailagic A, et al. Improving lesion segmentation for diabetic retinopathy using adversarial learning. *International Conference Image Analysis and Recognition, Lecture Notes in Computer Science*. Springer International Publishing, 2019, pp. 333–44. https://doi.org/10.1007/978-3-030-27272-2.

50. Deepa R, Narayanan NK. Detection of microaneurysm in retina image using machine learning approach. *International Conference on Innovative Trends in Information Technology*, 2020, pp. 1–5. https://doi.org/10.1109/icitiit49094.2020.9071522.

51. Mateen M, Wen J, Nasrullah N, Sun S, Hayat S. Exudate detection for diabetic retinopathy using pretrained convolutional neural networks. *Complexity* 2020;2020:1–11. https://doi.org/10.1155/2020/5801870.

52. Sambyal N, Saini P, Syal R, Gupta V. Modified U-Net architecture for semantic segmentation of diabetic retinopathy images. *Biocybern Biomed Eng* 2020;40(3):1094–109. https://doi.org/10.1016/j.bbe.2020.05.006.

8 An Embedded Solution for Real-Time Implementation of a Deep Learning Model for Malicious Breast Tumour Detection

S. Malarvizhi, R. Kayalvizhi,
H. Heartlin Maria, Revathi Venkatraman,
Shatanu Patil, and A. Maria Jossy

8.1 OVERVIEW OF BREAST CARCINOMA

Breast cancer, otherwise known as breast carcinoma or breast malignancy, is an illness that originates as a result of uncontrolled cell multiplication in the breast region. Several types of breast carcinoma exist, and each type is identified by its cell origin. Breasts are composed of a few major components, such as lobules, ducts, and connective tissue, and cancer can arise from any of these components. The lobules are generally presumed to be the glands responsible for milk production. Tubes that transfer the produced milk are known as ducts. Connective tissue surrounds the lobules and ducts and holds them together. The majority of breast malignancy can originate in the ducts and lobules. Breast cancer has the capability to grow outside the breast through blood and lymph arteries. Breast carcinoma affects women of all ages, although it is more common in those over the age of 50. Men can also be affected by breast carcinoma, although it is rare [1–3].

In 2018, a projected 2.08 million women worldwide were diagnosed with breast cancer. In addition, breast cancer accounted for around 24.2% of all malignancies in women. Breast cancer accounted for about one-quarter of all cancer in women. Cancer of the breast was reported as the second-most frequent malignancy in women in 2008, accounting for 115,251 cases. Breast cancer was still the most frequent malignancy in women in 2018, with 162,468 women diagnosed for the first time.

DOI: 10.1201/9781003363361-8

8.1.1   RISK FACTORS OF BREAST CARCINOMA

According to various research findings, there are various risk factors that increase the chances of breast cancer. These are some examples [4]:

(i) **Age:** Women beyond 55 years have a high chance of breast carcinoma.
(ii) **Sex:** Women are at a higher risk of being affected with breast carcinoma when compared to men.
(iii) **Genetic history:** If one's parents or a close relative has a history of breast cancer, one is at a higher risk of developing it.
(iv) **Smoking:** Tobacco usage has been related to several cancers, including breast cancer.
(v) **Consumption of alcoholic beverages:** According to research, drinking alcohol may raise your chance of developing some forms of breast carcinoma.
(vi) **Obesity:** Obesity may increase the probability of contracting breast carcinoma and its reoccurrence.
(vii) **Radiation exposure:** If one has previously had radiation therapy, especially for the head, neck, or chest, one is more likely to develop breast cancer.
(viii) **Hormone replacement:** People who have undertaken hormone replacement therapy (HRT) are often prone to developing breast cancer.

8.1.2   TREATMENT AND PROGNOSIS FOR BREAST CARCINOMA

Breast carcinoma can be treated in several ways [1]. Treatment is defined by the kind of breast cancer and its level of dissemination. Patients with breast cancer usually undergo more than one sort of therapy.

(i) **Surgery:** This is a medical procedure in which the malignant tissue is removed.
(ii) **Chemotherapy:** Cancer cells are shrunk or destroyed using certain drugs. The treatments might be pills that patients take, injections into their veins, or both.
(iii) **Hormone replacement:** This kind of treatment prevents malignant cells from getting the hormones required to grow.
(iv) **Biological treatment:** This treatment aids the body's immune system in attacking cancer cells or reduces the unfavourable effects of other cancer treatments.
(v) **Radiation therapy:** In this process, high-energy radiation is applied to eliminate cancer cells.

8.1.3   PROBLEM STATEMENT

The use of computers to assist radiologists in the capture, administration, and preservation of medical images, as well as in diagnosis, is widely established. Recently, computer algorithms that help radiologists detect probable anomalies in diagnostic radiological scans have been created and authorized for use in clinical practice.

However, the existing computer-aided design (CAD) systems for diagnosis focus on an analysis of any one of the available imaging modalities. But each modality is of significant importance. Therefore, from the observed gap, the idea is to develop a DL model that can both analyze and diagnose multi-modality breast images.

8.1.4 Salient Contributions of this Study

- An artificial intelligence (AI) solution developed and trained to predict breast cancer is multi-modality images.
- Development and implementation of a Field Programmable Gate Array (FPGA)-accelerated hardware platform for real-time breast cancer diagnosis.
- An improvement in the performance accuracy of breast cancer medical diagnosis.
- Reduction in power and time consumption to optimize the diagnostic process.
- Aiding radiologists, oncologists, and gynaecologists in fast and efficient decision-making, which is the need of the hour in cancer research.

8.2 ARTIFICIAL INTELLIGENCE IN BREAST CANCER DIAGNOSIS

Artificial intelligence is becoming more sophisticated at accomplishing what humans do, but does so rather more effectively, swiftly, and cheaply. Lately, the potential of AI has been increasingly vast for diagnostic purposes in the healthcare sector.

8.2.1 Latest Research in the Field

According to a significant new research study published [5], artificial intelligence is a viable tool for breast malignancy detection in mammogram screening. Mammography images collected through breast cancer screening programmes that are population-based greatly increase radiologists' workload. Artificial intelligence has been suggested as an automatic secondary expert for mammogram analysis, which might help to reduce this pressure. Although the technology has shown encouraging results in cancer detection, evidence of its usefulness in real-world screening conditions is limited.

Norwegian researchers conducted the largest study of its kind to date, comparing the findings of a widely viable AI system against the ground truth. Data from approximately 123,000 tests done on over 47,000 women across four different institutions as part of a BreastScreen Norway screening programme were included in the study.

The dataset included 752 cancers found during screening and 205 tumours discovered between rounds of screening. The AI programme calculated the likelihood of cancer on a scale of one to ten, with one being the least risky and ten representing the highest danger. AI scores of ten were obtained by 87.6% of screen-detected tumours and 44.9% of interval malignancies.

The researchers devised three criteria to assess the AI model's performance as a diagnostic tool. By employing a criterion corresponding to the average diagnosis rate of a radiologist, the proportion of tumours seen on film that were not picked up by the AI system was below 20%. While the AI model performed well, the survey's reliance on observational data suggests that more research is needed.

8.2.2 RELATED WORK ON DEEP LEARNING MODELS PROPOSED FOR THE DETECTION OF BREAST CANCER

Deep learning (DL) is an AI subclass that mimics how humans learn specific types of information. Deep learning is a key component of data science, along with statistics and predictive modelling. Deep learning is particularly valuable for data scientists who must gather, analyze, and interpret massive volumes of data; deep learning speeds up and simplifies this process. Various research studies have been carried out in breast cancer diagnosis using deep learning corresponding to different imaging modalities. This section addresses the latest literature in this field diagnosed using DL-based CAD systems and is categorized as per the screening modality preferred for diagnosis.

Shallu Sharma et al. [6] offered two machine learning algorithms for the automated classification of malignancy from histopathology datasets for breast cancer screening. The first method relies on handmade characteristics taken from the Hu moment, colour histogram, and textures. These features were being used to train conventional classifiers, whereas the latter system depends on transfer learning and employs pre-trained networks such as VGG and ResNet. The VGG-16 network incorporating linear SVM produced great accuracy in this situation.

Ashwaq Qasem et al. [7] devised a modified form of the Bees algorithm with the initialization of the selective best step to deliver an optimal ensemble pruning solution. Additionally, integrating ensemble models with equal weights reduces the group's effectiveness. In addition to the Random Star Best (RSB) step initialization, a weighted local majority-based voting method is suggested to solve this problem. Using a mammography imaging dataset provided by a hospital in Kuala Lumpur, the proposed technique to overcome ensemble clipping and fussy problems was evaluated. Using numerous assessment criteria, the results reveal that the proposed technique outperforms previous techniques in the field.

Ahmet et al. [8] suggested a breast MRI classifier based on the DL approach. Magnetic resonance imaging (MRI) has lately been utilized to identify breast cancer in order to reduce needless biopsies. MRI is the standard for recognizing and monitoring breast cancer tumours, as well as for interpreting lesioned areas. Convolutional neural networks (CNNs), on the other hand, have outperformed feature-based approaches in image classification and show promising results in medical imaging. MRI scans were used to classify lesions as either malignant or benign tumours using CNN. A multi-layer CNN architecture with online data augmentation was created using just pixel information. The CNN architecture was later taught and evaluated. The network's accuracy is 98.33%.

He Ma et al. [9] proposed the Fuz2Net, a groundbreaking deep learning network, to improve performance in recognizing carcinoma and non-carcinoma breast ultrasound tumour images, enabling rapid breast tumour screening. A second dataset of 100 breast tumour scans of cancerous and non-cancerous cases that had not been used in network training was used to evaluate the classification model. This fuzzy-based DL network resulted in 92% accuracy while classifying benign and malignant cases.

8.2.3 FPGA ACCELERATION FOR DEEP LEARNING

A field-programmable gate array (FPGA) is a reprogrammable logic gate hardware circuit. By overwriting a chip's settings, users can develop a bespoke circuit when the chip is deployed in the field (rather than only during the design or fabrication process). FPGA chips are very beneficial in machine learning and deep learning. Using FPGA for deep learning, for example, allows you to improve throughput and adjust processors to fit the particular demands of various deep learning architectures. Even if the use of deep learning in healthcare is increasing for a variety of applications, the acceleration of deep learning models remains an unexplored field. FPGAs are excellent accelerators for deep learning networks. Researchers are gradually introducing FPGA acceleration for DL in the healthcare industry. A few examples of such works are described below.

Siyu Xiong et al. [10] suggested a deep learning-based CAD system for brain tumour segmentation that was expedited utilizing FPGAs. When compared to standard computer systems, the proposed FPGA accelerator offers much higher performance and lower power consumption. The FPGA-dependent brain tumour segmentation accelerator is 5.21 and 44.47 times quicker than the graphics processing unit (GPU) and central processing unit (CPU) on the BraTS datasets, respectively. Furthermore, as compared to the GPU and CPU, the architecture achieves 11.22 and 82.33 times the energy efficiency.

Omiya Hassan et al. [11] proposed a digital hardware approach for detecting sleep apnea that uses a feed-forward model built on FPGA. The network was trained and evaluated with hyperparameters generated from an optimization approach that guarantees a succinct conceptual framework in minimal-power miniaturized complementary metal oxide semi-conductor (CMOS) circuits. A network trained using Adam Optimizer has an accuracy of roughly 88%. The results of the study can be incorporated into a system-on-a-chip (SoC) platform to create an artificial intelligence-driven sleep apnea detection device.

With these advancements and state-of-the-art technologies in mind, we have proposed an FPGA-accelerated ensemble deep learning model for breast cancer diagnosis for various imaging techniques.

8.3 METHODOLOGY AND ARCHITECTURAL DETAILS OF THE PROPOSED FLOW

The proposed method is an ensemble model comprising three deep learning networks, trained to diagnose multiple breast cancer imaging modalities such as mammogram, ultrasound, MRI, and histopathology. The developed ensemble model is accelerated using a Python productivity for ZYNQ (PYNQ) FPGA hardware board to optimize the performance. The proposed flow of the breast carcinoma binary classifier, which outputs the benign or malignant diagnosis of various imaging modalities, is shown in Figure 8.1.

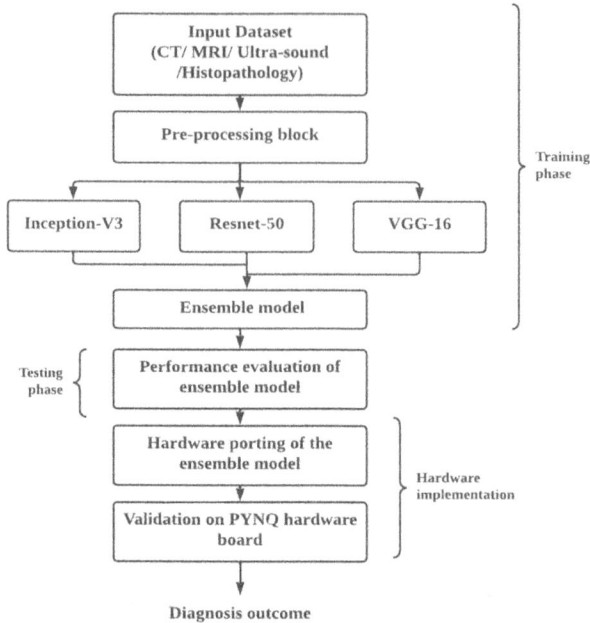

FIGURE 8.1   Proposed flow of test-bed approach of the breast cancer classification model.

(i) Dataset

The proposed model was trained and tested on benchmark mammogram, histopa-thology, MRI, and ultrasound datasets. The total available datasets were balanced equally and split in a ratio of eight-to-two for training and testing, respectively. Also, the developed model was later tested on real-time breast cancer cases from SRM Medical College, Hospital, and Research Centre, for which ethical clearance was obtained.

The benchmark breast ultrasound dataset used contained images from women aged 25 to 75. This information was gathered in 2018. There were 600 female patients in all. The dataset contained 780 photos, each of which was 500 × 500 pix-els in size. PNG files were used for the images. Original photos were shown with the ground truth images [12].

The benchmark MIAS database of mammograms used was lowered to a pixel edge of 200 microns and clipped and padded such that each picture was 1024 × 1024 pixels [13].

The benchmark histopathology dataset used contained a huge number of tiny pathological pictures to categorize. An image identifier was assigned to each file. The training labels which are in comma separated values (CSV) file format is the source of ground truth for the dataset in the train folder [14]. In the benchmark MRI data-set that was utilized, ages were classified as Healthy (Benign) or Sick (Malignant). Both categories comprised 700 MRI scan pictures of both healthy and ill people for training purposes. Both categories comprised 40 MRI scan pictures of both healthy and ill individuals for validation [15].

(ii) Preprocessing

Since the datasets used for training were benchmark datasets which were free from instrumental noise, de-noising was not applied to the training dataset. However, as the benchmark datasets were gathered from various sources, the dimensions of each dataset were different and, hence, the images were resized to 150×150 pixels before processing.

(iii) Transfer learning

The application of a previously learned model to a new issue is referred to as transfer learning in machine learning. In transfer learning, a computer uses prior task skills to increase generalization about a new task. Rather than starting from zero, we begin using patterns discovered through completing a similar activity. In computer vision, for example, neural networks are widely used to recognize edges in the first layer, forms in the intermediate layer, and task-specific properties in later layers. The early and intermediate layers are used in transfer learning, but only the latter layers are retrained. This aids in the use of the labelled data from the first project on which it was trained.

(iv) Ensemble model

After preprocessing, the dataset was then sent into the ensemble model for training. Ensemble modelling is a method in which numerous distinct models are developed to predict a result, either by utilizing many separate modelling techniques or by employing a combination of modelling algorithms. The ensemble model then combines each model's estimate, yielding a single final prediction for the unseen data. The dataset consisted of images of both cancerous and non-cancerous breast tumours and masses in order to train the ensemble model to classify both benign and malignant cases.

Inception V3 is a convolutional neural network-based deep learning model for picture classification. Inception V3 is an upgraded version of Inception V1, which was released in 2014 as GoogLeNet. As the name suggests, it was designed by a Google team.

VGG-16 is a 16-layer deep convolutional neural network. The network's pre-trained version is trained on over a million pictures from the ImageNet collection. The pre-trained network can categorize data into 1000 different item categories.

ResNet has numerous variants that follow the same idea but have different numbers of layers. The name ResNet-50 refers to a variant that may operate with 50 neural network layers. This network's pre-trained version is also trained on over a million photos from the ImageNet collection. The pre-trained network can classify input into 1000 unique item categories.

(v) Implementation of hardware board

The implemented ensemble model was accelerated using the PYNQ-Z2 board. The PYNQ-Z2 is an FPGA development board based on the ZYNQ XC7Z020 FPGA that has been rigorously built to support PYNQ, a new open-source framework that allows embedded programmers to explore the capabilities of Xilinx ZYNQ SoCs without having to create programming logic circuits.

The weights of each deep learning network of the ensemble model were saved in hierarchical file format (H5) and these H5 files were imported to the PYNQ board. The weight files of the saved model were then executed using the Python Jupyter platform available on the PYNQ API. The desired Python libraries such as OpenCV, Keras, TensorFlow, etc. were also installed on the PYNQ board, as per the DL model requirement. The test images were uploaded to the secure digital (SD) card of the PYNQ board for testing, and the time taken for the prediction of each case was monitored on the PYNQ board and was observed to be much faster than the time consumed for each prediction on CPU and GPU systems.

The subjective results of the simulation and comparative analysis performed on both software and hardware are provided elaborately in the following sections.

8.4 SOFTWARE PERFORMANCE ANALYSIS OF THE MODELS AND THEIR MODALITIES

In this section, the software simulation results of the three DL networks – namely VGG-16, ResNet-50, and Inception V3 – for each modality is discussed along with the ensemble model.

The models were trained using 25 epochs with an early stopping condition to avoid overfitting issues. Early stopping is an optimization approach that reduces overfitting while maintaining model correctness. The basic goal of early stopping is to terminate training before a model becomes overfit. The optimizer used for this process is Adam with a learning rate of 0.0001. The learning rate governs how quickly the model adjusts to a new circumstance. Smaller learning rates need more training epochs due to smaller changes in the weights with each update, whereas higher learning rates yield faster changes and require fewer training epochs.

(i) Magnetic resonance imaging

As observed from the accuracy and loss plots of Figure 8.2, it is evident that VGG-16 has resulted in better validation of MRI data classification than the other two networks. The confusion matrix in Figure 8.3 is used to extract the performance measures in Table 8.1. From Table 8.1, it is significant that the ensemble model has yielded better performance than the other individual networks. Precision is a measure of how many positive predictions were made by the model. For the MRI dataset, the precision of VGG-16 is next-best to the ensemble model.

Resnet-50

VGG-16

Inception V3

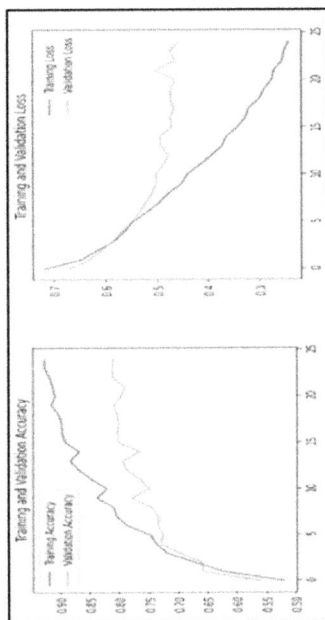

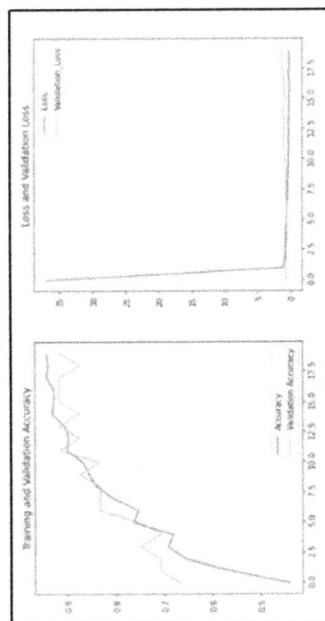

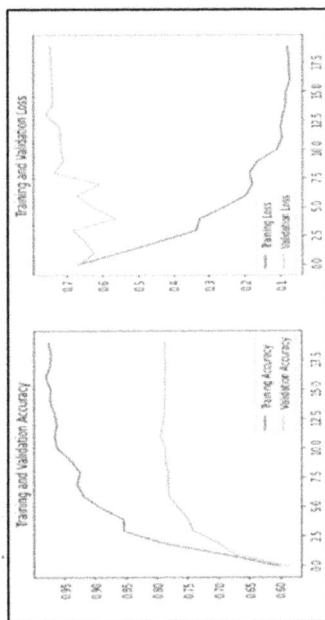

FIGURE 8.2 Loss and accuracy plots of MRI data classification.

(i) Ultrasound

As observed from the accuracy and loss plots of Figure 8.5, it is evident that ResNet-50 resulted in better validation of ultrasound data classification than the other two networks. The confusion matrix in Figure 8.4 is used to extract the performance measures in Table 8.2. From Table 8.2, it is significant that the ensemble model has yielded better performance than the other individual networks. For the ultrasound dataset, the precision of ResNet-50 is next-best to the ensemble model.

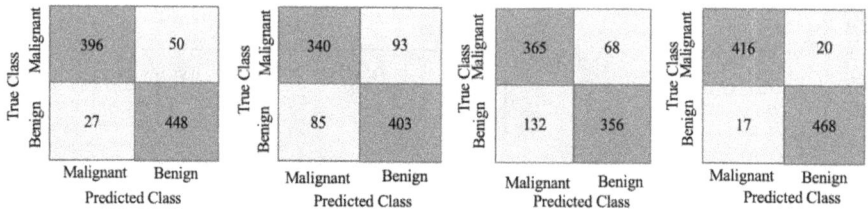

FIGURE 8.3   Confusion of MRI data classification.

TABLE 8.1
Performance Measures of MRI Data Classification.

Model	Class	Accuracy	Precision	Recall	F1 Score
VGG-16	Malignant	91.6	0.94	0.89	0.91
	Benign		0.90	0.94	0.92
ResNet-50	Malignant	80.6	0.80	0.79	0.79
	Benign		0.81	0.82	0.81
Inception V3	Malignant	78.2	0.73	0.84	0.78
	Benign		0.84	0.73	0.77
Ensemble	Malignant	95.9	0.96	0.95	0.95
	Benign		0.95	0.96	0.95

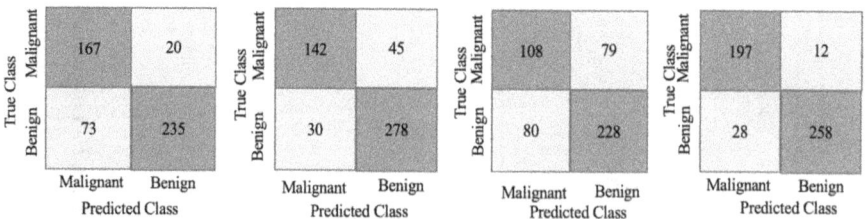

FIGURE 8.4   Confusion of ultrasound data classification.

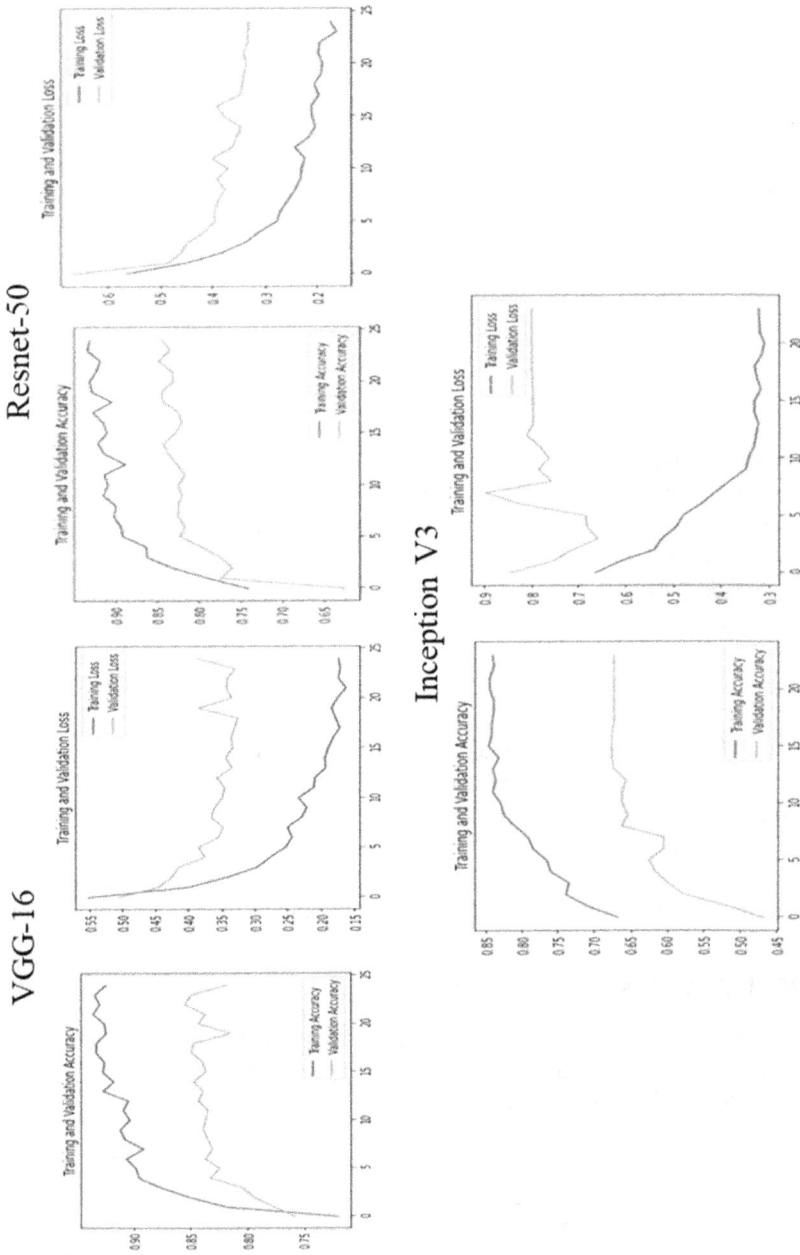

FIGURE 8.5 Loss and accuracy plots of ultrasound data classification.

TABLE 8.2

Performance Measures of Ultrasound Data Classification

Model	Class	Accuracy	Precision	Recall	F1 Score
VGG-16	Malignant	81.2	0.70	0.89	0.78
	Benign		0.92	0.76	0.83
ResNet-50	Malignant	84.8	0.83	0.76	0.79
	Benign		0.86	0.90	0.88
Inception V3	Malignant	67.8	0.57	0.57	0.56
	Benign		0.74	0.74	0.73
Ensemble	Malignant	91.9	0.88	0.94	0.91
	Benign		0.96	0.90	0.93

(ii) Histopathology

As observed from the accuracy and loss plots of Figure 8.6, it is evident that VGG-16 resulted in better validation of histopathology data classification than the other two networks. The confusion matrix in Figure 8.7 is used to extract the performance measures in Table 8.3. From Table 8.3, it is significant that the ensemble model has yielded better performance than the other individual networks. For the histopathology dataset, the precision of VGG-16 is next-best to the ensemble model.

(ii) Mammogram

As observed from the accuracy and loss plots of Figure 8.8, it is evident that ResNet-50 resulted in better validation of mammogram data classification than the other two networks. The confusion matrix in Figure 8.9 is used to extract the performance measures in Table 8.4. From Table 8.4, it is significant that the ensemble model has yielded better performance than the other individual networks. For the mammogram dataset, the precision of ResNet-50 is next-best to the ensemble model.

8.5   REAL-TIME TESTING RESULTS

In this section, the subjective results of hardware testing are provided. The hardware setup was tested using benchmark datasets as well as real-time datasets. The flow of the real-time testing is shown in Figure 8.10.

(i) Magnetic resonance imaging

In Figure 8.11, a clear visualization of the consecutive hardware deployment results of 16 MRI datasets is provided, where the "actual" label represents the ground truth and the "predicted" label represents the classification provided by the hardware. The

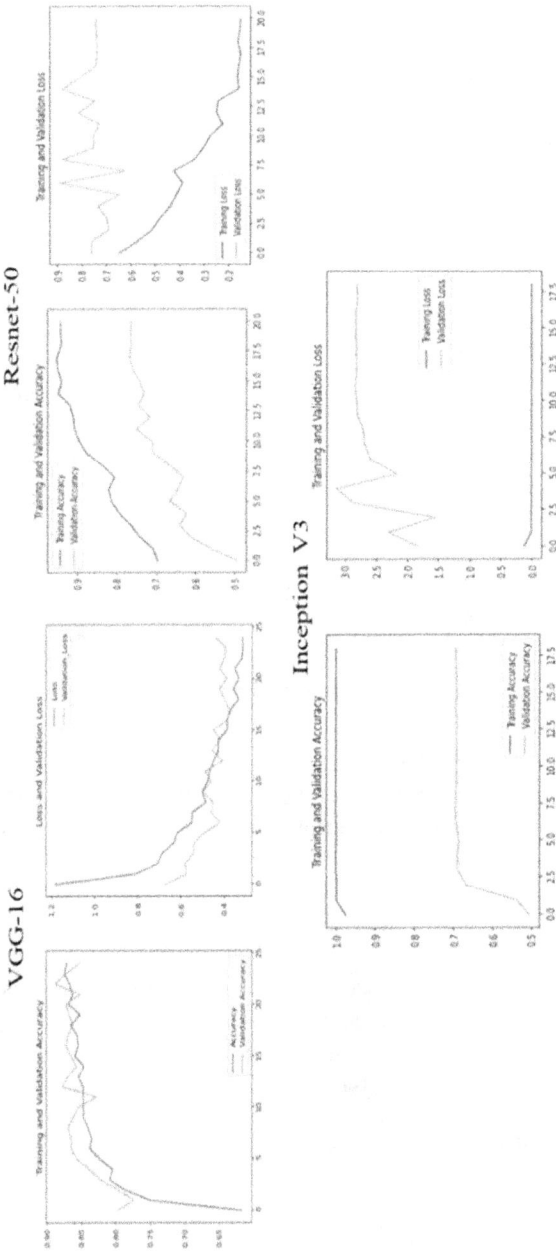

FIGURE 8.6 Loss and accuracy plots of histopathology data classification.

VGG-16		Resnet-50		Inception V3		Ensemble	
247	74	85	122	156	168	283	54
78	620	138	674	152	543	48	634

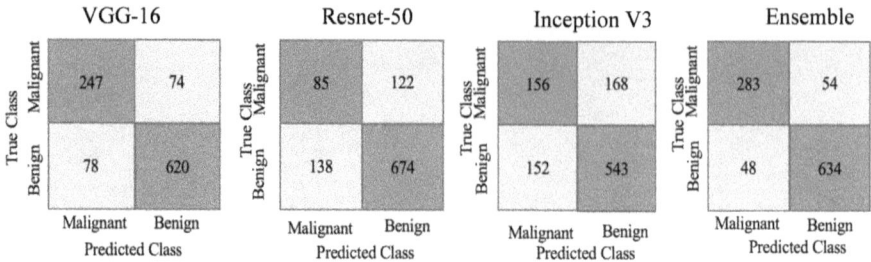

FIGURE 8.7   Confusion of histopathology data classification.

TABLE 8.3
Performance Measures of Histopathology Data Classification

Model	Class	Accuracy	Precision	Recall	F1 score
VGG-16	Malignant	85.0	0.76	0.77	0.76
	Benign		0.89	0.88	0.89
ResNet-50	Malignant	74.5	0.38	0.41	0.40
	Benign		0.S5	0.83	0.S4
Inception V3	Malignant	68.59	0.51	0.48	0.48
	Benign		0.76	0.78	0.77
Ensemble	Malignant	89.9	0.85	0.84	0.85
	Benign		0.92	0.93	0.92

hardware setup of the PYNQ board for MRI data classification is shown in Figure 8.12, and the time taken for each prediction was observed to be 10.62 milliseconds. Also, the power consumption of the setup was measured using a power meter and was found to be 3.4 watts.

(ii) Ultrasound

In Figure 8.13, a clear visualization of the consecutive hardware deployment results of 16 ultrasound datasets is provided, where the "actual" label represents the ground truth and the "predicted" label represents the classification provided by the hardware. The hardware setup of the PYNQ board for ultrasound data classification is shown in Figure 8.14 and the time taken for each prediction was observed to be 10.14 milliseconds. Also, the power consumption of the setup was measured using a power meter and was found to be 3.2 watts.

(iii) Histopathology

In Figure 8.15, a clear visualization of the consecutive hardware deployment results of 16 histopathology datasets is provided, where the "actual" label represents the

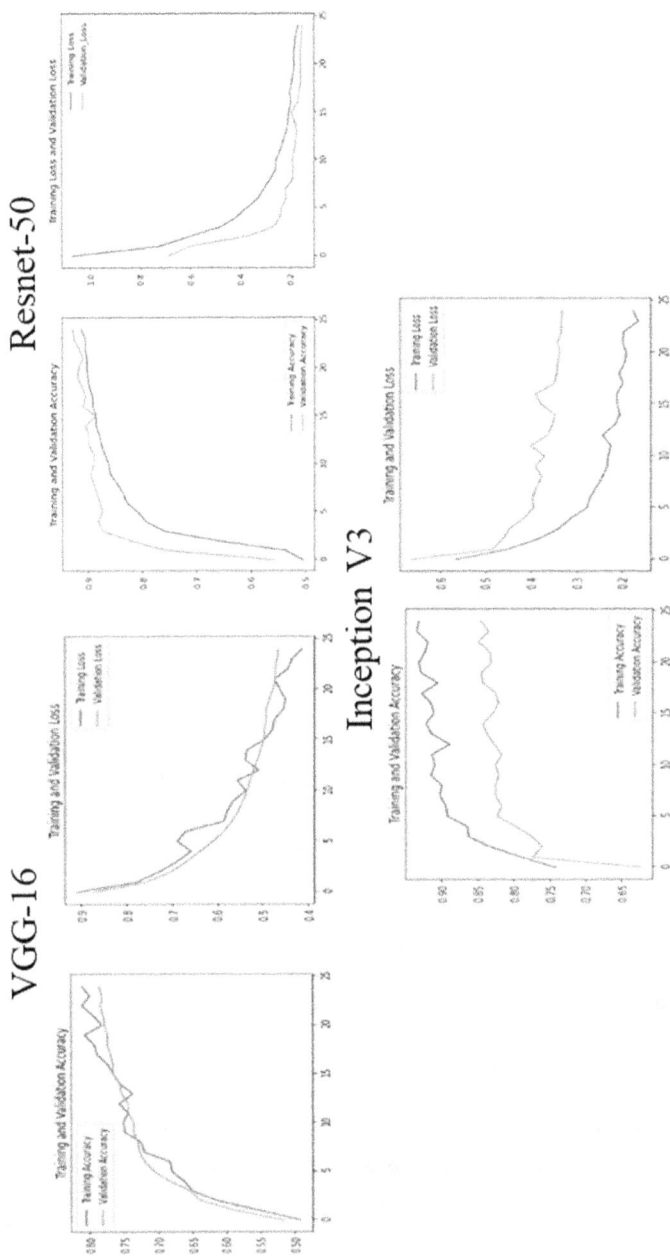

FIGURE 8.8 Loss and accuracy plots of mammogram data classification.

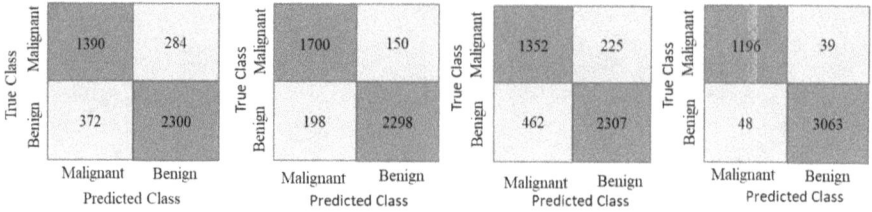

FIGURE 8.9   Confusion of mammogram data classification.

TABLE 8.4
Performance Measures of Mammogram Data Classification

Model	Class	Accuracy	Precision	Recall	F1 score
VGG-16	Malignant	84.9	0.78	0.83	0.80
	Benign		0.89	0.86	0.86
ResNet-50	Malignant	91.9	0.89	0.92	0.89
	Benign		0.94	0.92	0.93
Inception V3	Malignant	84.1	0.75	0.86	0.80
	Benign		0.92	0.83	0.87
Ensemble	Malignant	97.9	0.96	0.97	0.96
	Benign		0.98	0.98	0.98

ground truth and the "predicted" label represents the classification provided by the hardware. The hardware setup of the PYNQ board for histopathology data classification is shown in Figure 8.16, and the time taken for each prediction was observed to be 10.46 milliseconds. Also, the power consumption of the setup was measured using a power meter and was found to be 3.4 watts.

(iv) Mammogram

In Figure 8.17, a clear visualization of the consecutive hardware deployment results of 16 mammogram datasets is provided, where the "actual" label represents the ground truth and the "predicted" label represents the classification provided by the hardware. The hardware setup of the PYNQ board for mammogram data classification is shown in Figure 8.18, and the time taken for each prediction was observed to be 10.12 milliseconds. Also, the power consumption of the setup was measured using a power meter and was found to be 3.6 watts.

```
┌─────────────────────────────┐
│        Scanning unit        │
│  (Mammogram/ultra-sound/    │
│      histopathology/MRI)    │
└─────────────────────────────┘
              │
              ▼
┌─────────────────────────────┐
│    Picture Archiving and    │
│   Communication System      │
│           (PACS)            │
└─────────────────────────────┘
              │
              ▼
┌─────────────────────────────┐
│   Export the medical image  │
│  from PACS to the desktop in│
│     the desired format      │
│      (DICOM,JPG etc)        │
└─────────────────────────────┘
              │
              ▼
┌─────────────────────────────┐
│  Import the acquired image  │
│  onto the PYNQ hardware     │
│           board             │
└─────────────────────────────┘
              │
              ▼
┌─────────────────────────────┐
│  Run the neural network to  │
│   get the diagnosis results │
└─────────────────────────────┘
```

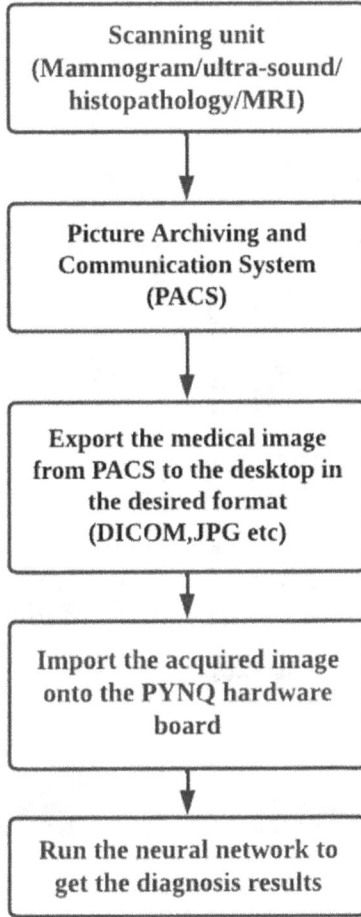

FIGURE 8.10   Flow diagram of real-time testing.

8.6 CONCLUSION

Early detection of breast carcinoma, followed by proper treatment, can reduce the mortality rate to a vast extent and thereby aid women around the globe. This artificial intelligence-based breast carcinoma classifier accelerated by the PYNQ hardware board is an efficient and significant method which contributes to breast cancer diagnosis. This method is an ensemble model which is based on multiple deep learning networks trained on multi-modality breast imagery, making it suitable for various forms of diagnostic purposes, such as early detection, localization, spread of cancer, and so on. The simulation results have revealed that, with FPGA acceleration, this

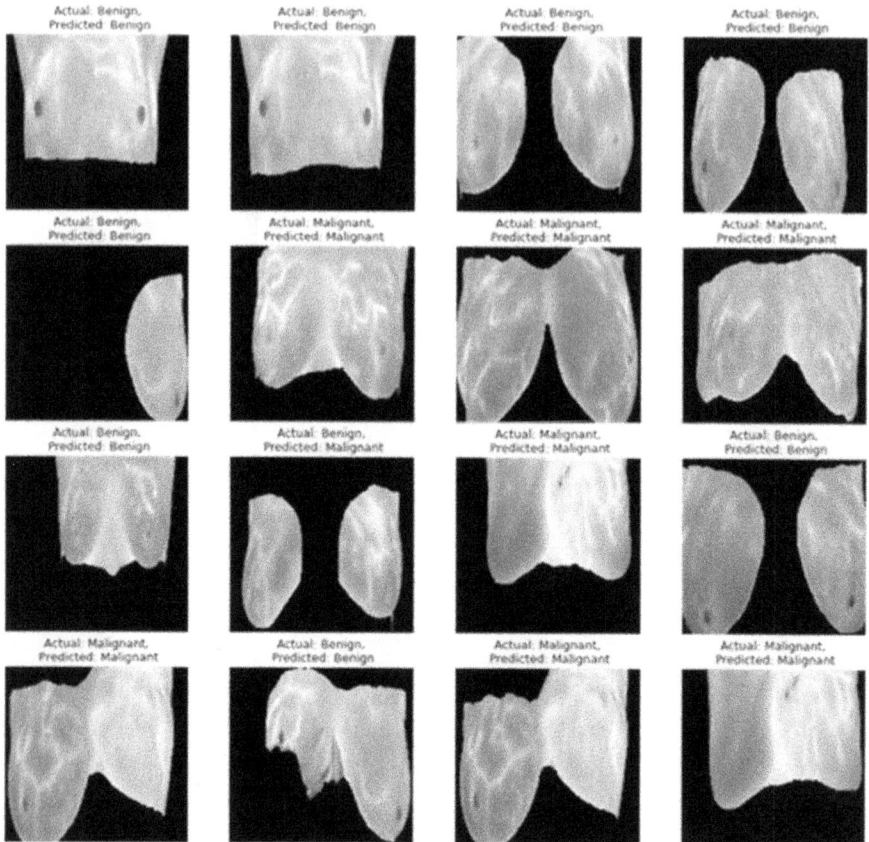

FIGURE 8.11 Hardware testing results of MRI dataset.

model can predict the diagnosis result in milliseconds. The average time taken by the ensemble model to diagnose an image is 10.40 milliseconds and the average power consumption required for this prototype is less than 3.4 watts. This form of rapid diagnostic prediction can aid radiologists, oncologists, and healthcare professionals as a means of a second confirmation in the diagnosis of breast cancer. In the future, we would like to focus on more subclassification of breast cancer and its staging to assist doctors further in the field.

ACKNOWLEDGEMENT

The authors would like to acknowledge Xilinx for sponsoring the hardware boards used in this study.

Funding

This work was funded by the Xilinx Women in Technology Fall Grant 2021.

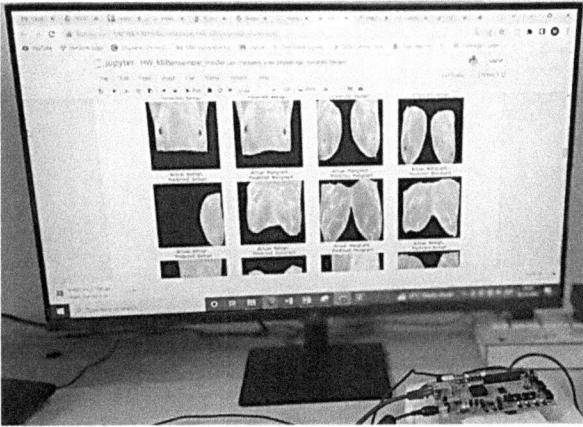

FIGURE 8.12 Hardware implementation setup of MRI dataset.

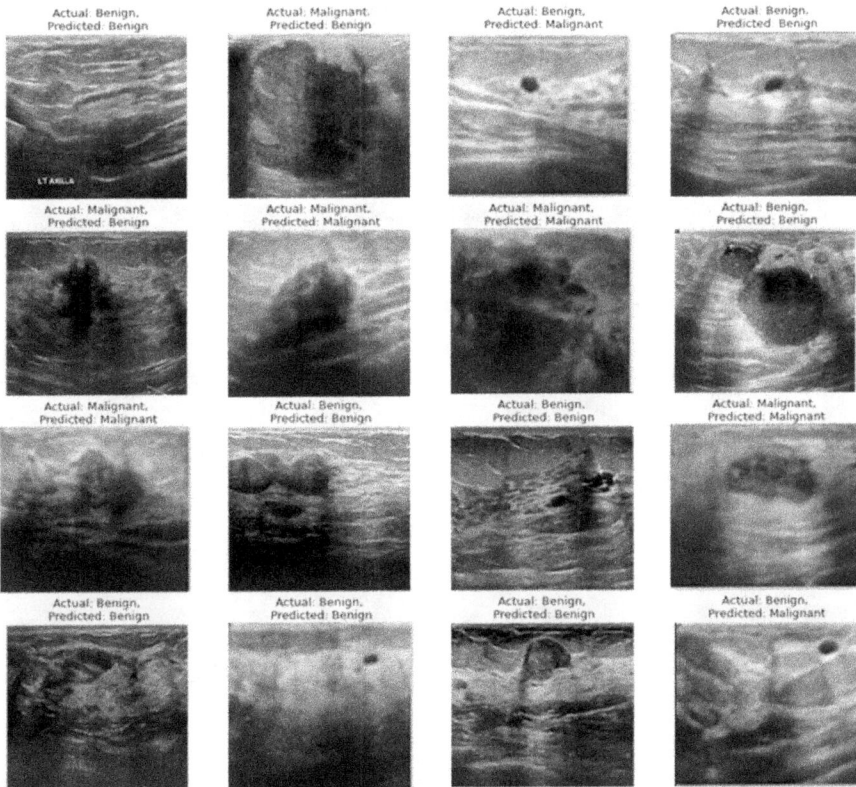

FIGURE 8.13 Hardware testing results of ultrasound dataset.

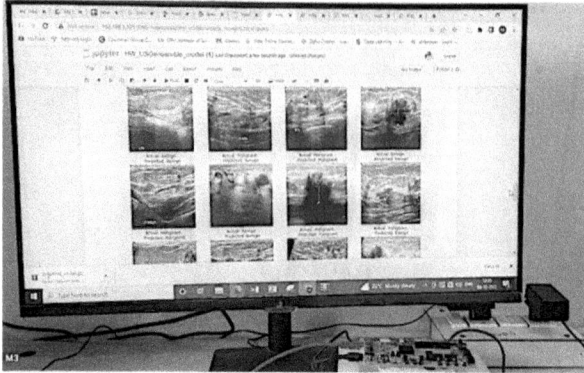

FIGURE 8.14 Hardware implementation setup of ultrasound dataset.

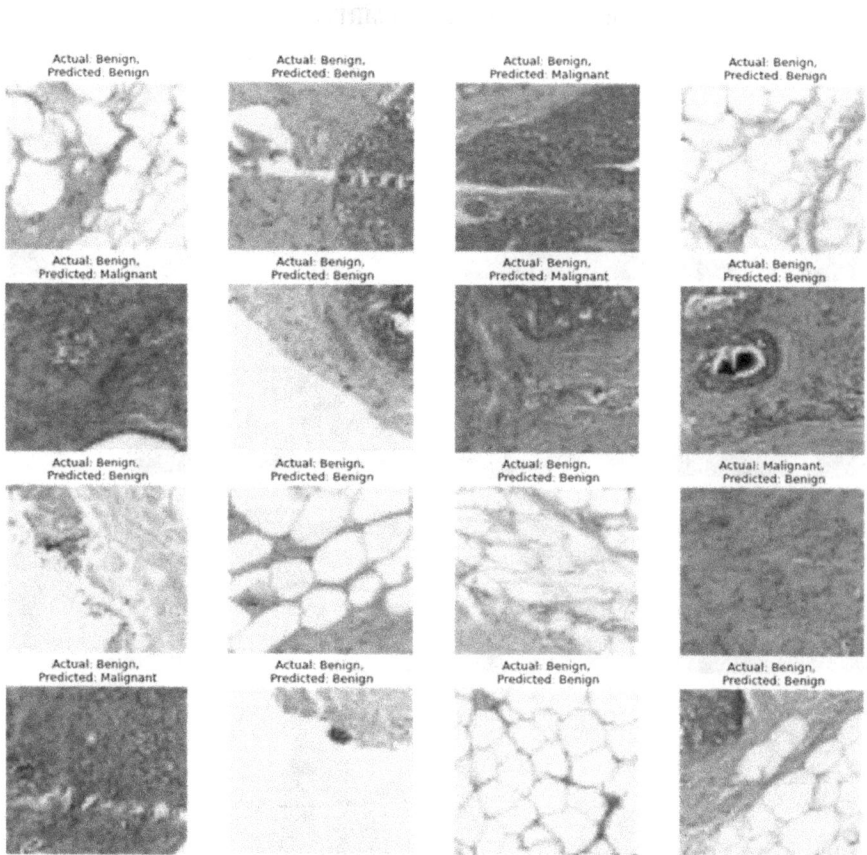

FIGURE 8.15 Hardware testing results of histopathology dataset.

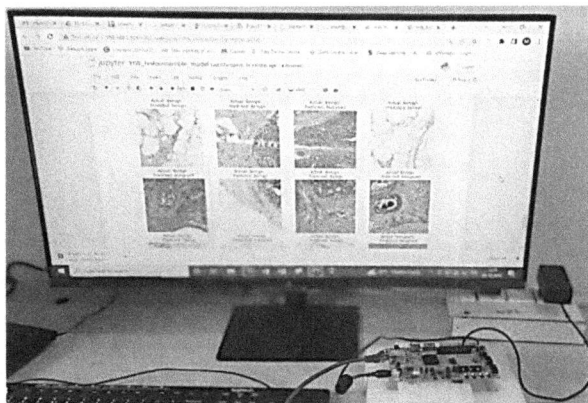

FIGURE 8.16 Hardware implementation setup of histopathology dataset.

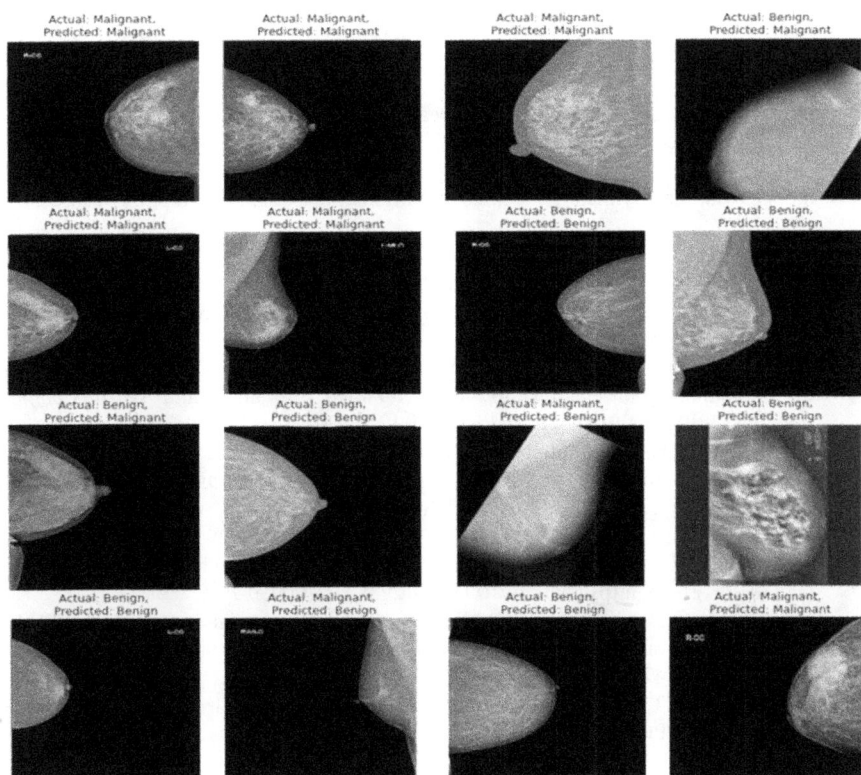

FIGURE 8.17 Hardware testing results of mammogram dataset.

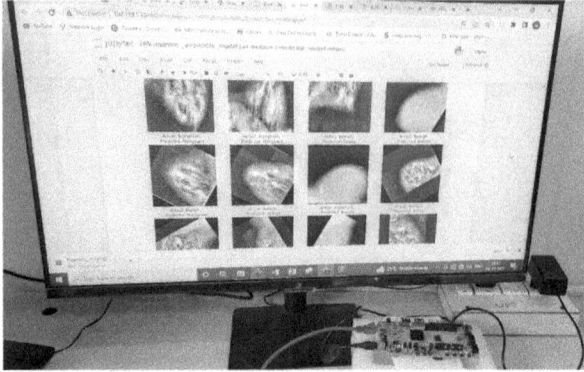

FIGURE 8.18 Hardware implementation setup of mammogram dataset.

REFERENCES

1. Centers for Disease Control and Prevention. (2020) Breast cancer: Things you should know. Retrieved from https://www.cdc.gov/cancer/breast/basic_info/what-is-breast -cancer.html.
2. https://my.clevelandclinic.org/health/diseases/3986-breast-cancer.
3. https://www.uicc.org/news/globocan-2020-new-global-cancer-data# Manage with L (2022) Breast cancer, 1–20.
4. https://www.mayoclinic.org/diseases-conditions/breast-cancer/symptoms-causes/syc -20352470.
5. https://www.radiologyinfo.org/en/info/screening-breast.
6. Sharma S, Mehra R (2020) Conventional machine learning and deep learning approach for multi-classification of breast cancer histopathology images—A comparative insight. *J Digit Imaging* 33(3):632–654. https://doi.org/10.1007/s10278-019-00307-y.
7. Qasem A, Sheikh Abdullah SNH, Sahran S, et al. (2022) An improved ensemble pruning for mammogram classification using modified Bees algorithm. *Neural Comput Appl* 34(12):10093–10116. https://doi.org/10.1007/s00521-022-06995-y.
8. Yurttakal AH, Erbay H, İkizceli T, Karaçavuş S (2020) Detection of breast cancer via deep convolution neural networks using MRI images. *Multimed Tool Appl* 79(21–22):15555–15573. https://doi.org/10.1007/s11042-019-7479-6.
9. Ma II, Tian R, Li H, et al. (2021) Fus2Net: A novel Convolutional Neural Network for classification of benign and malignant breast tumor in ultrasound images. *Biomed Eng Online* 20(1):1–15. https://doi.org/10.1186/s12938-021-00950-z.
10. Xiong S, Wu G, Fan X, et al. (2021) MRI-based brain tumor segmentation using FPGA-accelerated neural network. *BMC Bioinformatics* 22(1):1–15. https://doi.org/10.1186/ s12859-021-04347-6.
11. Hassan O, Paul T, Shuvo MMH, et al. (2022) Energy efficient deep learning inference embedded on FPGA for sleep apnea detection. *J Signal Process Syst* 94(6):609–619. https://doi.org/10.1007/s11265-021-01722-7.
12. Al-Dhabyani W, Gomaa M, Khaled H, Fahmy A (2020) Dataset of breast ultrasound images. *Data Brief* 28:104863. https://doi.org/10.1016/j.dib.2019.104863.

13. Moreira IC, Amaral I, Domingues I, et al. (2012) INbreast: Toward a full-field digital mammographic database. *Acad Radiol* 19(2):236–248. https://doi.org/10.1016/j.acra .2011.09.014.
14. https://www.kaggle.com/code/abhinand05/histopathologic-cancer-detection-using -cnns/data.
15. https://www.kaggle.com/datasets/uzairkhan45/breast-cancer-patients-mris.

9 Towards Robust Diagnosis of Alzheimer's Disease Using Ensemble Framework of Convolutional Neural Network and Vision Transformer

Poonguzhali Elangovan and Malaya Kumar Nath

9.1 INTRODUCTION

The brain is the most complicated organ in the human body. It is in charge of most bodily activities, such as processing, integrating, and coordinating sensory information from various sense organs. Hence, the normal and active functioning of the brain is critical in enabling daily activities. Some disorders, such as Alzheimer's disease (AD), schizophrenia (SZ), Parkinson's disease (PD), dementia, and brain tumours, can impair brain function. In developed countries, the pervasiveness of AD is estimated to affect 5% of people over the age of 65 and a staggering 30% of people over the age of 85 [1]. By 2050, it is expected that 0.64 billion individuals are going to be affected by this disease [2]. AD mainly affects the portion of the brain responsible for memory. It causes brain cells to deteriorate and, hence, AD patients experience memory loss in the early stages. People with AD lose their ability to respond to their surroundings as the disease progresses. They frequently misplace time and may misidentify family members as strangers. As a result, they may become aggressive or prone to wandering out of the house. In the advanced stage, AD eventually results in death by ruining the brain section liable for breathing and cardiac function. Hence, timely screening of AD is critical. Moreover, early diagnosis can save patients from unneeded pharmacologic therapies and their side effects. Alzheimer's disease is a catastrophic neurological dysfunction that impairs memory and cognitive abilities. The clinical manifestation of AD is the excessive production

DOI: 10.1201/9781003363361-9

of beta-amyloid [1]. Cell loss and damage occur as the hippocampus shrinks [3]. Due to this, neurons can no longer respond through synapses. This affects memory and thinking ability [1]. Owing to the unavailability of a cure for AD, the only way to slow cognitive decline is to remove amyloid from the brain [3]. However, due to the slow progression of AD, diagnosis at an early stage is quite challenging. Screening of AD is cumbersome, as symptoms occur at the final stage. Thus, effective diagnosis of AD is critical. Physical and neurobiological examinations, as well as a detailed history of the patient, are required for proper assessment of AD. Furthermore, imaging plays a dominant role in AD diagnosis. Neurologists have used magnetic resonance imaging (MRI) to visualize the structure and functionality of the brain. They ascertain AD signs and conduct various examinations to diagnose AD. Accurate diagnosis may be possible with these examinations. Appropriate medications can be recommended based on the stages of AD (such as moderate, mild, and very mild). Pathologies associated with AD can be detected in MRI images. This distinguishes the MRI modality as the notable one in AD diagnosis.

Clinical diagnosis of AD requires a trained expert and may be amenable to intra-/inter-observer errors due to the numerous control parameters involved. Furthermore, the imaging instruments employed are expensive and bulky. Though the pathological features are noticeable in the MRI images, clinical examination is a tedious process. Therefore, utilizing a computer-aided detection (CAD) technique for AD diagnosis is essential. Machine learning (ML) and deep learning (DL) are progressively being deployed to extract pertinent features from brain imaging data as technology advances. This research aims to boost the outcome of AD categorization using deep learning techniques. The following are the primary goals of this work:

- To investigate the performance of EfficientNet-B0 and vision transformers for the categorization of AD stages from MRI images.
- To illustrate the efficacy of classifiers like KNN, softmax, Bi-LSTM, and SVM towards the AD classification task.
- To explore the effectiveness of feature selection techniques like wavelet transform and principal component analysis (PCA).
- To propose a novel ensemble model based on a stacking technique to enhance overall performance.

The subsequent sections of the paper are structured as follows. Section 9.2 offers a quick overview of the existing work. The database and suggested approach are explained in Section 9.3. Sections 9.4 and 9.5 discuss the outcomes and conclusions, respectively.

9.2 RELATED WORK

Deep CNN learns effective attributes in a stratified manner. As a result, these networks are an excellent choice for image classification tasks such as glaucoma classification [4, 5], malaria parasite detection [6], breast cancer detection [7], and skin cancer detection [8]. Several algorithms have been developed in recent years for

AD classification using CNN. Authors have employed various models for effective feature extraction and classification. Either a 2D CNN or 3D CNN is employed in existing works. In some works [9–16], either a pre-trained model or own CNN is employed, whereas other works [17–19] deal with vision transformers (ViTs).

Payan et al. [10] have described an approach that uses a sparse autoencoder and 3D CNN. MRI images from patients over the age of 75 are used. The method captured the features using 3D-CNN. The authors reported satisfactory classification results among mild cognitive impairment (MCI), normal, and AD, with 89.5% accuracy. Classification of the healthy and AD in older adults using a two-stage pipeline is employed in Sarraf and Tofighi [20]. Significant preprocessing was done in the first stage to remove distortion from the data. Following that, a CNN model using LeNet and GoogLeNet was implemented. The authors have obtained an overall accuracy of 99.9% and 98.84% using structural functional magnetic resonance imaging (fMRI) and structural MRI data, respectively.

Maysam et al. [21] have incorporated the conditional deep triplet network to overcome the data scarcity in machine learning problems. The Siamese and triplet networks are investigated for the AD classification task. Features are extracted from MRI images using VGG-16 as the base model. The models were tested using 87 very mild dementia images, 167 normal images, 105 mild dementia images, and 23 moderate dementia images from the OASIS database. The authors have concluded that the conditional triplet model outperforms with an overall classification accuracy of 99.41%.

Investigation of ResNet and GoogLeNet for multiclass classification is carried out by Farooq et al. [12]. Suitable preprocessing is carried out prior to feature extraction. Based on the obtained probability scores, an input image is categorized into AD, normal, MCI, and late mild cognitive impairment (LMCI) classes. Authors have reported an accuracy of 98.8% and 97.9% in four-class and three-class classification tasks, respectively. Spasov et al. suggest a parameter-efficient 3D CNN to overcome the overfitting problem [11]. The detailed pertinent features from structural MRI images are extracted using 3D separable and grouped convolutions. An overall classification accuracy of 86% is reported in a subset of the Alzheimer's Disease Neuroimaging Initiative (ADNI) database (192 AD, 409 MCI, and 184 healthy controls (HC)).

Luo et al. proposed a compact 3D CNN model for binary classification [22]. Evaluation is carried out using MRI scans (34 normal and 47 AD patients) obtained from the ADNI database. Their work claims a recall of 100% and a specificity of 93%. Korolev et al. investigated the effectiveness of plain CNN and residual CNN for multi-classification tasks via binary classification [13]. The pre-trained VGG model is modified to develop the VoxCNN. The efficacy of the models is evaluated using MRI scans obtained from a subset of the ADNI database, comprising 50 AD, 43 LMCI, 77 early mild cognitive impairment (EMCI), and 61 normal cohort (NC). The authors have concluded that the classification of AD and NC produced better results with accuracies of 79% and 80% using VoxCNN and ResNet, respectively.

Hon et al. carried out an investigation of VGG-16, VGG-19, and Inception V4 [14]. Both naive learning and transfer learning techniques were employed for binary classification. The models were evaluated using 200 randomly-selected subjects from the OASIS database. The authors considered 6400 images with equal instances of AD and non-demented cases. They concluded that transfer-learned Inception V4 outperforms the others, with an accuracy of 96.12%. Ramzan et al. explore the effectiveness of ResNet-18 model for AD categorization [15]. Transfer learning is attempted for six-class classification tasks. The authors consider 138 subjects (25 cognitive normal (CN), 25 LMCI, 25 AD, 25 EMCI, 25 subjective memory complaints (SMC), and 13 MCI) from the ADNI database. Naive and transfer-learned models yield an accuracy of 97.92% and 97.88%, respectively. Geneedy et al. investigate the performance of 14-layered shallow CNN for global and local classification of AD using MRI scans [23]. The model is assessed using 6400 photos obtained from the OASIS-3 database. An accuracy of 99.68% is reported. A deep CNN based pipeline is developed by Islam et al. for AD classification [24]. Three various deep CNNs, each with a little modified structure, are adopted. The authors validate the models using structural MRI images from OASIS database and report an accuracy of 93.18%.

Recently, models based on Vision Transformer have demonstrated great promise in AD classification tasks. These models require a larger amount of data for better performance. Due to the practical difficulties in obtaining large amounts of medical data, cross-domain transfer learning is employed. Wang et al. have suggested a unique model: IGnet for AD detection [17]. The effectiveness of 3D CNN and transformer encoder are integrated into their work. The compact 3D CNN includes equal instances of convolutional and max pooling layers. Through this series of ten layers, pertinent features are extracted from MRI scans. A bi-layered transformer encoder is developed to extract the relevant information from the genetic sequence. The image embeddings from 3D CNN and genetic embeddings from the transformer encoder are integrated. This is then processed by a series of layers comprised of multi-layer perceptron (MLP) and fully connected layers. Finally, the class probabilities generated by the softmax layer are used to categorize the applied input into "normal" and "diseased" classes. The authors tested their model with the ADNI database and reported an overall accuracy of 83.78%.

In an approach proposed by Zhang et al., AD detection is performed by modified ViT and shallow 3D CNN [18]. A unique convolutional patch embedding (CPE) module and positional encoding method are incorporated into the vanilla ViT to develop a convolutional voxel vision transformer (CVVT). The proposed CVVT takes advantage of the inter-association of all voxels in the entire MRI scan. The compact 3D CNN (S3DCNN) includes four blocks. Each block comprises layers (such as 3D convolutional, 3D batch normalization, 3D max pooling, 3D leaky ReLU, and 3D dropout). The pertinent features extracted from the layers are further processed by a fully connected layer. This is then followed by softmax and classification layer for classification. Both the models are evaluated with MRI scans from the ADNI database. Findings represent an overall accuracy of 84% and 98% in CCVT and S3DCNN, respectively.

The majority of the existing research has concentrated on AD classification using pre-trained models. Furthermore, a subset of images is investigated in many of these works. Minimal work has been performed for AD classification using ViTs. This incited us to devise a novel method for classifying AD stages using deep CNN and ViT.

9.3　METHODOLOGY

Categorization of pertinent phases of AD from MRI images may assist in providing reliable medical care to symptomatic individuals. The potency of CNN and ViT are effectively combined in this research to categorize the MRI images as "very mild demented" (VMD), "moderate demented" (MOD), "non-demented" (ND), and "mild demented" (MD).

9.3.1　DATABASE

The third version of the open-access series of imaging studies (OASIS-3) database [25] is considered in this work. This dataset includes 6400 images, grouped into 4 classes based on the severity of AD. The images are in JPG format with a dimension of 176 × 208 pixels. The number of samples is depicted in Figure 9.1. The database consists of 14% MD samples, 1% MOD samples, 50% ND samples, and 35% VMD samples. The sample scans are depicted in Figure 9.2.

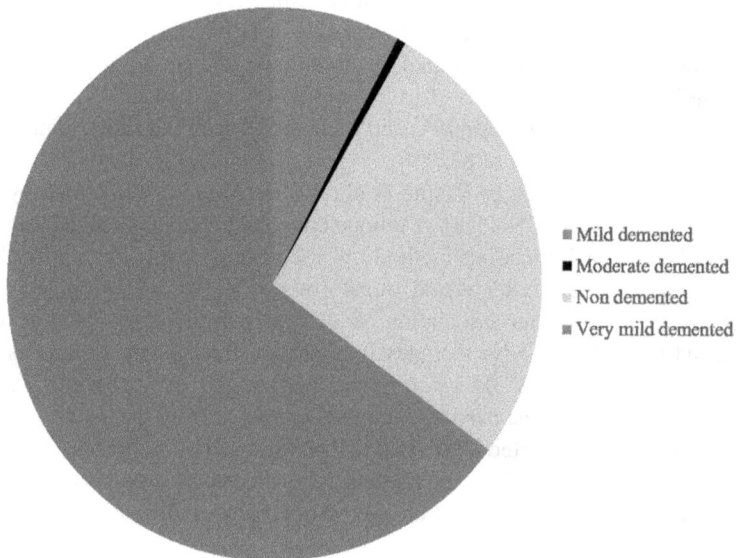

Mild demented
Moderate demented
Non demented
Very mild demented

FIGURE 9.1　Distribution of images in the dataset.

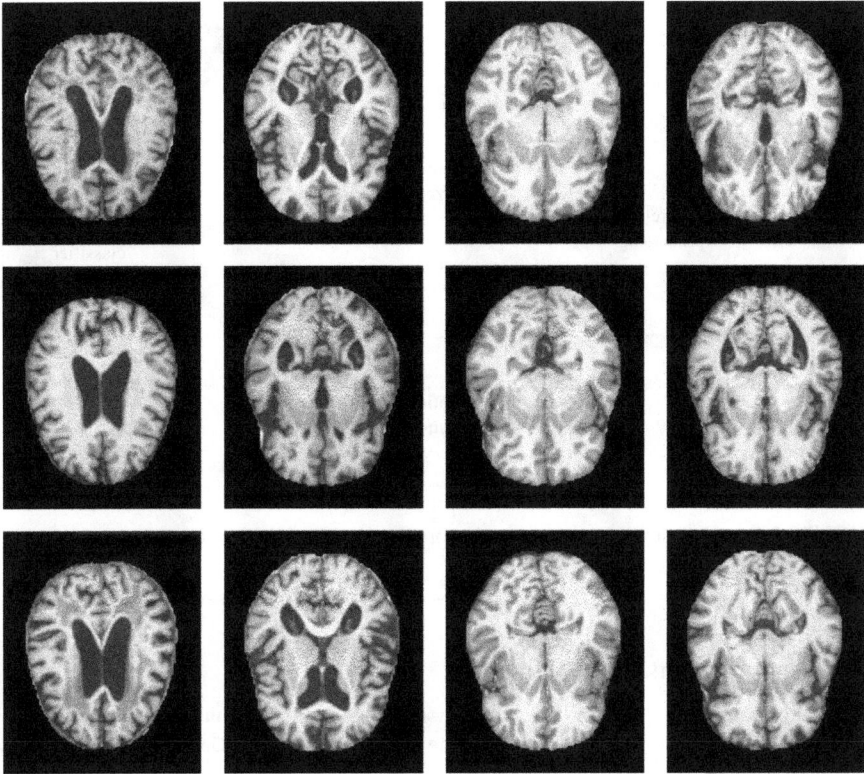

FIGURE 9.2 Sample MRI scans depicting various stages of AD. The MD and MOD images are visible in the first and second columns, respectively. A few ND and VMD images are represented in the third and fourth columns, respectively.

9.3.2 PROPOSED FRAMEWORK

The typical workflow of the suggested approach is illustrated in Figure 9.3. It has three primary modules: preprocessing, feature extraction and classification, and ensemble learning. The oversampling data-level technique and image resizing are carried out during preprocessing. The feature extraction and classification module extracts the pertinent attributes and classifies them using customized EfficientNet-B0 and customized ViT models. The best configurations from CNN and ViT are picked for further processing. To enhance the overall performance, ensemble learning is adopted in the final stage. This stage involves ensemble selection, probability averaging, and classification.

Preprocessing: Generally, deep CNN yield better outcomes with huge data. The data distribution confirms the presence of a class imbalance problem. To address this, an oversampling data-level technique is utilized. The training set images are

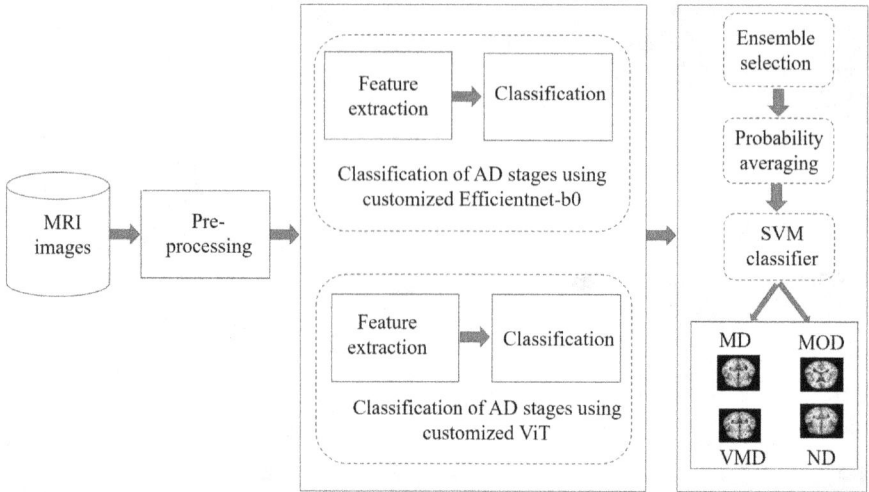

FIGURE 9.3   Workflow of the suggested approach for AD classification.

TABLE 9.1
Details of Augmentation Technique

Number of Images in Original Dataset	Step Size	Angle of Rotation	Number of Images in Generated Dataset
MD: 717	1	0 and 6	MD: 5019
MOD: 52	0.1	1 and 10	MOD: 5200
ND: 2560	1	0 and 1	ND: 5120
VMD: 1792	1	0 and 2	VMD: 5376

enlarged using a rotation augmentation technique to yield a balanced dataset. Table 9.1 depicts the details of the augmentation method with relevant parameters.

Classification using customized EfficientNet-B0: EfficientNet-B0 is trained with a larger number of samples from the ImageNet database. Due to this, the model learns descriptive image features effectively. Therefore, fine-tuning the model simplifies the learning process. The model is modified by tweaking the final layers. Figure 9.4 illustrates the attribute extraction using the EfficientNet-B0 model.

Feature extraction: EfficientNet models proposed by Tan et al. have garnered considerable interest because of the inclusion of the compound scaling technique [26]. It scales resolution, depth, and width evenly using a group of parameters represented by the following equations:

$$depth: d = \delta^{\theta} \tag{9.1}$$

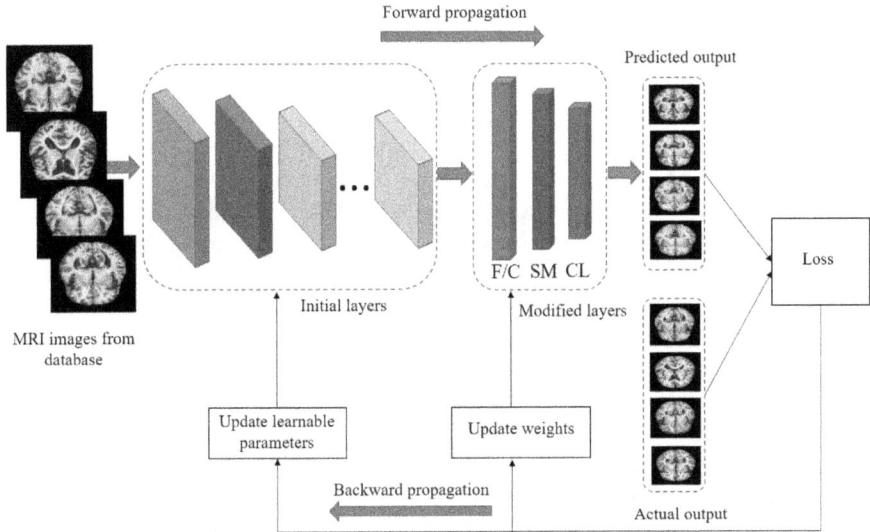

FIGURE 9.4   Pertinent attribute extraction using modified EfficientNet-B0 CNN.

$$width : w = \varphi^{\theta} \tag{9.2}$$

$$resolution : r = \zeta^{\theta} \tag{9.3}$$

where θ is a compound parameter and $\delta, \varphi,$ and ζ are the scaling parameters of individual dimensions. A grid search technique is employed to select the optimum values of coefficients by validating the constraints $\delta \; \varphi^2 \zeta^2 \approx 2$ and $\delta \geq 1, \varphi \geq 1, \zeta \geq 1$. The layers of the model are outlined in Table 9.2.

TABLE 9.2
Details of EfficientNet-B0 Model

Stage	Operator	Resolution	No. of Channels	No. of Layers
1	Conv $k3$	224×224	32	1
2	MIBConv1, $k3$	112×112	16	1
3	MIBConv6, $k3$	112×112	24	2
4	MIBConv6, $k5$	56×56	40	2
5	MIBConv6, $k3$	28×28	80	3
6	MIBConv6, $k5$	14×14	112	3
7	MIBConv6, $k5$	14×14	192	4
8	MIBConv6, $k3$	7×7	320	1
9	Conv $k1$/pooling/FC	7×7	1280	1

$k3$: 3×3, $k5$: 5×5, and $k1$: 1×1

Feature selection: Choosing robust features may aid in the effective categorization of AD stages. Haar wavelet transform and PCA are employed to accomplish this. First, the extracted features are decomposed using the Haar wavelet. Approximation and detail bands are provided by the decomposition. It is evident that the approximation band has a greater impact on AD characteristics. Thus, exploring only the low-frequency band may drastically decrease the number of attributes required for classification [27]. Secondly, PCA is utilized to obtain the valid attributes from the bands. Reconstruction of the attributes is carried out by zeroing the parameters of the detail band and unaltering the parameters of the approximation band. Then, PCA is employed to generate relevant attributes for categorization.

Classification: The appropriate selection of the classifier may significantly improve the outcome of AD categorization. The robust features are classified into four classes using the Bi-LSTM network [28]. This is a group of two LSTMs, with one taking the input sequence from beginning to end and the other taking the input sequence in reverse order.

Classification using customized ViT: This work employs the customized ViT for AD classification. This is accomplished through the use of the transfer learning approach. The ViT model utilized for the natural image task is fine-tuned for the AD classification stage. The basic representation of customized ViT is presented in Figure 9.5. The transformer encoder is a crucial component of ViT. It includes a clump of several equivalent layers. Each layer is made of multi-head attention and the MLP. Two Gaussian error linear unit (GELU) nonlinear layers are included in MLP. After layer normalization, a residual connection is used around each of the two sub-layers (Lnorm). The transformer accepts a sequence of N-embedded patches (L_p^i) and a special token (L_{sp}). Each patch embedding is appended with learnable position embeddings, mathematically represented by the following equations:

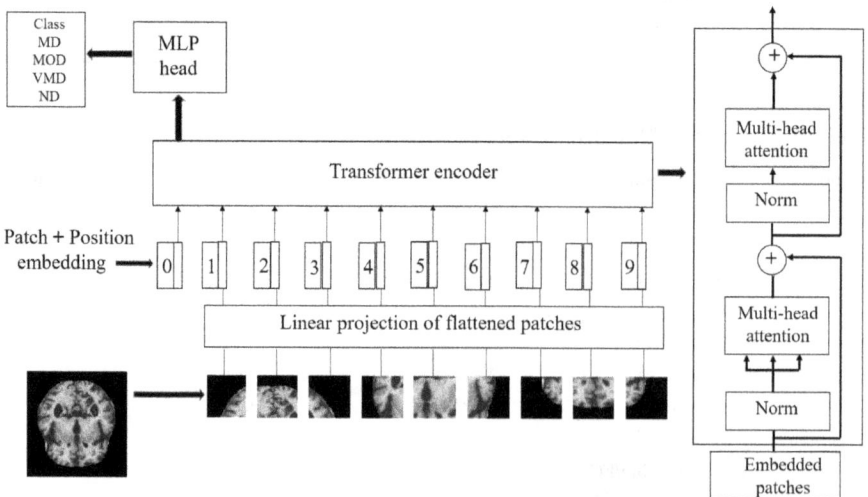

FIGURE 9.5 Extraction of pertinent features using customized ViT.

$$X_o = \left[L_{sp}; L_p^1; L_p^2; \ldots\ldots L_p^N \right] + L_{pos} \tag{9.4}$$

$$X_l^* = MSA(lnorm(X_{l-1})) + X_{l-1} \tag{9.5}$$

$$X_l = MLP(lnorm(X_l^*)) + X_l^* \tag{9.6}$$

$$Y = lmorm(X_0) \tag{9.7}$$

Ensemble learning:

Ensemble learning is predominantly employed to enhance performance as well as to improve robustness. In this work, a stacking ensemble technique is employed [29]. The best configuration of the EfficientNet-B0 model and the best ViT model are selected. The metric classification accuracy is considered for the selection process. The likelihood scores of the selected models are averaged using:

$$P_{Final}(B_k) = \left(\sum_{i=1}^{N} P_{s(i)}(B_k) \right) / N \tag{9.8}$$

where $P_{Final}(B_k)$ represents the ultimate likelihood score of B_k, k is the class indicator, $P_s(B_k)$ represents the likelihood score, and N denotes the total models used in the ensemble. Final prediction is performed using the SVM classifier.

9.4   EXPERIMENTAL FINDINGS

Throughout training, the preliminary layers of the model are preserved, whereas the end layers are customized to four-class tasks. Figure 9.6 depicts the amount of samples in unaugmented and generated databases. The model is trained with 5019 MD images, 5200 MOD images, 5120 ND images, and 5376 VMD images. Since the Adam optimizer [30] performs well for a majority of image classification tasks [31], it is employed with a learning rate of 0.0001. Experimentation is carried out with epochs of 20 and a batch size of 32. The trainable variables are modified to mitigate the cross-entropy loss specified by

$$loss = -\sum_{i=1}^{S} \sum_{j=1}^{C} t_{ij} \ln(p_{ij}) \tag{9.9}$$

where S is sample length, C is total classes, t_{ij} indicates target output, and p_{ij} indicates the predicted output. The model is evaluated with 1279 images (179 MD, 12 MOD, 640 ND, and 448 VMD) in different settings, which are mentioned below.

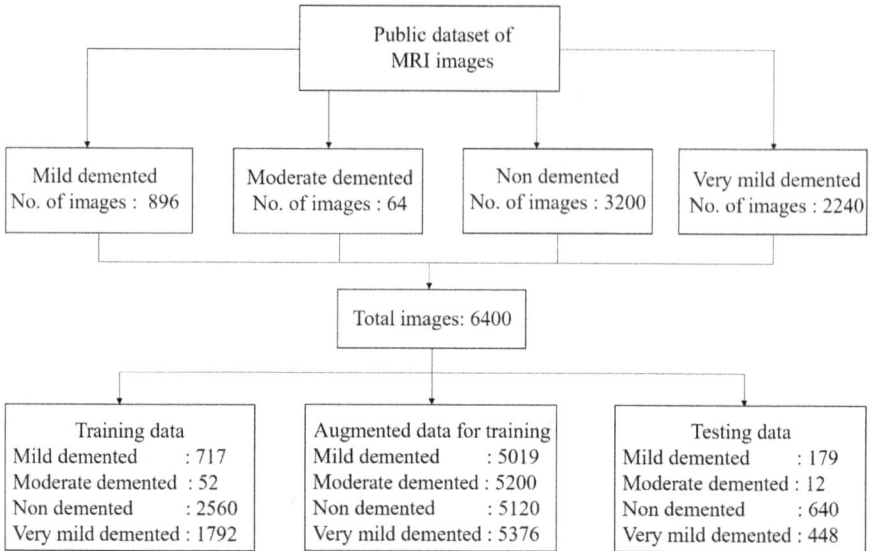

FIGURE 9.6 Distribution of images in the dataset. This dataset includes 896 MD, 64 MOD, 3200 ND, and 2240 VMD images.

- S1: The likelihood scores obtained from the softmax function are employed to categorize the images into different classes.
- S2 and S3: SVM and KNN classifiers are used to categorize the extracted features in settings S2 and S3, respectively. The attributes are acquired from the global average pooling layer.
- S4: The Bi-LSTM network is used in this setting. The model is assessed using pertinent attributes. Classification is carried out based on the likelihood scores acquired through the softmax function.
- S5, S6, and S7: These settings explore the efficacy of feature selection using the Haar wavelet transform. SVM, KNN, and Bi-LSTM are used to classify the transformed attributes in S5, S6, and S7 settings, respectively.
- S8, S9, and S10: The relevance of robust features for AD classification is analyzed in these settings. PCA is used to select robust features. SVM, KNN, and Bi-LSTM are used to classify robust features in settings S8, S9, and S10.

The following metrics are used to assess the efficacy of the various settings:

Accuracy (ACC):

This indicates the total samples predicted correctly by the model. It is specified as

$$ACC = \frac{TPM + TPMO + TPVM + TPN}{N} \qquad (9.10)$$

where $TPM, TPMO, TPVM$, and TPN represent the "mild demented" samples classified correctly, "moderate demented" image samples classified correctly, "very mild demented" samples classified correctly, and "non-demented" samples classified correctly, respectively. The overall samples are indicated by N.

Recall:

SEN_M, SEN_{MO}, SEN_{VM}, and SEN_N indicate the proportion of "mild demented" samples, "moderate demented" samples, "very mild demented" image samples, and "non-demented" samples correctly predicted by the model, respectively. It is calculated using

$$SEN_M = \frac{TPM}{TPM + FNM} \tag{9.11}$$

$$SEN_{MO} = \frac{TPMO}{TPMO + FNMO} \tag{9.12}$$

$$SEN_{VM} = \frac{TPVM}{TPVM + FNVM} \tag{9.13}$$

$$SEN_N = \frac{TPN}{TPN + FNN} \tag{9.14}$$

Experimentation is carried out with original and augmented databases. A classification accuracy of 71% is reported for the original samples. Due to the existence of data discrepancies among the classes, the model fails to capture the relevant attributes. Hence, there is a need for an oversampling data-level approach. The likelihood scores computed by the softmax function are employed for AD categorization in the softmax classifier. This setting (S1) correctly predicts 121 MD samples, 4 MOD samples, 531 ND samples, and 330 VMD samples. Table 9.3 demonstrates the metrics obtained by different settings.

An SVM classifier with a linear kernel is employed in settings (such as S2, S5, and S8), whereas a KNN classifier with a Euclidean kernel (with K-value of five) is employed in settings like S3, S6, and S9. SVM and KNN models are evaluated using 1280 extracted features in S2 and S3, respectively. Experimental findings indicate that SVM classifier outperforms KNN with 74.2% accuracy. A Bi-LSTM network is employed in settings like S4, S7, and S10. The model predicts MD images with 77% accuracy, MOD images with 41.6%, ND images with 84.3%, and VMD images with 75.8% accuracy.

The inclusion of a feature selection technique may substantially improve classifier performance. Wavelet transform is utilized to choose the useful attributes. The decomposition of attributes into approximation and detail coefficients is performed using a single-level Haar wavelet. As the approximation band contains significant information, only those features are considered. Thus, a total of 640 features are selected. SVM and KNN classifiers are evaluated with these features in S5 and S6, respectively. An accuracy of 79.5% and 78.3% are obtained in S5 and S6, respectively. The bi-LSTM network is evaluated with 640 features in the S7 setting. It

TABLE 9.3
Performance Metrics Obtained by Various Configurations

Classifiers	ACC	SEN_M	SEN_{MO}	SEN_{VM}	SEN_N
S1 (Softmax)	77.1	67.6	33.3	83	73.7
S2 (SVM)	74.2	44.7	50	72	89.7
S3 (KNN)	73.7	55.3	83.3	70.9	84.6
S4 (Bi-LSTM)	79.9	77	41.6	84.3	75.8
S5 (Haar + SVM)	79.5	78.2	33.3	83.5	75.4
S6 (Haar + KNN)	78.3	77.4	41.6	85.2	74.6
S7 (Haar + Bi-LSTM)	83.4	78.7	50	87.5	80.3
S8 (Haar + PCA + SVM)	82.4	77	50	92.1	71.4
S9 (Haar + PCA + KNN)	81.3	78.7	33.3	89	72.5
S10 (Haar + PCA + Bi-LSTM)	87.4	83.7	50	90.6	85.3

classifies the MD images with 78.7% accuracy, MOD images with 50% accuracy, ND images with 87.5% accuracy, and VMD images with 80.3% accuracy.

The settings S8, S9, and S10 demonstrate the potency of wavelet transform and PCA. The number of extracted features is lowered from 640 to 254. Evaluation of SVM and KNN classifiers with these attributes has achieved an accuracy of 82.4% and 81.3% in S8 and S9, respectively. It is evident that the S8 and S9 settings have lower computational complexity than the S2 and S3 settings.

Experimental evaluation of the Bi-LSTM model with 254 features has achieved an accuracy of 87.41%. This setting (S10) predicts the MD images with 83.7% accuracy, MOD images with 50% accuracy, ND images with 90.6% accuracy, and VMD images with 85.3% accuracy. According to the findings, the model accuracy improves when the classifiers are assessed with useful attributes rather than original attributes.

For customized ViT models, fine-tuning is carried out. The training is done in such a manner that patch embedding layers and classifiers are customized based on a four-class classification problem. The transformer encoder's parameters, on the other hand, remain unchanged. Three homogeneous ViTs with different model sizes (such as tiny [ViTT], small [ViTS], and base [ViTB]) are implemented in this work. Table 9.4 illustrates the metrics obtained by different ViTs. It is inferred that the small ViT

TABLE 9.4
Performance Metrics Obtained by Various ViTs

Classifiers	ACC	SEN_M	SEN_{MO}	SEN_{VM}	SEN_N
ViTT	87.4	82.1	41.6	89.6	84.2
ViTS	88.6	86	50	91.4	86.6
ViTB	86.8	83.7	50	89.5	85.2

model outperforms with an overall accuracy of 88.6%. This model correctly classifies 154 MD images, 6 MOD images, 585 ND images, and 388 VMD images.

An ensemble of the scores obtained by the C10 configuration and the ViTS model yields an accuracy of 90.38%. The final SVM classifier correctly predicts the MD images with 87.1% accuracy, MOD images with 41.6% accuracy, ND images with 92.9% accuracy, and VMD images with 89.2% accuracy.

Comparison with previous works:

The work suggested by Hon et al. [14], Farooq et al. [12], Ramzan et al. [15], Geneedy et al. [23], and Islam et al. [24] are considered for comparison. The pretrained models are implemented with the following hyperparameters:

- Batch size: 32
- Learning rate: 0.0001
- Maximum epochs:100
- Adam optimizer

Table 9.5 shows the metrics obtained by the different models. The model suggested by Geneedy et al. correctly predicts 1065 of 1279 images, yielding an accuracy of 83.3%. Experimental investigation of DenseNet-121, DenseNet-161, and DenseNet-169, as mentioned by Islam et al., yields the highest accuracy of 85.6% with the DenseNet-161 model. It is inferred from the findings that aggregating the outcomes of the three models using a majority voting ensemble technique improves accuracy by 2%. The final ensemble model correctly classifies 143 MD, 9 MOD, 571 ND, and 401 VMD images. This results in an accuracy of 87.8%. Investigating the performance of three deep CNNs (GoogLeNet, ResNet-18, and ResNet-152) suggested by Farooq et al. yields better predictions with the ResNet-152 model. Among 1279 images, 1085 images are correctly predicted, resulting in an accuracy of 84.8%. The effectiveness of residual connection in ResNet-18 is investigated by Ramzan et al. to predict AD disease from MRI images. The results show that this model correctly predicts 1070 of 1279 images. This yields an accuracy of 83.6%. Experimental investigation of VGG-16 and Inception V4, as mentioned by Hon et al., yields an

---

TABLE 9.5

Performance Analysis of Various Models in Comparison With Proposed Model

Author	ACC	SEN_M	SEN_{MO}	SEN_{VM}	SEN_N
Farook et al. [2017]	84.8	71.5	83.3	86.1	87.6
Hon et al. [2017]	84.6	74.3	83.3	85.9	86.7
Islam et al. [2018]	87.8	79.8	75	89.5	89.2
Ramzan et al. [2019]	83.6	70.9	75	86.2	86.2
Geneedy et al. [2023]	83.3	70.9	91.7	85.0	85.9
Proposed	90.4	97.1	41.6	89.2	92.9

overall accuracy of 82.64% and 84.6% in respective models. The architectural improvement of Inception V4 results in correctly predicting 1083 of 1279 images.

The findings demonstrate that the suggested model outperforms other extant methodologies. The suggested model may fail to capture the distinct features of MOD images because MOD images are distributed differently than the other three classes. As a result, the sensitivity of MOD images is quite a bit lower than that of existing approaches. However, when compared to other models, the suggested model effectively captures the features of MD, ND, and VMD images, resulting in a lower misclassification rate.

9.5 CONCLUSION

An effective framework for the categorization of AD stages using CNN and ViT is suggested in this work. Different classifiers are employed in various settings to classify the attributes obtained from the customized CNN. The effectiveness of each setting is evaluated on a dataset which includes 21,994 MRI images (5198 MD, 5212 MOD, 5760 ND, and 5824 VMD photos). It is evident that useful attributes acquired using PCA and wavelet transform results in notable performance improvement when categorized with a Bi-LSTM network. It is concluded that combining CNN and Bi-LSTM significantly improves the overall outcome of the AD classification task. Fine-tuning the customized small ViT model yields an overall accuracy of 88.6%. By integrating the performance of the best configuration of EfficientNet-B0 and the best ViT model using a stacking ensembling approach, improvement in accuracy is observed. Out of 1279 images, 1156 images are correctly predicted by the suggested approach. Thus, the suggested approach may assist neurologists in classifying the stages of AD.

BIBLIOGRAPHY

1. "World Alzheimer report 2018—The state of the art of dementia research: New frontiers." *Alzheimer's Disease International*, vol. 48, pp. 1–48, 2018.
2. R. Brookmeyer, E. Johnson, K. Ziegler Graham, and H. M. Arrighi, "Forecasting the global burden of Alzheimer's disease." *Alzheimer's and Dementia· The Journal of the Alzheimer's Association*, vol. 3, no. 3, pp. 186–191, Jul 2007.
3. S. S. Khan and G. S. Bloom, "Tau: The center of a signaling nexus in Alzheimer's disease." *Frontiers in Neuroscience*, vol. 10, pp. 1–5, Feb 2016.
4. P. Elangovan and M. K. Nath, "Glaucoma assessment from color fundus images using convolutional neural network." *International Journal of Imaging Systems and Technology*, vol. 31, no. 2, pp. 955–971, June 2021.
5. P. Elangovan, D. Vijayalakshmi, and M. K. Nath, "Detection of glaucoma from fundus images using pre-trained densenet201 model." *Indian Journal of Radio and Space Physics*, vol. 50, no. 1, pp. 33–39, March 2021.
6. P. Elangovan and M. K. Nath, "A novel shallow ConvNet-18 for malaria parasite detection in thin blood smear images." *SN Computer Science*, vol. 2, no. 5, pp. 1–11, Jul 2021.
7. S. Majumdar, P. Pramanik, and R. Sarkar, "Gamma function based ensemble of CNN models for breast cancer detection in histopathology images." *Expert Systems with Applications*, vol. 213, pp. 119022, Mar 2023.

8. V. Venugopal, J. Joseph, M. V. Das, and M. K. Nath, "An EfficientNet-based modified sigmoid transform for enhancing dermatological macro-images of melanoma and nevi skin lesions." *Computer Methods and Programs in Biomedicine*, vol. 222, pp. 106935, Jul 2022.

9. D. AlSaeed and S. F. Omar, "Brain MRI analysis for Alzheimer's disease diagnosis using CNN-based feature extraction and machine learning." *Sensors*, vol. 22, no. 8, pp. 1–14, 2022.

10. A. Payan and G. Montana, "Predicting Alzheimer's disease: A neuroimaging study with 3D convolutional neural networks." *CoRR*, vol. abs/1502.02506, pp. 1–9, Feb 2015.

11. S. Spasov, L. Passamonti, A. Duggento, P. Lio, N. Toschi, "A parameter efficient deep learning approach to predict conversion from mild cognitive impairment to Alzheimer's disease." *Neuroimage*, vol. 189, pp. 276–287, Apr 2019.

12. A. Farooq, S. Anwar, M. Awais, and S. Rehman, "A deep CNN based multi-class classification of Alzheimer's disease using MRI." In *2017 IEEE International Conference on Imaging Systems and Techniques (IST)*, Beijing, IEEE, pp. 1–6, Oct 2017.

13. S. Korolev, A. Safiullin, Y. Dodonova, and M. Belyaev, "Residual and plain convolutional neural networks for 3D brain MRI classification." *2017 IEEE 14th International Symposium on Biomedical Imaging (ISBI 2017), Melbourne, VIC, Australia*, pp. 835–838, Jan 2017. doi: 10.1109/ISBI.2017.7950647.

14. M. Hon and N. M.Khan, "Towards Alzheimer's disease classification through transfer learning." *In 2017 IEEE International conference on bioinformatics and biomedicine (BIBM)*, pp. 1166–1169, 2017. doi: 10.1109/BIBM.2017.8217822.

15. F. Ramzan, M. U. G. Khan, A. Rehmat, S. Iqbal, T. Saba, A. Rehman, and Z. Mehmood, "A deep learning approach for automated diagnosis and multi-class classification of Alzheimer's disease stages using resting-state fMRI and residual neural networks." *Journal of Medical Systems*, vol. 44, no. 2, pp. 1–16, Nov 2019.

16. H. A. Helaly, M. Badawy, and A. Y. Haikal, "Deep learning approach for early detection of Alzheimer's disease." *Cognitive Computing*, vol. 14, no. 2, pp. 1711–1727, 2022.

17. J. X. Wang, Y. Li, X. Li, and Z. H. Lu, "Alzheimer's disease classification through imaging genetic data with IGnet." *Frontiers in Neuroscience*, vol. 16, no. 846638, pp. 1–8, Mar 2022.

18. Z. Zhang and F. Khalvati, "Introducing vision transformer for Alzheimer's disease classification task with 3D input." *arXiv*, pp. 1–21, 2022.

19. Y. Lyu, X. Yu, D. Zhu, and L. Zhang, "Classification of Alzheimer's disease via vision transformer." In *The 15th International Conference on Pervasive Technologies Related to Assistive Environments (PETRA)*, Greece, ACM, pp. 463–468, Jun 2022.

20. S. Sarraf and G. Tofighi, "Classification of Alzheimer's disease structural MRI data by deep learning convolutional neural networks." *CoRR*, vol. abs/1607.06583, pp.1–14, 2016.

21. M. Orouskhani, C. Zhu, S. Rostamian, F. S. Zadeh, M. Shafiei, Y. Orouskhani, and U. R. Acharya, "Alzheimer's disease detection from structural MRI using conditional deep triplet network." *Neuroscience Informatics*, vol. 2, no. 4, pp. 100066, 2022.

22. S. Luo, X. Li, and J. Li, "Automatic Alzheimer's disease recognition from MRI data using deep learning method." *Journal of Applied Mathematics and Physics*, vol. 5, no. 9, pp. 1892–1898, Sep 2017.

23. M. Geneedy, H. Moustafa, F. Khalifa, H. Khater, E. AbdElhalim, L. Saunders, M. Suh, and K. Hasenstab, "An MRI-based deep learning approach for accurate detection of Alzheimer's disease." *Alexandria Engineering Journal*, vol. 63, pp. 211–221, Feb 2023.

24. J. Islam and Y. Zhang, "Brain mri analysis for Alzheimer's disease diagnosis using an ensemble system of deep convolutional neural networks" *Brain Informatics*, vol. 5, no. 2, pp. 1–14, 2018.

25. A. Chincarini, P. Bosco, P. Calvini, G. Gemme, M. Esposito, C. Olivieri, L. Rei, S. Squarcia, G. Rodriguez, R. Bellotti, "Local MRI analysis approach in the diagnosis of early and prodromal Alzheimer's disease." *NeuroImage*, vol. 58, pp. 469–480, 2011.

26. M. Tan and Q. V. Le, "Efficientnet: Rethinking model scaling for convolutional neural networks." *Clinical Orthopaedics and Related Research*, vol. abs/1905.11946, 2019.

27. M. K. Gar, G. Ravichandran, P. Elangovan, and M. K. Nath, "Analysis of diagnostic features from fundus images using multiscale wavelet decomposition." *ICIC Express Letters: Part B Applications*, vol. 10, no. 2, pp. 175–184, Feb 2019.

28. M. Schuster and K. K. Paliwal, "Bidirectional recurrent neural networks." *IEEE Transactions on Signal Processing*, vol. 45, no. 11, pp. 2673–2681, 1997.

29. P. Elangovan and M. K. Nath, "En-ConvNet: A novel approach for glaucoma detection from color fundus images using ensemble of deep convolutional neural networks." *International Journal of Imaging Systems and Technology*, vol. 32, no. 6, pp. 2034–2048, Nov 2022.

30. D. P. Kingma and J. Ba, "Adam: A method for stochastic optimization." CoRR, vol. abs/1412.6980, 2015, pp. 1–13.

31. P. Elangovan and M. K. Nath, "Performance analysis of optimizers for glaucoma diagnosis from fundus images using transfer learning." In *Lecture Notes in Electrical Engineering*, Singapore, Springer, vol. 749, pp. 507–518, May 2021.

10 RetinalAlexU-Net
Segmentation of the Retinal Vascular Network for the Diagnosis of Diabetic Retinopathy

A. Sathya Vani and D. Sumathi

10.1 INTRODUCTION

According to the International Diabetes Federation (IDF), 463 million people were living with diabetes mellitus (DM) in 2019, and this number is estimated to rise to 700 million by 2045 (*About Diabetes*, 2022). One of the most common factors leading to impaired eyesight in people of working age is diabetic retinopathy. Diabetes can result in a wide variety of abnormalities, the most common of which are diabetic retinopathy, diabetic nephropathy, and diabetic neuropathy (Saini et al., 2021). Diabetic retinopathy occurs when the diabetic condition affects the retina, while diabetic nephropathy and diabetic neuropathy occur when the diabetic condition affects the kidney, as shown in Figure 10.1. These diseases are the fundamental causes of vision impairment and blindness associated with the retina. Screening your retina is the best way to detect diabetic retinopathy in its earliest stages, well before any noticeable changes to your vision occur.

10.1.1 INTRODUCTION TO DIABETIC RETINOPATHY AND CLASSIFICATION

Diabetic retinopathy, sometimes known as DR, is characterized by microaneurysms, hemorrhages, or, in more severe cases, lesions that impair at least one eye, as shown in Figure 10.2.

Individuals who suffer from diabetes are at a significantly higher risk of DR, making it the secondary consequence that occurs most often. If a diagnosis is not made on time or a treatment intervention is not provided, it might lead to vision impairment, partial blindness, and other ocular issues. Therefore, gaining a grasp of the processes at play in DR is very important if one is interested in ensuring accurate diagnosis, evaluation, and treatment of this condition (Wang and Lo, 2018). Non-proliferative diabetic retinopathy (NPDR) and proliferative diabetic retinopathy

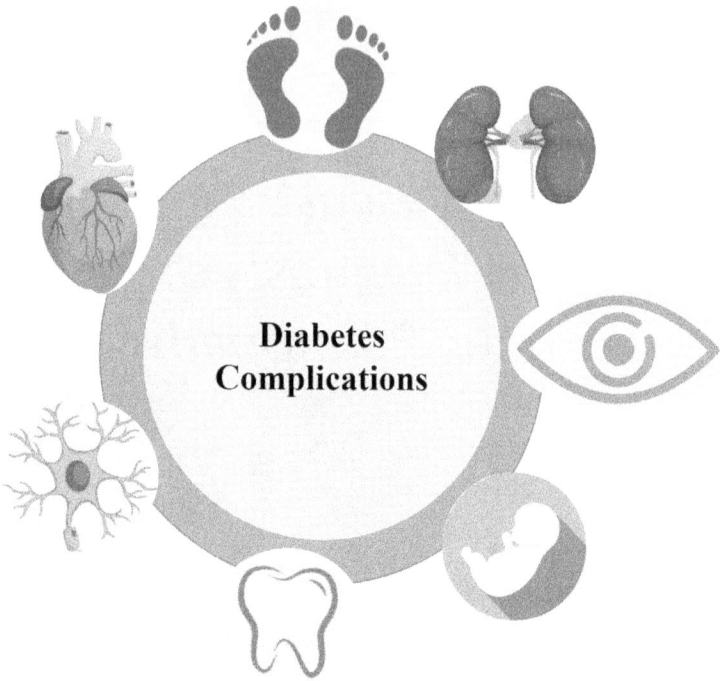

FIGURE 10.1   Major complications of diabetes.

(PDR) are the two primary categories that can be used to categorize diabetic retinopathy (Riaz et al., 2020). These categories are determined by the pathophysiology of microvascular aneurysms, pre-retinal vascularization, retinal hemorrhages,
intraretinal microvascular abnormalities, and other clinical patterns. PDR is distinguished as the abnormal formation of fibrous connective tissue on the retina's outer
layer, whereas NPDR is caused by lesions that develop within the retinal capillaries
as a consequence of edema, hemorrhage, microaneurysms of the blood vessels, and/
or capillary blockage. Both conditions can lead to vision loss in the affected eye.

Classification of DR

Non-proliferative diabetic retinopathy and proliferative diabetic retinopathy are the
two broad classifications that may be used to classify diabetic retinopathy, as shown
in Table 10.1.

    1. **Non-Proliferative Diabetic Retinopathy [NPDR]:** The early stage of the
       disease NPDR has minimal symptoms. NPDR patients have brittle retinal
       blood vessels that produce tiny bulges (Riaz et al., 2020). Fluid may flow
       into the retina, causing it to swell or bleed. This is also called background
       retinopathy. Non-proliferative retinopathy has three stages:
       a. **Mild NPDR:** In the early stages of the condition, small retinal blood
          vessels grow. These people have at least one microaneurysm (MA) but

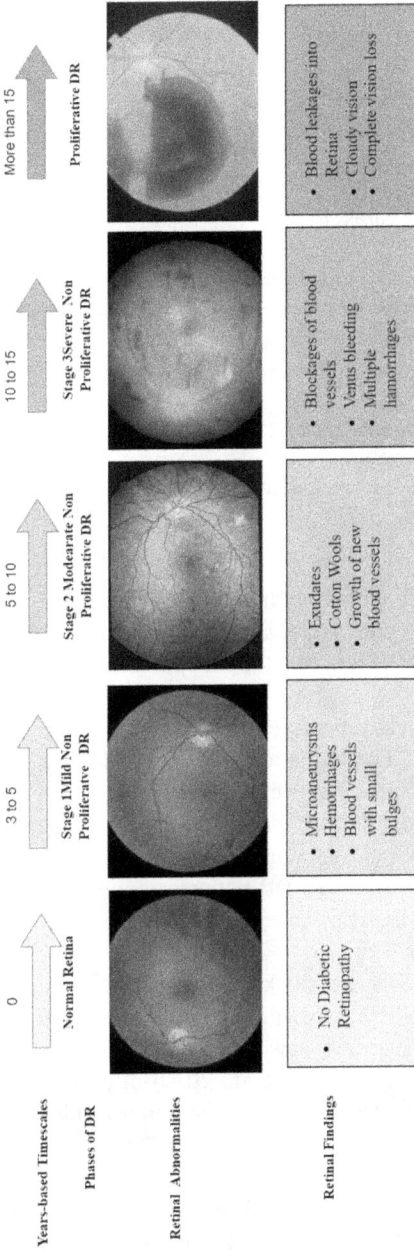

FIGURE 10.2 Classification of diabetic retinopathy with abnormalities found on year-based timelines.

TABLE 10.1

Clinical Examination Results of Diabetic Retinopathy

Diabetic Retinopathy	Results of a Clinical Examination
No apparent DR	No anomalies.
Mild Non-Proliferative DR	Only microaneurysms are being considered here.
Moderate Non-Proliferative DR	Microaneurysms include further signs (including hemorrhages, cotton wool spots, and hard exudates).
Severe (high-risk) Non-Proliferative DR	Moderate non-proliferative DR combined with any of the following: • Each of the four quadrants has more than 20 intraretinal hemorrhages. • Veins strongly beaded in at least two of the four quarters. • Intraretinal microvascular abnormalities (IRMA) in one quadrant. • No evidence of proliferative retinopathy.
Proliferative DR	Consistent with severe, non-proliferative DR, the following symptoms may be present: • Optical disc neovascularization (NVD) and/or systemic neovascularization (NVE). • A bleed in the vitreous or the membrane that covers the retina.

no other symptoms. A non-diabetic patient with one or more MAs in their eye should see their primary care physician for further testing. Hence, reporting small observations and noting their location will help doctors track sickness progression.

b. **Moderate NPDR:** As the condition advances, retinal veins enlarge and twist, compromising retinal health. The retina lacks oxygen and nutrients due to clogged blood vessels. Macula swelling may impair eyesight. These patients have hemorrhages or macular holes in one to three retinal quadrants with cotton-wool patches, hard exudates, or venous beading in one or more veins. Moderate NPDR patients should visit their doctor every six to eight months. They have a 12–27% probability of developing PDR in the following year.

c. **Severe NPDR:** Several blood vessels are blocked in the third stage. The retina cannot get blood from them. Growth factors are produced in certain retinal areas. The retina grows new blood vessels due to these stimuli. Intraretinal hemorrhages (Riaz et al., 2020) in at least two quadrants must not be accompanied by neovascularization, which would indicate PDR.

Proliferative Diabetic Retinopathy [PDR]: PDR appears late in this eye disease. PDR starves the retina and grows frail, abnormal blood vessels on or near the optic nerve or vitreous (the clear, gelatinous mass between the retina and lens) that might result in. Blurriness and loss of vision.. Some people have gotten PDR from NPDR and had vitreous or pre-retinal hemorrhage or disc or other neovascularization. These patients must be transferred to a retina specialist immediately for additional testing and treatment, and they must be seen regularly until their condition stabilizes.

In this work, a novel deep learning-based model is presented using RetinalAlexU-Net. The key contributions of this analysis are:

- The suggested RetinalAlexU-Net efficiently diagnoses diabetic retinopathy and thereby extracts retinal vessels. This approach reduces the time complexity and increases accuracy significantly.
- In contrast to existing works, RetinalAlexU-Net is robust enough to perform segmentation of retinal blood vessels.

The following sections of this chapter are structured as follows: Section 10.2 details the literature works with a brief description of existing algorithms. In Section 10.3, the methodology of the proposed algorithm is presented. The results and experimental setup of the algorithm are given in Section 10.4. Section 10.5 summarizes the work along with future possibilities.

10.2 LITERATURE SURVEY

We classify DR detection tasks into three groups based on their clinical relevance to (i) segmenting retinal blood vessels (Soomro et al., 2019); (ii) locating and segmenting the optic disc (Kumar et al., 2020); (iii) detecting and classifying lesions (Erciyas and Barışçı, 2021). In the sections that follow, we examine the latest advancements in DL-based methods for possible application to these tasks.

10.2.1 SEGMENTING RETINAL BLOOD VESSELS

Early diagnosis of retinal blood vessel alterations is crucial in preventing pathological retinal damage-induced vision impairment. Retinal blood vessels' low contrast, morphological variety against a noisy backdrop, and diseases like macular degeneration and inherited macular angiogenesis make segregating them challenging. Table 10.2 shows the different CNN-based blood vessel segmentation approaches.

Using random walk algorithms, Gao, J., et al. (2020) created an autonomous model for blood vascular centerline-based segmentation. Multiscale vascular enhancement, based on a Hessian matrix, projects structural vessels with the utmost intensity. The divergence of the normalized gradient vector field and random walk segmentation is used to assign labels to seed groups based on morphological differences and discover blood vessels in healthy and disturbed areas to extract the centerlines.

To automatically detect and distinguish blood vessels, Siva Sundhara Raja and Vasuki (2015) suggested removing the optic disc (OD) from the retina (Ting et al., 2020). After segmenting the OD area with an anisotropic diffusion filter, numerical dual semantic functioning is employed to locate blood vessels. Before vascularizing the retina, the optic disc was cropped off for blood vessel extraction, to increase segmentation accuracy.

TABLE 10.2

Description of Models for Lesion Detection for DR

Types	References	Methodologies	Datasets	Performance Metrics
Retinal Blood Vessels	Gao et al. (2020)	Multiscale vascular enhancement based on a Hessian matrix (MVEH).	STARE	SE: 75.8%, SP: 95.5%, ACC: 94.01%
	Siva Sundhara Raja and Vasuki (2015)	Anisotropic diffusion filter (ADF).	STARE	SE: 93.6%, SP: 98.9%, ACC: 94.94%
	Adarsh et al. (2020)	Convolutional autoencoder with dense residual paths (DRCE).	DRIVE	SE: 91.4%, SP: 95.4%, ACC: 92.8%
	Atteia et al. (2021)	The stacked autoencoder neural network with deep feature transfer learning (DTLENN).	IDRiD	SE: 97.5%, SP: 95.5%, ACC: 96.8%
Optic Disc	Shaikha and Sallow (2019)	Histogram template matching (HTM).	DIARETDB0	SE: 88.2%, SP: 90.24% ACC: 96%
	Bengani et al. (2021)	Convolutional autoencoder (CAE).	DRISHTI GS1	SE: 93.14%, SP: 95.39%, ACC: 96.4%
	Jadhav et al. (2020)	Deep belief network (DBN) and neural network (NN).	DIARETDB1	SE: 88.8%, SP: 92.4%, ACC: 92.4%
Microaneurysms &Hemorrhages	Long et al. (2020)	Machine learning approach (ML).	e-Ophtha MA	SE: 84.5%, SP: 89.9%, ACC: 87.1%
	Revathy et al. (2020)	Hybrid machine learning classifier.	Kaggle	SE: 81.19%, SP: 81.16%, ACC: 82

For medical picture segmentation, Adarsh et al. (2020) presented the dense residual path convolutional network. When a connection is skipped, the residual routes are filtered and are responsible for the segmentation produced by a U-effective net, which allows the network to collect more targeted data. Experiments performed on the DRIVE dataset (DRIVE Dataset, 2022) revealed significant improvements in semantic segmentation.

Atteia et al. (2021) suggested an approach that combines the effectiveness of stacked autoencoders for feature extraction and classification with convolutional neural networks previously trained to extract features. ResNet-50, SqueezeNet, Inception V3, and GoogLeNet, four well-known pre-trained deep networks, can retrieve many properties from a small input dataset (GoogLeNet, 2020). Next, a stacked autoencoder neural network selects the most informative features.

10.2.2 Locating and Segmenting the Optic Disc

Localization of the OD can elevate DR identification and classification due to its clear visibility. The first step in OD detection is localization, and the second is OD segmentation. The OD's location and borders are determined with the help of a few deep learning models, as shown in Table 10.2.

Shaikha and Sallow (2019) divided the optic disc region of interest (ROI) using a binary mask. The approach has generally used the centre of the OD and OD ROI rectangle dimensions. Histogram template matching found the centre of the OD, and the projected size of the OD ROI rectangle (N × N) determined the OD diameter. Database size determines rectangle size. Following that, the OD centre and ROI rectangle size determined a binary mask to segment the OD.

Bengani et al. (2021) provide a semi-supervised and transfer learning deep learning model for autonomous optic disc segmentation in retinal fundus pictures. A convolutional autoencoder (CAE) is trained to learn attributes from many unlabeled fundus photographs. The autoencoder (AE) recreates input images to learn characteristics from unlabeled photographs. After this, the pre-trained autoencoder network is segmented.

Jadhav et al. (2020) developed a three-level DR detection method based on blood vessels, optic discs, and retinal abnormalities. After preprocessing, the optic disc is segmented using the open-close watershed transform, the blood vessels are segmented using grey level thresholding, and abnormalities are segmented by analyzing three features simultaneously using top-hat transformation and Gabor filtering, and classifying images as normal, mild, moderate, or severe.

10.2.3 Clinical Manifestations of Microaneurysms (ME) and Hemorrhages (HE)

Long et al. (2020) developed a machine learning microaneurysm detection method using directed local contrast for early DR diagnosis (DLC). A better enhancement function was employed to improve and segment blood vessels after studying the Hessian matrix eigenvalues. After eliminating blood vessels, microaneurysm zones were identified by shape and components. The model separated the image into patches, gathered attributes from each patch to assess whether it was a microaneurysm, and then classified each patch.

Revathy et al. (2020) developed a hybrid classifier using a support vector machine, k-nearest neighbours, random forest, logistic regression, and multilayer perceptron network to categorize exudates, hemorrhages, and microaneurysms. Green channel extraction, masking, smoothing, and bitwise AND improve exudate estimations. Hemorrhages and microaneurysms are found by morphological methods like opening. Dilation and erosion occur here. Microaneurysms, hemorrhages, and exudates determine diabetic retinopathy.

10.3   METHODS AND MATERIALS

10.3.1   DR DETECTION METHODOLOGY

In this research, the proposed approach is named RetinalAlexU-Net, a deep learning-based vessel segmentation method having U-Net as its core architecture. In 2015, Ronneberger et al. introduced U-Net, a contracting and expanding route network, for biomedical segmentation, essentially composed of convolution layers, which provide the model the ability to recognize information automatically and adaptively. U-Net is being used as the foundational architecture because of its efficacy in pixel-level segmentation challenges, especially in the field of medical image analysis. Figure 10.3 shows our RetinalAlexU-Net. It is divided into three sections: encoding, bridge, and decoding.

RetinalAlexU-Net: The modified model makes an effort to retain the majority of the salient characteristics and architectural components as the original implementation of the U-Net design. However, a few improvements are made to the standard model to enhance the efficiency of the model, as well as to improve the speed and simplicity of the model and reduce its time consumption. RetinalAlexU-Net is a kind of encoding-decoding network architecture that relies on a single set of encoder and decoder blocks connected by an AlexNet bridge.

Encoder: The flow on the left, known as the contradiction path, contrasts with the provided flow on the right, which is known as the expansion path. The contradicting path is the typical convolutional network architecture, consisting of 3×3 convolutions replicated three times. The feature map that was produced as a result of the convolution process is then given to the rectified linear activation function (ReLU) layer, as shown in the equation below, which is then followed by the 2×2 max=pooling operation, which is done to minimize the overall size of the feature map. After each maximum pooling process is complete, downsampling is carried out, and, in parallel, feature channels are increased by double.

$$R(x) = \max(0, x) \tag{10.1}$$

Thereby,

$$\text{if } x < 0, R(x) = 0 \text{ and if}$$
$$x \geq 0, R(x) = x \text{ whereas x=Positive Value}$$

AlexNet Interconnectivity:

The bridge of the U-Net model is comprised of a simple AlexNet convolutional neural network. (Alom et al., 2018). This network has a total of five convolution

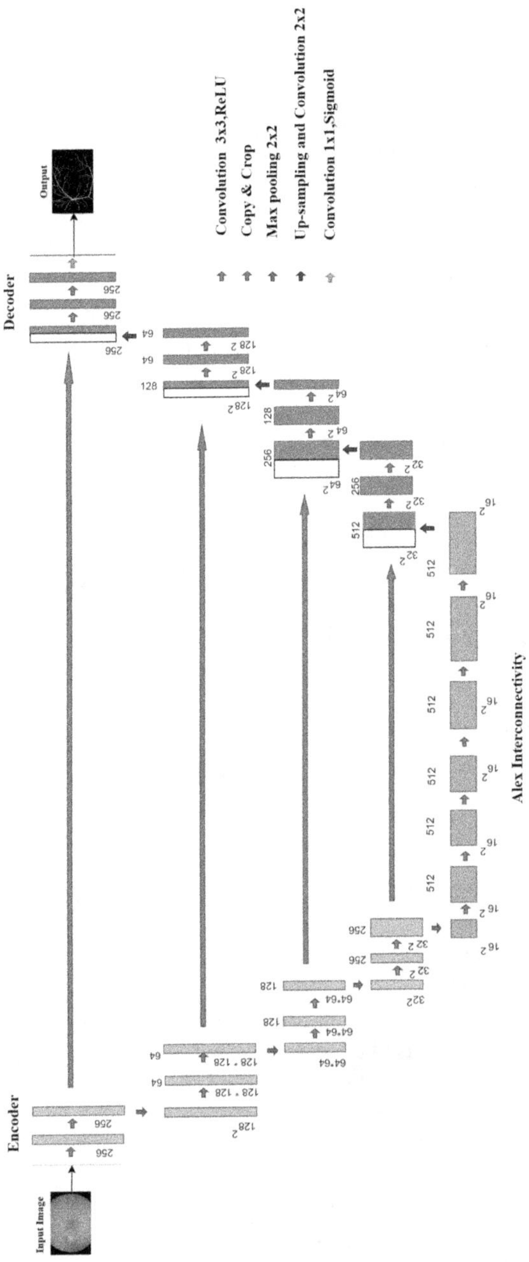

FIGURE 10.3 The proposed RetinalAlexU-Net architecture.

layers, some of which are followed by max-pooling layers, and it concludes with three fully connected layers that are combined with a softmax layer. AlexNet's connection mandates that the model gets the input data through the encoder's downsampling channel. The five convolutional layers in the network are composed of a collection of feature maps and kernels for extracting feature information, like edges, corners, and other angular characteristics. The term "convolution operation" refers to the procedure of sliding and overlaying the kernels across the entire image. The ReLU layer is inserted in AlexNet after each fully connected (FC) layer of the convolutional portion of the network. This network mitigates the overfitting issue by inserting a dropout layer after every FC layer.

Decoder: The decoder flow is the counterpart of the encoder flow, which uses downsampling, and consists of phases for upsampling of feature maps before proceeding to a convolution procedure with a kernel size of 2×2. Convolution results in a two-channel reduction in feature channels compared to their encoder equivalent. The ReLU activation function is utilized at the end of every stage of the convolutional layers. The suggested paradigm reduces the computational burden of the network, making its use simple and effective. This improves network training while transforming dense features into sparse features, which effectively makes the features more robust.

In addition, the model utilizes stochastic gradient descent (SGD). This is an optimization approach for training neural network models. To derive updated values for the model variables, this method has to compute gradients denoted by Equation 10.2 for each variable and carry out a parameter change for every single training sample $x^{(i)}$ and label $y^{(i)}$.

$$\theta = \theta - \eta . \Delta_\theta J(\theta; x^{(i)}; y^{(i)}) \tag{10.2}$$

Where:

θ = Model parameter.

η = The learning rate of the size of the steps we take in order to attain a (local) minimum.

$\Delta_\theta J(\theta)$ = Object function for parameters.

We utilized the binary cross-entropy loss function represented by Equation 10.3 throughout the training process because we used a sigmoid with a zero to one range.

$$\text{Cross Entropy} = \frac{1}{\sum_{T=1..M} y_{o,t} \log(p_o, t)} \tag{10.3}$$

For lowering the loss, which refers to the value that is assumed by the loss function, at the initial stage the learning rate of the Adam optimizer is set to 0.0005. Finally, we evaluated the outcome using Intersection over Union for the segmentation of the RetinalAlexU-Net and ground truth. The accuracy increases with the value of the Dice coefficient.

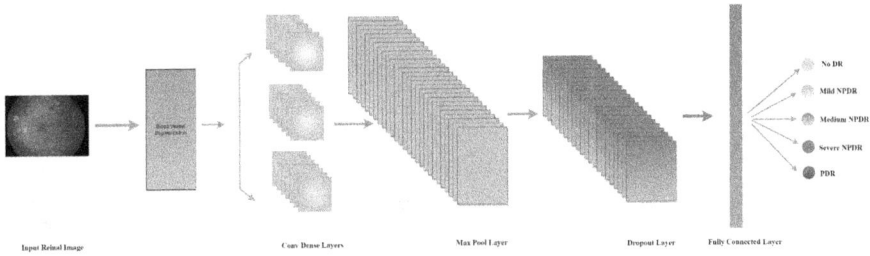

FIGURE 10.4   Classification of diabetic retinopathy based on deep neural networks.

Finally, diabetic retinopathy is classified by the retinal vascular network using the proposed RetinalAlexU-Net, as shown in Figure 10.4.

10.3.2   Datasets and Various Metrics of Performance

Retinal Fundus Images: Here, we summarize the most common performance metrics and standard datasets used in DR research. For training and evaluating the framework for algorithms used in different DR detection tasks, many datasets comprising retinal fundus pictures have been created. Listed below are several publicly available benchmark datasets that we will briefly discuss: Kaggle (Kaggle Dataset, 2022), MESSIDOR (Messidor Dataset, 2022), high resolution fundus (HRF), DRIVE (DRIVE Dataset, 2022).

KAGGLE: This data was given by EyePACS clinics and comprises several high-resolution retinal pictures captured in a variety of illumination situations. Expert ophthalmologists annotated each picture at the pixel level, and a DR grade between zero and four was applied to each image.

MESSIDOR: The Ministry of French Research and Defense supported this dataset's creation as part of the MESSIDOR research program. This data was obtained by three different ophthalmology clinics using a Topcon non-mydriatic retinography and a 45° field of view (FOV) colour video 3CCD camera. Image-level annotations for DR grades and macular edema risk were given by ophthalmologists.

HRF: The HRF database includes 45 high-resolution eye fundus pictures with a size of 3504×2336 pixels. These photographs were segmented by a group of professionals who work in the area of retinal image processing as well as clinicians from the ophthalmology clinics who participated in the research. To be more explicit, the dataset may be separated into 15 photos of healthy patients, 15 images of diabetic retinopathy patients, and 15 images of glaucoma sufferers. For each picture, there is an associated ground truth image as well as a mask with a determined field of view. In this study, we choose 41 photos at random for training purposes, and we use the remaining four images for testing purposes, to segment retinal vessels.

DRIVE: To facilitate comparative analyses of vascular segmentation in retinal pictures captured with a non-mydriatic Canon camera. Forty randomly chosen fundus photos are used: thirty-three don't exhibit any symptoms of DR, whereas seven indicate mild to severe early DR.

10.3.3 PERFORMANCE MEASURES

Metrics for evaluating DR detection techniques are defined below. Accuracy, sensitivity (recall), specificity (precision), F-score, receiver operating characteristic (ROC) curve, IoU, and the Dice similarity coefficient are all common metrics used to evaluate the efficiency of classification algorithms.

Accuracy: This metric measures the ratio of the proportion of properly categorized occurrences relative to the total number of occurrences. It is precisely defined as shown in Equation 10.4:

$$\text{Acc} = \frac{TP + TN}{TP + TN + FP + FN} \tag{10.4}$$

Sensitivity (SE): This statistic, shown in Equation 10.5, sometimes called the "true positive rate" or "recall", measures the percentage of correctly labelled positive instances.

$$\text{Recall}(SE) = \frac{TP}{TP + FN} \tag{10.5}$$

Specificity (SP): This metric is more often referred to as the true negative rate, and it is the fraction of negative cases that are correctly identified, as defined by Equation 10.6.

$$SP = \frac{TN}{TN + FP} \tag{10.6}$$

Precision (P): Often known as PPV (positive predictive value), this is a metric for determining how accurately positive occurrences are identified, as shown in Equation 10.7.

$$P = \frac{Tp}{Tp + FP} \tag{10.7}$$

Where:

TP (true positive) refers to the total amount of positive occurrences.

TN (true negative) is the total number of adverse occurrences.

FP (false positive) and FN (false negative) are numbers of positive and negative instances.

F-score (F): This is a combination of the two measures of precision and recall represented in Equation 10.8:

$$F = 2 * \frac{Precision + Recall}{Precision * Recall} \tag{10.8}$$

Intersection over Union (IoU): The ratio of the area of intersection to the sum of the areas of prediction and ground truth constitutes the IoU measure. It can be estimated as follows (Equation 10.9), where TP, FP, and FN are just areas or the number of pixels.

$$\text{IoU} = \frac{TP}{TP + FP + FN} \qquad (10.9)$$

10.4 EXPERIMENTAL RESULTS

This section provides the outcome performance assessment (*Performance Analysis*, 2022) of the suggested retinal blood vessels algorithm on the publicly accessible datasets (DRIVE, Kaggle, HRF, and MESSIDOR).

The dataset is composed of manually annotated blood vessel photographs that are called ground truth images. To assess the efficacy of recently developed vascular segmentation algorithms for the diagnosis of diabetic retinopathy, ground truth photographs are used.

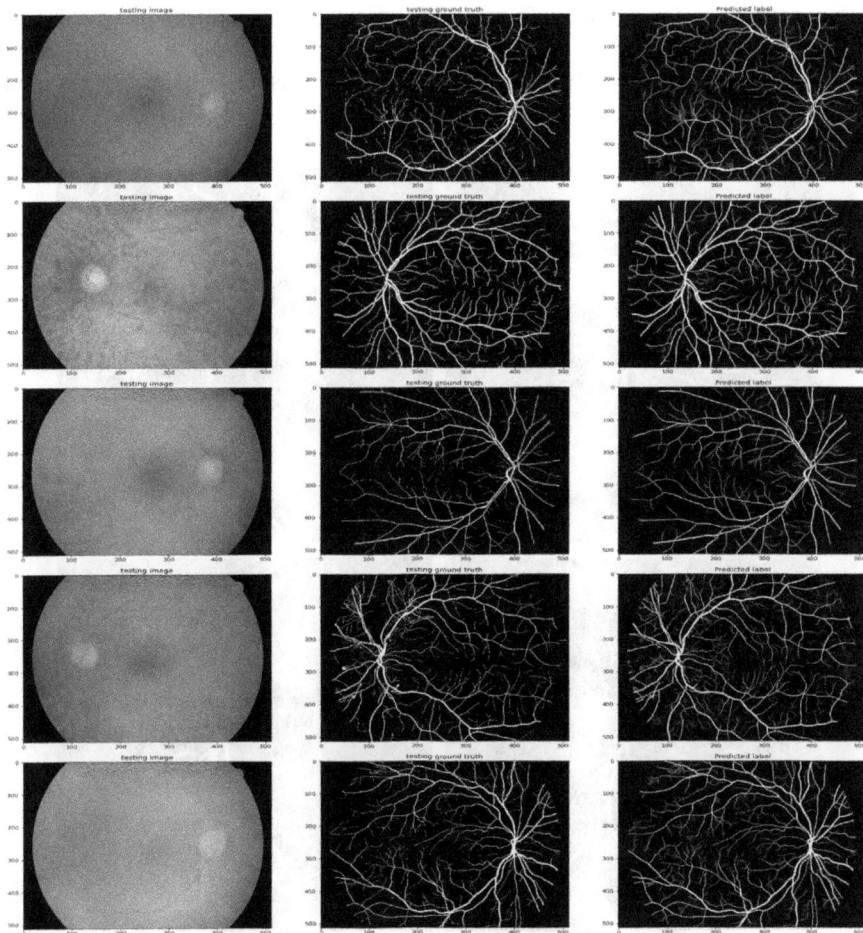

FIGURE 10.5 Classification of segmented retina using RetinalAlexU-Net architecture and comparison with their ground truth.

Despite this, the RetinalAlexU-Net network has performed very well, and the outcomes that have been accomplished are satisfactory. To offer a more precise rating, we will now look at the proposed procedure utilizing several different evaluation images. The findings of the diabetic retinal pathology detection are shown in Figure 10.5, which includes three divisions that show the raw data, ground truth image, and predicted segmentation outcomes, and Figure 10.6, which shows a retina predicted with DR and without DR by the RetinalAlexU-Net.

To accurately estimate retinal vascular segmentation and structural similarities, we adopted another measure, the IoU, which has been considered the gold standard for evaluating segmentation performance for several semantic segmentation challenges. The experimental outcomes state that the suggested methodology achieved a 0.97 IoU on the custom KDHF dataset, as shown in Figure 10.7.

In order to analyze the benefits of the proposed technology, RetinalAlexU-Net is compared to prior methods. Figure 10.8 compares the segmentation results of RetinalAlexU-Net to current models on all metrics that were used in our studies. As shown in Figure 10.8, for diabetic retinopathy prediction using segmentation of blood

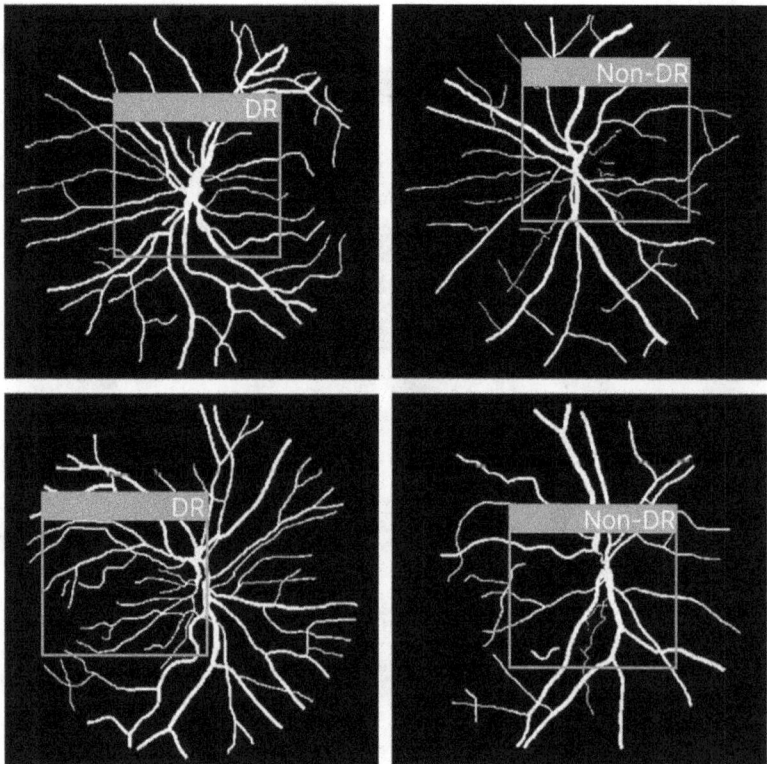

FIGURE 10.6 Diabetic retinopathy and non-diabetic vasculopathy identification using segmented vasculature.

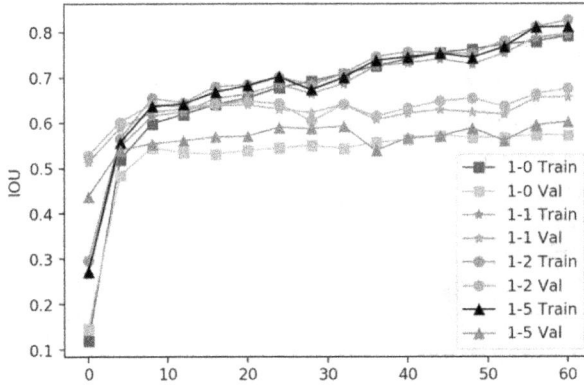

FIGURE 10.7 IoU evaluation results of proposed RetinalAlexU-Net.

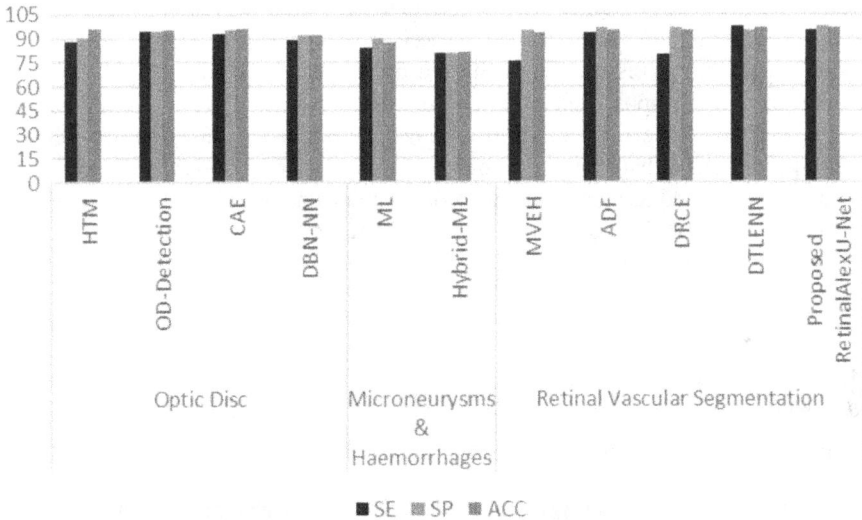

FIGURE 10.8 Performance comparison of proposed model with existing models.

vessels, our final proposed model, RetinalAlexU-Net. achieved the best performance on several metrics, including ACC, SP, and SE. Table 10.3 shows RetinalAlexU-Net achieved outstanding results compared to other models.

Finally, experimental results in Figure 10.8 show that retinal blood vessel segmentation significantly improves the results of the classification of diabetic retinopathy.

TABLE 10.3
RetinalAlexU-Net Performance Results

RetinalAlexU-Net Performance Metrics	Percentage (%)
Intersection over Union	0.971
Accuracy	0.966
F1-Score	0.967
Precision	0.979
Specificity	0.979
Sensitivity	0.954

10.5 CONCLUSION

In this study, an automated diagnostic method for retinal blood vessels is based on the process of segmentation. Classification and diagnosis of DR severity rely heavily on the accurate segmentation of blood vessels. Automated segmentation and detection of retinal blood vessels were achieved using the suggested RetinalAlexU-Net architecture. The proposed method achieves 0.96 ACC and 0.97 IoU in a customized dataset for its corresponding ground truth images. The suggested model has shown performance that is superior to that of prior research. However, the approach currently being used has certain constraints and does not provide the optimum outcomes for all kinds of datasets. In the future, the researchers may expand the framework to enhance accuracy over a wide range of datasets, use images of the retinal fundus, and target early diagnosis of additional eye problems, such as glaucoma and cataracts.

REFERENCES

About diabetes., 2022, October. https://idf.org/aboutdiabetes/what-is-diabetes/facts-figures .html,12.

Adarsh, R., Amarnageswarao, G., Pandeeswari, R. and Deivalakshmi, S., 2020, March. Dense residual convolutional auto encoder for retinal blood vessels segmentation. In *2020 6th International Conference on Advanced Computing and Communication Systems (ICACCS)* (pp. 280–284). IEEE.

Alom, M.Z., Taha, T.M., Yakopcic, C., Westberg, S., Sidike, P., Nasrin, M.S., Van Esesn, B.C., Awwal, A.A.S. and Asari, V.K., 2018. *The History Began from Alexnet: A Comprehensive Survey on Deep Learning Approaches.* arXiv Preprint ArXiv:1803.01164.

Atteia, G., Abdel Samee, N. and Zohair Hassan, H., 2021. DFTSA-net: Deep feature transfer-based stacked autoencoder network for DME diagnosis. *Entropy*, 23(10), p. 1251.

Bengani, S., 2021. Automatic segmentation of optic disc in retinal fundus images using semi-supervised deep learning. *Multimedia Tools and Applications*, 80(3), pp. 3443–3468.

Diabetic retinopathy: An historical assessment, 2022, December 8. https://drkalantzis.gr/files /pdf/DiabeticRetinopathy.pdf.

DRIVE dataset, 2022, November 13. https://paperswithcode.com/dataset/drive.

Erciyas, A. and Barışçı, N., 2021. An effective method for detecting and classifying diabetic retinopathy lesions based on deep learning. *Computational and Mathematical Methods in Medicine*, 2021.

Gao, J., Chen, G. and Lin, W., 2020. An effective retinal blood vessel segmentation by using automatic random walks based on centerline extraction. *BioMed Research International*, 2020.

GoogleNet, 2022, November 18. https://towardsdatascience.com/deep-learning-googlenet -explained-de8861c82765.

Jadhav, A.S., Patil, P.B. and Biradar, S., 2020. Analysis on diagnosing diabetic retinopathy by segmenting blood vessels, optic disc and retinal abnormalities. *Journal of Medical Engineering and Technology*, 44(6), pp. 299–316.

Kaggle dataset, 2022 October 24. https://www.kaggle.com/datasets/mariaherrerot/ eyepacspreprocess.

Kumar, S., Adarsh, A., Kumar, B. and Singh, A.K., 2020. An automated early diabetic retinopathy detection through improved blood vessel and optic disc segmentation. *Optics and Laser Technology*, 121, p. 105815.

Long, S., Chen, J., Hu, A., Liu, H., Chen, Z. and Zheng, D., 2020. Microaneurysms detection in color fundus images using machine learning based on directional local contrast. *BioMedical Engineering Online*, 19(1), pp. 1–23.

Messidor dataset, 2022 October 16. https://www.adcis.net/en/third-party/messidor/.

PerformanceAnalysis, 2022 October 25. https://medium.com/@xaviergeerinck/artificial -intelligence-how-to-measure-performance-accuracy-precision-recall-f1-roc-rmse -611d10e4caac.

Revathy, R., Nithya, B.S., Reshma, J.J., Ragendhu, S.S. and Sumithra, M.D., 2020. Diabetic retinopathy detection using machine learning. *International Journal of Engineering Research and Technology*, 9(6), pp. 2278–0181.

Riaz, H., Park, J., Choi, H., Kim, H. and Kim, J., 2020. Deep and densely connected networks for classification of diabetic retinopathy. *Diagnostics*, 10(1), p. 24.

Saini, D.C., Kochar, A. and Poonia, R., 2021. Clinical correlation of diabetic retinopathy with nephropathy and neuropathy. *Indian Journal of Ophthalmology*, 69(11), p. 3364.

Shaikha, H.K. and Sallow, A.B., 2019, April. Optic disc detection and segmentation in retinal fundus image. In *2019 International Conference on Advanced Science and Engineering (ICOASE)* (pp. 23–28). IEEE.

Siva Sundhara Raja, D. and Vasuki, S., 2015. Automatic detection of blood vessels in retinal images for diabetic retinopathy diagnosis. *Computational and Mathematical Methods in Medicine*, 2015.

Soomro, T.A., Afifi, A.J., Zheng, L., Soomro, S., Gao, J., Hellwich, O. and Paul, M., 2019. Deep learning models for retinal blood vessels segmentation: A review. *IEEE Access*, 7, pp. 71696–71717.

Ting, D.S., Foo, V.H., Tan, T.E., Sie, N.M., Wong, C.W., Tsai, A.S., Tan, G.S., Lim, L.S., Yeo, I., Wong, D.W. and Ong, S.G., 2020. 25-years trends and risk factors related to surgical outcomes of giant retinal tear-rhegmatogenous retinal detachments. *Scientific reports*, 10(1), pp. 1–8.

Wang, W. and Lo, A.C., 2018. Diabetic retinopathy: pathophysiology and treatments. *International Journal of Molecular Sciences*, 19(6), p. 1816.

11 Decoding EEG Signals to Generate Images Using GANs

Ritik Naik, Kunal Chaudhari,
Ketaki Jadhav, and Amit Joshi

11.1 INTRODUCTION

Humans have always been curious to comprehend the imaginings happening inside the human brain. With the advent of artificial intelligence (AI) technology and brain imaging techniques, it has been possible to build computation models to capture the human brain's imagination. Millions of neurons process the perceived visual stimuli, constituting the brain signals. These brain signals are generally recorded using brain-imaging techniques like magnetic resonance imaging (MRI) and functional magnetic resonance imaging (fMRI). Some non-invasive techniques like magnetoencephalography (MEG) and electroencephalography (EEG) are also used for the same purpose. Each method has its own merits and demerits. The scalp surface area of the brain is used in recording EEG signals. EEG signals are classified on the basis of signal frequencies corresponding to different visual stimuli. These brain signals can be decoded by means of deep learning methods and further used to generate images of objects visualized by the subject.

Recent developments in the field of deep learning have enabled fast and efficient operations in the healthcare domain. Various deep learning techniques, like convolutional neural networks (CNN), long short-term memory (LSTM), autoencoders, and others, are used to extract features from encoded brain signals. These extracted features are used by generative adversarial networks (GANs) in order to generate realistic images. This technology can assist patients with disabilities and those suffering from paralysis. Patients will be able to better express their thoughts and emotions with the help of this technology. This can also prove to be helpful to medical practitioners for improved diagnosis.

Reconstructing and generating images from EEG signals has become one of the trending topics in recent years. EEG signals and images cannot be translated using traditional approaches. Various deep learning architectures decode the features from raw EEG signals, which are subsequently fed to GANs for image reconstruction [1]. Image reconstruction from brain signals is largely carried out with the use of fMRI and EEG data. Some early works include a deep convolutional generative adversarial

DOI: 10.1201/9781003363361-11

network (DCGAN) for learning latent space. Seeliger et al. used this DCGAN along with their own complex loss function for predictive models [2]. As the brain-computer interface (BCI) is used for recording EEG signals, it's critical to understand the BCI system in detail. Almabrok Essa and Hari Kotte discussed different ways of acquiring and processing brain signals and classification methods used over a period of time. It concludes that extracted features from EEG signals are precise when time-domain parameters are used [3]. Some approaches have attempted to "read the mind" using neuroadaptive technologies that include modelling a user's mindset with corresponding brain signals. For this purpose, a novel modelling approach combining neuroadaptive brain interfacing with a generative neural network has been proposed by Kangassalo et al. [4]. There is a longstanding challenge to differentiate visual words from each other in reference to their induced stimuli. Few approaches analyze the way in which EEG signals can be used to decode and reconstruct visual words [5]. Earlier GAN-based methods were unable to achieve fine fidelity and naturalness. A Bayesian visual reconstruction method based on GAN was proposed by Qiao et al. that uses a generator of a pre-trained BigGAN model to improve the quality of generated images [6]. However, this research topic is not limited only to human experimentation. Hayashi, Ryusuke, and Hayaki Kawata have attempted image reconstruction by a brain-machine interface using the brain signals of a monkey, depending on its neural activity [7]. Some methods have also attempted to use statistical techniques for EEG feature extraction and achieved good accuracy. An adversarial autoencoder that combines the advantages of GANs and variational autoencoders (VAE) was modified and used along with statistical techniques for feature extraction by Chaurasiya et al. [8]. Efforts have been made to generate target and non-target images for EEG signals using a novel conditional GAN-based approach for image reconstruction and performed an analysis of the conditional GAN model with EEG, EEG, and noise as inputs [9]. Sometimes unwanted noise is introduced while recording EEG signals. Depending on the changing points of the signals, a finite amplitude frequency transformation method is introduced. Without using any preprocessing techniques, this work successfully classified different types of biomedical signals [10]. Generally, EEG signals are affected by unforeseen noise due to heartbeat, eye movements, and head muscle movements. Hence, a GAN-based denoising method for noise removal from multichannel EEG signals is proposed by An et al. that attempts to limit EEG signal range to detect unusual EEG signals [11]. With huge advances happening in this domain, an overview of various image reconstruction methods is helpful for researchers. A study done by Rakhimberdina et al. provides an analysis of various methods based on evaluation metrics, architectural design, and benchmark datasets. It gives a detailed comprehensive analysis for researchers [12]. Despite considerable progress in this field, there exists little variety among the reconstructed images. There is a need to address the gap between fidelity and the diversity of generated images by scaling up GANs and training them on multiple categories. A work done by Brock et al. has discovered some instabilities regarding large-scale GANs and analyzed them empirically [13]. It has been observed that adding more structure to the latent space in GANs with a specialized cost function enhances the image quality. Odena et al. introduced auxiliary conditional generative adversarial networks (AC-GAN) and has generated more diverse and globally consistent images [14]. There is a technique that has tried to boost the accuracy of EEG data classification by using EEG recorded during both perception tasks and imagination tasks. With the help of the attention module and Sinc-EEGNet, it attempts to enhance the understandability of neural networks [15]. Transfer learning is the application of previously learned knowledge and abilities to solve closely related problem-solving cases. Deep neural network (DNN) algorithms, domain adaptation, subspace learning, and improved common spatial patterns (CSP) algorithms are the four frequently used methods in transfer learning for analyzing EEG signals. In the review proposed by Wan et al., the strengths, weaknesses, applications, and challenges of the mentioned transfer learning techniques are discussed [16]. Deep learning methods for EEG signal feature extraction help to detect brain diseases and different psycho-neuro disorders. These methods assist in better understanding human emotions. A review by Praveena et al. provides a broad perspective on the applications of deep learning architectures like recurrent neural networks (RNNs), CNNs, autoencoders, and others in the analysis of signals [17].

This work attempts to visualize the human imagination from EEG signals using deep Learning methods. To generate images, features from the EEG signals need to be extracted first. The extracted features are fed to the generator of the GAN. These features act as conditions on the generator to generate a corresponding image.

This work aims to provide improved implementation of:

1. Feature extractors for EEG signals.
2. Image classifiers.
3. GANs for generating images of digits and characters.

The rest of this chapter is organized across different sections. Section 11.2 discusses the literature review in detail, followed by a proposed methodology in Section 11.3. Results and discussions regarding the presented approach are analyzed in Section 11.4. At last, Section 11.5 discusses conclusions about the proposed approach.

11.2   LITERATURE REVIEW

Brain signal analysis and feature extraction are compelling topics in the biomedical research domain. Combining them with the recent developments in the deep learning field like CNNs and GANs, it is now feasible to generate realistic images using the features extracted from the brain signals.

Tirupattur et al. have encoded EEG signals with deep learning architecture and used them as conditioning to generate images. They have carried out experiments on three different domains of input, namely digits, characters, and objects, and demonstrated that their GAN architecture can generate images of a specific class conditioned on EEG patterns [18]. Shen et al. have demonstrated that combining multiple DNN layers enhances the quality and generalizability of generated images. They have also been able to reconstruct artificial shapes along with natural images with the use of a deep generative network (DGN) [19]. Jiao et al. have proposed a two-staged decoding framework comprising a visual-guided EEG classification stage and a visual-guided image generation stage. They have achieved better decoding results by employing visual representations acquired from deep learning models in the computer vision domain [20]. Fu et al. have proposed an AC-GAN that uses emotional information from corresponding EEG signals to generate facial expressions [21]. Mishra et al. have increased EEG classification accuracy by using distance metric learning via a Siamese network with triplet loss. They have also proved the benefit of minimizing the number of channels by using a correlation-based channel selection strategy [22]. St-Yves et al. have observed that the quality of reconstructed images depends on the denoising of voxels and that reconstruction variability depends on the accuracy of the encoding model. They have concluded that the activity patterns can be used to denoise and compress the raw EEG signals [23]. Strohm et al. used the eye fixations of the subject for the reconstruction of facial images. They devised the reconstruction of images as a similarity-scoring task between neural attention maps and human eye fixations [24]. Gaziv et al. have introduced a self-supervised approach that gives better results in large-scale semantic categorization of fMRI data. With self-supervised training on huge amounts of data, they have improved the quality of the reconstructed images and classification accuracies [25]. Shen et al. achieved the best performance by using three-loss functions for training their image reconstruction model. Both perceptual and adversarial losses are important for their image reconstruction model [26]. Li et al. have proposed a cross-modal semi-supervised method for generating images that addresses the modality gap problem by learning semantic features from the non-image modality [27]. Some researchers have attempted to generate real-time images from brain signals. Rashkov et al. proposed a closed-loop BCI system that can potentially generate real-time images from EEG features [28]. At times, electrocorticography (ECoG) signals are also being used along with EEG signals. Date et al. have attempted to reconstruct images using ECoG signals and have highlighted the significance of the temporal dynamics of ECoG signals [29].

Generally, CNNs are used to decode brain signals. However, some approaches have attempted to use LSTM models for the same task. Kavasidis et al. have proposed a deep learning framework consisting of an LSTM encoder for EEG signal classification and a decoder that maps these features onto images. They have tested two approaches, namely GANs and VAEs, for the decoder, and concluded that GANs surpass VAEs in generating realistic images, however they lack fine details [30]. Palazzo et al. have used an LSTM layer for preprocessing and decoding raw EEG signals. These decoded signals are then used to generate realistic and diverse images using conditional GANs [31]. Khare et al. proposed a conditional progressive generative adversarial network (cProGAN) to reconstruct perceived images. Their model showed an improvement in inception score (IS) as compared to other approaches and is able to produce decent images [32]. Jolly et al. have developed a common encoder for different tasks so that features of the superficially different tasks can be extracted using it. They have experimented with CNNs, autoencoders and gated recurrent units (GRUs) [33].

Some approaches have utilized autoencoders for image generation. Qiao et al. proposed an alternating autoencoder and observed that two converse autoencoders are obtained by integrating the encoder and decoder in different orders [34]. Bethge et al. have developed an EEG2Vec model with a conditional variational autoencoder for encoding raw EEG signals that act as input to a feed-forward neural network for emotion classification [35]. Ren et al. have built a dual-variational autoencoder/generative adversarial network (D-VAE/GAN) model that integrates the benefits of both VAE and GANs and generates more realistic visual stimuli [36].

Various statistical methods are used to preprocess raw EEG signals in order to achieve better classification accuracy and generate high-quality images. Du et al. have presented a deep generative multiview model (DGMM) that uses two view-specific generators for modelling the statistical relationships between the image and the fMRI signals [37]. Mishra et al. attempted to refine EEG data by proposing a correlation-based approach that showed significant improvement in EEG classification accuracy [38]. Yilmaz et al. have increased classification performance by making a few changes in their baseline signal transformation [39].

In general, EEG signals contain many unwanted features. Yao et al. have introduced a GAN-based autoencoder approach to remove undesirable features from EEG signals and have opened the door to many potential applications [40]. They have further improved the accuracy of their feature filter, which retains the desired features by discarding most of the unwanted features [41]. George et al. have presented techniques for data augmentation for decoding brain signals using neural networks. They have proved that frequency recombination and noise addition improve the decoding performance as compared to unaugmented approaches [42].

GANs are an integral part of image generation methods. Ever since their introduction, they have made many remarkable accomplishments in image generation. Goodfellow et al. have introduced a technique called generative adversarial network in which two neural networks, namely the generator and discriminator, compete against one another to become more accurate in their predictions and generate new data based on the training data [43]. Radford et al. have introduced DCGAN and highlighted that, for supervised tasks, the generator and discriminator can be used as feature extractors [44]. Mirza et al. proposed a conditional GAN. When given an input of a label and a random array, a conditional GAN generates data corresponding to the given label and has a similar structure to that of the training data [45]. Arjovsky et al. presented an approach that increases learning stability and discards problems like mode collapse and gives meaningful learning curves for debugging and hyperparameter searches [46]. Salimans et al. introduced an evaluation metric called inception score for testing the quality of generated images [47]. Zhang et al. generated photo-realistic images conditioned on text descriptions. They introduced a two-staged approach in which stage one generates images from text descriptions and stage two increases the quality of the images [48].

Attempts have been made to turn the visualization of brain signals into a reality. But current EEG feature encoders lack the potential to extract meaningful features from brain signals and, hence, EEG classification accuracy is not very good. Also, improvements can be made in the methods for generating images from extracted features. This work aims to provide a better approach for feature extraction from EEG signals and generate imagined images using the extracted features.

11.3 PROPOSED METHODOLOGY

This work generates images from EEG signals using GANs. It focuses generation of images from EEG data corresponding to digits and characters. It begins by first encoding the features of EEG data. This is done to use only the extracted features from the data, instead of using the raw EEG data, which generally contains a lot of noise. These extracted features are then given as input to the generator of the GAN, along with noise. The generator's output is given to the discriminator and image classifier. The discriminator learns to discriminate between real and fake samples and the classifier predicts the class of the generated image. This is to ensure that the generator learns to generate images that resemble real images and belong to the correct class. Figure 11.1 depicts the entire flow of the proposed approach.

This approach is divided into three phases, namely feature encoding, image classification, and image generation. These phases are discussed in detail below.

11.3.1 FEATURE ENCODING

To create robust encoding of the features of EEG data, this work makes use of a CNN. The CNN can capture contextual information from the data. The CNN also enables learning features from different channels by parameter sharing. Different models for the classification of EEG data have been trained and the most promising architecture is demonstrated in Figure 11.2. The architecture for the CNN encoder model consists of multiple Convolutional2D and Convolutional1D layers along with max pooling and batch normalization, followed by three fully connected (FC) layers. Convolution across the time axis and the channel axis is applied to enable the model to learn features throughout the time steps, as well as across different channels. The activation function used throughout the layers is a leaky rectified linear unit (LeakyReLU). The final fully connected layer has ten neurons with a softmax activation function which classifies data. The stochastic gradient descent optimizer with a learning rate of 1e-4 and momentum of 0.92 is used to train this model for 200 epochs with a 128 batch size.

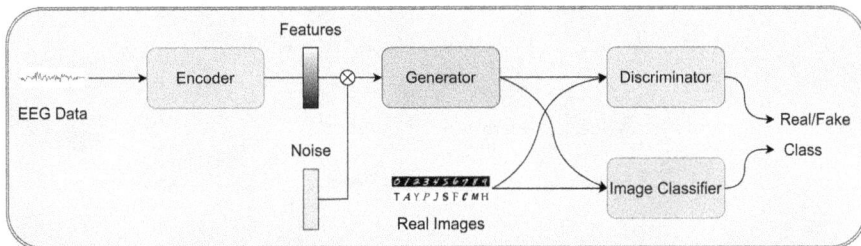

FIGURE 11.1 Complete flow of the proposed approach

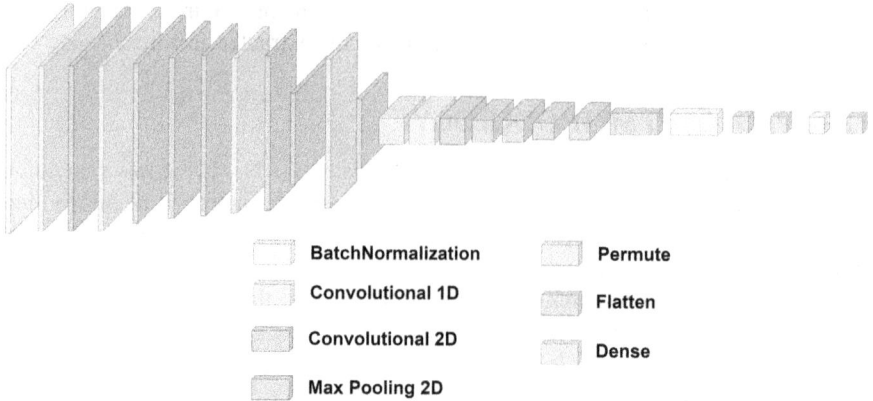

	BatchNormalization		Permute
	Convolutional 1D		Flatten
	Convolutional 2D		Dense
	Max Pooling 2D		

FIGURE 11.2 Architecture of EEG classifier

After training the model on the classification task, the output of the last batch normalization layer is used as the encoded features for EEG signals. These features are used as input to the GAN model.

11.3.2 IMAGE CLASSIFICATION

In image classification, in order to predict the class for an input image, the model must learn the weights. It seems to be a trivial task for humans but might not be that easy for a computer. But advancements in deep learning have made it possible. CNNs have shown exceptional results in learning the spatial dependencies of the input image using its convolution operations. To perform image classification, a deep convolutional neural network is designed. The architecture for this model is displayed in Figure 11.3. It comprises Convolutional2D layers along with max pooling and dropout. The filter size of each convolution layer is 3×3 and the number of filters is 16, 32, 64, 128, 256, and 512. Dropout layers act as regularizers and switch off

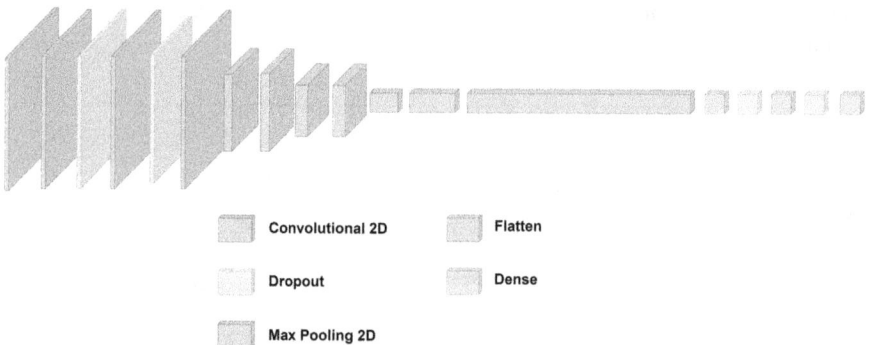

	Convolutional 2D		Flatten
	Dropout		Dense
	Max Pooling 2D		

FIGURE 11.3 Architecture of image classifier

some neurons of the model for better learning. For both datasets, the same architecture is used because this work focuses only on digits and characters which appear to be fundamentally similar. Ten classes for digits as well as for characters are considered in this work. For the activation function, rectified linear unit (ReLU) is utilized throughout all layers of the model and the last layer has softmax as the activation function. This model is trained with Adam as the optimizer on both datasets for 100 epochs with batch sizes of 32.

These trained classifiers for digits and characters are saved and later used along with a discriminator to train the GAN model.

11.3.3 IMAGE GENERATION

GANs are used to generate images from encoded EEG features. A GAN comprises two models: a generator and a discriminator. Each competes against the other to learn to capture the features and variations from the dataset. The generator $G(z;\theta g_g)$ learns a distribution (p_g) to map the input noise (z) from space (p_z) to target space (p_{data}) with parameters θg_g. The input x is classified as real or fake using the discriminator $D(x;_d)$. $D(x)$ indicates the probability that x comes from p_{data} instead of p_g. The following equation represents the objective function for the entire GAN model [43].

$$\min_{G} \max_{D} V\left(D,G\right) = E_{x\sim pdata}\left[logD\left(x\right)\right] + E_{z\sim pz}\left[log\left(1-D\left(G\left(z\right)\right)\right)\right]$$

(11.1)

This work proposes two GAN architectures, each for digits and characters. The digit GAN includes a digit generator and a digit discriminator. The digit generator takes EEG encodings as input along with noise and learns to generate realistic images. By taking generated images and real images as input, the digit discriminator performs the task of classifying generated images as real or fake. The image classifier discussed in the previous subsection is used along with the discriminator in this stage and predicts the class to which the generated image belongs. This helps in the training of the generator to generate real images which belong to the correct class. Digit generator architecture contains a combination of fully connected layers along with batch normalization, Convolutional2D, and upsampling. LeakyReLU activation is used across all the layers. The digit discriminator architecture contains Convolutional2D layers followed by max Pool layers and one fully connected layer. Figures 11.4 and 11.5 show the architecture of the digit generator and digit discriminator. An Adam optimizer having 5e-5 as a learning rate is used to train the digit GAN model for 120 epochs with a batch size of 100.

The character GAN works in the same manner as the digit GAN. The character generator takes EEG feature encodings along with noise and generates character images. The character discriminator takes these generated images along with real images and then classifies the generated images as real or fake. The architecture of the character generator comprises fully connected layers followed by batch normalization, convolution, and Convolution2DTranspose. The activation function used is

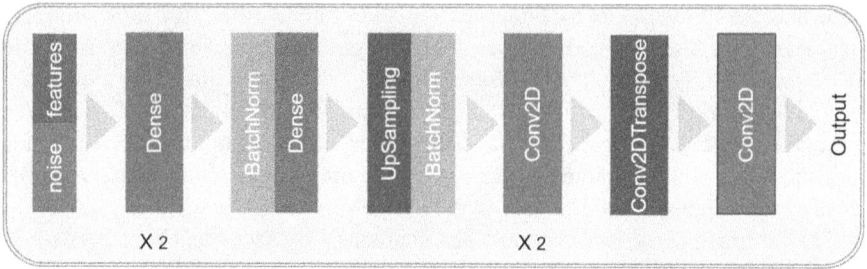

FIGURE 11.4   Architecture for digit generator

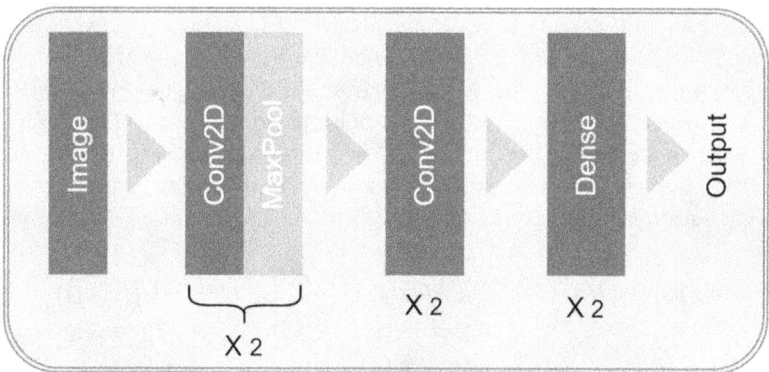

FIGURE 11.5   Architecture for digit discriminator

LeakyReLU. The character discriminator architecture comprises Convolutional2D layers followed by max pool and Gaussian noise layers. Adding Gaussian noise to the discriminator helps stabilize the training and enables the GAN to generate sharper images. Figures 11.6 and 11.7 show the architecture of the character generator and the character discriminator. The Adam optimizer with 5e-5 as the learning rate is used to train the character GAN model for 200 epochs with a batch size of 100.

The summarized algorithm of the approach is given below.

Algorithm:
  for number of epochs **do**
        for number of mini-batches **do**

- Sample mini-batch of b EEG signals from dataset $\{s^{(1)}, s^{(2)}, ..., s^{(b)}\}$
- Pass these sampled signals through EEG feature encoder to get their encodings $\{e^{(1)}, e^{(2)}, ..., e^{(b)}\}$ respectively
- Sample mini-batch of b noise samples $\{n^{(1)}, n^{(2)}, ..., n^{(b)}\}$
- Pass this sampled noise and encodings to the generator

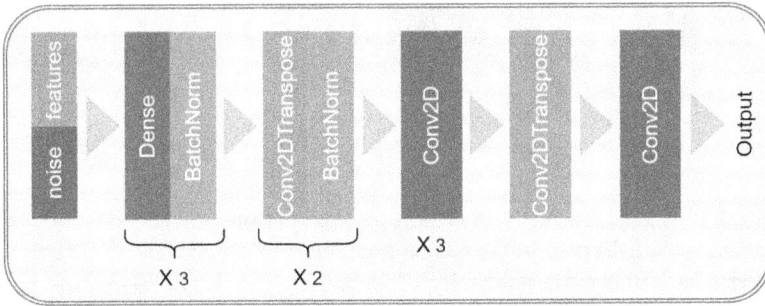

FIGURE 11.6   Architecture for character generator

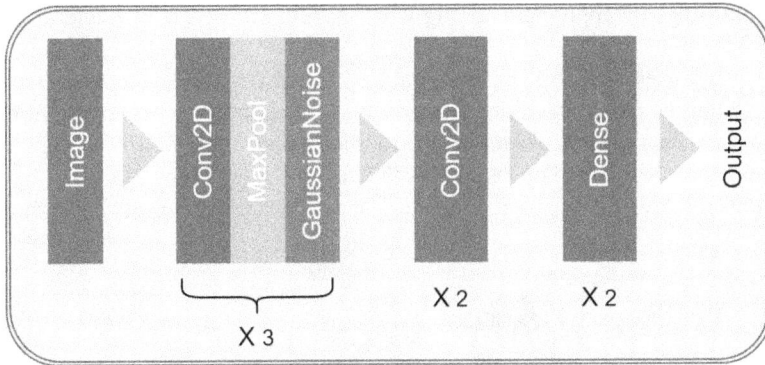

FIGURE 11.7   Architecture for character discriminator

- Generator concatenates the noise with encodings to get $\{n^{(1)}e^{(1)}, n^{(2)}e^{(2)}, ..., n^{(b)}e^{(b)}\}$ and uses it to generate mini-batch of b fake images $\{f^{(1)}, f^{(2)}, ..., f^{(b)}\}$
- Sample mini-batch of b examples of corresponding real images $\{x^{(1)}, x^{(2)}, ..., x^{(b)}\}$ from target distribution $p_{data}(x)$
- Update the discriminator through optimizer based on real and fake images
- Update the generator through optimizer

    end for
end for

11.4   RESULTS AND DISCUSSION

Experimental setup, performance parameters used to evaluate the above models, and achieved results are discussed in this section.

11.4.1   EXPERIMENTAL SETUP

The proposed work uses a publicly accessible dataset. Kumar et al. [49] originally produced this dataset and Tirupattur et al. [18] preprocessed it. Kumar et al.

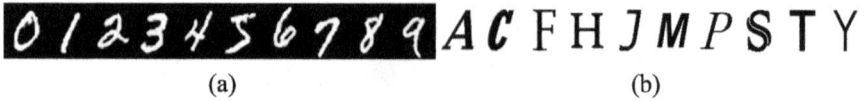

(a)   (b)

FIGURE 11.8 Dataset images with ten classes – (a) MNIST dataset (b) Char74K dataset

conducted an experiment with 23 volunteers aged between 15 and 40 years. A total of 30 images, with 10 images from each digit, character, and object, were shown to volunteers. Each image was shown for 10 seconds, with a gap of 20 seconds between successive recordings. Then, volunteers were asked to imagine those images. Their imaginations were recorded as EEG signals with the Emotiv EPOC+ sensor, consisting of 14 channels and a frequency of 128 Hz. Tirupattur et al. preprocessed these EEG recordings by applying a sliding window with an overlap of 8 and a window size of 32.

This work uses digit and character datasets for EEG signals without any preprocessing from the above-mentioned dataset by Tirupattur et al. The original images for digits and characters are taken from Modified National Institute of Standards and Technology (MNIST) [51] and Char74K [52] as shown in Figure 11.8.

Details regarding the dataset, hardware, and software configuration are shown in Table 11.1.

11.4.2 PERFORMANCE PARAMETERS

The performance of the proposed model on different parameters is analyzed in this section.

11.4.2.1 Model Accuracy

Classification models are evaluated using an accuracy metric. This metric represents a percentage of correct predictions performed by a classification model.

11.4.2.2 Inception Score (IS)

Inception score is an objective measure that helps to judge the quality of images generated using GANs. IS evaluates generated images based on two parameters: quality

TABLE 11.1
Experimental Setup

System Configurations	GPU	NVIDIA Tesla V100 GPU
	System RAM	256 GB
	Framework	TensorFlow (TF)
	Digits	**Characters**
Dataset	MNIST [51]	Char74K [52]
No. of Classes	10	10
Image Dimensions (pixel)	28 × 28	64 × 64 (Reshaped)

and diversity. To examine the quality of images generated with the proposed GAN model, the IS is calculated using the TensorFlow-GAN (TF-GAN) library.

Following are some of the most effective metrics aside from the inception score that are used for the evaluation of images generated by GANs. Implementations of the following three parameters, as given by Müller et al. [50], are used in this work.

11.4.2.3 Peak Signal-to-Noise Ratio (PSNR)

This ratio signifies the quality of the generated image as compared with the original image. It is the ratio of maximum pixel power of an original image to noise between original and generated image.

11.4.2.4 Structural Similarity Index Measure (SSIM)

SSIM is an evaluation metric which calculates the resemblance between two images. It compares images based on the three key features of luminance, contrast, and structure.

11.4.2.5 Root Mean Square Error (RMSE)

RMSE shows the closeness between observed data points and values predicted by the model. It performs an evaluation based on the deviation between values.

11.4.3 RESULT

After training and testing the above architecture on the digit and character datasets, the following results were obtained.

11.4.3.1 Feature Encoding

Features of EEG signals for the digit and character datasets are encoded using CNNs, as discussed in Section 11.3.1. The trained EEG classifier was tested on the test dataset for digits and characters. EEG classification accuracy of 75.06% for the digits and 73.09% for the character dataset is achieved by this work.

This work has compared EEG classification accuracy with the EEG classification accuracy of the Kumar et al. [49] and Tirupattur et al. [18] models for the digits and characters datasets. As demonstrated in Table 11.2, the proposed EEG classifier shows an improvement in accuracy.

TABLE 11.2
EEG Classification Accuracy Comparison

Dataset	Accuracy (%)		
	Kumar et al. [49]	Tirupattur et al. [18]	Proposed Method
Digits	68.45	72.88	75.06
Characters	66.91	71.18	73.09

TABLE 11.3

Image Classification Accuracy for Different Datasets

Dataset	Accuracy (%)
Digits	99.44
Characters	99.46

11.4.3.2 Image Classification

The image classifier is trained using a deep convolutional neural network, as discussed in Section 11.3.2, and has achieved an image classification accuracy of 99.44% for the digit dataset, while the character dataset gave an accuracy of 99.46%, as mentioned in Table 11.3.

11.4.3.3 Image Generation

The trained image classifier from Section 11.3.2 is used along with the discriminator of the GAN. By making use of this trained GAN, images are generated for both the digit and character datasets from their EEG signals. The output images of the proposed GAN are shown in Figure 11.9.

For the digit dataset, generated images of digits were evaluated using an additional evaluation metric – namely IS – using the TF-GAN library, and obtained a value of 9.88. The generated images are evaluated using different evaluation metrics, as discussed in Section 11.4.2. Values obtained for these metrics for digits and character datasets are in Table 11.4.

This work has generated images of digits and characters using the features extracted from the corresponding EEG recordings. The EEG feature encoder

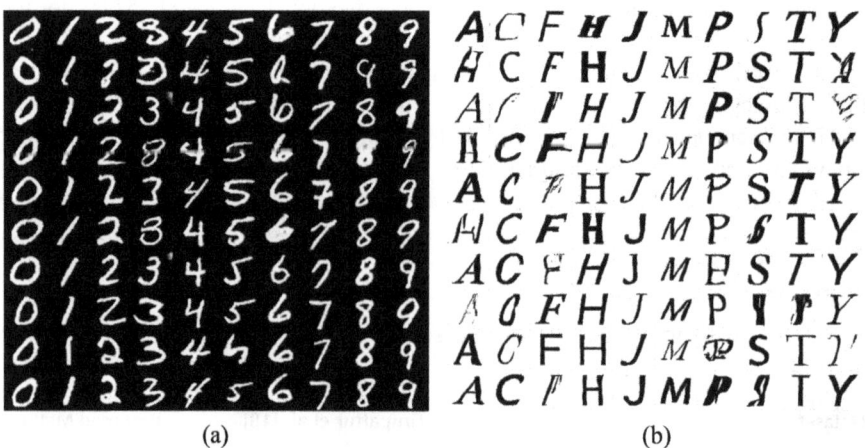

(a)   (b)

FIGURE 11.9 Images generated by proposed GAN for EEG signals – (a) Digits (b) Characters

TABLE 11.4

Different Evaluation Metrics for the Proposed GAN

Dataset	Evaluation Metric		
	PSNR	SSIM	RMSE
Digits	34.41	0.6481	0.0194
Characters	32.66	0.7266	0.0237

is developed using CNN architecture to classify EEG signals. This EEG feature encoder achieves higher classification accuracy, which helps to capture better features from EEG signals. After that, the deep convolutional neural network is trained and used to classify images. The discriminator uses this image classifier for better learning. The proposed GAN generates realistic images of digits and characters. However, this work is limited to the digit and character categories.

11.5 CONCLUSION AND FUTURE WORK

This work has introduced an approach to generate realistic images from brain signals. In this approach, features from the EEG signals are extracted to get important information from them and these extracted features and original images are used as input for training the GAN. The trained GAN model makes use of EEG signals as input to generate realistic images, thus correctly interpreting human thoughts. The accuracy of the EEG encoder has been instrumental in the generation of realistic images. The proposed model has achieved an EEG classification accuracy of 75.06% and 73.09% for the digit and character datasets, respectively. This model has been successful in achieving higher accuracy for EEG classification.

This work has attempted to generate realistic images of digits and characters. It can be further improved to visualize entire words or sentences rather than a single character. There is still scope for further improvement by trying different models which can classify EEG signals more accurately. Attempts can also be made to improve the quality of the generated images. This work can be further extended to generate realistic images of various objects, as well as scenarios using their corresponding EEG signals.

ACKNOWLEDGEMENT

We are thankful to the Department of Computer Engineering and IT, COEP Tech, for providing the GPU server facility to implement this work. This facility was established under TEQIP-III (A World Bank Project).

REFERENCES

1. Yang, Delong, et al. "The survey of image generation from EEG signals based on deep learning." In *2021 International Symposium on Biomedical Engineering and Computational Biology*, 2021.
2. Seeliger, Katja, et al. "Generative adversarial networks for reconstructing natural images from brain activity." *NeuroImage* 181 (2018): 775–785.
3. Essa, Almabrok, and Hari Kotte. "Brain signals analysis based deep learning methods: Recent advances in the study of non-invasive brain signals." arXiv preprint arXiv:2201.04229 (2021).
4. Kangassalo, Lauri, Michiel Spapé, and Tuukka Ruotsalo. "Neuroadaptive modelling for generating images matching perceptual categories." *Scientific Reports* 10(1) (2020): 14719.
5. Ling, Shouyu, et al. "How are visual words represented? Insights from EEG-based visual word decoding, feature derivation and image reconstruction." *Human Brain Mapping* 40(17) (2019): 5056–5068.
6. Qiao, Kai, et al. "BigGAN-based Bayesian reconstruction of natural images from human brain activity." *Neuroscience* 444 (2020): 92–105.
7. Hayashi, Ryusuke, and Hayaki Kawata "Image reconstruction from neural activity recorded from monkey inferior temporal cortex using generative adversarial networks." In *2018 IEEE International Conference on Systems, Man, and Cybernetics (SMC)*. IEEE, 2018.
8. Chaurasiya, R. K., S. K. Arvind, and Saket Garg. "Adversarial autoencoders for image generation from standard EEG features." In *2020 First International Conference on Power, Control and Computing Technologies (ICPC2T)*. IEEE, 2020.
9. Lee, Yonggun, and Yufei Huang. "Generating target/non-target images of an RSVP experiment from brain signals in by conditional generative adversarial network." In *2018 IEEE EMBS international conference on Biomedical & Health Informatics (BHI)*. IEEE, 2018.
10. Hatipoglu, Bahar, Cagatay Murat Yilmaz, and Cemal Kose. "A signal-to-image transformation approach for EEG and MEG signal classification." *Signal, Image and Video Processing* 13(3) (2019): 483–490.
11. An, Yang, Hak Keung Lam, and Sai Ho Ling. "Auto-denoising for EEG signals using generative adversarial network." *Sensors* 22(5) (2022): 1750.
12. Rakhimberdina, Zarina, et al. "Natural image reconstruction from fMRI using deep learning: A survey." *Frontiers in Neuroscience* 15 (2021): 795488.
13. Brock, Andrew, Jeff Donahue, and Karen Simonyan. "Large scale GAN training for high fidelity natural image synthesis." arXiv preprint arXiv:1809.11096 (2018).
14. Odena, Augustus, Christopher Olah, and Jonathon Shlens. "Conditional image synthesis with auxiliary classifier gans." In *International Conference on Machine Learning*. PMLR, 2017.
15. Shimizu, Hirokatsu, and Ramesh Srinivasan. "Improving classification and reconstruction of imagined images from EEG signals." *PLOS ONE* 17(9) (2022): e0274847.
16. Wan, Zitong, et al. "A review on transfer learning in EEG signal analysis." *Neurocomputing* 421 (2021): 1–14.
17. Merlin Praveena, D., D. Angelin Sarah, and S. Thomas George. "Deep learning techniques for EEG signal applications–a review." *IETE Journal of Research* 68(4) (2022): 3030–3037.

18. Tirupattur, Praveen, et al. "Thoughtviz: Visualizing human thoughts using generative adversarial network." *Proceedings of the 26th ACM international conference on Multimedia*, 2018.

19. Shen, Guohua, et al. "Deep image reconstruction from human brain activity." *PLOS Computational Biology* 15(1) (2019): e1006633.

20. Jiao, Zhicheng, et al. "Decoding EEG by visual-guided deep neural networks." *IJCAI* (2019).

21. Fu, Boxun, et al. "Conditional generative adversarial network for EEG-based emotion fine-grained estimation and visualization" *Journal of Visual Communication and Image Representation* 74 (2021): 102982.

22. Mishra, Rahul, and Arnav Bhavsar. "EEG classification for visual brain decoding via metric learning." *Bioimaging* (2021).

23. St-Yves, Ghislain, and Thomas Naselaris. "Generative adversarial networks conditioned on brain activity reconstruct seen images." In *2018 IEEE International Conference on Systems, Man, and Cybernetics (SMC)*. IEEE, 2018.

24. Strohm, Florian, et al. "Neural Photofit: Gaze-based mental image reconstruction." In *Proceedings of the IEEE/CVF International Conference on Computer Vision*, 2021.

25. Gaziv, Guy, et al. "Self-supervised natural image reconstruction and large-scale semantic classification from brain activity." *NeuroImage* 254 (2022): 119121.

26. Shen, Guohua, et al. "End-to-end deep image reconstruction from human brain activity." *Frontiers in Computational Neuroscience* (2019): 21.

27. Li, Dan, Changde Du, and Huiguang He. "Semi-supervised cross-modal image generation with generative adversarial networks." *Pattern Recognition* 100 (2020): 107085.

28. Rashkov, Grigory, et al. "Natural image reconstruction from brain waves: A novel visual BCI system with native feedback." *bioRxiv* (2019): 787101.

29. Date, Hiroto, et al. "Deep learning for natural image reconstruction from electrocorticography signals." In *2019 IEEE International Conference on Bioinformatics and Biomedicine (BIBM)*. IEEE, 2019.

30. Kavasidis, Isaak, et al. "Brain2image: Converting brain signals into images." In *Proceedings of the 25th ACM International Conference on Multimedia*, 2017.

31. Palazzo, Simone, et al. "Generative adversarial networks conditioned by brain signals." In *Proceedings of the IEEE International Conference on Computer Vision*, 2017.

32. Khare, Sanchita, et al. "NeuroVision: Perceived image regeneration using cProGAN." *Neural Computing and Applications* 34(8) (2022): 5979–5991.

33. Jolly, Baani Leen Kaur, et al. "Universal EEG encoder for learning diverse intelligent tasks." In *2019 IEEE Fifth International Conference on Multimedia Big Data (BigMM)*. IEEE, 2019.

34. Qiao, Kai, et al. "Reconstructing natural images from human fMRI by alternating encoding and decoding with shared autoencoder regularization." *Biomedical Signal Processing and Control* 73 (2022): 103397.

35. Bethge, David, et al. "EEG2Vec: Learning affective EEG representations via variational autoencoders." arXiv preprint arXiv:2207.08002 (2022).

36. Ren, Ziqi, et al. "Reconstructing seen image from brain activity by visually-guided cognitive representation and adversarial learning." *NeuroImage* 228 (2021): 117602.

37. Du, Changde, et al. "Reconstructing perceived images from human brain activities with Bayesian deep multiview learning." *IEEE Transactions on Neural Networks and Learning Systems* 30(8) (2018): 2310–2323.

38. Mishra, Rahul, Krishan Sharma, and Arnav Bhavsar "Visual brain decoding for short duration EEG signals." In *2021 29th European Signal Processing Conference (EUSIPCO)*. IEEE, 2021.

39. Yilmaz, Bahar Hatipoglu, Cagatay Murat Yilmaz *et al.* "Diversity in a signal-to-image transformation approach for EEG-based motor imagery task classification." *Medical and Biological Engineering and Computing* 58(2) (2020): 443–459.

40. Yao, Yue, Jo Plested, and Tom Gedeon. "A feature filter for EEG using Cycle-GAN structure." In *International Conference on Neural Information Processing.* Springer, 2018.

41. Yao, Yue, Josephine Plested, and Tom Gedeon. "Information-preserving feature filter for short-term EEG signals." *Neurocomputing* 408 (2020): 91–99.

42. George, Olawunmi, et al. "Data augmentation strategies for EEG-based motor imagery decoding." *Heliyon* 8(8) (2022): e10240.

43. Goodfellow, Ian, et al. "Generative adversarial networks." *Communications of the ACM* 63(11) (2020): 139–144.

44. Radford, Alec, Luke Metz, and Soumith Chintala. "Unsupervised representation learning with deep convolutional generative adversarial networks." arXiv preprint arXiv:1511.06434 (2015).

45. Mirza, Mehdi, and Simon Osindero. "Conditional generative adversarial nets." arXiv preprint arXiv:1411.1784 (2014).

46. Arjovsky, Martin, Soumith Chintala, and Léon Bottou. "Wasserstein generative adversarial networks." *International Conference on Machine Learning.* PMLR, 2017.

47. Salimans, Tim, et al. "Improved techniques for training gans." *Advances in Neural Information Processing Systems* 29 (2016).

48. Zhang, Han, et al. "Stackgan: Text to photo-realistic image synthesis with stacked generative adversarial networks." In *Proceedings of the IEEE International Conference on Computer Vision,* 2017.

49. Kumar, Pradeep, et al. "Envisioned speech recognition using EEG sensors." *Personal and Ubiquitous Computing* 22(1) (2018): 185–199.

50. Müller, Markus U., et al. "Super-resolution of multispectral satellite images using convolutional neural networks." arXiv preprint arXiv:2002.00580 (2020).

51. LeCun, Yann, et al. "Gradient-based learning applied to document recognition." *Proceedings of the IEEE* 86(11) (1998): 2278–2324.

52. De Campos, Teófilo Emídio, Bodla Rakesh Babu, and Manik Varma. Character recognition in natural images VISAPP (2) 7.2 (2009).

12 Mental Health Disorder through Electroencephalogram Analysis using Computational Model

Kiran Waghmare and Meenakshi Malhotra

12.1 INTRODUCTION

A World Health Organization (WHO) special initiative for mental health – Universal Health Coverage for Mental Health – was announced by the WHO in 2019 (Agudelo-Toro and Neef, 2013), with the mandate to provide 100 million people in 12 priority countries with quality and affordable mental health care over the next ten years (Soufineyestani et al., 2020). The WHO defines health as physical, mental, and social well-being (Soufineyestani et al., 2020). Ramadan states that "[h]ealth is a state of complete physical, mental, and social well-being and not merely the absence of disease or infirmity". The WHO report indicates that approximately 450 million people worldwide suffer from at least one psychological disorder or mental health disorder (MHD), and one in every four people suffers from one or more symptoms at some point in their lives (Titchkosky, 2015). WHO statistics state that 2.3 billion people worldwide suffer from depression, 60 million from bipolar disorder, and 23 million from schizophrenia (Newson et al., 2017). An estimated one in 160 people suffer from autism spectrum disorders, 5–7% of adolescents suffer from attention deficit hyperactivity disorder (ADHD) (Waghmare et al., 2018), and 15% of adults over 60 suffer from a mental illness (Newson and Thiagarajan, 2019). The traditional MHD follows the ICD-11 diagnostic classification system (Organization, 1997). The medical practitioner investigates MHDs with classical interviews, which are based on self-reported symptoms. Each mental illness has its unique collection of symptoms, including physical, emotional, cognitive, and behavioural manifestations (Newson and Thiagarajan, 2019). However, subjective assessments are prone to recall and response bias for patients. The researchers have sought to develop new methods for successful clinical diagnosis and treatment of MHDs. One such method is the non-invasive technique of electroencephalography (EEG) used in deciphering and

DOI: 10.1201/9781003363361-12

extrapolating the results to identify MHDs, both psychological and neurological, which is used with the brain-computer interface (BCI). The detection of mental activity patterns and their manipulation with external devices can be done by computer algorithms based on BCI. EEG is one of the imaging technologies and artificial intelligence (AI) can be utilized in machine learning techniques (Liv, 2021) to classify EEG-based BCI (Shruti et al., 2016).

The structure of this chapter is as follows: Section 12.2 discusses the types of EEG signals and the frequency bands associated with them. Section 12.3 explains the signal acquisition techniques with its time-frequency domain analysis. Section 12.4 gives an idea of reviewed preprocessing and classification techniques used with EEG signals. Section 12.5 reviews the computational modelling challenges with mental health disorders. Section 12.6 represents the results of various reviewed articles and provides our conclusion and future work directions.

12.2   MATERIAL AND METHODS

BCI technology provides users with the power to control computer applications using their thoughts alone (Liv, 2021). The term BCI was coined to represent a novel way of utilizing computers, in which commands are received directly from the user's brain rather than through nerves and muscles or other sections of the body like the neurological system (Waghmare et al., 2018b). It requires real-time signal processing to analyze the EEG brainwave. Therefore, BCI is a system of artificial intelligence capable of detecting patterns in brain signals (Nicolas-Alonso and Gomez-Gil, 2012; Akilandeswari and Nasira, n.d.). A system like this would increase the quality of life for people with severe physical and mental limitations as well as reduce the cost of critical care (Hramov et al., 2021; Al-Qazzaz et al., 2014; Shoka et al., 2019).

In BCI techniques, special devices are used to capture brain neuron signals (Waghmare et al., 2018b). There are three different methods for signal acquisition, as shown in Figure 12.1: invasive BCI signal acquisition, non-invasive BCI signal acquisition, and partially invasive BCI signal acquisition (Newson et al., 2017). The brain neurons transmit ionic currents and supply flow inside and across neuronal assemblies. The intracellular currents are the primary currents in cells. Secondary currents encircle the primary currents and exchange electric charges with the extracellular currents (Agudelo-Toro and Neef, 2013; Newson et al., 2017). With a spatial resolution of ten millimetres and a temporal resolution of approximately zero, EEG electrical measurements (Newson et al., 2017; Jeong et al., 2020), magnetic measurements (Mills, 2005), and metabolic measurements (Agudelo-Toro and Neef, 2013; Mills, 2005; Newson et al., 2017) play key roles. EEG electrical measurement of non-invasive brainwave signals is portable during EEG signal acquisition, but MEG and fMRI are non-portable (Agudelo-Toro and Neef, 2013; Mills, 2005; Newson et al., 2017; Agarwal et al., 2020).

The following section focuses on one of the non-invasive EEG techniques and the different frequency spectrums of EEG.

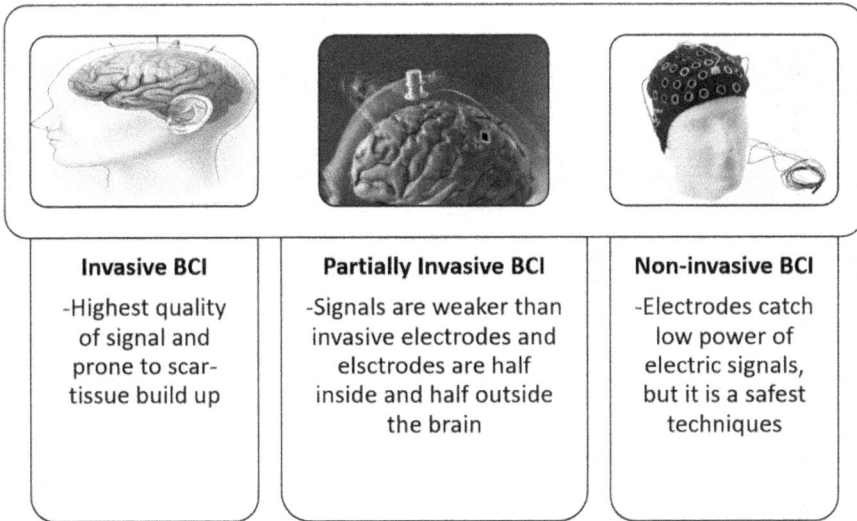

Invasive BCI	Partially Invasive BCI	Non-invasive BCI
-Highest quality of signal and prone to scar-tissue build up	-Signals are weaker than invasive electrodes and elsctrodes are half inside and half outside the brain	-Electrodes catch low power of electric signals, but it is a safest techniques

FIGURE 12.1   Types of BCI for signal acquisition.

12.2.1   EEG FREQUENCY SPECTRUMS

Hans Berger coined the term EEG in 1924 after he successfully recorded the first human EEG (Reaves et al., 2021). Brainwave activity is measured using frequencies observed in the brain as a result of normal brain activity. In addition, EEG can be used to diagnose neurological disorders like epilepsy, tumours, sleep disorders, and inflammations of the brain. The advancement of neuroscience research has developed BCI (Agarwal et al., 2020; Roohi-Azizi et al., 2017). Most EEG facts are accrued in terms of precise frequencies. Through the addition of electrodes, the brain signals can be localized (Titchkosky, 2015). Ethos is generally classified into 10-10 or 10-20 systems, where electrodes are placed at specific distances from each other. Neuronal electric activity is recorded non-invasively using a tiny metallic plate, i.e., electrodes inside the scalp referred to as EEG electrodes. The voltages, which are in the microvolts (μV) range, must be meticulously recorded and digitized before being saved and examined on a computer (Akilandeswari and Nasira, n.d.). Electrodes, amplifiers, an A/D converter, and a recording device make up the EEG recording system. For the A/D converter to more correctly digitalize the EEG signal, the amplifiers process the analogue signal after the electrodes collect the signal from the scalp (Liv, 2021). The EEG is made up of both frequency-based and time-based signals. This range of frequency ranges is known as delta (δ), theta (θ), alpha (α), beta (β), and gamma (γ). Table 12.1 summarizes the characteristics of these brainwaves (Teplan, 2002; Mills, 2005). The details of brainwaves and associated brainwave disorders can be correlated with their brain activity and its effect.

TABLE 12.1

Details of EEG Brainwaves, Their Frequency Range, Brain-Related Activities Involved in Brain Parts, and Mental Health Disorders Associated with Brainwaves Can be Studied Using EEG Signals.

Name	Brainwave	Frequency Range	Brain-Involved Activity	Effect	MHD Detection
Gamma waves		>40 Hz	Higher levels of mental function, such as fear, problem-solving, perception, and consciousness	Self-control, epiphany, highest level of consciousness, intelligence, and sentiments of unity	Mood disorders, major depression, bipolar disorder
Beta waves		13–39 Hz	Active focus, arousal, cognition, and/or paranoia as well as active, busy, or anxious thinking	Concentration, arousal, alertness, motivation, problem-solving	Anxiety, obsessiveness, sleep difficulties, hyperactivity
Alpha waves		7–13 Hz	Drowsiness, pre-sleep and awake, REM sleep, dreams, and relaxation (when awake)	Creativity, flow state, focus, learning, and serotonin boost	Anxiety, depression
Theta waves		4–7 Hz	NREM sleep, profound meditation, or relaxation	Addiction assistance, healing, REM sleep, inner calm, and deep meditation	Anxiety Dementia

(Continued)

TABLE 12.1
(Continued)

Name	Brainwave	Frequency Range	Brain-Involved Activity	Effect	MHD Detection
Delta waves		<4 Hz	Loss of body awareness during a deep sleep without dreams	Access to the subconscious, pain alleviation, dreamless NREM sleep. bodily awareness is lost	Parasomnias, insomnia, sleep disorders, ADHD, brain injuries
Mu waves		8–12 Hz	Sensorimotor rhythm, Mu rhythm, sensorimotor rhythm	Enormous numbers of synchronized electrically active neurons, most likely of the pyramidal type	Autism

The comparison of dynamical properties of different brainwaves, frequency range, brain-involved activity, frequency effect, physiological and pathological brain states, and associated MHD is mentioned in Table 12.1. Seizure activity showed the strongest evidence of nonlinear deterministic dynamics. Therefore, in analyzing the EEG data for any computational modelling, signal acquisition plays an important role. The signal acquisition can be of two types: wired and wireless. The general practice done by neurologists is to use electrode-based wired 10-20 systems. Similarly, for various BCI applications, wireless signal acquisition devices are also used (Waghmare et al., 2018b), as shown in Table 12.1.

12.3   EEG SIGNAL ACQUISITION

Various EEG signal acquisition devices are available on the market to acquire and analyze brainwaves. The professional will use different devices, depending on the requirements of the EEG applications. With a NeuroSky Mind Wave device, a Bayesian t-test, and various regression analyses, Tafhim Bin Nasir et al. measured the power spectrum of students' brainwaves to determine their level of attention in the classroom (Hramov et al., 2021; Roohi-Azizi et al., 2017). The RMS manufacturers designed a high-quality EEG machine with 24 channels at an affordable price. Using a 16-channel headset or cap, the open-source brain-computer interface (OpenBCI) analyzes the electrical activity of the human body (Jeong et al., 2020), including the heart (ECG), skeletal muscles (EMG), and the brain (EEG) (Newson et al., 2017; Zotev et al., 2014). Using a total of 14 sensors, plus an additional two, EMOTIV EPOC uses a high-resolution, wireless neuroheadset to tune into brain electrical signals in real time and recognize the user's thoughts, feelings, and facial expressions (Nicolas-Alonso and Gomez-Gil, 2012; Hramov et al., 2021; EMOTIV solution, 2020). It has various key features like wirelessly connecting, rechargeable batteries, motion sensors, saline-based electrodes, and EEG channels with a fast setup (EMOTIV solution, 2020). Muse is a multi-sensor meditation tool that offers real-time data on your heart rate, breathing, and physical activity to assist you in developing a regular meditation routine (Agarwal et al., 2020). In Mahsa Soufineyestani et al., the various data collection devices, their types, applications, and EEG sensor would correlate a specific task (Surya et al., 2017) with their technical, specifications, battery life, and limitations discussed (Akilandeswari and Nasira, 2014). Also, the details of the EEG device with its neurological applications are mentioned in detail (Soufineyestani et al., 2020).

The selection of the channels for EEG analysis is the most crucial step after the device is prepared. EEG is recorded in neurospecialist clinics by 10-20 electrode placement technique of 19 electrodes (Waghmare et al., 2018b; Al-Qazzaz et al., 2014), primarily for clinical reasons (Hramov et al., 2021). The International EEG and Clinical Neurophysiology Society advise using the scalp electrode placement method known as the International 10-20 System (IFSECN) (Alotaiby et al., 2015). The EEG of patients was recorded in specialized clinical units using 10-20 electrodes for clinical applications. This 10-20 electrode placing system is of international standards. In such studies, the non-invasive method is used to trace EEG signals. The cap consists of 14, 16, 32, or 64 electrodes and is used with patients in various hospitals. The electrodes of the 10-20 system are named Fp1, Fp2, F7, F3, Fz, F4, F8, A1, T3, C3, Cz, C4, T4, A2, T5, P3, Pz, P4, T6, O1, and O2 (Nicolas-Alonso and Gomez-Gil, 2012) and are situated in the frontal, temporal, occipital, and parietal lobes (Agudelo-Toro and Neef, 2013; Soufineyestani et al., 2020; Alotaiby et al., 2015). EEG data signal processing must start as soon as the EEG signal acquisition is complete.

12.4 DATA PROCESSING AND FEATURE SELECTION

Data preprocessing involves transforming data from its original form into a format that is better suited for analysis and user comprehension. To get EEG data closer to the real brain impulses, preprocessing typically comprises removing noise from the data. The preprocessing steps need to reduce noise in EEG signals for better results. It is also important in this step to determine the frequency and channel from the EEG produced by a large number of electrodes (Waghmare et al., 2018). The EEG is made to capture electrical activity in the brain, which represents brain activity. Physiological and non-physiological artefacts are two categories of recorded movements that are not brain-originating. External sources provide additional physiological artefacts (Shoka et al., 2019). The various algorithms were efficiently used for preprocessing and classification based on the time-frequency domain, as shown in Table 12.2.

12.4.1 Time-Frequency Domain

In time-frequency analysis, a valuable tool for creating controllers and feedback devices is time-frequency analysis, which takes into account the non-stationary nature of EEG data and provides a temporal indication of various aberrations with the feature of the time (Collazos-Huertas et al., 2020; Newson and Thiagarajan, 2019; Titchkosky, 2015). A crucial but difficult stage in the processing of EEG data is the removal of artefacts (Zotev et al., 2014). Less than half of the research addresses artefact removal, with more than 80% concentrating on manual removal since they have a deep understanding of the issue (Alotaiby et al., 2015). Among the most popular methods for removing artefacts are ICA and discrete wavelet transform (DWT). However, several of these studies have placed a strong emphasis on the use of time-frequency analysis, which minimizes artefacts by better resolving the input signal, by analyzing it in both the time and frequency domains (Titchkosky, 2015). It is frequently utilized to work more effectively with intrinsically non-stationary signals using EEG data and wavelet transformations (WT) (Collazos-Huertas et al., 2020). In Kaur and Kaur et al., EEG is based on electrical activity recorded as the event-related potentials (ERP) at various places across the brain. These signals are typically non-stationary and time-varying. Various signal processing techniques such as a computer-aided method for EEG classification using the fractional linear prediction (FLP) technique can be used to analyze EEG data with maximum accuracy. Instead of using typical models employing integer-order derivatives, fractional

TABLE 12.2
Domain Analysis with Feature Extraction

Feature Domain	Feature Extraction Method	Advantages	Disadvantages	Methods for EEG Signal Feature Extracted
Time (D'Sa et al., 2016) (Newson et al., 2017) (Olias et al., 2019) (Newson et al., 2017)	Linear prediction (LP)	High spatial resolution	Low sampling rate, greater loss of photons	Event-related potentials (ERP)
	Independent component analysis (ICA)	High penetration depth	The tool is bigger	information on signal strength (mean, standard deviation, first difference, second difference, entropy, ANOVAs)
		Most accurate separation of absorption and scattering	Stabilization/coding required	Features of Hjorth (activity, mobility, complexity)
			The most sophisticated system is more expensive	Fractal dimension (FD)
Frequency (Newson et al., 2017) (Turganbayeva, 2021) (Auboiroux et al., 2020)	Fast Fourier transform (FFT)	High sampling rate	Can be susceptible to noise	High-order crossing (HOC)
	Short-time Fourier transform (STFT)	Relatively accurate separation of absorption and scattering	Moderate penetration depth-sensitive loss of photons	Band power
	Spectrogram			High-order spectra (HOS)
	Autoregressive method (ARM)			
	Eigenvector			

(Continued)

TABLE 12.2
(Continued)

Feature Domain	Feature Extraction Method	Advantages	Disadvantages	Methods for EEG Signal Feature Extracted
Time-Frequency (Ahuja et al., 2017) (Newson et al., 2017) (Auboiroux et al., 2020)	Wiger Ville distribution	Gives the feasibility of examining great continuous segments of EEG signal	It deals mostly with the idea of stationary, therefore the preprocessing module requires a windowing process	Combination of time and frequency features
	Scalogram Hilbert-Huang spectrum Discrete wavelet transform (DWT) Wavelet packet decomposition (WPD)	Analyze clean signals for good results	Due to gradient ascent computation, it is a bit slow	
Spatial-Time-Frequency (Shruti et al., 2016) (Auboirouxet al., 2020)	In multielectrode analysis, spatial dimension is calculated by the geometrical position of the electrodes	When analyzing the small data segments, spatial analysis based on the AR model is beneficial	Extracted features	Can be dependent on each other

derivatives were effectively employed to model many physical processes. The focus on one-parameter fractional linear prediction demonstrates that the proposed model is just a specific instance of the traditional first-order linear prediction. The fractional derivative operator is given in Equation 12.1:

$$_aD_t^\alpha x(t) = \lim_{h \to 0} \frac{1}{h^\alpha} \sum_{j=0}^{K=\left[\frac{t-a}{h}\right]} (-1)^j \binom{\alpha}{j} x(t - jh)$$

(12.1)

Where:

K = the integer part of the fraction $(t{-}a)/h$
a and t = lower and upper terminals of differentiation,
$\alpha \in R$ = the arbitrary real order of the fractional derivative,
h = step size,
t, a = the number of terms.

12.4.2 INDEPENDENT COMPONENT ANALYSIS

Hérault, Jutten, and Ans proposed an iterative real-time algorithm when they initially introduced independent component analysis (ICA) in the 1980s The objective of ICA is to extract from the data relevant information or source signals (a set of measured mixed signals). Image, stock, or audio formats are all possible for this data. Consequently, ICA has been applied to extract source signals in many different applications. ICA is also regarded as a dimensional reduction method if it can eliminate or keep a single source. This process, which is also known as filtering, can remove or filter some signals (Collazos-Huertas et al., 2020).

12.4.3 PRINCIPAL COMPONENT ANALYSIS

Principal component analysis (PCA) is frequently used to reduce the size of large datasets so they can be broken down into smaller variables that contain most of the information. Accuracy suffers when the dataset's variables are reduced, but the trick to lowering dimensions is to exchange some accuracy for simplicity. The easier the dataset is to examine and visualize, the faster and easier it is for machine learning algorithms to analyze the data (EMOTIV), and the less need there is to process irrelevant factors.

12.4.4 DIFFERENTIAL WINDOW

A differential window (DW) is applied to easily distinguish seizures from electrical signals. DW is added to the EEG recordings to produce more audible signals

(Kaur et al., 2018). Signals from EEGs run through a Butterworth filter with a cut-off frequency of 60 hertz (Waghmare and Reeja, 2019), which eliminates noise and all other distortions. Time-frequency orthogonal WFBs are used to put the signals together (Kumar et al., 2020; Hamad et al., 2017).

12.4.5 Discrete Wavelet Transform

After preprocessing the EEG signal, different methods are utilized to extract various aspects of EEG brainwaves and then the EEG data has been preprocessed. The most often-used method is based on DWT nonlinear characteristics like sample and estimated entropy. Peak voltage, rising and falling voltages, slopes, and line length are morphological traits. The nonlinear energy operator (NLEO) is useful for detecting extra-terrestrial life (Sharmila and Geethanjali, 2016). With discrete wavelet transform-based features extraction, entropy, min, max, mean, median, standard deviation, variance, skewness, energy, and relative entropy are the ten features that will be collected from the EEG signal to assist the classifier in accurately detecting epilepsy (Gaikwad and Kshirsagar, 2014; Shoka et al., 2019; Sharmila and Geethanjali, 2016; Reeja et al., 2021). Traits are unique functions to understand neural activity in the brain and help in diagnosing anomalies (Auboiroux et al., 2020; Olias et al., 2019; Kotov et al., 2017). In addition, various algorithms have been developed to visualize brain activity using reconstructed images from EEG. Each domain has its advantages and problems, and each method can be best depending on the information you want to extract. Time analysis can distinguish between normal and abnormal wave contours in the EEG signal, helping to identify the presence or absence of brain rhythms. In some cases, the time method cannot provide important functions. In such cases, spectral analysis provides additional information that resolves the main frequency present in the egg signal. In this case, the methods used are a fast Fourier transform (FFT) a short-time Fourier transform (STFT), a spectrum diagram, and a self-regression (ARM), and the extracted main characteristics are tape power and high (Auboiroux et al., 2020). STFTs, or spectrograms of neural signals, usually provide better results because short-time windows are used by dividing the data into smaller time intervals. For aperiodic signals, time-frequency conversion is typically used for signal decomposition and provides a lot of important information. Spatial reference methods enhance local activity, filter noise measured from different electrodes, and help estimate the variance of EEG information. A set of features needs to be extracted from EEG signals to recognize and detect EEG signals (Akilandeswari and Nasira, n.d.). Therefore, brainwave feature specification, band pattern, and noise removal techniques need to be coupled with high-dimensional reduction. Generally, PCA or ICA is used to reduce dimensions (Liv, 2021). The various EEG wave classification taxonomy is discussed and a comparative accuracy analysis of the various algorithms is generated by (Waghmare and Reeja 2019).

12.5 CHALLENGES WITH COMPUTATIONAL MODELLING OF MENTAL HEALTH DISORDERS

As is the standard of healthcare practice, the development of MHD diagnoses is categorically supported by phenomenological research (Roohi-Azizi et al., 2017). According to the International Classification of Disorders (ICD-10), clinicians evaluate overt and obvious signs and symptoms and provide category diagnoses based on which symptoms they fall within (Ravan et al., 2023; Organization, 1997). This descriptive nosology simplifies communication, yet, it is constrained by potentially insufficient impartiality because it relies on clinician observation and/or the patients or informants presenting concerns (Waghmare and Reeja, 2019). Furthermore, the current method excludes psychopathology, as symptom variability within the same disorder category, as well as homogeneity among illnesses, is common. As data-driven methodologies for examining neurological and molecular pathways, such as the Research Domain Criteria initiative of the National Institute of Mental Health have recently been used as a diagnostic aid, symptom-focused diagnosis has been discovered to limit the focus of treatment to symptom relief only (Roohi-Azizi et al., 2017; Kaur et al., 2018; Surya et al., 2017; Ravan, 2015). Machine learning (ML) employs out-of-sample estimation to offer personalized information and potentially achieve high clinical translation results. It does this by utilizing previously unseen data (test data), which was not part of the model training process with the initial dataset (training data). This approach differs from traditional statistical methods like null hypothesis testing (e.g., G-test, ANOVA), as it does not provide a separate explanation but, instead, retroactively focuses on estimating and identifying group differences within the sample. This methodology has been employed in the study by Olbert and Gala in 2015.

The study covers various mental health disorders, including anxiety, bipolar disorder, obsessive-compulsive disorder (OCD), depression, anxiety disorders, panic disorders, phobias, epilepsy, and more. This wide range of disorders is discussed in the research (Teplan, 2002).

Bell et al., Chawla et al., D'Sa et al., and Hiremath and Wale conducted studies on stress (Bell et al., 2008), mood swings (Newson et al., 2017), and addiction (D'Sa et al., 2016) that state that patients suffer from fear, anger, and hatred, and never recover from these adverse symptoms (Hiremath and Wale, 2017). This instigates the process of overthinking, stress, addiction, and negative attitudes in patients. Kodakandla et al. mentioned that 76% of cases suffered from mental illness, of which 31% were psychological and not taking any treatment. The symptom of anxiety is prevalent in most cases (Kodakandla et al., 2016). Nebhinani et al. and Ram et al. mentioned that depression with suicidal tendencies was observed in the younger generation (Nebhinani et al., 2017). Among the patients, 15% were negatively labelled with MHD, 23% showed suicidal attention-seeking behaviour, and the rest of the patients were stubborn and quickly changed their minds (Ram et al., 2017). Kalra and Gulati et al. mentioned that 29–65% of MHD patients (Kalra, 2012) are easily identified with their behaviour and social reactions (Gulati et al., 2014).

Bell et al., Joshi et al., and Surekha et al. mentioned that epilepsy disorders are the majority observed in the younger generation, which indicates low IQ levels, anxiety, and depression in patients suffering from epilepsy (Joshi et al., 2012). Approximately 36% were not aware that epilepsy is a brain disorder and is a cause of mental illness. Other causative factors like birth defects, blood disorders, and family history were not known to the study subjects. There is a need for awareness about the treatment and psychological impact of epilepsy in such patients (Agudelo-Toro and Neef, 2013). Abraham et al., and Thakur and Olive mentioned nomophobia or fear factors in the younger generation, which leads to panic attacks or suicidal tendencies. These symptoms are found in approximately 37% of people (Nebhinani et al., 2017) who lack knowledge and treatment available for this MHD, which may lead to loss of life.

12.6 RESULTS AND DISCUSSION

The classification algorithms are classified into linear classifiers, neural network classifiers, nonlinear Bayesian classifiers, and nearest neighbour classifiers (Waghmare and Reeja, 2019; Mumtaz et al., 2018). The most popular artificial neural network (Agudelo-Toro and Neef, 2013) is used for the emotional identification of human beings. The accuracy, sensitivity, and specificity of the support vector machine (SVM) algorithm used to examine the emotional quotient in Shahabi and Moghimi et al. (2016) were 93.7%, 80.43%, and 83.04%, respectively. In the discussion by Handojoseno et al. of integrated spatial, spectral, and temporal features of the EEG signals (Handojoseno et al., 2013), wavelet coefficients were used for the input of an multilayer perceptron and a K-nearest neighbour classifier (Shi et al., 2007), with 87% sensitivity and 73% accuracy, as shown in Figure 12.2.

The study of classification algorithms for various neurological mental health disorders is mentioned in Figure 12.2. This can improve the accuracy of diagnosis and can improve quality of life. Also, classification algorithms play an important role in feature selection. The MHD symptoms and MHD most-affected age group each play a vital role in predicting analysis. Early prediction can provide remedial solutions for the triggering cause of MHD. The studies into MHD detection with triggering symptoms in particular age groups are as follows:

Etzersdorfer, Chawla, Gulati, and Agarwal et al., discussed the study of younger age patients who deal with psychiatric MHD patients. The study specifies that the most-involved age group is approximately 20 years old. Such patients deal with various symptoms like fear factors, mood swings, obsessiveness, and addiction. The D'Sa et al. study is about addiction in psychiatric disorders which involves subjects aged 20 ±2 years. Also, Kodakandla, Ahuja, Hiremath, and Wale's study observes anxiety and neurological disorders like epilepsy, depression, adjustment problems, and so on. The involved age group is about 20 years old, as shown in Figure 12.3.

(a) Distribution of accuracy, sensitivity and specificity of Parkinson's disorder

(b) Distribution of accuracy, sensitivity and specificity of Autism disorder

(c) Distribution of accuracy, sensitivity and specificity of Depression disorder

(d) Distribution of accuracy, sensitivity and specificity of Dimentia disorder

(e) Distribution of accuracy, sensitivity and specificity of ADHD's disorder

Distribution of accuracy, sensitivity and specificity of Schizophrenia's disorder

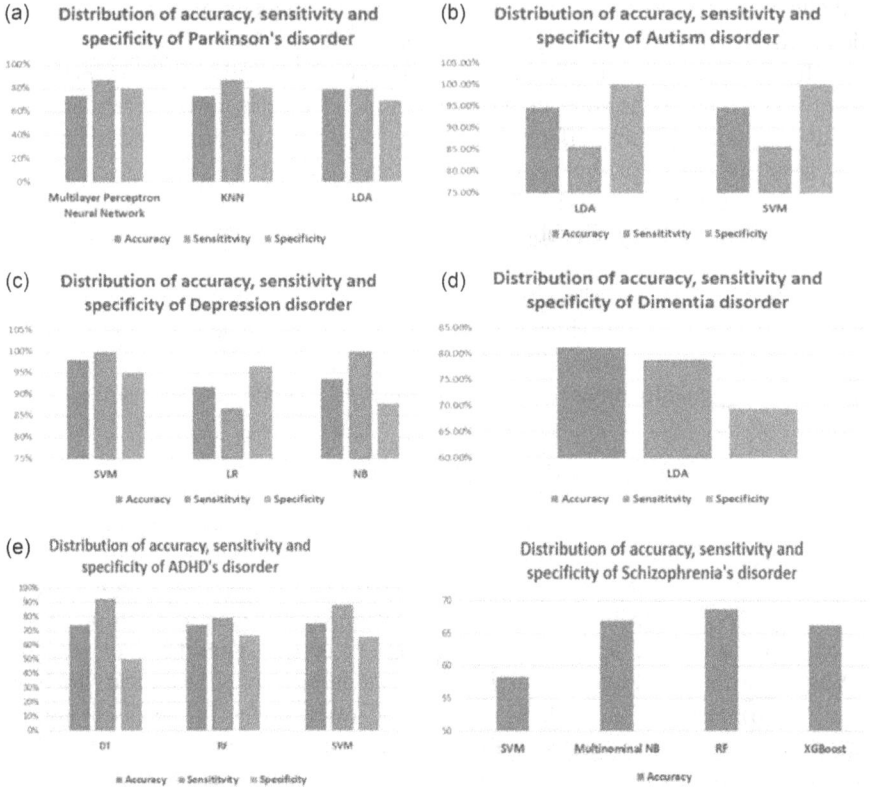

FIGURE 12.2 The study of classification algorithms of various neurological mental health disorders. Figure 12.2.a The distribution of accuracy, sensitivity, and specificity for Parkinson's disorder using MPP, KNN, and LDA. Figure 12.2.b Autism disorder using SVM and LDA. Figure 12.2.c Depression disorder using SVM, LR, and NB. Figure 12.2.d Dementia disorder using LDA. Figure 12.2.e ADHD disorder using DT, RF, and SVM. Figure 12.2.f Schizophrenia disorder using SVM, multi-nominal NB, RF, and XGBoost.

12.7 CONCLUSION

This study discusses the types of EEG brainwaves, the EEG frequency spectrum of different waves, signal acquisition, preprocessing, and classification techniques used in various MHDs. The selection of brainwave devices is mainly based on portable capabilities, channels, electrodes, and reinforced quality signals. The leading focus of the literature review was to identify the triggering symptoms of various MHDs and their classification accuracy using computational modelling for EEG waves. The majority of the case studies included the young generation, both normal and suffering from MHDs. Studies have shown that advanced preprocessing filtering and postprocessing classifiers can be applied to draw accurate conclusions about the presence and symptoms of MHDs. Future research directed towards the

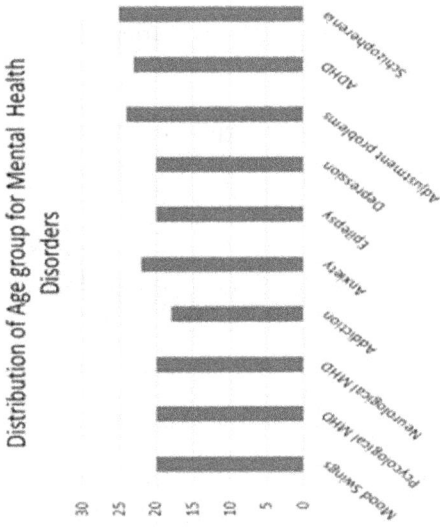

Reference	Mental Health Disorder	Age
Chawla et al., 2012 (90)	Mood Swings	20
Gulati et al., 2014 (79)	Psychological MHD	20
Aggarwal et al., 2016 (92)	Neurological MHD	20
D'Sa et al., 2016	Addiction	18
Kodabandla et al., 2016 (81)	Anxiety	22
Sarefa et al., 2016	Epilepsy	20
Ahuja et al., 2017	Depression	20
Hiremath & Wale, 2017 (74)	Adjustment problems	24
Grazioli et al., 2023(99)	ADHD	23
Bae et al., 2022(98)	Schizophrenia	25

FIGURE 12.3 The predictive study on MHD symptoms and age group for triggering parameters.

computational modelling of MHDs with accurate algorithms and methodological advances can improve the accuracy of disease diagnosis. The accurate diagnosis of MHDs using improved algorithms for multiple MHD classifications will help to improve the quality of life for patients.

Author Contributions: All authors have made a substantial contribution to the study and manuscript preparation.

Funding: This research received no external funding.

Conflicts of Interest: No potential conflict of interest was reported by the authors.

REFERENCES

Agarwal, M., Venkateswaran, S. K., and Sivakumar, R. (2020). Human-in-the-loop RL with an EEG wearable headset: On effective use of brainwaves to accelerate learning. *WearSys 2020 - Proceedings of the 6th ACM Workshop on Wearable Systems and Applications, Part of MobiSys 2020*, 25–30. https://doi.org/10.1145/3396870.3400014

Agudelo-Toro, A., and Neef, A. (2013). Computationally efficient simulation of electrical activity at cell membranes interacting with self-generated and externally imposed electric fields. *Journal of Neural Engineering, 10*(2). https://doi.org/10.1088/1741-2560/10/2/026019

Ahuja, K. K., Dhillon, M., Juneja, A., and Sharma, B. (2017). Psychosocial Intervention mental illness stigma among Indian college students. *Psychosocial Intervention, 26*(2), 103–109. http://doi.org/10.1016/j.psi.2016.11.003

Akilandeswari, K., and Nasira, G. M. (n.d.). Swarm optimized feature selection of EEG signals for brain-computer interface. *International Journal of Computational Intelligence and Informatics, 4*(1), 44–53.

Akilandeswari, K., and Nasira, G. M. (2014). Bagging of EEG signals for brain computer interface. *Proceedings - 2014 World Congress on Computing and Communication Technologies, WCCCT 2014*, 71–75. https://doi.org/10.1109/WCCCT.2014.42

Al-Qazzaz, N. K., Ali, S. H. B. M., Ahmad, S. A., Chellappan, K., Islam, M. S., and Escudero, J. (2014). Role of EEG as biomarker in the early detection and classification of dementia. *Scientific World Journal, 2014*. https://doi.org/10.1155/2014/906038

Alotaiby, T., El-Samie, F. E. A., Alshebeili, S. A., and Ahmad, I. (2015). A review of channel selection algorithms for EEG signal processing. *EURASIP Journal on Advances in Signal Processing, 2015*(1). https://doi.org/10.1186/s13634-015-0251-9

Auboiroux, V., Larzabal, C., Langar, L., Rohu, V., and Mishchenko, A. (2020). Space – time – frequency multi-sensor analysis for motor cortex localization using magnetoencephalography. *Sensors (Basel), 20*(9), 2706.

Bell, C. J., Shenoy, P., Chalodhorn, R., and Rao, R. P. N. (2008). Control of a humanoid robot by a noninvasive brain-computer interface in humans. *Journal of Neural Engineering, 5*(2), 214–220. https://doi.org/10.1088/1741-2560/5/2/012

Collazos-Huertas, D. F., Álvarez-Meza, A. M., Acosta-Medina, C. D., Castaño-Duque, G. A., and Castellanos-Dominguez, G. (2020). CNN-based framework using spatial dropping for enhanced interpretation of neural activity in motor imagery classification. *Brain Informatics, 7*(1). https://doi.org/10.1186/s40708-020-00110-4

D'SA, J. R., Shetty, S., V., S., Sahu, S., Prabhakar, S., Kundapur, R., and Kiran, K. G. (2016). Awareness of alcohol among adolescents and young adults of Mangalore. *Journal of Health and Allied Sciences NU, 06*(01), 042–044. https://doi.org/10.1055/s-0040-1708615

Gaikwad, S. R., and Kshirsagar, S. S. (2014). A review: Analysis of EEG Signal based brain-computer Interface. *International Journal of Science and Research.* www.ijsr.net

Gulati, P., Das, S., and Chavan, B. S. (2014). Impact of psychiatry training on attitude of medical students toward mental illness and psychiatry. *Indian Journal of Psychiatry*, *56*(3), 271–277. https://doi.org/10.4103/0019-5545.140640

Hamad, A., Hassanien, A. E., Houssein, E. H., and Fahmy, A. A. (2017). Feature extraction of epilepsy EEG using discrete wavelet transform. *2016 12th International Computer Engineering Conference, ICENCO 2016: Boundless Smart Societies*, 190–195. https://doi.org/10.1109/ICENCO.2016.7856467

Handojoseno, A. M. A., Shine, J. M., Nguyen, T. N., Tran, Y., Lewis, S. J. G., and Nguyen, H. T. (2013). Using EEG spatial correlation, cross frequency energy, and wavelet coefficients for the prediction of Freezing of Gait in Parkinson's disease patients. *Proceedings of the Annual International Conference of the IEEE Engineering in Medicine and Biology Society, EMBS*, 4263–4266. https://doi.org/10.1109/EMBC.2013.6610487

Hiremath, L. C., and Wale, G. R. (2017). Assessment of the knowledge and attitude regarding adjustment problems among nursing students. *Asian Journal of Nursing Education and Research*, *7*(3), 423. https://doi.org/10.5958/2349-2996.2017.00084.2

Hramov, A. E., Maksimenko, V. A., and Pisarchik, A. N. (2021). Physical principles of brain–computer interfaces and their applications for rehabilitation, robotics and control of human brain states. *Physics Reports*, *918*, 1–133. https://doi.org/10.1016/J.PHYSREP.2021.03.002

Jeong, J. H., Shim, K. H., Kim, D. J., and Lee, S. W. (2020). Brain-controlled robotic arm system based on multi-directional CNN-BiLSTM network using EEG signals. *IEEE Transactions on Neural Systems and Rehabilitation Engineering*, *28*(5), 1226–1238. https://doi.org/10.1109/TNSRE.2020.2981659

Joshi, H., Mahmood, S. E., Bamel, A., Agarwal, A., and Shaifali, I. (2012). Perception of epilepsy among the urban secondary school children of Bareilly district. *Annals of Indian Academy of Neurology*, *15*(2), 125–127. https://doi.org/10.4103/0972-2327.94996

Kalra, G. (2012). Talking about stigma towards mental health professionals with psychiatry trainees: A movie club approach. *Asian Journal of Psychiatry*, *5*(3), 266–268. https://doi.org/10.1016/J.AJP.2012.06.005

Kaur, K., Kaur, C., Tarandeep, Bhatia, K. (2018). *Demystifying Big Data Analytics Techniques*. www.tjprc.org

Keerthi Kumar, M., Parameshachari, B. D., Prabu, S., and Ullo, S. L. (2020). Comparative analysis to identify efficient technique for interfacing BCI system. *IOP Conference Series: Materials Science and Engineering*, *925*(1). https://doi.org/10.1088/1757-899X/925/1/012062

Kodakandla, K., Nasirabadi, M., and Pasha, M. S. (2016). Attitude of interns towards mental illness and psychiatry: A study from two medical colleges in South India. *Asian Journal of Psychiatry*, *22*, 167–173. https://doi.org/10.1016/j.ajp.2016.06.008

Kotov, R., Waszczuk, M. A., Krueger, R. F., Forbes, M. K., Watson, D., Clark, L. A., Achenbach, T. M., Althoff, R. R., Ivanova, M. Y., Michael Bagby, R., Brown, T. A., Carpenter, W. T., Caspi, A., Moffitt, T. E., Eaton, N. R., Forbush, K. T., Goldberg, D., Hasin, D., Hyman, S. E., Miller, J. D., Moffitt, T. E., Morey, L. C., Mullins-Sweatt, S. N., Ormel, J., Patrick, C. J., Regier, D. A., Rescorla, L., Ruggero, C. J., Samuel, D. B., Sellbom, M., Simms, L. J., Skodol, A. E., Slade, T., South, S. C., Tackett, J. L., Waldman, I. D., Waszczuk, M. A., Widiger, T. A., Wright, A. G. C., and Zimmerman, M. (2017). The hierarchical taxonomy of psychopathology (HiTOP): A dimensional alternative to traditional nosologies. *Journal of Abnormal Psychology*, *126*(4), 454–477. https://doi.org/10.1037/abn0000258

Liv, N. (2021). *Recommended citation recommended citation NEUROLAW: Brain-Computer Interfaces*, *15*(1). https://ir.stthomas.edu/ustjlpp; https://irstthomas.edu/ustjlpp/vol15/iss1/9

Mills, K. R. (2005). The basics of electromyography. *Neurology in Practice, 76*(2), 32–35. https://doi.org/10.1136/jnnp.2005.069211

Mumtaz, W., Ali, S. S. A., Yasin, M. A. M., and Malik, A. S. (2018). A machine learning framework involving EEG-based functional connectivity to diagnose major depressive disorder (MDD). *Medical and Biological Engineering and Computing, 56*(2), 233–246. https://doi.org/10.1007/s11517-017-1685-z

Nebhinani, N., Jagtiani, A., Chahal, S., Nebhinani, M., and Gupta, R. (2017). Medical students' attitude toward suicide prevention: An exploratory study from North India. *Medical Journal of Dr. D.Y. Patil University, 10*(3), 277–280. https://doi.org/10.4103/MJDRDYPU.MJDRDYPU_277_16

Newson, J. J., and Thiagarajan, T. C. (2019). EEG frequency bands in psychiatric disorders: A review of resting state studies. *Frontiers in Human Neuroscience, 12*(January), 1–24. https://doi.org/10.3389/fnhum.2018.00521

Newson, J. J., Thiagarajan, T. C., Walter, M., Surya, M., Jaff, D., Stilwell, B., Schubert, J., Tit, T., Aubrecht, K., Liv, N., Nicolas-Alonso, L. F., Gomez-Gil, J., Keerthi Kumar, M., Parameshachari, B. D., Prabu, S., Ullo, S. L., Hassanien, A. E., Azar, A. T., Agudelo-Toro, A., and Networks, A. N. (2017). Medical students' attitude toward suicide prevention: An exploratory study from North India. *Indian Journal of Psychiatry, 10*(1), 277–280. https://doi.org/10.1109/TNSRE.2019.2905894

Nicolas-Alonso, L. F., and Gomez-Gil, J. (2012). Brain computer interfaces, a review. *Sensors, 12*(2), 1211–1279. https://doi.org/10.3390/s120201211

Olbert, C. M., and Gala, G. J. (2015). Supervenience and psychiatry: Are mental disorders brain disorders? *Journal of Theoretical and Philosophical Psychology, 35*(4), 203–219. https://doi.org/10.1037/teo0000023

Olias, J., Martin-Clemente, R., Sarmiento-Vega, M. A., and Cruces, S. (2019). EEG signal processing in mi-bci applications with improved covariance matrix estimators. *IEEE Transactions on Neural Systems and Rehabilitation Engineering, 27*(5), 895–904. https://doi.org/10.1109/TNSRE.2019.2905894

Ram, D., Chandran, S., H, B. (2017). Suicide and depression literacy among health professions students in tertiary care centre in South India. *Journal of Mood Disorders, 5*, 1. https://doi.org/10.5455/jmood.20170830064910

Ravan, M., Noroozi, A., Sanchez, M. M., Borden, L., Alam, N., Flor-Henry, P., and Hasey, G. (2023). Discriminating between bipolar and major depressive disorder using a machine learning approach and resting-state EEG data. *Clinical Neurophysiology, 146*, 30–39.

Reaves, J., Flavin, T., Mitra, B., and Mahantesh, K. (2021). *Assessment and Application of EEG: A Literature Review Journal of Applied Assessment and Application of EEG: A Literature Review.* August.

Reeja, S. R., Cherian, R., Waghmare, K., and Jothimani (2021). EEG signal-based human emotion detection using an artificial neural network. In *Handbook of Decision Support Systems for Neurological Disorders*, 107–124. https://doi.org/10.1016/B978-0-12-822271-3.00007-4

Roohi-Azizi, M., Azimi, L., Heysieattalab, S., and Aamidfar, M. (2017). Changes of the brain's bioelectrical activity in cognition, consciousness, and some mental disorders. *Medical Journal of the Islamic Republic of Iran, 31*(1), 307–312. https://doi.org/10.14196/mjiri.31.53

Shahabi, H., and Moghimi, S. (2016). Toward automatic detection of brain responses to emotional music through analysis of EEG effective connectivity. *Computers in Human Behavior, 58*, 231–239.

Sharmila, A., and Geethanjali, P. (2016). DWT based detection of epileptic seizure from EEG signals using naive Bayes and k-NN classifiers. *IEEE Access, 4*, 7716–7727. https://doi.org/10.1109/ACCESS.2016.2585661

Shi, Y., Ruiz, N., Taib, R., Choi, E., and Chen, F. (2007). Galvanic skin response (GSR) as an index of cognitive load. *Conference on Human Factors in Computing Systems - Proceedings*, 2651–2656. https://doi.org/10.1145/1240866.1241057

Shoka, A., Dessouky, M., El-Sherbeny, A., and El-Sayed, A. (2019). Literature review on EEG preprocessing, feature extraction, and classifications techniques. *Menoufia Journal of Electronic Engineering Research*, 28(1), 292–299. https://doi.org/10.21608/mjeer.2019.64927

Shruti, A., Singh, S., and Kataria, D. (2016). Knowledge, attitude and social distance practices of young undergraduates towards mental illness in India: A comparative analysis. *Asian Journal of Psychiatry*, 23, 64–69. https://doi.org/10.1016/J.AJP.2016.07.012

Soufineyestani, M., Dowling, D., and Khan, A. (2020). Electroencephalography (EEG) technology applications and available devices. *Applied Sciences (Switzerland)*, 10(21), 1–23. https://doi.org/10.3390/app10217453

Sureka, R. K., Saxena, S., Rijhwani, P., Chaturvedi, S., and Charan, A. (2016). Knowledge, attitude and practice of epilepsy among undergraduate medical and nursing students in Rajasthan. *Journal of Evolution of Medical and Dental Sciences*, 5(98), 7166–7169. https://doi.org/10.14260/jemds/2016/1622

Surya, M., Jaff, D., Stilwell, B., and Schubert, J. (2017). The importance of mental well-being for health professionals during complex emergencies: It is time we take it seriously. *Global Health Science and Practice*, 5(2), 188–196. https://doi.org/10.9745/GHSP-D-17-00017

Teplan, M. (2002). Fundamentals of EEG measurement. *Measurement Science Review*, 2(2), 1–11.

Titchkosky, T. (2015). Life with dead metaphors: Impairment rhetoric in social justice praxis. *Journal of Literary & Cultural Disability Studies*, 9(1), 1–18.

Waghmare, K. J., Professor, A., and Bosco, D. (2018a). Analysis of EEG neurofeedback using brain machine interface, *SWAYAM-2018, Conference Proceeding*, 23–26.

Waghmare, K. J., and Reeja, S. R. (2019). A computational intelligence paradigm with human computer interface learning. *International Journal of Innovative Technology and Exploring Engineering*, 9(2S), 384–389. https://doi.org/10.35940/ijitee.b1032.1292s19

World Health Organization. (1997). Implementation of the international statistical classification of diseases and related health problems, tenth revision (ICD-10). *Epidemiological Bulletin*, 18(1), 1–4.

13 Machine Learning Techniques in ECG Data Analysis for Medical Applications

S. Daphin Lilda and R. Jayaparvathy

13.1 INTRODUCTION

Healthcare being a major area of focus, there are many factors that are to be considered, out of which accurate and early prediction are the most important factors. The global mortality rate for deaths caused by cardiovascular disease (CVDs) is higher when compared to deaths caused by brain disorders [1]. CVDs including stroke, ischemic heart disease, myocardial infarction, and a number of other conditions caused by the abnormality or malfunctioning of the cardiac condition contribute to a high rate of global mortality [2]. The early detection of CVDs can reduce mortality, as the affected patients can be assisted with counselling and medications.

An electrocardiogram (ECG) is a quick, painless, and non-invasive treatment that records the heart's electrical activity [3]. The ECG can be used in combination with other exams to track and identify various cardiac diseases. Knowing the source of the heartbeat is crucial in order to interpret a cardiac failure from the ECG signal. An ECG segment, or a heartbeat, includes a PQRST segment. The sinoatrial node (SA), considered the pacemaker of the heart, is responsible for generating the P wave. The atrioventricular node (AV) generates the QRS wave. The P wave, QRS complex, and T wave in an ECG segment symbolize atrial depolarization, ventricular depolarization, and ventricular repolarization, respectively. For instance, if a P wave is lacking, atrial depolarization is absent, and this condition is called an atrial standstill. Junctional or ventricular tachycardia is indicated by P waves that combine in the QRS complexes [4, 5]. The identification of various cardiac problems is made feasible by carefully examining these ECG signals and identifying slight differences.

Nowadays, artificial intelligence (AI) and machine learning (ML) techniques are used in almost all real-world applications, creating a pervasive automated environment. Instead of spending their time on information search and entry in the medical field, machine learning enables healthcare professionals to concentrate solely on patient treatment and care.

DOI: 10.1201/9781003363361-13

The various machine learning techniques and algorithms that are currently employed in the prediction of heart disease from ECG signals are covered in this chapter. This chapter discusses ways the ventricular late potential (VLP), which appears on ECG data, might be used to predict cardiac disease. One of the main goals of machine learning-based prediction systems for healthcare is the development of models that can be used to predict health. This contributes to the reduction of disease severity and, consequently, mortality. The general flowchart for a healthcare management system based on machine learning is given in Figure 13.1. The main step in the machine learning pipeline is collecting data for the ML model's training. The accuracy of the prediction is dependent on the data size and characteristics used to train the model. Various denoising approaches are used to eliminate noise from the data, which is then followed by feature extraction and feature selection, where the optimum features are chosen from the extracted features. To predict diseases, these chosen features are input into a variety of classification algorithms. The expected values are observed, and, depending on the severity, decisions are made on whether to seek immediate medical supervision or to continue taking the recommended regular medications.

The prediction technique for a system with an ECG signal as input involves the prediction of abnormalities from deviations that occur in the ECG. Each of the

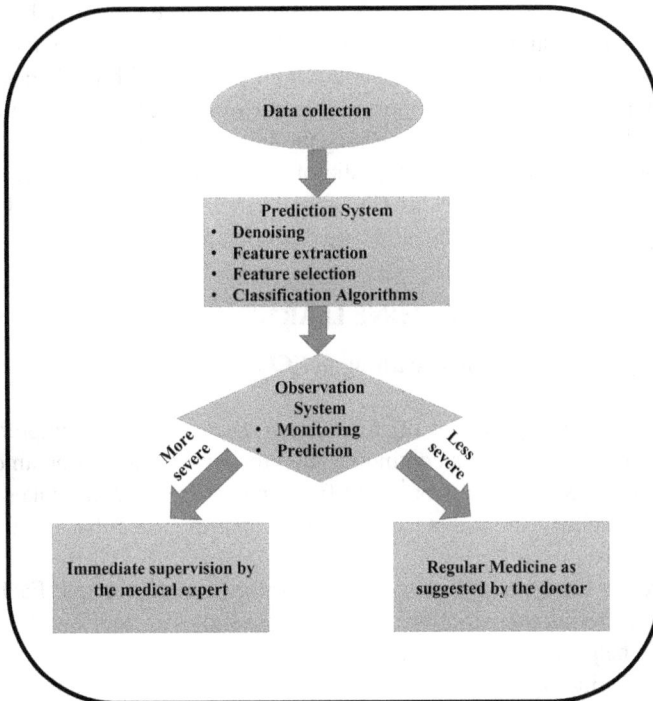

FIGURE 13.1   Flowchart for machine learning-based healthcare management system

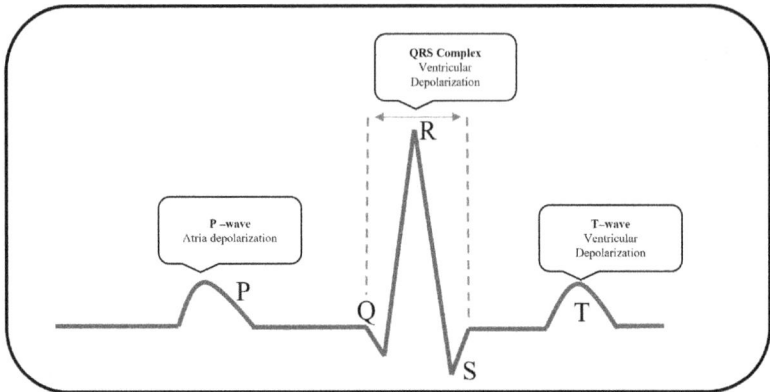

FIGURE 13.2 General ECG heartbeat – PQRST segment

elements in the PQRST segment has a particular significance in the cardiac cycle and any deviation may contribute to some type of abnormality. Careful examination of these deviations is an important factor in the prediction of particular CVDs. Manually locating deviations may not give accurate results, whereas an automatic prediction system using ML techniques is used to produce more reliable results. A segment of the ECG signal consisting of the PQRST segment is given in Figure 13.2.

Early CVD prediction and treatment are both possible with meticulous analysis of ECG signals, which lowers the mortality rate. However, there will be a number of mistakes made when manually deciphering the signals to identify the various CVDs, owing to the non-stationary characteristic of the ECG data. Therefore, to analyze ECGs for the existence of various CVDs and circumvent the limits of manually interpreting the ECG signals, an automatic detection method is crucial.

13.2 THE NEED FOR MACHINE LEARNING IN ECG ANALYSIS

The main objectives of machine learning in ECG analysis are:

- To maximize the amount of information extracted from comprehensive ECG signals. By using a continuous monitoring system, a large amount of data for the ML model is obtained from the patients, which makes it possible to identify the minute variations or abnormalities that occur in the ECG signal.
- To predict the type of disease from the information extracted. Each CVD is related to minute variations in the ECG signal extracted. The ML-based system helps in identifying the type of disease.
- To determine the disease's severity. The severity of the abnormality that occurred has a direct link with the amount of deviation on the ECG signal using the pretrained ML model.

- The ML-based system enables the early prediction of diseases and thus enables giving immediate treatment based on the severity, thereby reducing the mortality rate.

13.3 THE PROCESS INVOLVED IN MACHINE LEARNING-BASED ECG CLASSIFICATION

The steps involved in ML-based ECG classification are discussed below.

13.3.1 DENOISING

The extracted original ECG signals have a lot of interference, with multiple noise signals. Appropriate denoising techniques are required to extract the original ECG signals from these noisy signals. For accurate and reliable analysis of the signals to predict various diseases, signals devoid of noise are essential. The most important noises in the ECG signal are electromyographic (EMG)/muscle artifact [6, 7], baseline wander (BW) [8, 9] and power line interferences (PLI) [10]. Several denoising techniques are used to remove the above-discussed noises from ECG signals. The traditionally used denoising techniques are the adaptive filtering method [11], principal and independent component analysis [12], and fuzzy wavelet denoising [13]. Discrete wavelet transform (DWT) and empirical mode decomposition (EMD) are found to be the most effective denoising techniques and are discussed in detail.

- **Discrete wavelet transform (DWT):** In DWT, it is important to define the optimal function for a particular ECG signal [14]. For instance, Ho et al. utilized the wavelet energy to calculate the necessary wavelet coefficients, and then a sub-band smoothing filter is applied to further reduce noise [15]. The number of wavelet decomposition layers has an impact on the denoising effect. The mother wavelet product and the wavelet coefficients are combined linearly to represent the signal in DWT. The fundamental principle of WT is the breakdown of a signal into several frequency level coefficients. Determining how signals behave in various frequency ranges may be done using the basic capacity to analyze signals in various frequency bands and scales. The signal is broken down into specific information using DWT, making it possible to analyze the signal at various frequency bands and resolutions [16, 17]. The precision of the denoising process is dependent on some factors, including DWT's wavelet function, the choice of the threshold approach and the DWT decomposition level. The mathematical representation of continuous wavelet transform (CWT) is given as:

$$CWT\left(a,b;x\left(t\right),\psi\left(t\right)\right)=\int_{-\infty}^{\infty}x\left(t\right)\frac{1}{a}\psi^{*}\left(\frac{t-b}{a}\right)dt \qquad (13.1)$$

where $x(t)$ is the original signal, $\psi(t)$ is the analyzing function (wavelet), a is a scale parameter, and b is a position in time. DWT is the discrete representation of CWT. DWT is the most commonly used technique for the denoising of ECG signals.

- **Empirical Mode Decomposition (EMD):** For processing nonlinear and non-stationary signals, empirical mode decomposition (EMD) is a versatile and efficient decomposition technique that offers a number of advantages [18]. Any complex signal can be decomposed into a few intrinsic mode functions (IMFs) by using the EMD approach. The fundamental principles of the Fourier transform and wavelet transform of signal decomposition are incorporated into EMD. EMD demonstrates the self-adaptability property by decomposing the signal based on its own time scale without the need for a basis function. EMD is appropriate for all sorts of signals because it does not require a basis function. IMFs should meet the following two conditions:

  i) The number of zero crossings or the total number of extrema should be equal or must have a maximum difference of one.
  ii) The average between the upper and lower envelopes must always be zero.

The aggregate of the decomposed IMFs and the resulting residual signal is therefore used to represent the original signal that was decomposed using EMD. A wider range of information would be available and the denoising performance might be improved with the use of EMD.

13.3.2 FEATURE EXTRACTION

For better analysis of the obtained raw data, they are converted to unmodified information in terms of numerical values called features. The process of obtaining these features is termed feature extraction. This feature information is easier to analyze using various ML techniques, and they are found to provide better and satisfactory results. The most distinctive aspects of signals are found through feature extraction, making machine learning's classification stage easier to employ.

- **Morphological Features Extraction:** ECG signals are resolved into heartbeats, representing a cardiac cycle; P, Q, R, S, and T are the smaller functional standard waves that make up a heartbeat. A heartbeat also consists of inter-wave time segments called the PR interval, QRS complex, QT interval, and ST segment. The values of these morphological features in terms of amplitude and time can be used as features to detect normal and abnormal conditions [19].
- **Statistical Features Extraction:** It may be necessary in some circumstances to measure the signal's fluctuations with regard to its time, position,

and frequency. SFE approaches provide the mean, standard deviation, variance, kurtosis measures, and skew measurements of the provided medical data in certain circumstances. With these measurements, medical professionals may analyze the signal and, on their advice, the signal's qualities are extracted.

13.3.3 FEATURE SELECTION

The size of the medical record volume makes processing the entire record challenging and time-consuming. In the medical sector, saving a patient's life depends on speed. Here, choosing which features to use is a necessary effort. Various feature selection techniques can be utilized, depending on the patient test result pattern or the medical record pattern [20].

- **The filter methods:** The filter method calculates the significance of the characteristic, which indicates the feature's capacity for class distinction. Lower-ranked characteristics are eliminated based on the determined relevance value. The feature's ability to distinguish between the various groups is indicated by its significance. A few of the filter methods which use the ranking methods are Euclidian distance, one-way analysis of variation (ANOVA) test, T-test, chi-squared test (χ^2), correlation-based feature selection (CFS), ReliefF method, information gain method, and minimum redundancy maximum relevance (MRMR) method.
- **The wrapper-based method:** This method chooses the best features instead of the most relevant collection of features. This technique takes into account various feature combinations. The best subset of features is chosen after these combinations have been analyzed and contrasted with other feature combinations. The subset of features is selected in a greedy way based on a backward elimination process, by which the dependency between the features and the subset of features is maintained. The most commonly used wrapper-based methods are recursive feature elimination (RFE), backward and forward elimination, and sequential forward selection (SFS).
- **Embedded methods:** The above-listed advantages of the filter-based method and wrapper-based method are combined in embedded methods. Algorithms with built-in feature selection strategies put these methods into practice. Among the best-known examples of these approaches are regression techniques like LASSO and RIDGE, which have built-in penalization procedures to reduce overfitting.

13.3.4 CLASSIFIERS AND PREDICTORS

The classification of various diseases from the ECG signal and the prediction of the severity of the condition is based on the automatic detection method and classification is based on many machine learning (ML) techniques. The ML methods for the

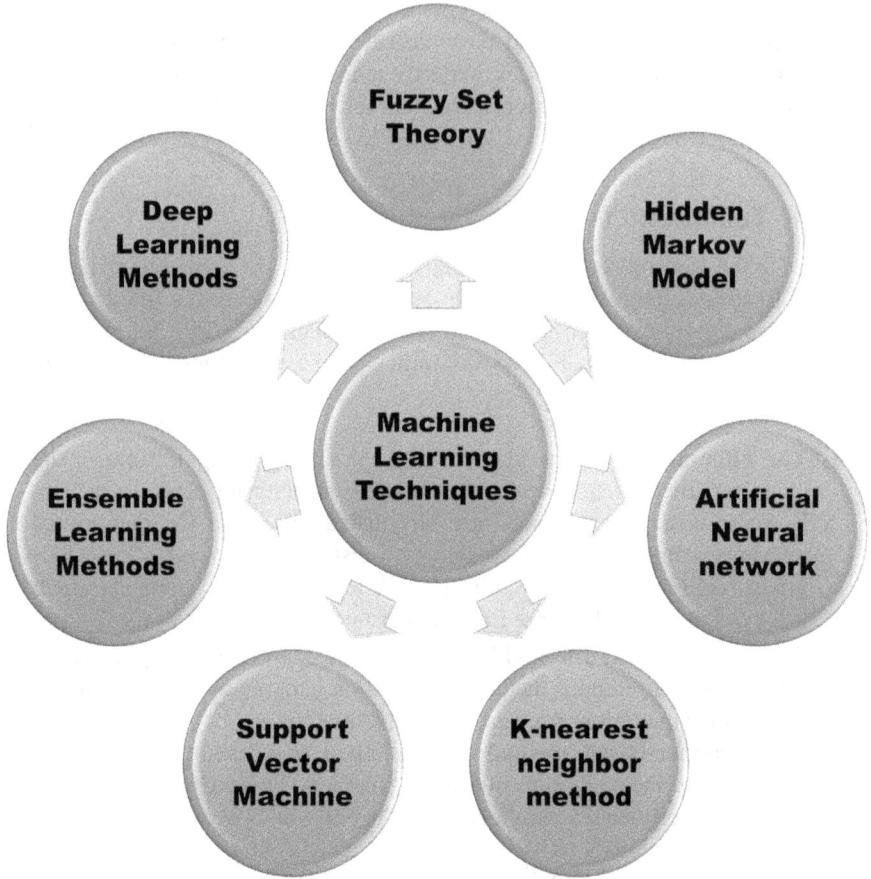

FIGURE 13.3   Various machine learning methods for CVD prediction

computerized ECG analysis and diagnosis are given in Figure 13.3 and discussed below.

- **Fuzzy set theory:** The fuzzy-based approach uses membership functions and smooth variables for ECG analysis and abnormality prediction [21]. Modifications were done to the fuzzy algorithms and different methods, such as fuzzy clustering neural network algorithm [22] and fuzzy-based decision tree [23] were incorporated for better performance.
- **Hidden Markov model (HMM):** The HMM is frequently utilized in applications that require knowledge acquisition from ECG signal segments. Andreao et al classified the ECG signal utilizing the HMM's capabilities for heartbeat detection and segmentation [24]. With a maximum sensitivity of 99.79% for the classification of normal and diseased heartbeats, this approach was proven to work well.

- **Artificial neural network:** It is vital to employ automated approaches for the precise identification of cardiac problems since analyzing ECG signal patterns for diagnosis takes a considerable amount of time and effort. With many layers of grouped and interconnected processing nodes known as neurons and changeable weighted linkages, neural networks (NNs) are a specific type of machine learning algorithm created to replicate the neurological function system. Their goal is to handle a specific categorization problem inside the aggregated neurons as a whole. NNs are effective because they can extract data structures and identify patterns without the assistance of a specialist. Sao et al. proposed a diagnosis method for cardiac arrhythmias utilizing an artificial neural network classifier [25]. Anuradha et al. proposed ANN-based classifier combined with wavelet-based back propagation algorithm was used in the categorization of the abnormal and normal ECG signals [26]. In the paper, artificial neural network models-based cardiac arrhythmia disease diagnosis from ECG signal data, the ANN was combined with the static back propagation technique and momentum learning rule [27]. Several other modifications were done with the ANN for the effective classification of the ECG signals in classification of arrhythmic ECG data using machine learning techniques and ECG signal analysis and classification using data mining and artificial neural networks [28, 29].
- **K-nearest neighbour (KNN) method:** K-nearest neighbour is a search algorithm in which inference is based on the comparison made from the training data and a predefined sampled value for different disorders of the heart [30]. By taking into account the least distance from a dataset that contains the input value and a set of reference values, classification is performed. Various abnormality classification of the ECG signals is done using KNN and various modified KNN algorithms in order to produce better performance [31–33].
- **Support vector machine (SVM):** The SVM classifier, which is based on the statistical learning theory, is one of the mostly widely used ML approaches for ECG signal classification. In [34], SVMs are used to classify time series of heartbeats. The SVM classifier, which detects ECG data with a low signal-to-noise ratio, offers superior functionality to neural network-based classifiers, according to the researchers. For better classification performance, a lot of modifications are being done to the SVM classifier and are widely used in the classification of different types of CVDs [35–38].
- **Ensemble learning methods:** The outputs of the individual classifiers of the above-discussed ML algorithms are assessed to create the final prediction, and thus ensembles of classifiers are recommended to improve predictive accuracy by integrating many classifiers. Various ensemble classifiers, such as bagging, boosting, gradient boosting, and extreme gradient boosting, are used in the classification of various CVDs. Miao et al. [39] proposed the adaptive boosting algorithm which was found to produce precise classification and prediction of coronary heart disease. Stacked ensemble classifiers [40] and a number of reliable and accurate CVD classifications are done using various ensemble methods [41–45].

TABLE 13.1
Confusion Matrix

Samples	Normal ECG Signal (Predicted Value)	Abnormal ECG Signal (Predicted Value)
Normal ECG signal (Actual value)	True positive (TP)	False negative (FN)
Abnormal ECG signal (Actual value)	False positive (FP)	True negative (TN)

- **Deep learning methods:** Deep learning (DL) is the study of extracting information from data, generating predictions, making wise decisions, or, put differently, identifying complex patterns from a set of training data. Deep learning methods are used in automated ECG classification to improve efficiency. The performance efficiency of the system can be easily improved by modifying the layers used in the DL system or by increasing the samples used to train the model. The commonly used DL methods in the classification of ECG signals are deep belief network (DBN), convolutional neural network (CNN), gated recurrent unit (GRU), restricted Boltzmann machines (RBM), and long short-term memory (LSTM) [46–55].

13.3.5 PERFORMANCE EVALUATION

The performance evaluation is done to measure the efficiency of the system [56]. For binary classification, the optimal solution for evaluation during classification is defined by the confusion matrix. The actual and predicted values are compared using the confusion matrix by the machine learning model. The confusion matrix for a binary CVD classification is given Table 13.1. The evaluation metrics used to analyze the performance of the model and the focus of the evaluation are listed in Table 13.2.

13.4 VENTRICULAR LATE POTENTIAL (VLP) DETECTION USING MACHINE LEARNING TECHNIQUES

Ventricular late potentials can be seen in the beginning of the ST segment and at the end of QRS complexes. Due to their small amplitude, Ventricular Late Potentials are high frequency signals that are difficult to spot on an ECG. A direct correlation between the incidence of VLPs and arrhythmia, which can result in death by cardiac arrest, has been demonstrated in studies. VLPs are high frequency signals that are seen at the tailing end of QRS complexes and occasionally extend into the ST segment. Their frequency ranges from 40 to 250 Hz, and their voltage ranges from 1 to 20 V. The following are the requirements for late potential on a signal average ECG (SA-ECG) signal [57].

- Filtered QRS duration must be higher than 114 milliseconds.
- Terminal QRS (RMS) voltage should be less than 20 microvolts.
- Low-amplitude signal of a value less than 40 microvolts should occur for a duration greater than 38 milliseconds.

TABLE 13.2
Evaluation Metrics

Evaluation Metrics	Formula	Focus of Evaluation
Accuracy (ACC)	$\dfrac{TP+TN}{TP+FN+FP+TN}$	The percentage of the precise predictions made is known as accuracy.
Sensitivity (SN)	$\dfrac{TP}{TP+FN}$	The percentage of positive samples that are correctly categorized is known as sensitivity.
Specificity (SP)	$\dfrac{TN}{FP+TN}$	The percentage of negative samples that are correctly categorized is known as specificity.
Precision (P)	$\dfrac{TP}{TP+FP}$	Precision is the proportion of positive patterns within a positive class that are accurately predicted.
Recall (R)	$\dfrac{TP}{TP+FN}$	The percentage of positive samples that are correctly categorized is known as recall.
F-score	$\dfrac{2*p*r}{p+r}$	The harmonic mean of the recall and precision values is represented by the F-score.

The VLP may be considered an important prediction factor in post-infarction patients to avoid CVDs. The VLPs have been detected by using the wavelet-based decomposition technique [58, 59], various time-frequency representations (TFR), which include the Wigner-Ville (WV), short-time Fourier transform (STFT), and Choi-Williams (CW) distributions [60], and the ant colony optimization (ACO) technique [61]. Although VLPs are crucial in the prevention of arrhythmias, their detection is still not widely employed. It is possible to identify VLPs using EMD. The signal is broken down by EMD into a number of oscillatory functions known as intrinsic mode functions (IMFs). VLPs can occasionally be obscured by the cardiac signal's noise or the QRS complex. Due to the EMD-based technique's capacity to retrieve morphologically complete information, these hidden VLPs are clearly visible. The detection of VLPs using the EMD described in the paper entitled "An efficient machine learning based ventricular late potential detection and classification technique for cardiac healthcare" [62] is covered in this section.

The process involved in the detection of VLPs using the EMD is given in Figure 13.4. The VLPs are easily detected from a signal average ECG (SAECG) signal [63]. The signal averaging of N-beats is done to obtain the SAECG signal. Before the averaging of the ECG signals used for analysis, which are obtained from the PhysioNet open-access databases, they are subject to a filtering process [64]. The ECG signals for the normal and VLP-based signals were obtained from the Fantasia database and MIT Arrhythmia databases, respectively. In order to minimize the noise, nonlinear filters are used to preprocess the signals. The band-pass Butterworth filter is used for this purpose. The filtered signal is subject to a matched filter for the beat alignment of the ECG signal [65].

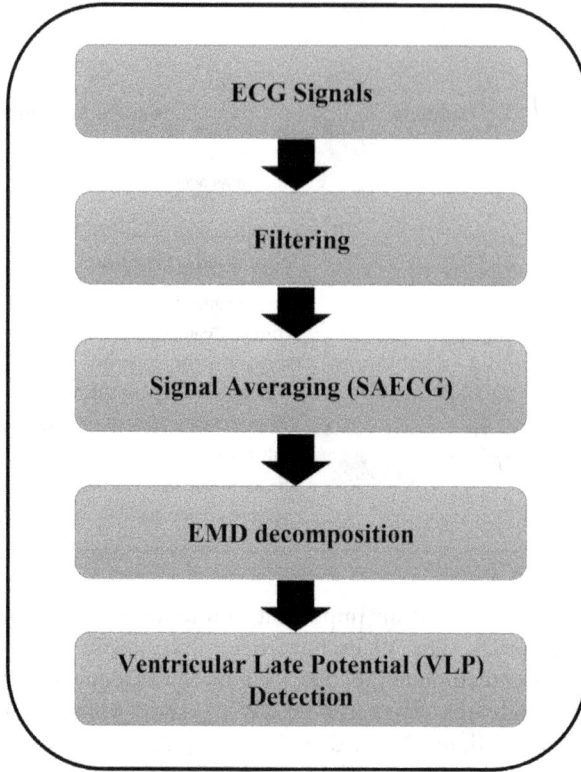

FIGURE 13.4 Detection of VLP using EMD

The SAECG signal is obtained by calculating the mean of the aligned beats obtained using the matched filter. Equation 13.2 represents the SAECG signal obtained from an ECG signal consisting of N-beats.

$$SAECG = \frac{1}{N} \sum_{i=1}^{N} s_i \qquad (13.2)$$

Where s_i is the ith beat of any ECG signal. This shows the output obtained by averaging the consecutive beats of the matched filter output signal.

The PhysioNet database is used to obtain the ECG signals. The MIT Arrythmia database is used to get ECG signals with VLP, while the Fantasia database is used to provide normal ECG signals. The original ECG signal from the MIT Arrythmia database is displayed in Figure 13.5. Figure 13.6 displays the SAECG signal that was produced after the ECG signal was filtered and beats were aligned.

After applying EMD to the acquired SAECG signal, IMFs and residuals are obtained. The EMD of the SAECG signal obtained from an abnormal ECG signal is shown in Figure 13.7. The existence of VLP is indicated by low-amplitude signals

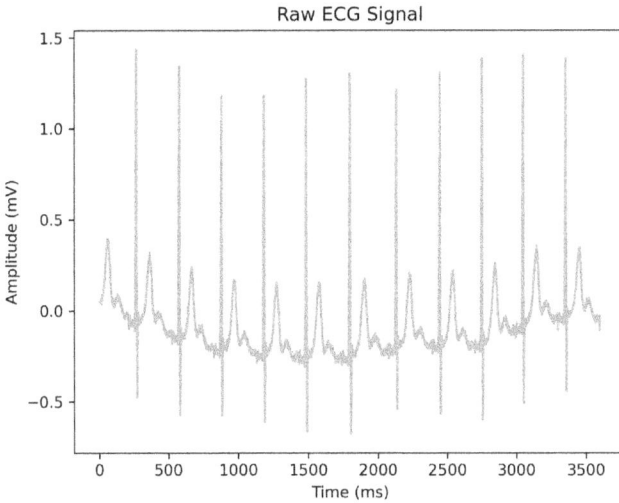

FIGURE 13.5 Raw abnormal ECG signal

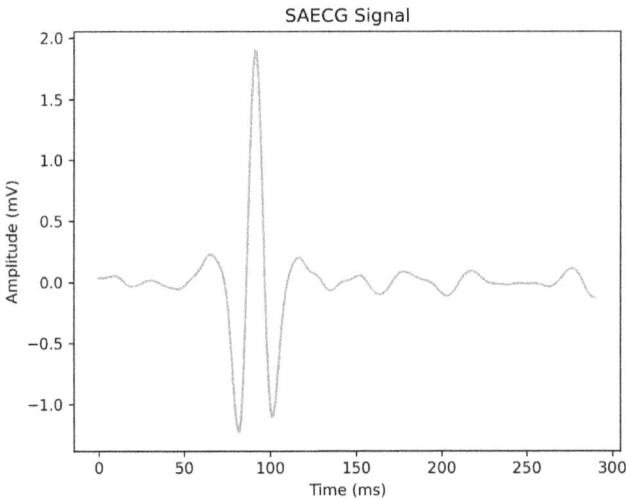

FIGURE 13.6 SAECG of abnormal ECG signal

in the residue signal at the end of the QRS complex. The need for the occurrence of the VLP signal is indicated by the presence of signals with an amplitude of less than 20 microvolts that occur at the end of the QRS complex and linger for more than 38 milliseconds. As a result, Figure 13.7 shows that the resulting residue contains VLP.

In Figure 13.8, the IMFs obtained by the decomposition of the normal ECG signal where there are no continuous low-amplitude signals present indicate there are no

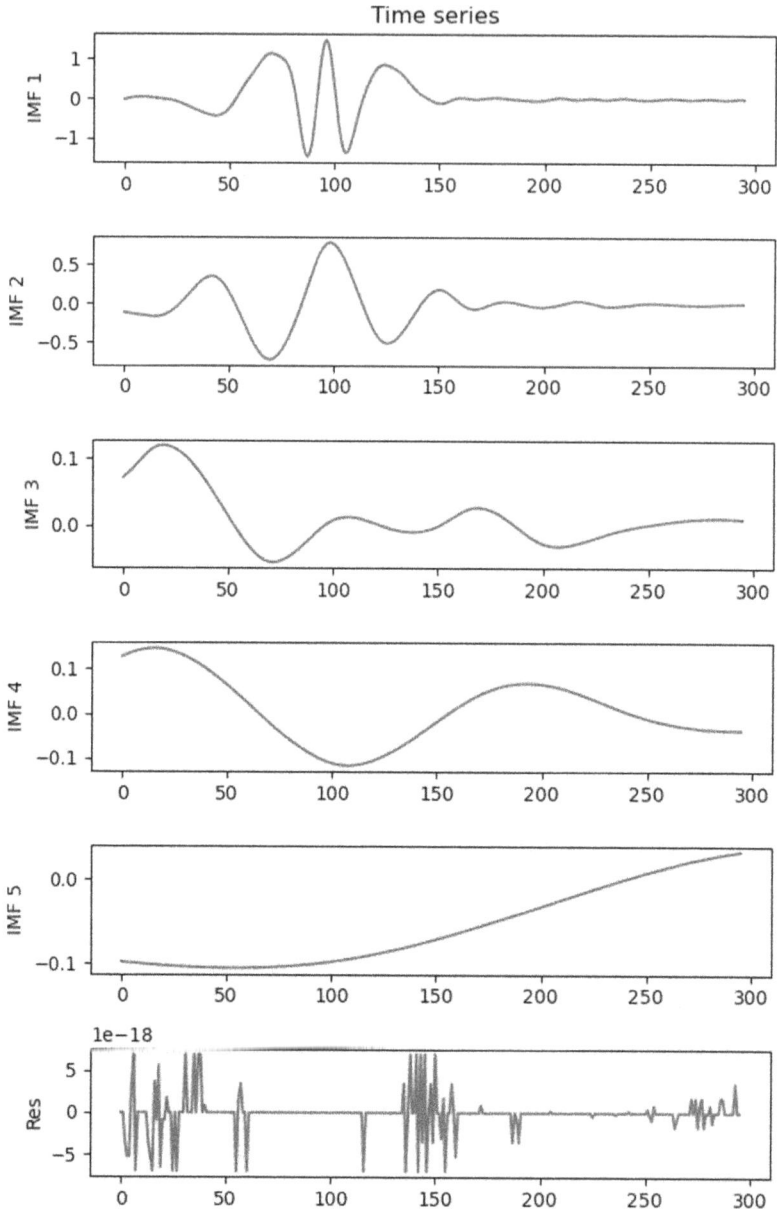

FIGURE 13.7 EMD applied to abnormal ECG signal

VLP present. The power spectrum of obtained IMFs is plotted and three features, namely mean, spectral entropy, and peak amplitude, are extracted.

The feature selection was done on the extracted features based on a ranking method, a one-way ANOVA test [66]. The Fisher's discrimination index (F) and

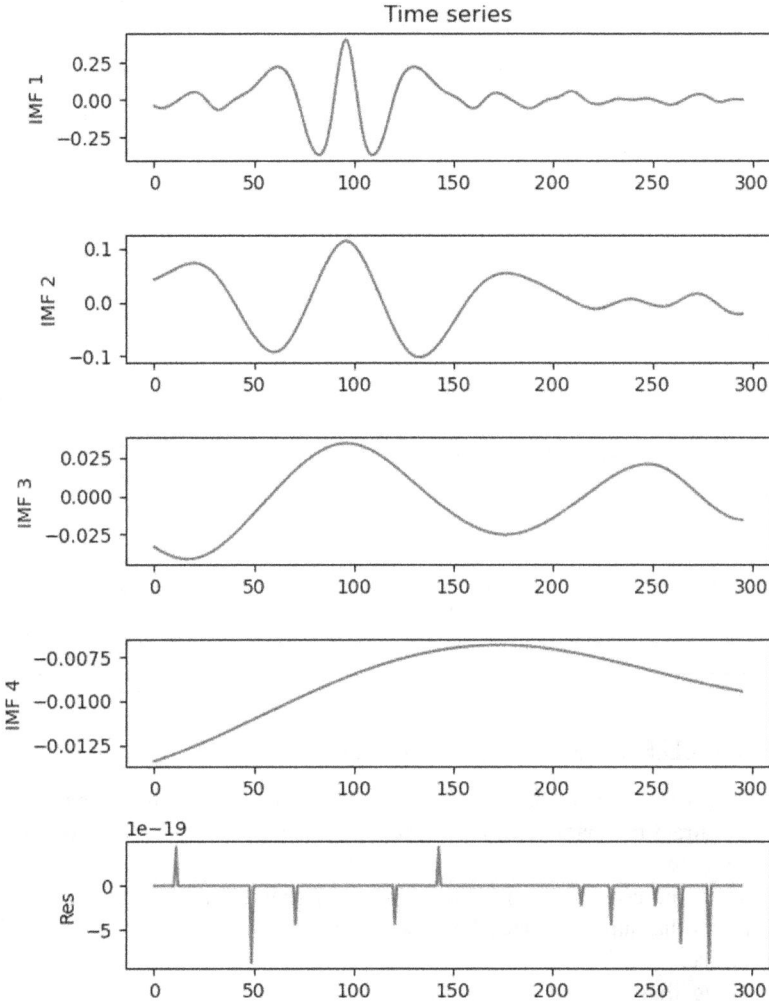

FIGURE 13.8   EMD applied to normal ECG signal

probability (p) were used to determine the potential for discrimination of the features and, based on the values of F and p, the features were sorted in descending and ascending order, respectively. The different classifiers receive the ranking features one at a time as input. The comparison of the outcomes with the current and existing works is shown in Table 13.3. It is observed that the suggested strategy yields superior outcomes.

Thus, the proposed method analyzes the ECG waveform, extracts these low-amplitude signals using the EMD method and classifies the normal and abnormal signals based on the bagging and boosting classifiers.

TABLE 13.3
Performance Evaluation Comparison

Technique Used	Performance Evaluation	
Wavelet transform and ANN [59]	ACC	78
	SP	77
	SP	80
Wigner-Ville distribution [60]	SP	86.31
	SN	83.1
Wavelet transform and ACO [61]	SP	95.24
	SN	94.12
Wavelet decomposition and SVM [67]	ACC	98.82
	SP	94.04
	SN	99.71
Wavelet decomposition and SVM [68]	ACC	98.35
	SP	98.36
	SN	98.33
Wavelet decomposition and quadratic discriminant [69]	ACC	98
Empirical mode decomposition with bagging and AdaBoost [62]	ACC	98.93
	SP	98.62
	SN	99.84

13.5 CHALLENGES IN ML-BASED ECG ANALYSIS

1. Intensity of care is reduced due to a lack of direct monitoring of the patients. The direct personal care of patients by medical experts is reduced, which may increase the risk for the patients. The number of visits may be reduced due to the continuous monitoring of the patients, but this may hide side effects that have occurred because monitoring is done only for a specific disease.

2. Wrong diagnosis during long-term monitoring may happen, due to the need for long-term continuous monitoring and the huge amounts of data required, which necessitates that the patient wear the device for a substantial period of time. Any careless action by the patient may lead to a loss of data or a wrong prediction being made. Sometimes, irregularities of data may occur, which may subside the crucial symptoms that have occurred in the patients.

3. The data acquired by the continuous monitoring of patients is given with the trust that data confidentiality will be maintained. But the reality is that it is not possible to rely on the medical expert alone to maintain the data confidentially. The medical history of the patient becomes known to a number of people, disturbing the patient's personal space.

4. A huge volume of data is collected from the patients. In times of emergency, it is required to segregate the critical data from the normal data. But this huge volume of data sometimes makes the extraction process very slow.
5. The machine learning algorithms used in predicting diseases may sometimes create a lot of conflicts between the medical expert and the researcher in terms of the analysis that is being done by the medical experts to predict the diseases.
6. Due to continuous monitoring, the external noises being introduced in the ECG and the artifacts due to various parameters, such as stress and anxiety, which are not filtered by the denoising techniques, can sometimes be misinterpreted as CVDs, leading to wrong predictions being made.

13.6 CONCLUSION

ML-based ECG analysis enables the continuous monitoring of the patient, helping medical experts to locate any abnormality in the ECG and thereby predict the presence of a particular CVD. Based on the severity of the abnormality detected, immediate treatment is given to the patients by medical experts, which can reduce mortality to a great extent. The manual prediction of disease from the ECG, which is time-consuming, is reduced by using the ML-based technique. The ML-based approach to ECG analysis will be an effective approach in post-CVD affected patients. These systems are trained using the existing data, making it much easier and less tense for the medical experts and the patients who are under examination.

A method to detect the ventricular late potential (VLP) using the ML-based system is discussed in this chapter. The VLP signals are considered important parameters in the detection of CVDs. In post-MI patients, VLPs can be used to notice factors in the ECG signal to avoid sudden cardiac death. Though VLPs play a significant role in the CVD characterization process, the detection process is not widespread. In this work, an EMD-based detection of VLPs is proposed. This method, along with an automatic detection phase, can be used for clinical applications. Using machine learning methods to create an automated ECG analysis system will help physicians more effectively diagnose a disease and suggest appropriate remedies at an early stage, thereby enhancing treatment and reducing mortality.

REFERENCES

1. Carroll, W. M. (2019). The global burden of neurological disorders. *The Lancet Neurology*, 18(5), 418–419. https://doi.org/10.1016/S1474-4422(19)30029-8
2. Kyu, H. H., Abate, D., Abate, K. H., Abay, S. M., Abbafati, C., Abbasi, N., & Breitborde, N. J. (2018). Global, regional, and national disability-adjusted life-years (DALYs) for 359 diseases and injuries and healthy life expectancy (HALE) for 195 countries and territories, 1990–2017: A systematic analysis for the Global Burden of Disease Study 2017. *The Lancet*, 392(10159), 1859–1922. https://doi.org/10.1016/S0140-6736(18)32335-3
3. World Health Organization (2000). Global health estimates: Deaths by cause. Age, sex and country, 2012, 2014.

4. Acharya, U. R., Bhat, P. S., & Niranjan, U. C. (2002). Comprehensive visualization of cardiac health using electrocardiograms. *Computers in Biology and Medicine*, 32(1), 49–54. https://doi.org/10.1016/S0010-4825(01)00029-4

5. Richardson, J., Haywood, L. J., Murthy, V. K., & Harvey, G. (1971). A mathematical model for ECG wave forms and power spectra. *Mathematical Biosciences*, 12(3–4), 321–328. https://doi.org/10.1016/0025-5564(71)90026-5

6. Clifford, G. D., Azuaje, F., & Mcsharry, P. (2006). ECG statistics, noise, artifacts, and missing data. *Advanced Methods and Tools for ECG Data Analysis*, 6(1), 18.

7. Friesen, G. M., Jannett, T. C., Jadallah, M. A., Yates, S. L., Quint, S. R., & Nagle, H. T. (1990). A comparison of the noise sensitivity of nine QRS detection algorithms. *IEEE Transactions on Bio-Medical Engineering*, 37(1), 85–98. https://doi.org/10.1109/10.43620

8. Van Alste, J. A., & Schilder, T. S. (1985). Removal of base-line wander and power-line interference from the ECG by an efficient FIR filter with a reduced number of taps. *IEEE Transactions on Bio-Medical Engineering*, 12(12), 1052–1060. https://doi.org/10.1109/TBME.1985.325514

9. Levkov, C., Mihov, G., Ivanov, R., Daskalov, I., Christov, I., & Dotsinsky, I. (2005). Removal of power-line interference from the ECG: A review of the subtraction procedure. *BioMedical Engineering Online*, 4(1), 1–18.

10. Frölich, L., & Dowding, I. (2018). Removal of muscular artifacts in EEG signals: A comparison of linear decomposition methods. *Brain Informatics*, 5(1), 13–22.

11. Martens, S. M., Mischi, M., Oei, S. G., & Bergmans, J. W. (2006). An improved adaptive power line interference canceller for electrocardiography. *IEEE Transactions on Bio-Medical Engineering*, 53(11), 2220–2231. https://doi.org/10.1109/TBME.2006.883631

12. Łęski, J. M., & Henzel, N. (2005). ECG baseline wander and powerline interference reduction using nonlinear filter bank. *Signal Processing*, 85(4), 781–793. https://doi.org/10.1016/j.sigpro.2004.12.001

13. Romero, I., Geng, D., & Berset, T. (2012, September). Adaptive filtering in ECG denoising: A comparative study. In *Computing in Cardiology*. IEEE, pp. 45–48.

14. Chawla, M. P. S. (2009). A comparative analysis of principal component and independent component techniques for electrocardiograms. *Neural Computing and Applications*, 18(6), 539–556.

15. Ho, C. Y. F., Ling, B. W. K., Wong, T. P. L., Chan, A. Y. P., & Tam, P. K. S. (2003). Fuzzy multiwavelet denoising on ECG signal. *Electronics Letters*, 39(16), 1163–1164. https://doi.org/10.1049/el:20030757

16. Aqil, M., Jbari, A., & Bourouhou, A. (2017). ECG signal denoising by discrete wavelet transform. *International Journal of Online Engineering*, 13(9), 51–68.

17. Singh, B. N., & Tiwari, A. K. (2006). Optimal selection of wavelet basis function applied to ECG signal denoising. *Digital Signal Processing*, 16(3), 275–287. https://doi.org/10.1016/j.dsp.2005.12.003

18. Huang, N. E., Shen, Z., Long, S. R., Wu, M. C., Shih, H. H., Zheng, Q., & Liu, H. H. (1998). The empirical mode decomposition and the Hilbert spectrum for nonlinear and non-stationary time series analysis. *Proceedings of the Royal Society of London. Series A: Mathematical, Physical and Engineering Sciences*, 454(1971), 903–995. https://doi.org/10.1098/rspa.1998.0193

19. Oweis, R. J., & Al-Tabbaa, B. O. (2014). QRS detection and heart rate variability analysis: A survey. *Biomedical Science and Engineering*, 2(1), 13–34.

20. Jović, A., Brkić, K., & Bogunović, N. (2015, May). A review of feature selection methods with applications. In *2015 38th International Convention on Information and Communication Technology, Electronics and Microelectronics (MIPRO)* (pp. 1200–1205). https://doi.org/10.1109/MIPRO.2015.7160458

21. Lei, W. K., Li, B. N., Dong, M. C., & Vai, M. I. (2007). AFC-ECG: An adaptive fuzzy ECG classifier. In *Soft Computing in Industrial Applications: Recent Trends* (pp. 189–199). Springer Berlin Heidelberg.

22. Ceylan, R., Özbay, Y., & Karlik, B. (2009). A novel approach for classification of ECG arrhythmias: Type-2 fuzzy clustering neural network. *Expert Systems with Applications*, 36(3), 6721–6726. https://doi.org/10.1016/j.eswa.2008.08.028

23. Chen, Y. L., Wang, T., Wang, B. S., & Li, Z. J. (2009). A survey of fuzzy decision tree classifier. *Fuzzy Information and Engineering*, 1(2), 149–159. https://doi.org/10.1007/s12543-009-0012-2

24. Andreao, R. V., Dorizzi, B., & Boudy, J. (2006). ECG signal analysis through hidden Markov models. *IEEE Transactions on Bio-Medical Engineering*, 53(8), 1541–1549. https://doi.org/10.1109/TBME.2006.877103

25. Sao, P., Hegadi, R., & Karmakar, S. (2015, April). ECG signal analysis using artificial neural network. In *International Journal of Science and Research, National Conference on Knowledge, Innovation in Technology and Engineering* (pp. 82–86).

26. Anuradha, B., & Reddy, V. V. (2008). ANN for classification of cardiac arrhythmias. *ARPN Journal of Engineering and Applied Sciences*, 3(3), 1–6.

27. Jadhav, S. M., Nalbalwar, S. L., & Ghatol, A. A. (2012). Artificial neural network models based cardiac arrhythmia disease diagnosis from ECG signal data. *International Journal of Computer and Applications*, 44(15), 8–13.

28. Vishwa, A., Lal, M. K., Dixit, S., & Vardwaj, P. (2011). Clasification of arrhythmic ECG data using machine learning techniques. *IJIMAI*, 1(4), 67–70.

29. Gupta, K. O., & Chatur, P. N. (2012). ECG signal analysis and classification using data mining and artificial neural networks. *International Journal of Emerging Technology and Advanced Engineering*, 2(1), 56–60.

30. Jayalalith, S., Susan, D., Kumari, S., & Archana, B. (2014). K-nearest neighbour method of analysing the ECG signal (to find out the different disorders related to heart). *Journal of Applied Sciences*, 14(14), 1628–1632. https://ui.adsabs.harvard.edu/link_gateway/2014JApSc..14.1628J/doi:10.3923/jas.2014.1628.1632

31. Saini, I., Singh, D., & Khosla, A. (2013). QRS detection using K-Nearest Neighbor algorithm (KNN) and evaluation on standard ECG databases. *Journal of Advanced Research*, 4(4), 331–344. https://doi.org/10.1016/j.jare.2012.05.007

32. Yang, F., Du, J., Lang, J., Lu, W., Liu, L., Jin, C., & Kang, Q. (2020). Missing value estimation methods research for arrhythmia classification using the modified kernel difference-weighted KNN algorithms. *BioMed Research International*, 2020. https://doi.org/10.1155/2020/7141725

33. Venkatesan, C., Karthigaikumar, P., & Varatharajan, R. J. M. T. (2018). A novel LMS algorithm for ECG signal preprocessing and KNN classifier based abnormality detection. *Multimedia Tools and Applications*, 77(8), 10365–10374. https://doi.org/10.1007/s11042-018-5762-6

34. Kampouraki, A., Manis, G., & Nikou, C. (2008). Heartbeat time series classification with support vector machines. *IEEE Transactions on Information Technology in Biomedicine: A Publication of the IEEE Engineering in Medicine and Biology Society*, 13(4), 512–518. https://doi.org/10.1109/TITB.2008.2003323

35. Dohare, A. K., Kumar, V., & Kumar, R. (2018). Detection of myocardial infarction in 12 lead ECG using support vector machine. *Applied Soft Computing*, 64, 138–147. https://doi.org/10.1016/j.asoc.2017.12.001

36. Ge, Z., Zhu, Z., Feng, P., Zhang, S., Wang, J., & Zhou, B. (2019, October). ECG-signal classification using SVM with multi-feature. In *2019 8th International Symposium on Next Generation Electronics (ISNE)* (pp. 1–3). IEEE. https://doi.org/10.1109/ISNE .2019.8896430

37. Thilagavathy, R., Srivatsan, R., Sreekarun, S., Sudeshna, D., Priya, P. L., & Venkataramani, B. (2020, February). Real-time ECG signal feature extraction and classification using support vector machine. In *2020 International Conference on Contemporary Computing and Applications (IC3A)* (pp. 44–48). IEEE. https://doi.org /10.1109/IC3A48958.2020.233266

38. Raj, S., & Ray, K. C. (2017). ECG signal analysis using DCT-based DOST and PSO optimized SVM. *IEEE Transactions on Instrumentation and Measurement*, 66(3), 470–478. https://doi.org/10.1109/TIM.2016.2642758

39. Miao, K. H., Miao, J. H., & Miao, G. J. (2016). Diagnosing coronary heart disease using ensemble machine learning. *International Journal of Advanced Computer Science and Applications*, 7(10), 30–39.

40. Yakut, Ö., & Bolat, E. D. (2022). A high-performance arrhythmic heartbeat classi- fication using ensemble learning method and psd based feature extraction approach. *Biocybernetics and Biomedical Engineering*, 42(2), 667–680. https://doi.org/10.1016/j .bbe.2022.05.004

41. Peimankar, A., Jajroodi, M. J., & Puthusserypady, S. (2019, October). Automatic detection of cardiac arrhythmias using ensemble learning. In *TENCON 2019-2019 IEEE Region 10 Conference (TENCON)* (pp. 383–388). IEEE. https://doi.org/10.1109/ TENCON.2019.8929348

42. Dalal, F., & Ingale, V. V. (2021, October). Arrhythmia identification and classifica- tion using ensemble learning and convolutional neural network. In *2021 2nd Global Conference for Advancement in Technology (GCAT)* (pp. 1–8). IEEE. https://doi.org/10 .1109/GCAT52182.2021.9587596

43. Puvar, P., Patel, N., Shah, A., Solanki, R., & Rana, D. (2021). Heart disease detection using ensemble learning approach. *International Research Journal of Engineering and Technology(IRJET)*, 8, 2395–0072.

44. Shi, H., Wang, H., Huang, Y., Zhao, L., Qin, C., & Liu, C. (2019). A hierarchical method based on weighted extreme gradient boosting in ECG heartbeat classification. *Computer Methods and Programs in Biomedicine*, 171, 1–10. https://doi.org/10.1016/j .cmpb.2019.02.005

45. Wong, A. W., Sun, W., Kalmady, S. V., Kaul, P., & Hindle, A. (2020, September). Multilabel 12-lead electrocardiogram classification using gradient boosting tree ensem- ble. In *2020 Computing in Cardiology* (pp. 1–4). https://doi.org/10.22489/CinC.2020 .128

46. Al-Huseiny, M. S., Abbas, N. K., & Sajit, A. S. (2020). Diagnosis of arrhythmia based on ECG analysis using CNN. *Bulletin of Electrical Engineering and Informatics*, 9(3), 988–995. https://doi.org/10.11591/eei.v9i3.2172

47. Burger, A., Qian, C., Schiele, G., & Helms, D. (2020). An embedded CNN implementa- tion for on-device ECG analysis. In *2020 IEEE International Conference on Pervasive Computing and Communications Workshops (PerCom Workshops)*, (pp. 1–6). IEEE. https://doi.org/10.1109/PerComWorkshops48775.2020.9156260

48. Wasimuddin, M., Elleithy, K., Abuzneid, A., Faezipour, M., & Abuzaghleh, O. (2021). Multiclass ECG signal analysis using global average-based 2-D convolutional neural network modeling. *Electronics*, 10(2), 170. https://doi.org/10.3390/electronics10020170

49. Avanzato, R., & Beritelli, F. (2020). Automatic ECG diagnosis using convolutional neu- ral network. *Electronics*, 9(6), 951. https://doi.org/10.3390/electronics9060951

50. Sayantan, G., Kien, P. T., & Kadambari, K. V. (2018). Classification of ECG beats using deep belief network and active learning. *Medical and Biological Engineering and Computing*, 56(10), 1887–1898. https://doi.org/10.1007/s11517-018-1815-2

51. Pandey, S. K., Janghel, R. R., Dev, A. V., & Mishra, P. K. (2021). Automated arrhythmia detection from electrocardiogram signal using stacked restricted Boltzmann machine model. *SN Applied Sciences*, 3(6), 624. https://doi.org/10.1007/s42452-021-04621-5

52. Polanía, L. F., & Plaza, R. I. (2018). Compressed sensing ECG using restricted Boltzmann machines. *Biomedical Signal Processing and Control*, 45, 237–245. https://doi.org/10.1016/j.bspc.2018.05.022

53. Hou, B., Yang, J., Wang, P., & Yan, R. (2019). LSTM-based auto-encoder model for ECG arrhythmias classification. *IEEE Transactions on Instrumentation and Measurement*, 69(4), 1232–1240. https://doi.org/10.1109/TIM.2019.2910342

54. Çınar, A., & Tuncer, S. A. (2021). Classification of normal sinus rhythm, abnormal arrhythmia and congestive heart failure ECG signals using LSTM and hybrid CNN-SVM deep neural networks. *Computer Methods in Biomechanics and Biomedical Engineering*, 24(2), 203–214. https://doi.org/10.1080/10255842.2020.1821192

55. Lynn, H. M., Pan, S. B., & Kim, P. (2019). A deep bidirectional GRU network model for biometric electrocardiogram classification based on recurrent neural networks. *IEEE Access*, 7, 145395–145405. https://doi.org/10.1109/ACCESS.2019.2939947

56. Hossin, M., & Sulaiman, M. N. (2015). A review on evaluation metrics for data classification evaluations. *International Journal of Data Mining & Knowledge Management Process*, 5(2), 1.

57. Xue, Q., & Reddy, B. S. (1997). Late potential recognition by artificial neural networks. *IEEE Transactions on Bio-Medical Engineering*, 44(2), 132–143. https://doi.org/10.1109/10.552243

58. Wu, S., Qian, Y., Gao, Z., & Lin, J. (2001). A novel method for beat-to-beat detection of ventricular late potentials. *IEEE Transactions on Bio-Medical Engineering*, 48(8), 931–935. https://doi.org/10.1109/10.936369

59. Zandi, A. S., & Moradi, M. H. (2006). Quantitative evaluation of a wavelet-based method in ventricular late potential detection. *Pattern Recognition*, 39(7), 1369–1379. https://doi.org/10.1016/j.patcog.2006.01.012

60. Orosco, L. L., & Laciar, E. (2009). Analysis of ventricular late potentials in high resolution ECG records by time-frequency representations. *Latin American Applied Research*, 39(3), 255–260.

61. Subramanian, A. S., Gurusamy, G., & Selvakumar, G. (2012). A new ventricular late potential classification system using ant colony optimization. *Journal of Computer Science*, 8(2), 259.

62. Daphin Lilda, S., Jayaparvathy, R., & Balaji, A. (2022). An efficient machine learning based ventricular late potential detection and classification technique for cardiac healthcare. *Concurrency and Computation: Practice and Experience*, 34(26), e7279. https://doi.org/10.1002/cpe.7279

63. Gatzoulis, K. A., Arsenos, P., Trachanas, K., Dilaveris, P., Antoniou, C., Tsiachris, D., & Tousoulis, D. (2018). Signal-averaged electrocardiography: Past, present, and future. *Journal of Arrhythmia*, 34(3), 222–229. https://doi.org/10.1002/joa3.12062

64. Goldberger, A. L., Amaral, L. A., Glass, L., Hausdorff, J. M., Ivanov, P. C., Mark, R. G., & Stanley, H. E. (2000). PhysioBank, PhysioToolkit, and PhysioNet: Components of a new research resource for complex physiologic signals. circulation, 101(23), e215–e220. https://doi.org/10.1161/01.CIR.101.23.e215

65. Da Poian, G., Rozell, C. J., Bernardini, R., Rinaldo, R., & Clifford, G. D. (2017). Matched filtering for heart rate estimation on compressive sensing ECG measurements. *IEEE Transactions on Bio-Medical Engineering*, 65(6), 1349–1358. https://doi.org/10.1109/TBME.2017.2752422

66. Gamage, J., & Weerahandi, S. (1998). Size performance of some tests in one-way ANOVA. *Communications in Statistics – Simulation and Computation*, 27(3), 625–640. https://doi.org/10.1080/03610919808813500

67. Guaragnella, C., Rizzi, M., & Giorgio, A. (2019). Marginal component analysis of ECG signals for beat-to-beat detection of ventricular late potentials. *Electronics*, 8(9), 1000. https://doi.org/10.3390/electronics8091000

68. Giorgio, A., Rizzi, M., & Guaragnella, C. (2019). Efficient detection of ventricular late potentials on ECG signals based on wavelet denoising and SVM classification. *Information*, 10(11), 328. https://doi.org/10.3390/info10110328

69. Fagan, X., Ivanko, K., & Ivanushkina, N. (2021). Detection of ventricular late potentials in electrocardiograms using machine learning. In *Advances in Computer Science for Engineering and Education* III 3 (pp. 487–497). Springer International Publishing. https://doi.org/10.1007/978-3-030-55506-1_44

14 Heartcare Assistance System

A Machine Learning-Based Cardiovascular Risk Monitoring Tool (CRMT)

A. Kannammal, E. Chandra Blessie,
S. Barath Vignesh, and P. Kanishk

14.1 INTRODUCTION

Among various life-threatening diseases, heart disease has received much attention in medical research. Diagnosing heart disease is a challenging task that can offer automated prediction of a patient's heart condition so that further treatment can be effective. The diagnosis of heart disease is usually based on the patient's signs, symptoms, and physical examination. A major challenge facing healthcare organizations such as hospitals and medical centres is providing quality services at an affordable cost. Factors that enhance blockage are called risk factors. These risk factors can be categorized as non-controllable and controllable risk factors. Some important factors are age, gender, and heredity.

The dataset for heart prediction has both numerical and categorical data. Before further processing, cleaning and filtering are applied to these data in order to filter out irrelevant data from the database. Data mining is used to automatically attain diagnostic norms and support medical experts to make the diagnostic process more reliable. The reason for predictions in data mining is to discover trends in patient data to improve their healthcare.

A random forest is an ensemble classifier that combines bagging and random feature selection. The random forest algorithm contains numerous decision trees and the outcome is a class which is the mode of the class of individual trees [1]. It is one of the few classifiers which provides high accuracy compared to others. It provides a very accurate classification for numerous datasets, specifically for the cardiovascular disease dataset [2].

The application can determine the exact hidden knowledge, i.e., the patterns and relationships associated with heart diseases, from the historical database of heart

DOI: 10.1201/9781003363361-14

diseases [3]. It can also answer complex queries with the help of a chatbot for quick remedial action; therefore, it may be useful to make intelligent clinical decisions for patients with health risks [4].

14.2   PROBLEM STATEMENT

Heart disease is one of the greatest causes of morbidity and mortality among the world's population. Data-mining methods are a means of bringing out important and hidden information from large amounts of available data. A health database usually consists of inaccurate information. Therefore, decision-making using inaccurate data becomes a complex and challenging task. In the medical field, machine learning can be used to diagnose, detect, and predict various diseases. ML plays a very important role in uncovering hidden discrete patterns and thus analyzing the given data. After analyzing the dataset, ML methods help in cardiovascular risk prediction and early diagnosis. The main goal of the cardiovascular risk monitoring tool (CRMT) is to provide patients with a tool for early detection of cardiac risk and for corrective measures using a chatbot.

14.3   LITERATURE SURVEY

UpToDate [5] is an evidence-based smartphone clinical tool that provides the latest clinical evidence and includes over 9000 physician topics, 5000 drug topics, practice change updates, etc. This app is very useful in bedside Evidence-Based Medicine (EBM) practice and is very useful for integrating test results with clinical information [6, 7]. At a community hospital, internal medicine residents reported UpToDate as their most frequently used evidence-based resource. Phua and Lim [5] conducted a survey on the use of evidence-based resources by residents of a tertiary care hospital in Singapore with an institutional subscription to UpToDate. Most users (93.4%) found it useful and would recommend UpToDate to their colleagues, and for about three-fifths of them, using UpToDate led to changes in patient management decisions.

Smartphone-based medication reference apps can be a useful evidence-based resources at the point of care, as shown by Richardson and Burdette [8] in their example of the use of Epocrates [8] in the practice of evidence-based medicine during hospitalization. A survey of Personal Digital Assistant (PDA) use by practice nurses reported that medication reference apps were the most useful of all apps and that 92% of PDA users surveyed used Epocrates.

Smartphones can also be used in the diagnosis and treatment process using a software application. A simple smartphone app for eye professionals is a visual acuity test. For example, EyeChart [1] is an iPhone app that includes a Snellen [9] eye chart for measuring visual acuity. A similar application is the EyePhone, which includes a test for distance, a test for near visual acuity, a colour test, an Amsler grid, and a pupil measurement test. The DizzyFIX app [10] guides the physician through the Epley manoeuvre, a series of precise head and body positions that are the primary treatment for benign paroxysmal positional vertigo.

In some articles, the Modified Directly observed Therapy National Library of Medicine (MDoT NLM) project has been referred to by its original name, "PubMed on Tap" [11], which is different from the "PubMed on Tap" for iPhone. MDoT is a client-server application in which a software client (available for Palm OS and the Windows Mobile platform) sends a simple text query to an intermediary server (called the MD on Tap server), which formats the query into appropriate search terms for the selected search engine (Essie, PubMed/MEDLINE, or Google) [12] and returns the search results to the client application.

14.3.1 GAP ANALYSIS

Unlike other solutions, the CRMT system mainly focuses on acquiring live heart rate (BPM) data and uses it to analyze and predict the existence of cardiac risk [13]. It also provides a visual dashboard for tracking, storing and viewing the medical records of cardiac risk patients [14, 15]. The CRMT system not only focuses on problem identification but also quick remedial measures for cardiac risk patients [16] using a chatbot.

14.4 METHODOLOGY

14.4.1 DATA COLLECTION

The most critical goal of data collection is to ensure that rich and reliable data are collected for statistical analysis in order to make data-driven research decisions. This dataset has 11 common features, making it the largest heart disease dataset available for research to date.

14.4.2 DATA PREPROCESSING

Data preprocessing can refer to the manipulation or shedding of data before it is used to ensure or increase performance and is an important step in the data-mining process. It also includes handling of missing values. Some of the data preprocessing steps taken are removal of unwanted columns, fixing structural errors, managing outliers, and label encoding.

14.4.3 DATA VISUALIZATION

14.4.3.1 Exploratory Data Analysis

Exploratory data analysis (EDA) is an important system for using summaries and graphical presentations for preliminary data analysis to uncover patterns, reveal complexity, hypothesis tests, and hypothetical assumptions. EDA is often used to determine what data can be released without formal modelling and to obtain additional information about the collection of data and how they interact with each other. It can also help us determine whether the mathematical processes we are considering for data analysis are appropriate.

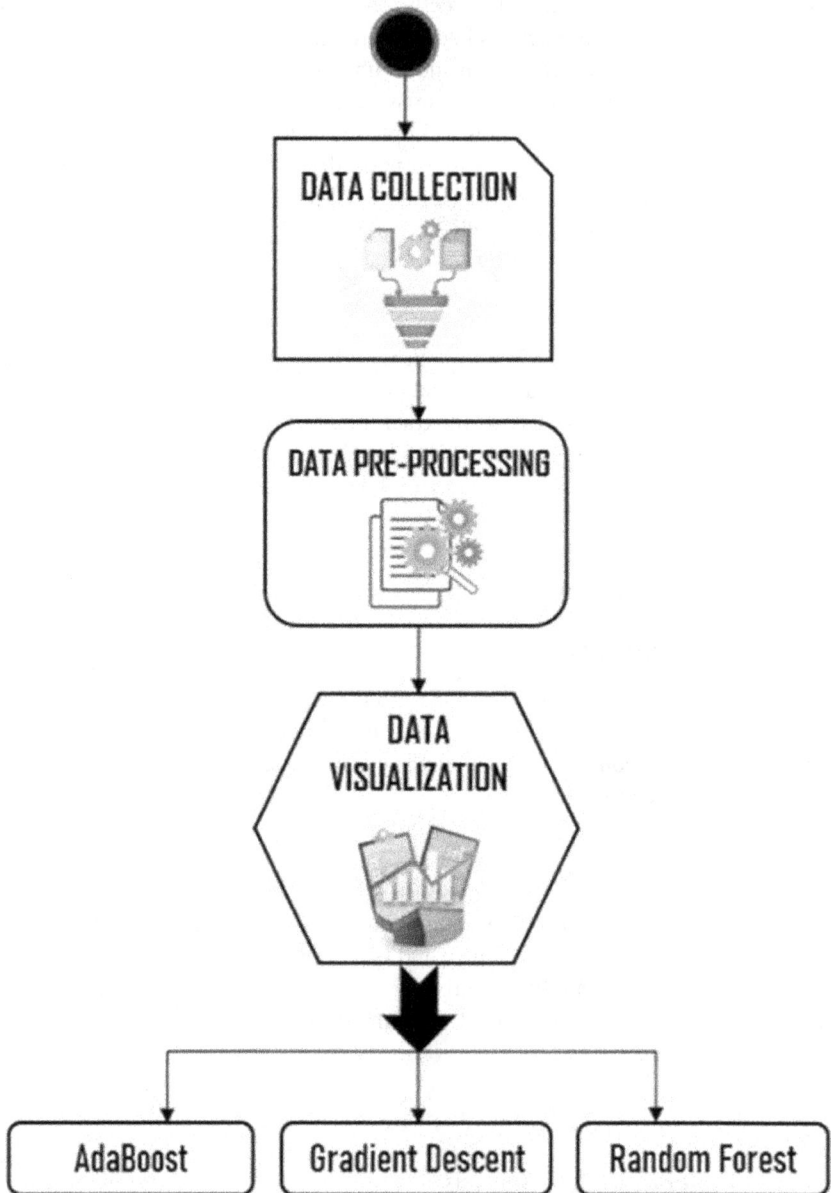

FIGURE 14.1   Heart risk classifier architecture

14.4.3.2 Visuals used for data analysis

It can be seen from Figure 14.2 that the cholesterol feature of people aged 50 to 60 reaches a maximum. Also, the cholesterol feature is directly proportional to the age feature [17]. It is clear from Figure 14.3 that columns like ST_Slope, ExerciseAngina,

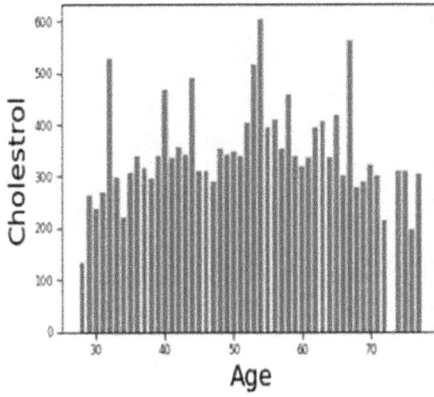

FIGURE 14.2 Bar graph on cholesterol and age

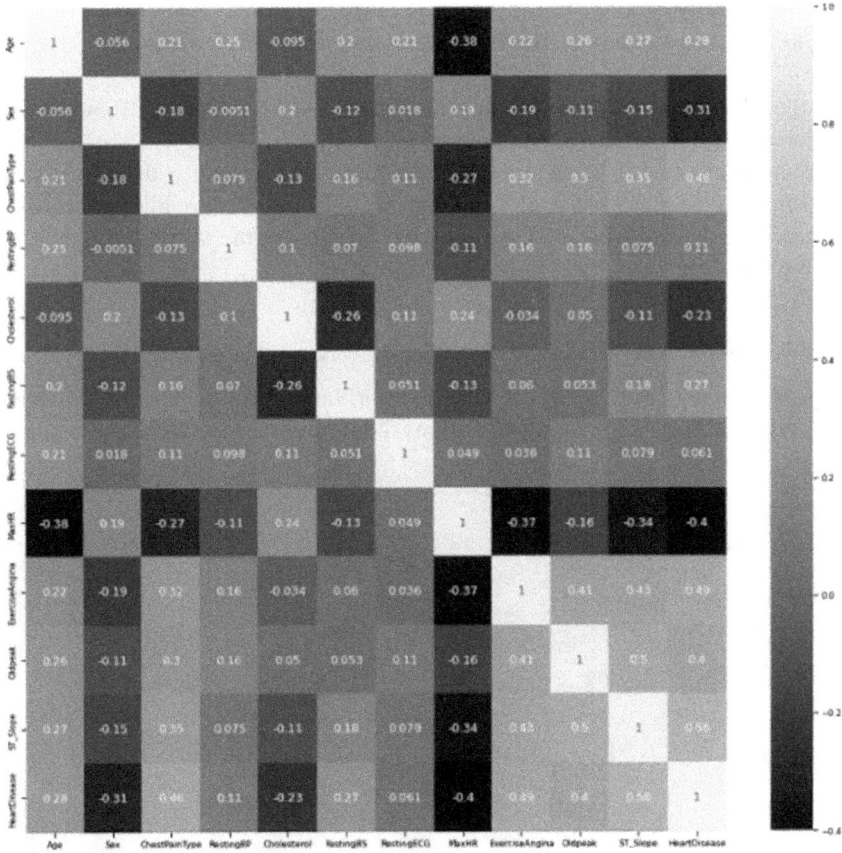

FIGURE 14.3 Correlation plot for all features

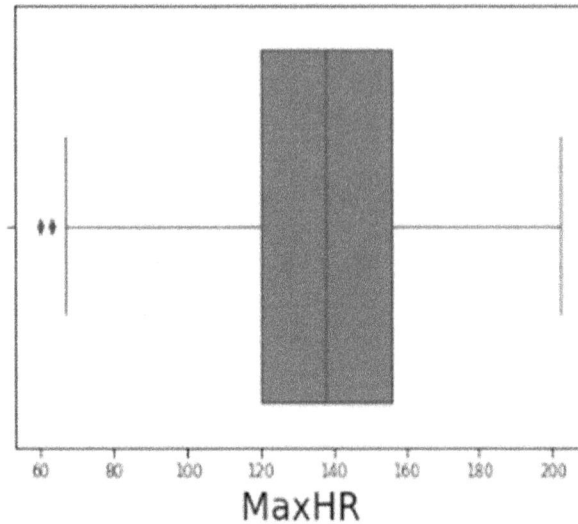

FIGURE 14.4 Histogram representing frequency of records based on age

ChestPainType, and Oldpeak are some of the important features that show a direct relationship with heart disease prediction.

From Figure 14.4, it is apparent that the number of people with heart disease peaks in the age range of 55 to 65 years and that older people have higher chances of heart disease. From Figure 14.5, we can detect outliers in the MaxHR columns and also remove them.

14.4.4 AdaBoost

AdaBoost is a statistical classification meta-algorithm used in conjunction with many other types of machine learning algorithms to improve performance. The output of

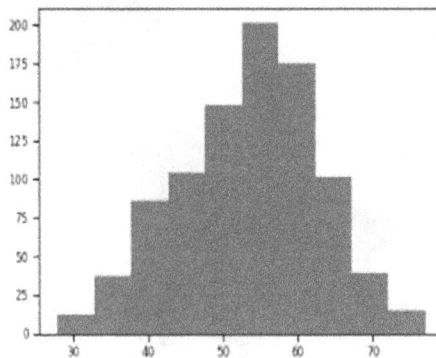

FIGURE 14.5 Box plot on MaxHR to detect and remove the outlier

the other learning algorithms ("weak learners") is combined into a weighted sum that represents the final output of the boosted classifier. Usually, AdaBoost is used for two-label classification, although it can be generalized to multiple classes or bounded intervals on the real line. Each learning algorithm tends to suit some types of problems better than others and usually has many different parameters and configurations that need to be adjusted before it achieves optimal performance on a dataset.

14.4.5   GRADIENT BOOSTING

Gradient boosting is an efficient algorithm in machine learning. It is known that errors in machine learning algorithms are generally classified into two categories: bias errors and deviation errors. Since gradient boosting is one of the boosting algorithms, it is used to minimize the bias error of the model. The basic estimator for the gradient boost algorithm is fixed and that is the decision stump. The gradient boosting algorithm can be used to predict not only a continuous target variable (as a regressor) but also a categorical target variable (as a classifier).

14.4.6   RANDOM FORESTS

The random forest (RF) algorithm is one of the most widely used classification approaches. The RF algorithm was used in the identification and probability calculation. RF consists of numerous decision trees. Each decision tree provides a vote that indicates a decision about a label class. The RF method bends with bagging and random feature selection.

There are three important tuning parameters in random forest. They are the total number of trees (n tree), the value of minimum node size, and the total number of features used in splitting each node.

Randomization is used to select the best node to split, which helps in constructing individual trees in a random forest.

14.5   TOOLS AND TECHNOLOGIES

14.5.1   APPLICATION DEVELOPMENT

14.5.1.1   Flutter

Flutter is an open-source framework from Google for building innovative, well-structured cross-platform applications from a single code base. Flutter is a software development kit (SDK) and portable user interface (UI) for building attractive, natively compiled mobile web and desktop applications from a single code base. Flutter works with existing code, is used by developers and institutes around the world, and is free and open-source. Flutter offers an outsized array of benefits for both marketers and developers.

14.5.1.2 Dart

Dart can be a programming language intended for consumer development such as web and mobile applications. It is developed by Google and can even be used to create server and desktop applications. With JavaScript-like syntax, Dart could also be a typed object-oriented programming language that focuses on front-end development.

14.5.1.3 Kommunicate

Kommunicate is a chatbot builder used to create custom chatbots. It's a simple, intuitive and easy-to-use interface wrapped around powerful conversational artificial intelligence (AI). We can create natural language processing- (NLP-) based support bots and conversational workflows without any code. Kommunicate provides a buildConversation function to directly create and start a chat, saving you the extra steps of authentication, creation, initialization, and startup. For building native interfaces for iOS and Android, CRMT used Flutter (Google SDK) as our framework with Dart as the primary programming language, in order to develop a fast app on any platform.

14.5.2 Backend Development

14.5.2.1 Mongo DB

MongoDB Atlas is a fully managed cloud database that handles all the complexity of deploying, managing, and healing your deployments on your chosen cloud service provider (AWS, Azure, and GCP). MongoDB Atlas is the most efficient way to deploy, run, and scale MongoDB.

14.5.2.2 FastAPI

FastAPI is a Python framework and toolkit that allows developers to use a REST interface to call commonly used functions to implement applications. It is accessible via a REST API to call common building blocks for the application. FastAPI is the fastest Python framework compared with Go and Node.js. ASGI enables the FastAPI to support concurrent and asynchronous code.

14.5.3 Server Deployment

14.5.3.1 Heroku Server

Heroku is a container cloud platform as a service (PaaS). Developers suggest Heroku to deploy, manage, and scale modern applications as it is elegant, flexible, and easy to use, Heroku offers developers the easiest way to bring their apps to market. Heroku also provides custom-built packages where developers can deploy applications in any other programming language. Applications running on Heroku typically have unique domain names that are used to route HTTP requests to the correct container.

14.6 CRMT SYSTEM PROCESS

14.6.1 DATA INFORMATION

14.6.1.1 Data Source – Heart Prediction Model

The CRMT dataset used for developing the detection models was taken from the University of California Irvine (UCI) repository [18] and has been converted into a comma-separated file. In this dataset, five heart datasets are combined with more than 11 common features, making it the largest heart disease database ever available for research purposes. The five datasets from different regions used to treat it are 305 observations from Cleveland, 296 observations from Hungary, 133 observations from Switzerland, 203 observations from Long Beach, Virginia, and 269 observations from the Stalag (heart) dataset. The attributes used are **Age**, which describes the age of the patient; **Sex**, which describes the gender of the patient (M: male, F: female); **ChestPainType**, which identifies the types of chest pain the user experiences; **RestingBP**, which tells the blood pressure when the user is at rest; **Cholesterol**, which indicates the cholesterol level of the user; **FastingBS**, which tells the sugar level of the user; **RestingECG**, which indicates the electrocardiogram when the user is at rest; **MaxHR**, which finds the maximum heart rate attained for the user; **ExerciseAngina**, which is also called exercise-induced angina and categorizes whether the user induced angina or not; **Oldpeak**, which finds the oldest peak attained by the patient; **ST_Slope**, which indicates when the user is at peak exercise under an ST segment; and **HeartDisease**, which is the output class which helps in finding whether or not the person has heart risk [4].

14.6.1.2 Authentication Database

The CRMT system has two tables used for registration and medical records. This helps to store the user's personal and medical information and allows the user to get the information to perform the program login. It is built on a No-SQL framework using MongoDB. The schematic definition of the two tables in the database is given in Figure 14.6 below.

14.6.1.3 Module Description

A program module is a class that represents a business application. Specifically, it contains the data model associated with the task and the specific code to perform the task. The program consists of six core modules that help patients track medical records and identify cardiac risk factors and treatment options.

Figure 14.7 shows five major modules present in the application, listed as follows:

- Authentication module
- Risk prediction
- Heart BPM estimator
- Dashboard
- Chatbot

Medical Record	
Fields	**Type**
Object_Id	int
Age	int
RestingBP	int
Cholestral	int
FastingBS	int
MaxHR	int
Oldpeak	int
Gender	string
ChestPainType	string
restingECG	string
exerciseAngina	string
st_slope	string
heartDisease	int
User_ID	int
created_at	timestamp

User	
Fields	**Type**
Object_Id	int
Username	string
Email	string
Password	string
Phone	int
User_ID	int
created_at	timestamp

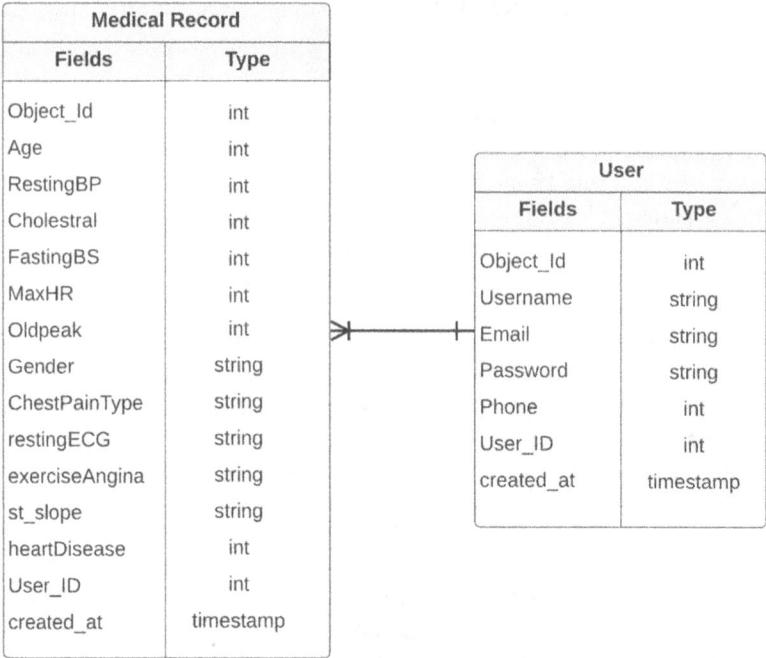

FIGURE 14.6   Schema diagram

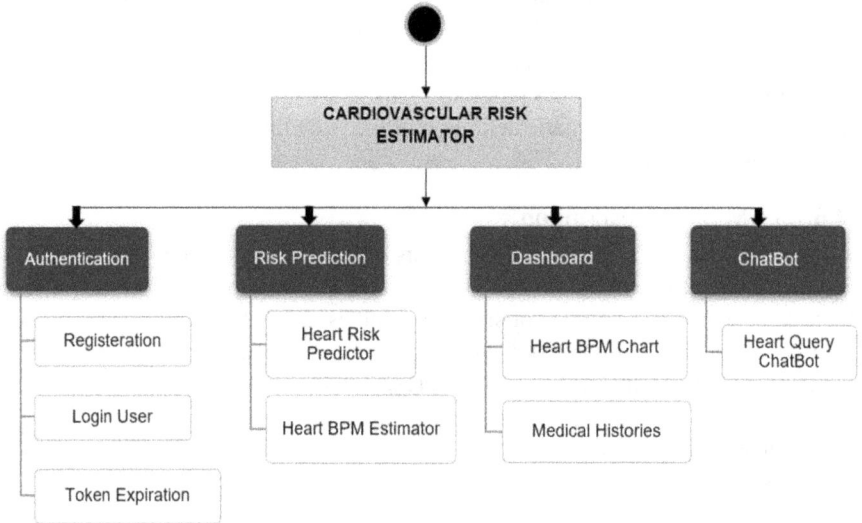

FIGURE 14.7   CRMT process

14.6.1.3.1 Authentication Module

This application enables the user to create an individual account with the help of register and login pages. The authentication module will be present at the start of the application. Once the user enters the application, they must register the details in the given sign-up form. The MongoDB stores the registration details and helps the user log in to the application using the login form. FastAPI acts as a validator to check whether the given login details match the existing database.

Figures 14.8 and 14.9 show the format of the sign-in page and sign-up page.

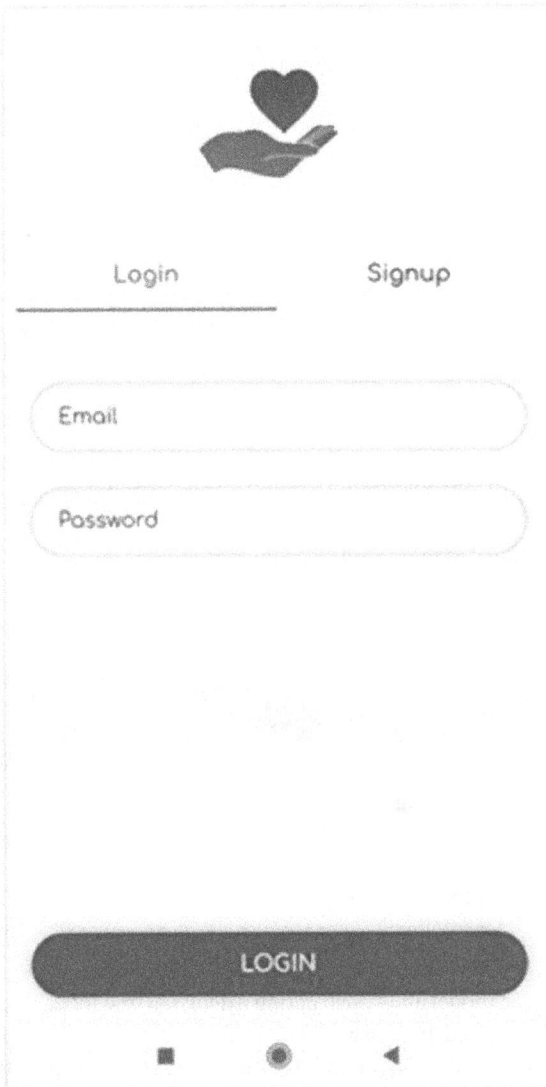

FIGURE 14.8 Sign-in page

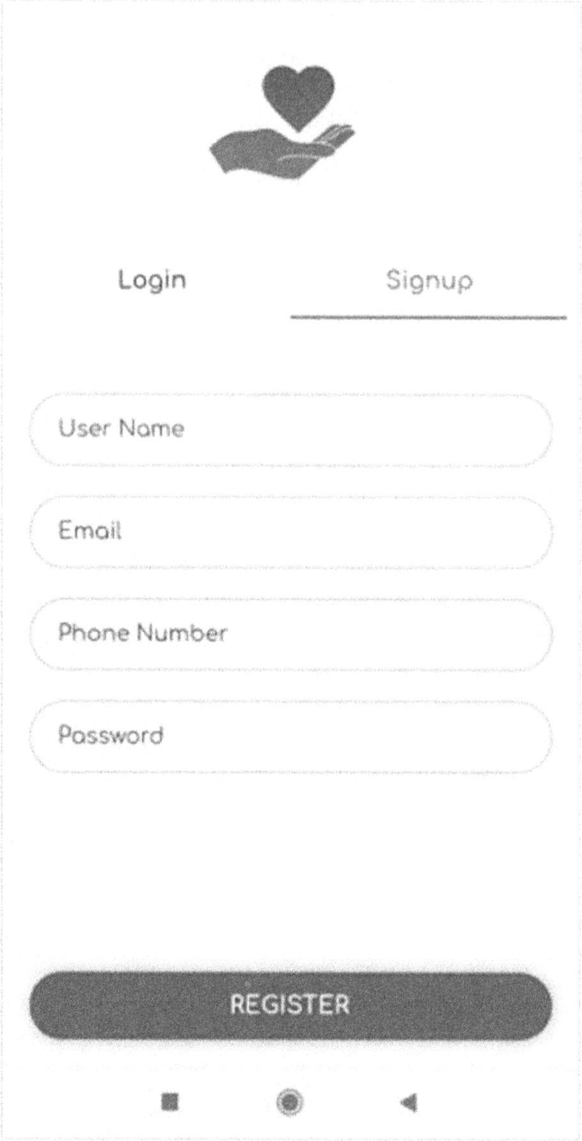

FIGURE 14.9   Sign-up page

14.6.1.3.2   Risk Prediction

Training data into the model and constructing a decision tree for each sample acquires a prediction result from each decision tree. Then, converting the model into a pickle model, allows us to save the model and to minimize lengthy re-training. This model is used in Flutter, in order to predict the risk of heart disease of an individual by getting an input of age, blood pressure, cholesterol, sugar, etc., as shown in Figures 14.10 and 14.11. Once the account has been created by the user, the user is requested to fill in the above values in the application. After the values have been filled, the ML model predicts the current state of the user, and the record is stored in the application for visual aid purposes.

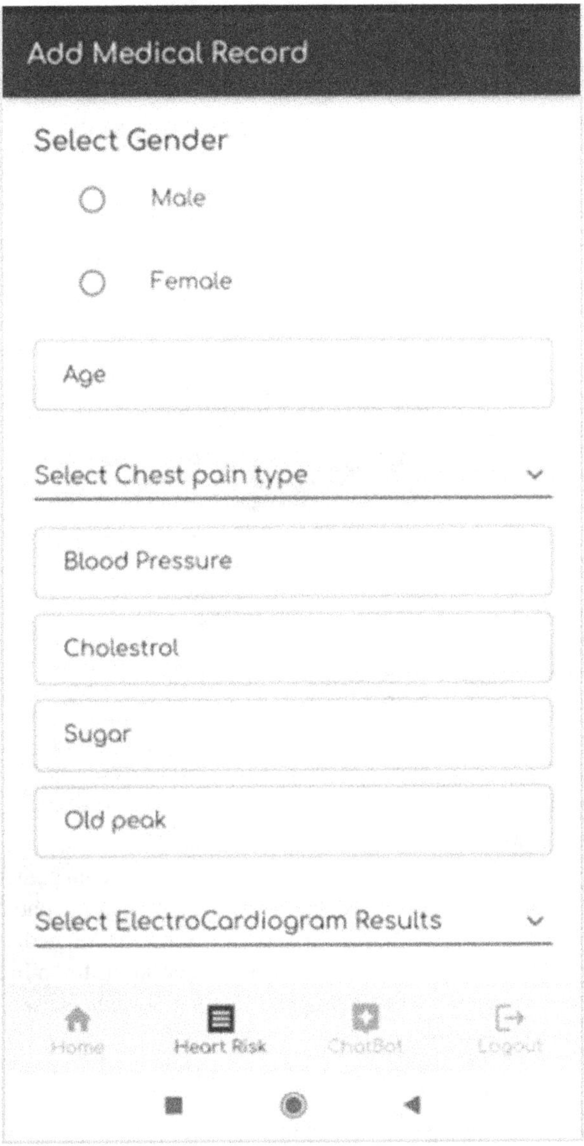

FIGURE 14.10   Add medical record

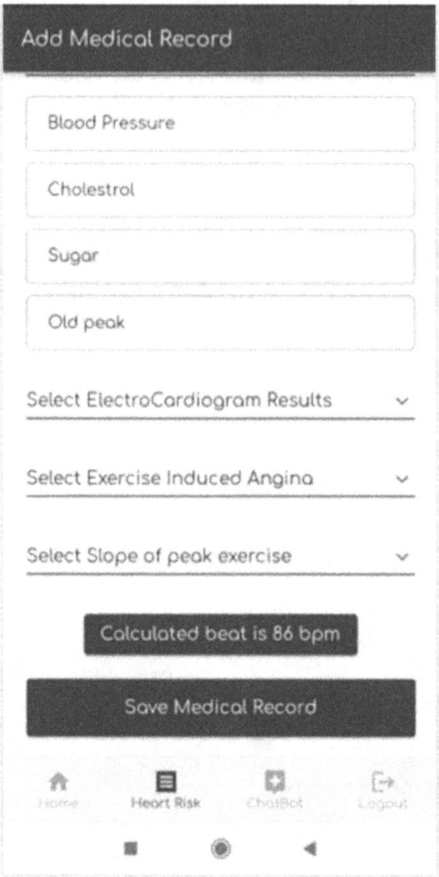

FIGURE 14.11   Add medical record

14.6.1.3.3 Heart BPM Estimator

This application helps the user fetch their live heart BPM rate with the help of a Flutter plugin called heart_bpm. The heart BPM is captured via camera and flash in the smartphone shown in Figures 14.12 and . Heart BPM acts as one of the features for predicting the user's heart risk [19]. In order to complete the medical records, the application requires the user to place their index finger on the torch light for 15 to 20 seconds in order and calculate the BPM. The calculated value is used for prediction and visualization purposes.

14.6.1.3.4 Dashboard

Dashboard reports are one-page images of live results and how they work against key metrics. They provide decision-makers with quick and easy-to-understand information and real-time analysis that helps improve decision-making. This application's

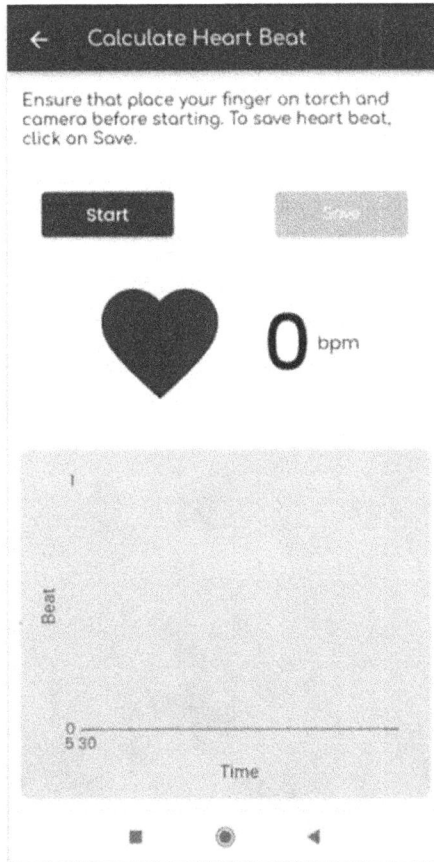

FIGURE 14.12 BPM estimator

dashboard consists of bar graphs representing BPM calculated on a daily basis, to find how BPM varies from day to day, and of medical history, which gives the overall picture of the user's health. It also enables the user to edit and update previous medical records in order to maintain data integrity.

Figure 14.14 is the BPM bar chart, which shows the daily heartbeat. Figures 14.15 and 14.16 show the list of medical histories.

14.6.1.3.5 Chatbot

The chatbot acts as a provider of remedial measures or solutions to users who have a high chance of suffering a heart attack, which is shown in Figures 14.17 and 14.18. Once the predictor module predicts the existence of heart risk for the user, the application redirects the user to the chatbot module. The chatbot is developed using kommunicate, which provides instant remedies before consulting a medical expert or hospital.

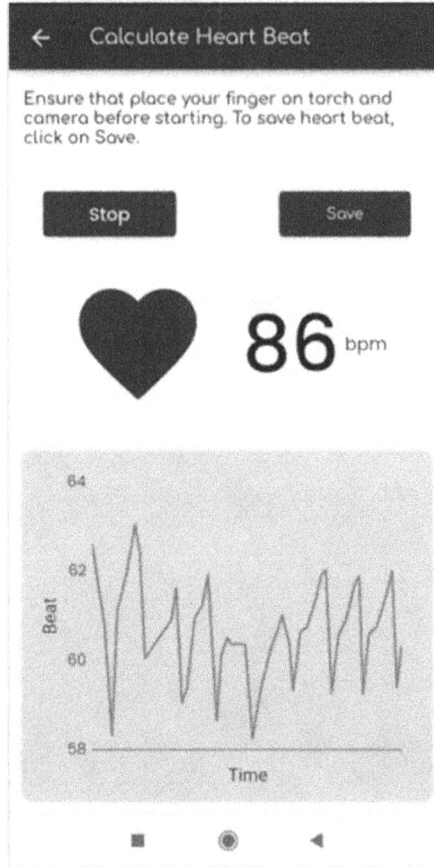

FIGURE 14.13   BPM estimator

14.7   EXPERIMENTAL ANALYSIS

14.7.1   COMPARATIVE STUDY

A comparative study helps in building an analytical and comprehensive approach for applying legal reasoning. This research helps to find the best approach to deploy the application. Analysis is done on various classification algorithms such as AdaBoost, gradient descent, and random forest. It is evident from Table 14.1 that the random forest classifier outperforms other classification algorithms with a maximum accuracy rate of 96.5% and is therefore adopted for further evaluation.

14.7.2   RESULTS AND DISCUSSIONS

14.7.2.1   Hyperparameter Tuning using GridSearchCV

GridSearchCV is a hyperparameter tuning process to determine the optimal value for a given model. The performance of the model is highly dependent on the value

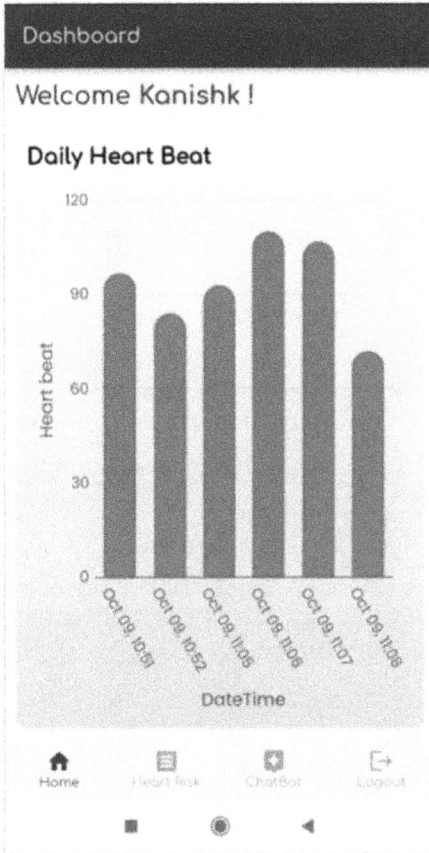

FIGURE 14.14   BPM bar chart

of the hyperparameters. Note that the best value for the hyperparameter cannot be known in advance; we must try all possible values to find the optimal value. GridSearchCV is used to automate the tuning of hyperparameters. GridSearchCV is a function included in the scikit-learn (or SK-learn) model_selection package. Some arguments used in GridSearchCV are estimator, params_grid, signature, cv, expression, and n_jobs. After running hyperparameter tuning on all three algorithms, the test data accuracy of the random forest classifier model performed better than the other two algorithms, and this model was adopted for the next evaluation step.

14.7.3 Performance Metrics

14.7.3.1 Precision

Precision is defined as the ratio of positive samples classified as correct (true positive) to the total number of positive samples (correct or incorrect). Precision helps to visualize the reliability of machine learning models in classifying the model as positive.

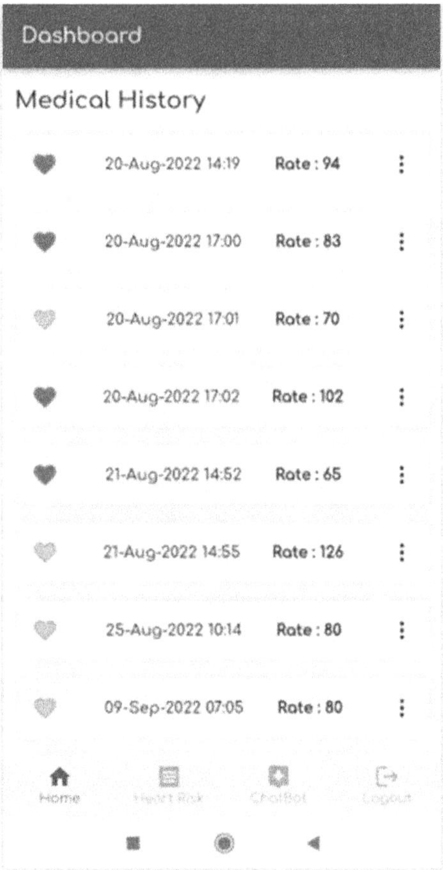

FIGURE 14.15 List of medical histories

14.7.3.2 Recall

Recall is calculated as the number of positive samples classified as positive to the total number of positive samples. Recall measures the ability of the model to detect positive samples. The higher the recall, the more positive samples are found. Negation does not depend on the number of negative sample classifications. Additionally, recall will be one if the model classifies all positive samples as positive.

In this model, it is important to remember that there is no error (100% recall) because it helps to predict the heart risk of the user with a better level of accuracy. The recall is 93.4%, which means that there is a 6.6% chance of the user being at risk of heart failure. The system can also adjust the performance evaluation criteria to reduce the error rate and increase the return rate.

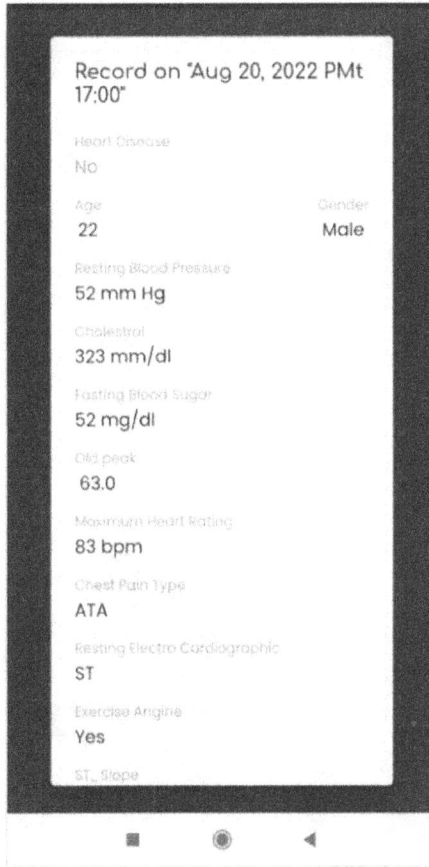

FIGURE 14.16   Medical history

14.7.3.3   Precision and Recall Tradeoff

The precision and recall tradeoff is used when changing the threshold to determine whether a class is positive or negative. Remember to increase or decrease to adjust accuracy.

From Figure 14.19, it is evident that when the recall is increased, precision will be decreased. By increasing the recall to one, the precision value is decreased to 0.7. Therefore, the recall is being increased by setting up the right threshold value.

14.7.3.4   Setting Threshold Value

In order the increase the recall value, the threshold value needs to be tuned. The current threshold value of the model is 0.2. From Figure 14.20, it is evident that the threshold value should be negative three to increase the value back to one. The model is evaluated based on the new threshold value.

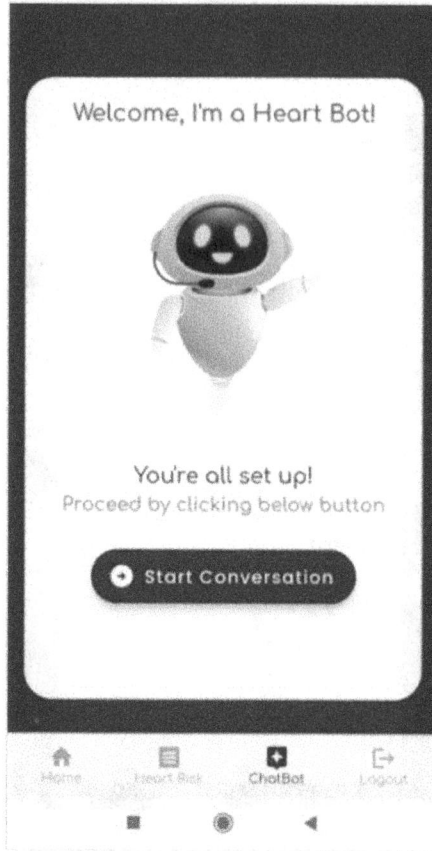

FIGURE 14.17   Chatbot home page

14.8   EVALUATING METRICS AND RESULTS

14.8.1   CONFUSION MATRIX

Confusion matrix is a table used to describe the performance of a classification algorithm. The confusion matrix visualizes and shortens the classification algorithm. Also known as an error matrix, a summary table is used to evaluate the performance of a classification model.

From Figure 14.21, it is known that the presence of a false negative (FN) is zero and it also achieves the recall of one. Hence, the model works error-free and works efficiently for all heart-risk patients.

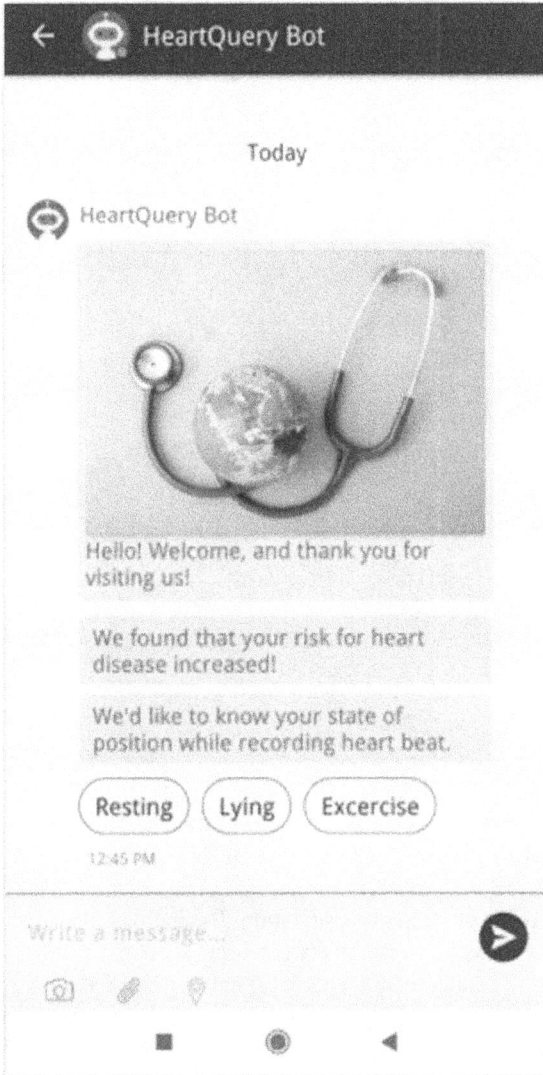

FIGURE 14.18 Heart query chatbot

TABLE 14.1
Comparison Chart

	Precision (%)	Recall (%)	Accuracy (%)
AdaBoost	93.3	90.1	88.5
Gradient Descent	91.7	87.4	92.9
Random Forest	94.1	92.7	96.5

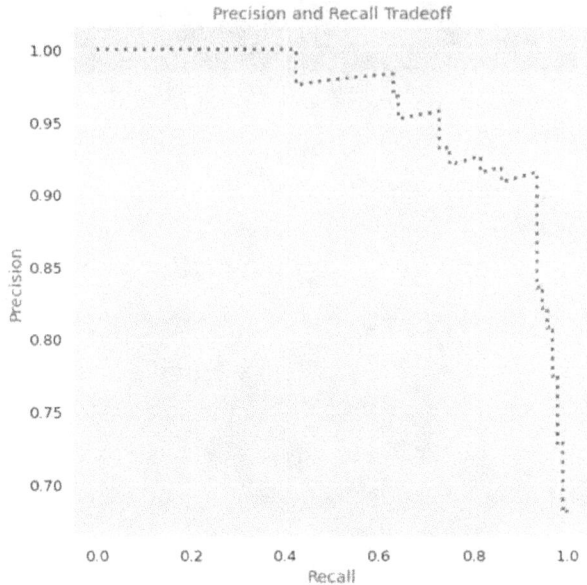

FIGURE 14.19   Precision and recall tradeoff

14.8.2   Area Under Curve - Receiver Operating Characteristic (AUC-ROC) Curve

The AUC-ROC curve is a performance measurement graph used in classification problems by adjusting the threshold values. ROC is also referred to as the probability curve and AUC describes the degree or measure of separability. The higher the AUC, the better the model is at binary classification. By analogy, the higher the AUC, the better the model is at distinguishing between users with and without heart risk.

From Figure 14.22 and the AUC score, we can see that the model is excellent and has an AUC near to one, which means it has a good measure of separability.

14.8.3   CRMT System Outcome

The CRMT system provides a valuable solution to the user using the chatbot functionality. A chatbot (conversational AI) is an automated program that generates human conversation through text messages, voice chats, or both. Experts predict that cost savings from healthcare chatbots will reach $11 billion globally by 2023. It learns to do that based on a lot of inputs and natural language processing (NLP) to provide a better user experience. Often referred to as virtual agents or intelligent virtual assistants, these NLP chatbots help human agents by taking over

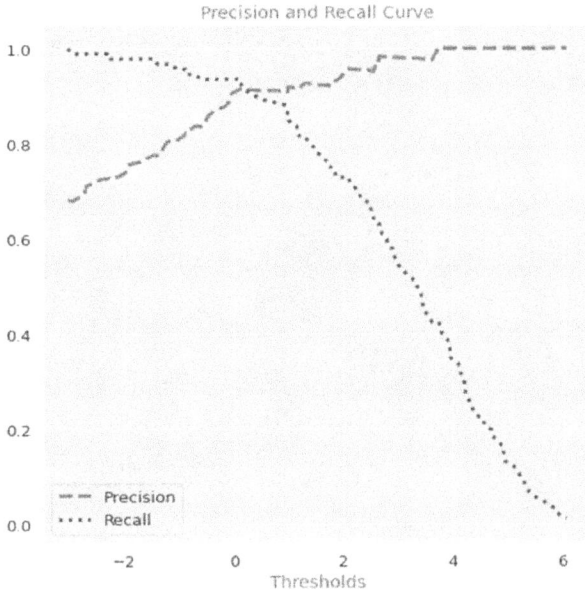

FIGURE 14.20   Precision and recall curve

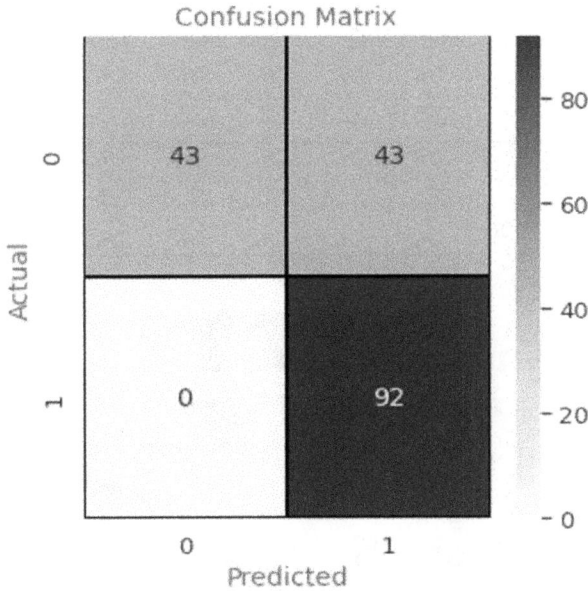

FIGURE 14.21   Confusion matrix

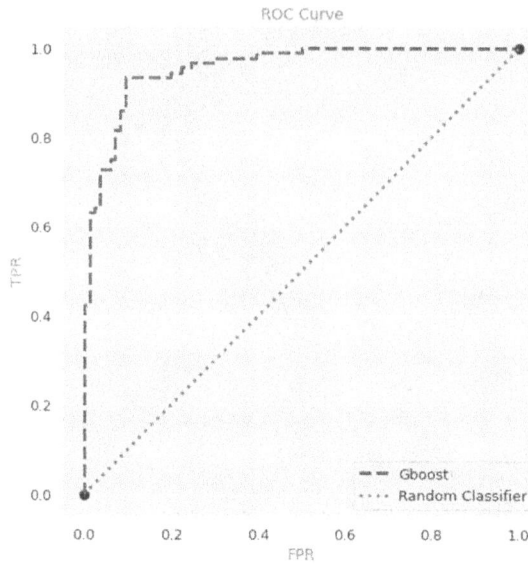

FIGURE 14.22 ROC curve and AUC score

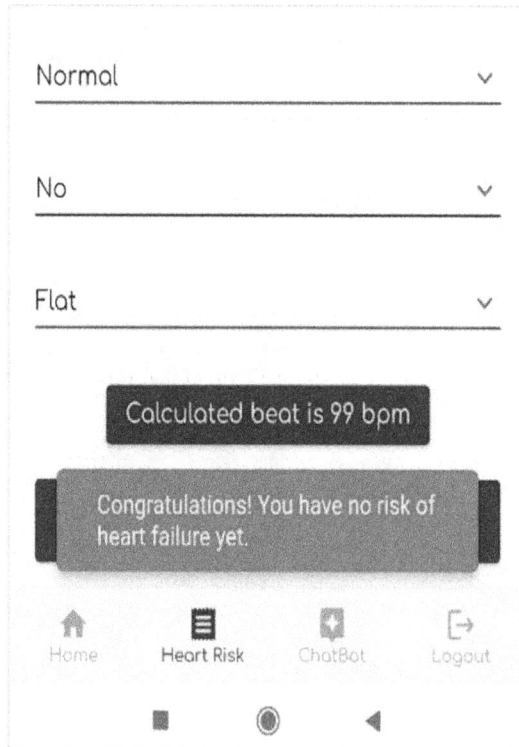

FIGURE 14.23 Risk prediction

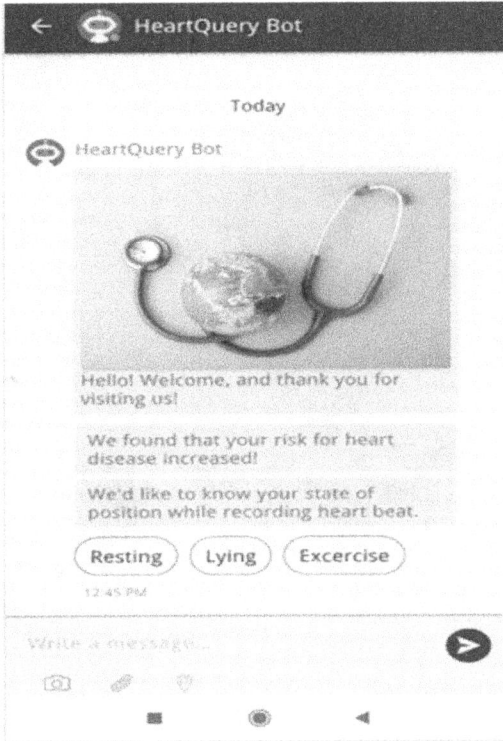

FIGURE 14.24   Heart query chatbot

repetitive and time-consuming communications. The CRMT system is developed using Kommunicate, which provides instant remedies before consulting a medical expert or hospital.

Once the required details have been filled by the patient, the CRMT System predicts the existence of heart risk for the user who has been redirected to the chatbot for quick remedies.

Figure 14.23 shows the prediction of heart risk by the CRMT system and Figure 14.24 gives us the mobile interface and working of chatbot for a simple query from a user who has been diagnosed with heart risk.

The user can also visit the chatbot interface without being diagnosed as a risk patient [20]. The query window or the chatbot interface starts asking basic questions and will suggest to the user a few tips for being healthy in daily life

Figure 14.25 shows the chatbot window for a user who hasn't been diagnosed with the presence of heart risk. Chatbots can leverage feedback to make smarter decisions and improve their practices.

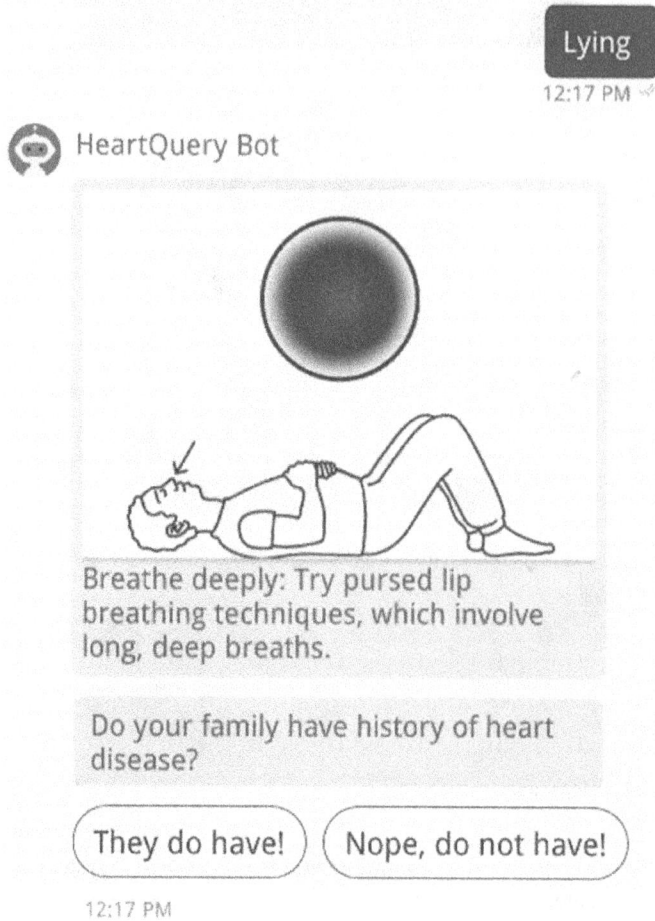

FIGURE 14.25   Heart query chatbot – sample query

14.9 CONCLUSION

In this research paper, we developed an efficient approach for the prediction of heart disease using random forest. Data mining plays an important role in the prediction of heart disease. Applying random forest has improved accuracy in the prediction of heart disease compared to other algorithms. Our proposed approach achieved an accuracy of 96.5% for the heart dataset. The introduction of chatbots serves as an important and quick decision-making tool for immediate solutions before seeking medical help. This application serves as the best solution, mainly for heart patients to track their medical condition on a daily basis, and also for doctors to monitor the previous medical records via the application itself. Machine learning blended with chatbots provides the best combination for predicting risk and providing remedial measures to a great extent.

14.10 FURTHER ENHANCEMENTS

- With the assistance of medical experts, chatbots can be further developed to suggest medicines before reaching the hospital.
- Providing the doctor's contact details in order to book appointments.
- Providing route maps in order to reach the hospital and also suggestions of medical centres available.
- Making the CRMT system a doctor-friendly application in order to track the medical records of the patients, to help in providing accurate medications and to improve the health of the patients.

REFERENCES

1. Pope L, Silva P, Almeyda R. I-phone applications for the modern day otolaryngologist. *Clinical Otolaryngology.* 2010;35(4):350–4. DOI: 10.1111/j.1749-4486.2010.02170.x.
2. Conroy RM, Pyorala K, Fitzgerald AP, et al. Estimation of ten-year risk of fatal cardiovascular disease in Europe: The SCORE project. *European Heart Journal.* 2003;24(11):987–1003.
3. Cushman M, Arnold AM, Psaty BM, et al. C-reactive protein and the 10-year incidence of coronary heart disease in older men and women: The cardiovascular health study. *Circulation.* 2005;112(1):25–31.
4. [NCEP-ATPIII]. National Cholesterol Education Program – Adult Treatment Panel III. Expert Panel on Detection, Evaluation, and Treatment of High Blood Cholesterol in Adults. Executive summary of the third report of the national cholesterol education program (NCEP) expert panel on detection, evaluation, and treatment of high blood cholesterol in adults (adult treatment panel III). *JAMA.* 2001;285:2486–97.
5. Phua J, Lim TK. How residents and interns utilise and perceive the personal digital assistant and UpToDate. *BMC Medical Education.* 2008;8:39. DOI: 10.1186/1472-6920-8-39.
6. D'Agostino RB, Sr, Grundy S, Sullivan LM, et al. Validation of the Framingham coronary heart disease prediction scores: Results of a multiple ethnic groups investigation. *JAMA.* 2001;286(2):180–7.
7. Deepa R, Sandeep S, Mohan V. Abdominal obesity, visceral fat and type 2 diabetes–Asian Indian phenotype. In: Mohan V, Rao GHR, editors. *Type 2 Diabetes in South Asians: Epidemiology, Risk Factors and Prevention.* New Delhi: Jaypee Brothers Medical Publishers (P) Ltd, 2006, pp. 138–52.
8. Richardson WS, Burdette SD. Practice corner: Taking evidence in hand. *Evidence-Based Medicine.* 2003;8:4. DOI: 10.1136/ebm.8.1.4.
9. Brindle PM, McConnachie A, Upton MN, et al. The accuracy of the Framingham risk-score in different socioeconomic groups: A prospective study. *British Journal of General Practice.* 2005;55(520):838–45.
10. Cappuccio FP, Oakeshott P, Strazzullo P, et al. Application of Framingham risk estimates to ethnic minorities in United Kingdom and implications for primary prevention of heart disease in general practice: Cross sectional population based study. *BMJ.* 2002;325:1271. Erratum in: *BMJ.* 2003;327(7420):919.
11. Hauser SE, Demner-Fushman D, Ford G, Thoma GR. PubMed on tap: Discovering design principles for online information delivery to handheld computers. *Studies in Health Technology and Informatics.* 2004;107:1430–1433.
12. Anooj PK. Clinical decision support system: Risk level prediction of heart disease using Weighted fuzzy rules. *Journal of King Saud University, CIS.* 2012;24:27–40.

13. Chow CK, Naidu S, Raju K, et al. Significant lipid, adiposity and metabolic abnormalities amongst 4535 Indians from a developing region of rural Andhra Pradesh. *Atherosclerosis*. 2007. Epub ahead of print.

14. Enas E, Senthilkumar A. Coronary artery disease in Asian Indians: An update and review, *The Internet Journal of Cardiology*. 2001;1(2).

15. Greenland P, Smith SC, Grundy SM. Improving Coronary Heart Disease risk Assessment in Asymptomatic People: Role of Traditional Risk Factors and Noninvasive cardiovascular Tests. *Circulation*. 2001;104(15):1863–7.

16. Cobb FR, Kraus WE, Root M, et al. Assessing risk for coronary heart disease: Beyond Framingham. *American Heart Journal*. 2003;146(4):572–80.

17. Detrano J, Janosi A, Steinbrunn W, et al. International application of new probability algorithm for the diagnosis of CAD. *The American Journal of Cardiology*. 1989;64(5):304–10.

18. https://archive.ics.uci.edu/ml/datasets/Heart+Disease.

19. Enas EA, Garg A, Davidson MA, et al. Coronary heart disease and its risk factors in first-generation immigrant Asian Indians to the United States of America. *Indian Heart Journal*. 1996;48(4):343–53.

20. Deepa M, Farooq S, Datta M, et al. Prevalence of metabolic syndrome using WHO, ATPIII and IDF definitions in Asian Indians: The Chennai Urban Rural Epidemiology Study (CURES-34). *Diabetes/Metabolism Research and Reviews*. 2007;23(2):127–34.

15 Parameter Estimation of Real-Time NCS Signal Acquired Using Designed Neurostimulator to Develop Microcontroller-Based Healthcare Support System

Amarprit Singh, Lachit Dutta, Anil Hazarika,
Champak Talukdar, and Manabendra Bhuyan

15.1 INTRODUCTION

Increasing health incidents and costs associated with prolonged non-communicable diseases such as cancer, cardiovascular diseases, and diabetes mellitus (DM) are today's most prominent healthcare challenges [1–3]. It is an obvious fact that the global population is increasing at a very rapid rate [4]. As a consequence, it was estimated that the number of diabetic-related complications is projected to rise to 366 million by 2030 all over the world [1], as a result of which approximately 90–95% of the global population will suffer from type two diabetes [5]. DM primarily affects the peripheral nervous system, resulting in peripheral nerve disorders in up to 50% of the patients [6]. However, prolonged DM results in diabetic neuropathy (DN), which can cause severe impairment of tiny fibres, loss of sensation, muscle weakness, and autonomic nerve damage, resulting in functional loss of end organs such as the liver, kidney, stomach, etc. [7]. On the contrary, sensory polyneuropathy is a length-dependent disorder commonly evident in neuromuscular adjunctive related to sensory neurons [8]. Early sensory symptoms are numbness and paresthesia in the toes, which gradually become more acute over time and often appear in the fingertips in later stages. Some patients develop distal weakness along with foot and leg pain with the advent of more advanced sensory manifestations [9]. Therefore,

DOI: 10.1201/9781003363361-15

diagnosis of DN through the proper acquisition of nerve conduction study (NCS) signal and estimation of nerve parameters for detection of abnormal features at the disease's initial stage is essential for preventing severe complications such as foot ulcers and limb loss.

Diagnosis of DN requires proper acquisition, pre- and postprocessing of NCS signal from the underlying nerve, and analysis of subsequent features contained in the signal for necessary evaluation [10, 11] (Figure 15.1). A neurostimulator with an appropriate design setting is used to convey electrical pulses to the nerve under examination to revive the functional loss of the impaired nerve. From the recording site that has the diagnostic nerve's vital information, the associated NCS signals are captured [12]. Motor DN is diagnosed using several nerve measures, including motor nerve conduction velocity (MNCV), proximal latency (PML), distal latency (DML), and compound muscle action potentials (CMAP) [13–16]. Numerous decision support systems that integrate fuzzy, support vector machines, linear discriminant analysis, and neural networks are used in this context for neuromuscular diagnosis applications [15–19]. For instance, Singh et al., an optimum neural network approach is implemented in a peripheral interface controller (PIC) microcontroller for online nerve parameter estimation and diagnosis after being derived from a MATLAB simulation utilizing a dataset for nerve diagnostics. Meesad et al. [17], "if, then" rules are used to detect diseases when linguistic data are converted into fuzzy variables, which proposes a hybrid fuzzy-neural network-based decision support system. Using the patient's demographic information and clinical factors, a multi-category support vector machine (MSVM) is developed by Kazemi et al. in [18] to predict the severity of diabetic peripheral neuropathy, which is then split into four categories. After that, three kernel functions, viz. radial basis function (RBF), linear, and polynomial, are utilized to predict the class of disease using the one-against-all and one-against-one approaches of MSVM. Furthermore, a study conducted by Fioretti et al. in [19] focuses on detecting neuropathy in asymptomatic subjects with the help of linear discriminant analysis, which could be embedded in a user-friendly interface for

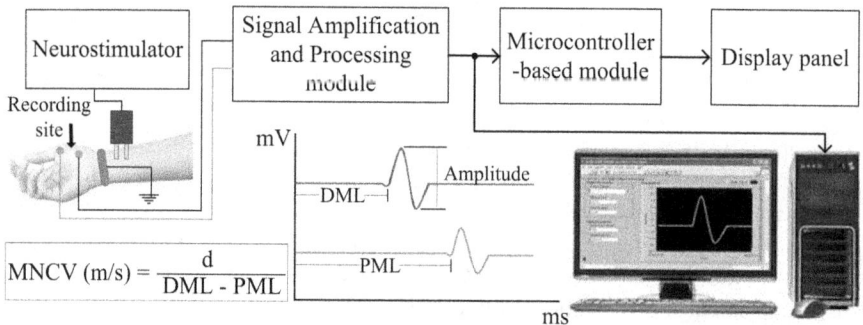

FIGURE 15.1 Block diagram of embedded setup for NCS signal recording with PC interfacing and recorded typical signature profile of NCS signal. Here, MNCV indicates motor nerve conduction velocity, d is the distance amidst the distal and proximal stimulation sites, and DML and PML denote the distal and proximal latency.

clinical application. However, among these methods, neural networks and support vector machines are found to be useful for embedded design platforms specifically because of their great adaptability to noise, higher accuracy, repeatability and testability, and compatibility [15, 20–22]. Therefore, the utility and dependence of such devices to manage smart diagnosis without the involvement of clinicians are marked by effective signal processing techniques, competent data acquisition modules, and feasible machine learning algorithms included in health monitoring devices.

Throughout the years, the challenges of proper management and treatment of patients suffering from nerve ailments with typical diagnosing techniques highlight the necessity for new and inventive approaches to confer healthcare to patients [23–25]. Conventional clinical approaches for disease diagnosis are carried out with the help of sophisticated laboratory types of equipment under the supervision of trained personnel. They are expensive, time-consuming, and exert a high-cost burden upon the patient [26–28]. Moreover, detecting, diagnosing, and preventing the disease requires complete development of the symptoms so that the change in responses is noticeable for necessary evaluation by the neurophysiologist. Such delays in diagnosis severely affect one's well-being and deteriorates life expectancy. Also, disease prevention through early detection and diagnosis of critical health changes could save millions of dollars annually [29, 30]. In this context, advanced information and communication techniques have developed personalized, low-cost, and user-friendly healthcare solutions to address the abovementioned issues [31–34]. In addition, the onset of next-generation inexpensive, robust, and unobtrusive bio-embedded healthcare devices integrated with advanced electronic circuitry has potentially led to early and automatic detection of critical health changes for necessary disease prevention [35, 36]. These devices are equipped with data collection modules to acquire responses from the body and the ability to learn the deviations of individuals' physiological parameters from the expected baseline. Also, along with embedded high-performance signal processing algorithms to explore the severity of the disease autonomously, such devices provide health alarms and subsequently inform the physician for medical assistance [36]. Moreover, in the last couple of years, technological advances have witnessed continuous improvement in low-power microelectronics, fabrication methods, and compact packaging techniques for device miniaturization [37–40]. As a result, evolution in micro- and nanofabrication, compact and portable device designs, and advanced machine learning algorithms for continuous disease management have propelled the development of intelligent health monitoring devices (IHMD) with a user-friendly interface for continuous vigilance of physiological markers for early diagnosis of diseases.

IHMDs integrated with advanced sensors incorporate high-performance machine learning algorithms employing traditional medical knowledge capable of self-assessment of disease are gaining enormous attention in today's healthcare scenario [41–44]. Such devices are low-cost, consume less power, are portable, are easy to handle, and offer high scalability to minimize predominant constraints for recording, processing, and estimating physiological parameters in the real-time domain [45]. The core of IHMD is a microcontroller (μC-)based data acquisition module that collects biomedical signals from the sensors via a wired link and then estimates the physiological markers for necessary diagnosis. Some prominent examples of specific systems include LiveNet [46], a distributed mobile platform for long-time health monitoring based on data processing in real time, streaming, and context classing. A wireless communication channel and wired local area network are used by the real-time wireless physiological data collection and monitoring system known as RTWPMS [47] to track the temperature, blood pressure, and heart rate of elderly patients. RTWPMS makes it easier for the nursing centre's medical team to keep track of the patient's physiological changes in real time. A microcontroller (μC-) based wearable multi-parameter ambulatory physiological monitoring system called Life Guard [48] is reported for space and terrestrial applications. It continuously records electrocardiogram signals employing two standard leads and measures the respiratory rate, haemoglobin oxygen saturation, body temperature, three axes of acceleration, and blood pressure. Chien et al. in [49], developed a portable wireless system for measuring physiological signals is proposed. It records phonocardiograms, electrocardiograms, and body temperature using bluetooth technology and personal digital help. A wearable device for managing home care activities of children with brain injuries such as nocturnal apnea is demonstrated by Tura et al. in [50]. It employs a multimedia card for storing measured information and is integrated with bluetooth wireless radio-communication technology for transmitting recorded data such as blood oxygen saturation, heart rate, respiration rate, and patient quantity of movement to a personal computer (PC) at a prescribed time. These healthcare support systems employ high-performance microelectronic systems fused with advanced sensing technologies to perform health monitoring in real-life scenarios [51]. Supporting the above statement, we derive our motivation to provide a comprehensive study and analysis of nerve conduction study signals for extraction, processing, and estimation of nerve parameters. Another motivation of the work is to embed a learning-based model, such as neural network, trained using a pre-diagnosed dataset to provide a better and more reliable decision on neuropathy. The main contribution of this study is as follows:

1. Design and development of a voltage-controlled neurostimulator module to provide stimulus to the nerve under diagnosis for proper generation of the NCS signal.
2. Processing of the NCS signal using a signal conditioning module consisting of various design stages such as pre-amplifiers, high- and low-pass filters, and post-amplifiers.
3. Performance analysis of the signal conditioning module by studying the efficiency of the designed filter stages in removing the noise artifacts using fast Fourier transform (FFT) of a synthetic signal and a real-time NCS signal.
4. Parameter estimation of the acquired NCS signal and real-time decision-making on the status of the nerve under examination using a PIC microcontroller. The microcontroller is fed with an optimal NN algorithm trained in MATLAB using a pre-diagnosed dataset for better accuracy of the diagnosis outcomes.

We contrive the originality of the proposed framework with its ability to record and process the NCS signal with an affordable, reliable, and efficiently designed electronic platform incorporating a microcontroller-based decision-making module capable of providing a real-time decision on nerve diagnosis. While doing so, we have stressed more on the signal processing stage incorporating filters for proper acquisition of the nerve signals with minimal noise interference. To be precise, we measure the signal parameters from healthy subjects to validate the performance of the designed framework to prove its efficacy while using it in a real-time scenario. In particular, the proposed framework is capable of providing point-of-care diagnosis and can be used by any layman for self-assessment of the underlying median nerve.

15.2 FRAMEWORK

Figure 15.2 shows the framework of the proposed design setup, which comprises (a) a neurostimulator for nerve stimulation (Block A), (b) a signal conditioning circuit for signal amplification and processing (Block B), (c) an optimal neural network obtained from a pre-diagnosed dataset which is to be embedded in μC for instigating decision-making capability for disease diagnosis, and (d) a μC-based nerve parameter estimation and decision module. In the following sections, a detailed elaboration of each module of the proposed framework is provided.

15.2.1 Neurostimulator Module

Diagnosis of a nerve requires proper stimulation of the underlying nerve so that significant features can be extracted to ensure the nerves' normal functioning. The voltage-controlled neurostimulator (VCN) acts as a stimulating platform for obtaining physiological nerve impulses from the diagnostic nerve site of the patients with the use of silver-silver chloride (Ag-AgCl) surface-disc electrodes. The VCN aims to

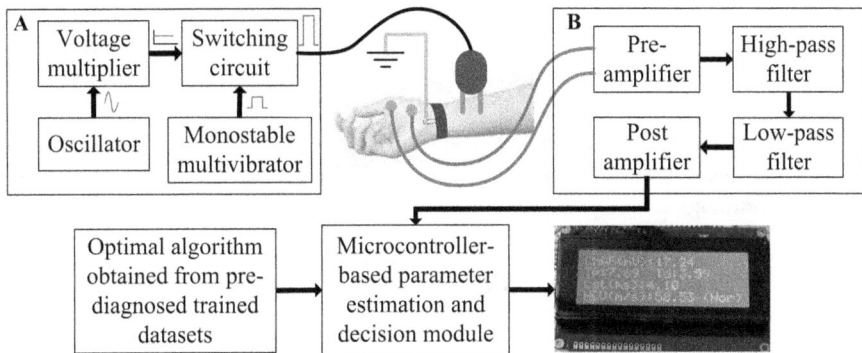

FIGURE 15.2 Block diagram of the proposed design setup. Block A and Block B represent VCN and signal conditioning modules, respectively. The display panel indicates the estimated NCS parameters and the diagnosis decision for a particular subject examined. Here, (Nor) represents the normal nerve status under examination.

produce stimulating pulses of a definite duration that are applied to the nerve under examination for depolarization of the nerve membrane. It results in the generation of CMAP due to the propagation of action potential along the nerve length [52–54]. The pulse voltage that the VCN generates could be incremented or decremented for a particular subject to obtain a proper undistorted NCS waveform to study various nerve parameters. Such stimulation pulse for proper NCS signal acquisition has voltage or current intensity that significantly excites all the muscle fibres along the nerve. The technique is referred to as supramaximal stimulation (SS), and the corresponding NCS signal recorded is termed the supramaximal response (SR). Unlike conventional stimulators used for nerve diagnosis that employ bulky equipment and operate on a 220-volt mains AC supply, the proposed VCN is compact and portable and can be designed to operate on a battery-based DC source. Moreover, it is affordable, consumes less power, and can function using two nine-volt lithium-ion (Li-ion) batteries for approximately 12 hours without any performance degradation. Figure 15.2, Block (A) represents the proposed VCN.

The design framework of VCN consists of a Wein bridge oscillator circuit which acts as a core of the VCN. It generates a proper sinusoidal signal when tuned at the resonant frequency. Moreover, the Wein bridge circuit offers excellent features, such as easy-to-tune, low distortion, and good stability at resonant frequency ($fc = 1/2\pi RC$) [55]. Furthermore, the circuit produces a phase shift of zero degrees at the resonant frequency to satisfy the Barkhausen criterion. The oscillator's output is supplied to the voltage multiplication stage, which boosts the voltage level to achieve SR. The voltage multiplier is a cascading stage consisting of diodes and capacitors that convert the oscillator's sinusoidal voltage to a constant DC voltage and raise the voltage level, depending upon the cascaded blocks added [15]. In the next stage, a monostable multivibrator is designed using a 555 timer integrated circuit (IC). The purpose of the monostable multivibrator is to control and keep the stimulating pulse duration within the safety limit of 50–1000 milliseconds [56], to avoid any skin irritation or skin burn caused by the application of overvoltage for a longer duration. A potentiometer is employed to control the intensity of the generated voltage while delivering stimulating pulses to the nerve under investigation. Finally, the switching circuit consisting of a transistorized circuit in a common emitter configuration is the last stage of the VCN, which acts as an ON-OFF switch in conveying the controlled voltage pulses for nerve diagnosis, as shown in Figure 15.2. Taking into account the safety guidelines for nerve testing, the developed VCN generates 5 milliamperes of output current and a voltage of 0–70 volts [56].

15.2.2　Signal Conditioning Module

Most biomedical circuits for healthcare applications require proper acquisition and transmission of biosignals picked up from the body via sensor probes. This put a strong emphasis on sensing methodology along with reliable and robust processing of biosignals to deliver high readability of the acquired signal. In such cases, the most prominent task in the analogue domain is necessary to signal preprocessing and filtering of noise artifacts. The NCS signals are typically of low magnitude (in millivolts or microvolts) and contaminated with electromagnetic (EM) and power line interference (PLI) disturbances, which causes undesirable frequencies to coincide with the signal frequency and makes it difficult to extract useful signal information. Therefore, the signal conditioning module plays an imminent role in processing the recorded signal through various design stages. Three electrodes, viz. active, reference, and ground, are used to record NCS signals: the ground electrode and the active electrode are placed at the site of signal recording, while the reference electrode is positioned at the wrist to minimize signal acquisition distortion [15]. Figure 15.2, block (B) shows the signal conditioning module that includes the pre-amplifier, high- and low-pass filters, and post-amplifier stage.

15.2.2.1   Pre-Amplifier

Usually, the NCS signal acquired employing the surface-disc electrodes is of low amplitude (millivolts or microvolts). As a result, a pre-amplification stage is incorporated as the basic building block of the signal conditioning module for necessary amplification to make the signal feasible for further processing. A basic amplifier generally used as the pre-amplifier in biomedical circuits is the instrumentation amplifier (IA) which can be employed to boost the signal levels extracted differentially from the body. An IA is a high-end differential amplifier characterized by a high-common mode rejection ratio, high input impedance, low drift, low noise, and high open-loop gain [55]. Such an amplifier is the basis of biomedical signal measurements such as recording of the electrical activity of the heart (ECG, PCG, EKG, etc.), muscles (EMG), as well as of brain (EEG). All these signals are of low magnitude, high-common mode noise, and relatively high output impedance [56] and therefore require high-gain IA for good readability. The following equation can be used to adjust the gain of an instrumentation amplifier:

$$G = 1 + \frac{50k}{R_g} \tag{15.1}$$

where, R_g is the gain adjustment resistor. Most commonly, IAs are available in the form of a monolithic IC package. A few examples are ADXXX series IA by Analog Devices and INAXXX series IA by Texas Instruments. These are FET-based IAs available in the form of surface mount devices (SMD) or dual in-line packages (DIP) and are robust, versatile, and easy to use with diverse biomedical applications [57].

15.2.2.2   Filters and Post-Amplifier

As stated earlier, biomedical signals acquired from the body are usually overlapped with unwanted frequencies from various external sources. Therefore, in the context of retrieving meaningful information regarding the physiological state of the body, filtering such undesired spectral ranges associated with desired signal content is of primary importance. A filter is an electrical circuit that removes unwanted frequency components to improve the spectral composition of the signal. Moreover, filters are often used to improve the signal power in specific bands, thereby improving the signal-to-noise ratio (S/N). Filters are usually composed of passive circuit elements connected in a specific fashion to filter noise in a particular segment of the frequency range. It serves as an essential part of the signal acquisition pipeline and can be used at any point in the signal processing stages to enhance the meaningful signal information and suppress noise artfacts. Given the requirement of a filter to remove high- or low-frequency noise without distorting or attenuating the original signal frequency, many filter designs meet the pass-band or stop-band criterion. A first-order Butterworth filter circuit is shown in Figure 15.3a. It consists of single R and C components connected in parallel. This filter circuit can be further extended to create higher-order filters with steeper roll-offs, as shown in Figure 15.3b. However, in doing so, a buffer amplifier is incorporated between RC stages to prevent the loading effects from the preceding stage. The performance of first- and fourth-order Butterworth filters is well understood with their ability to remove noise from the signal. This is accomplished by applying a 20 hertz sinusoidal signal contaminated with the noise produced by LabVIEW (Figure 15.4a) to each of the filter circuits of

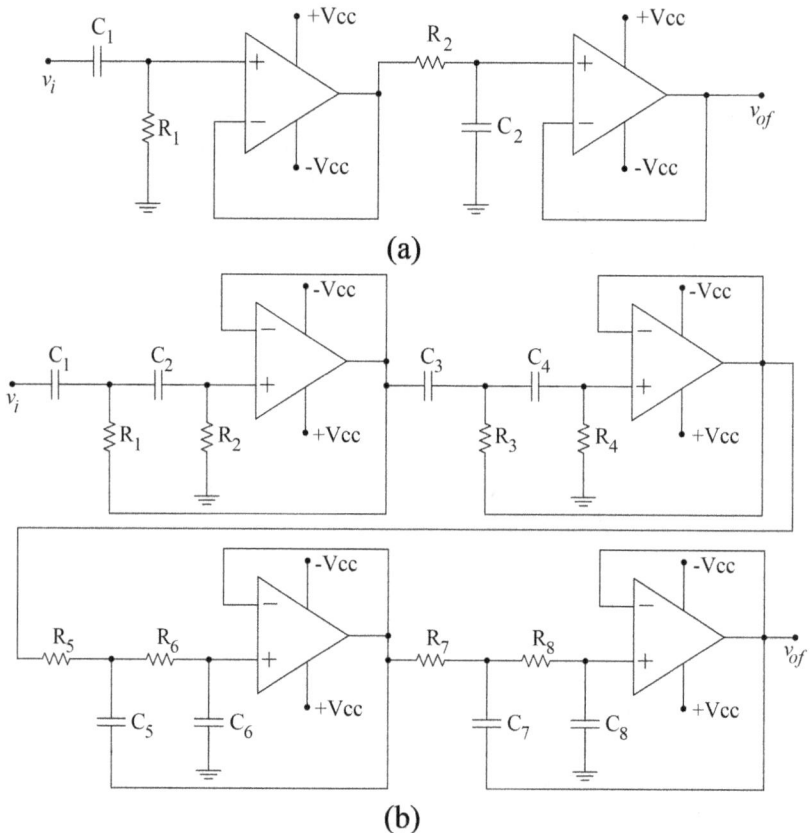

FIGURE 15.3　(a) First-order and (b) fourth-order Butterworth bandpass filters.

Figures 15.3a and 15.3b. It has been observed from Figures 15.4b and 15.4c that a considerable noise reduction is achieved as we go for higher-order filters. This is further justified with the help of fast Fourier transforms (FFT) spectrum of first- and fourth-order filtered sinusoidal signals. This indicates a corresponding reduction in the power spectral density of noise for higher-order filters, as shown in Figures 15.4e and 15.4f.

Aside from the interesting fact that the CMAP waveforms are resistant to changes in the high-frequency filter, it is essential to note that the meaningful frequency content of CMAP is found between two hertz and ten kilohertz [56]. Additionally, it has been experimentally proven that a rise in the low-pass filter's corner frequency causes the NCS signal to weaken [15, 56]. Therefore, the cut-off frequencies of the high- and low-pass filters are adjusted at two hertz and three kilohertz, respectively, for minimum attenuation using the following equation:

$$f_c = \frac{1}{2\pi\sqrt{(R_1 R_2 C_1 C_2)}} \tag{15.2}$$

The roll-off factor for the first-order high- and low-pass filters in unity gain mode is plus or minus six decibels per octave. Therefore, fourth-order Butterworth filters with an increased roll-off factor of plus or minus 24 decibels per octave are used to acquire the NCS signal more smoothly and with less noise. Furthermore, the performance of the first- and fourth-order Butterworth filters has been analyzed

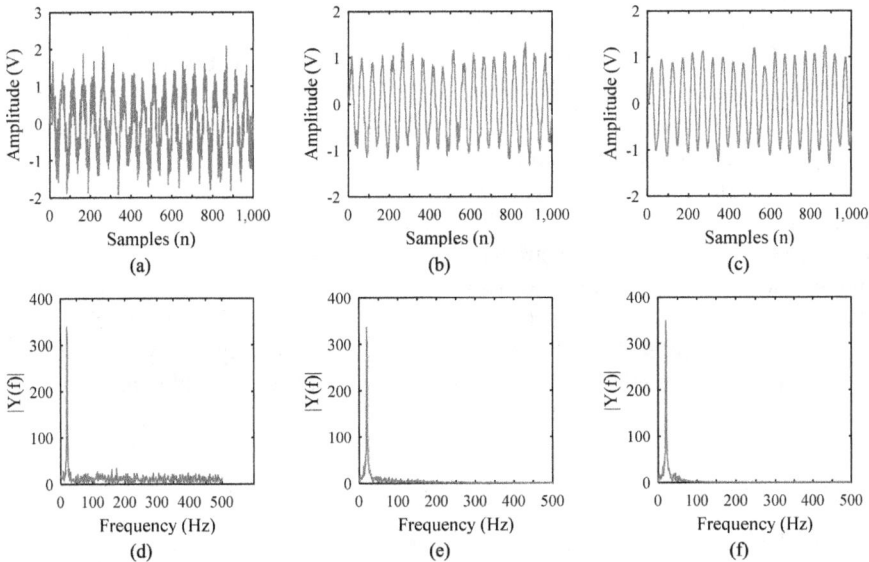

FIGURE 15.4 (a) 20 hertz (Hz) sinusoidal signal with LabVIEW generated noise, (b) first-order filtered sinusoidal output, (c) fourth-order filtered sinusoidal output, (d) the FFT spectrum of (a), (e) the FFT spectrum of (b), and (f) the FFT spectrum of (c).

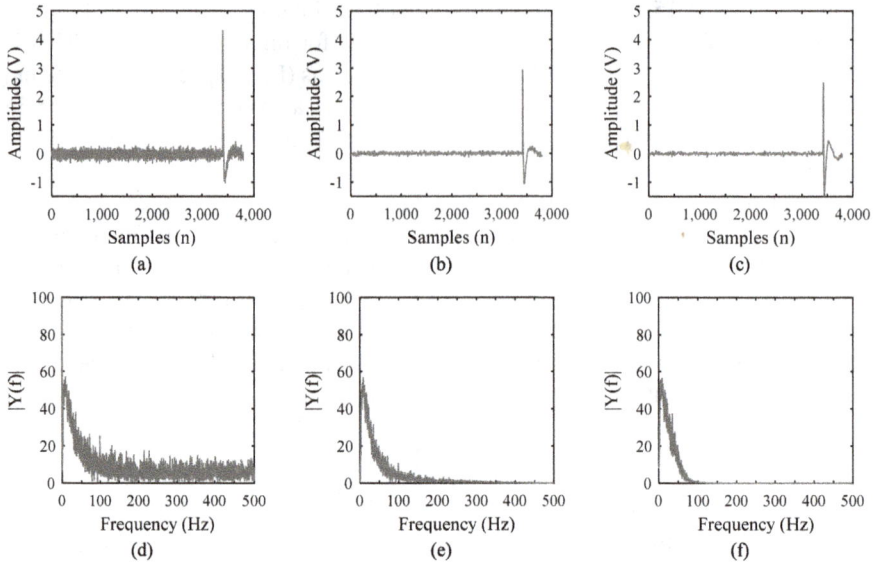

FIGURE 15.5   (a) Noisy NCS signal, (b) first-order filtered NCS signal, (c) fourth-order filtered NCS signal, (d) the FFT spectrum of (a), (e) the FFT spectrum of (b), and (f) the FFT spectrum of (c).

by considering a noisy NCS signal shown in Figure 15.5a. It is clearly understood from Figures 15.5b and 15.5c that, on increasing the filters' order, considerable noise reduction is observed with an SNR of 90.2% and 94.6%, respectively. Moreover, the FFT spectrum of the NCS signals (Figures 15.5d–f) further evinces the noise reduction capability of the designed filters.

The measurement of NCS parameters requires proper signal acquisition by the µC-based module so that an accurate evaluation of NCS signal parameters can be done. However, it has been noted that occasionally the pre-amplification stage is insufficient to raise the signal strength to a point where the µC can detect it, making it impossible to estimate proximal motor delay [15]. Therefore, to overcome this design pitfall, a post- amplification stage is incorporated. The post-amplification stage is the last stage of the signal conditional module and typically consists of a non-inverting DC-coupled high-gain amplifier that increases signal gain so that the µC can read the NCS signal easily.

15.2.3   ARTIFICIAL NEURAL NETWORK-BASED CLASSIFICATION

Artificial neural networks (ANNs), sometimes known as neural networks (NNs), are computational mathematical systems or models that are loosely based on the neural network of the human brain [58]. Artificial neurons, also known as nodes, are a common component of NN structures. These nodes are densely linked with one another and work together to perform massive parallel data processing computations and

create knowledge-based representations [59]. The ability to represent non-linear processes, immunity to noise in data processing, the capability to learn and adapt new
data, and the ability to handle imprecise fuzzy information are only a few ways that
NN outperforms other multidimensional analysis systems [60]. A straightforward
NN structure is depicted in Figure 15.6 and consists of an input layer, a hidden layer,
and an output layer. The number of neurons in the input layer is typically equal to the
number of features used, whereas the number of nodes in the output layer depends
on the number of classes to be recognized. For the optimum NN model performance,
the hidden layer should be made up of many layers of neurons or a single layer of
neurons with any number of neurons.

NNs are classified as feed-forward (FF) and recurrent/feedback networks based
on the architecture or how the neurons are interconnected. Again, FF networks
are networks without loops, whereas recurrent networks are networks with loops

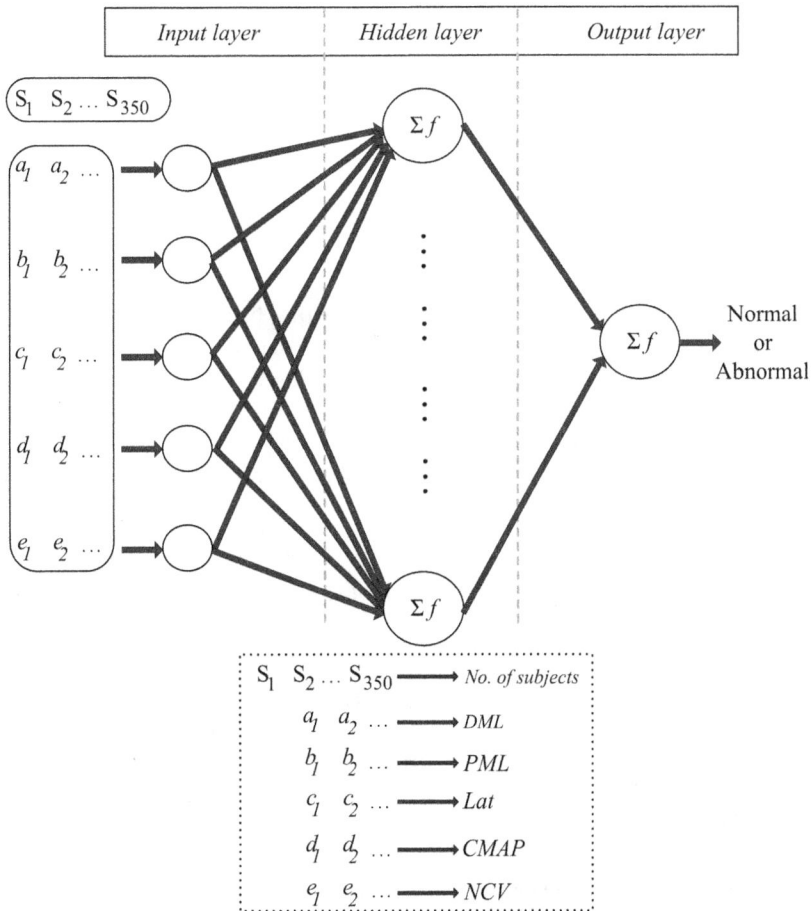

FIGURE 15.6 Representation of the NN model with input features and number of layers.

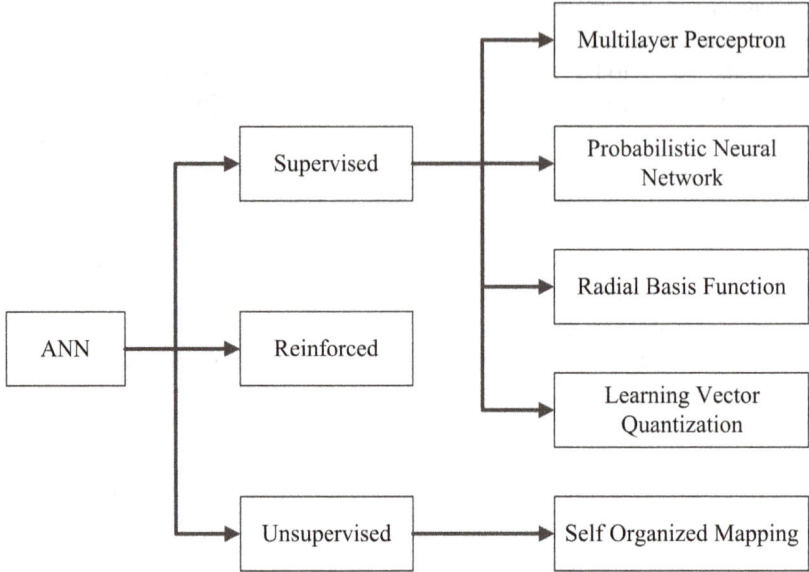

FIGURE 15.7 Classification of FF and recurrent/feedback neural network architecture.

because of feedback connections. A complete overview of the NN taxonomy of FF and recurrent networks is shown in Figure 15.7.

This study uses a three-layered FF network with a backpropagation (BP) algorithm, with each layer connected back-to-back to the previous layer. Due to its simplicity and shown performance, using a three-layered backpropagation neural network (BPNN) with a feed-forward structure contributes to a high level of accuracy when linear and sigmoid activation functions are employed in the output and hidden layers [20]. This offers excellent compatibility for µC-based designs. The following equations are used to train the network using the BP algorithm:

$$U_k(t) = \sum_{j=1}^{n} w_{j,k}(t) x_j(t) + b_{o,k}(t) \tag{15.3}$$

$$Y_k(t) = \phi(U_k(t)) \tag{15.4}$$

where, $x_j(t)$ is the jth value of input at time t, $w_{j,k}(t)$ is the assigned weight by the kth neuron to the jth value of input at time t, b_k is the kth neuron bias at time t, and $Y_k(t)$ is the kth neuron output at time t.

Gradient descent with adaptive learning rate backpropagation (GDA) is used to train the NN. Using an adjustable learning rate, this learning function changes the weights and bias matrices in accordance with gradient descent [61]. The adaptive learning rate is in charge of maintaining a steady learning process while maintaining large learning step sizes. Additionally, the learning rate affects how complicated the local error surface is. The new weights and biases are first computed using the NN's output and errors, and then they are calculated again using the ongoing learning rate. The modified weights are then used to estimate the new outputs and errors. The new weights and biases are rejected during the procedure if the estimated new error is greater than the previous error by a predetermined ratio (usually 1.04). Additionally, multiplying by 0.7 reduces the learning rate in order to prevent the retention of additional weights and biases. If the old error is greater than the new error, the learning rate is once more raised by a factor of 1.05. The learning rate is increased throughout this operation to a certain level so that the network can learn without experiencing a significant rise in error. Finally, a nearly ideal learning rate for the immediate terrain is achieved. When a higher learning rate results in stable learning, the learning rate is raised. Additionally, the learning rate decreases until stable learning are maintained when it is high enough to ensure a decrease in the learning rate.

The weight adjustment or learning process used in the iterative GDA method to reduce the error (e_k) between the desired and actual output of the network is denoted as:

$$e_k = (y - v_k) y_k (1 - y_k) \tag{15.5}$$

$$w_{j,k}(t+1) = w_{j,k}(t) - \mu(t) \frac{\delta e_k}{\delta w_{j,k}} \tag{15.6}$$

where ($y_k - \hat{y}_k$) gives the desired output deviation from the actual output.

15.2.4 SIGNIFICANCE OF NN IN DISEASE DIAGNOSIS

NN's classification, detection, and prediction power are prominent in disease diagnosis. The decision-making capability of the NN must be tested upon an independent dataset to govern the NN algorithm's efficacy in forecasting accurate outcomes. Five individual parameters often determine the predictive power of NN in medical applications:

$$\text{Sensitivity} : S_n = \frac{P_C}{P_T} \tag{15.7}$$

$$\text{Specificity} : S_p = \frac{N_C}{N_T} \tag{15.8}$$

$$\text{Accuracy} : A_c = \frac{P_C + N_C}{P_T + N_T} \tag{15.9}$$

$$\text{Positive predictive value} : PPV = \frac{P_T}{P_C + N_I} \tag{15.10}$$

$$\text{Negative predictive value}: NPV = \frac{N_T}{N_C + P_I} \qquad (15.11)$$

where the measures are described as:

P_C = Subject with disorder correctly predicted as diseased; P_I = Subject with disorder incorrectly predicted as diseased; P_T = Total number of diseased individuals; N_T = Total number of healthy individuals; N_C = Healthy subjects correctly predicted; N_I = Healthy subjects incorrectly predicted.

The statistical performance matrices of an NN classification are defined by Equations 15.7 and 15.8, which quantify sensitivity and specificity. Sensitivity analyzes the likelihood or percentage of true positive cases correctly categorized, whereas specificity assesses the likelihood or percentage of real negative cases correctly recognized. While PPV and NPV are the likelihood that a patient will be identified as diseased when a disorder is predicted, and NPV is the likelihood that a patient will be identified as negative in the case of a negative test result. Accuracy measures the probability or percentage of correct cases (correct positive and correct negative) rightly classified.

15.2.5 Dataset Description

A clinical dataset named NCS_{GNRC} is gathered from the Guwahati Neurological Research Centre (GNRC) hospital to train, test, and validate the NN algorithm. The dataset mentioned above, which consists of signal parameters from 350 participants (normal: 200, abnormal: 150, age group: 20–65 years, mean: 40 ± 4.87), is taken into consideration in order to create an appropriate learning model. Additionally, the institutional review board approved the dataset's use in diagnostic research. Next, three sub-datasets are formed by dividing the NCS_{GNRC} dataset such that 40%, 30%, and 30% of the NCS_{GNRC} dataset is chosen as the training set, testing set, and validation set. The normalized parameters are made to fall between zero and one.

15.2.6 NN Implementation in μC

The recording and processing of the physiological features depend on proper NCS acquisition and standard medical evaluation to develop a portable NCS system that meets the requirements of the end-user in a real-world scenario. Each characteristic feature retrieved from the NCS signal has a different confidence level. Therefore, each feature is combined into a single matrix of individual features for thoroughly evaluating the disease diagnosis using machine learning. In order to create an appropriate learning model using MATLAB R2015a, the NCS_{GNRC} dataset is obtained and classified as previously indicated. An FFBP network comprising three layers is considered with activation functions, as discussed in Section 15.2.3, along with the GDA technique to evaluate the matrices. According to the number of input features extracted from the NCS signal, the input layer is configured with five neurons. Depending on the normal and abnormal class for decision, the output layer is assigned one neuron. On the other hand, the hidden layer is assigned three and four neurons to find the best model. The network structure that provides the best weights and bias based on the mean square error (MSE) convergency is decided through the repetitive iteration method. The classification accuracy of the NN models produced using three and four was found to be 94.32% and 97.65%, respectively. Therefore, an NN model with four hidden neurons is considered for implementation in μC to achieve maximum accuracy in decision-making for NCS diagnosis. To ensure an improved diagnostic matrix of the prognostic system, examination of biomedical performance measures like S_n, S_p, PPV, and NPV are also evaluated [14]. While PPV and NPV are relative factors linked to S_n and S_p, S_e and S_p determine the extent of abnormal (subjects with disorders) and normal (healthy) subjects, respectively. The FFBP model's approximations for S_n, S_p, PPV, and N PV are found to be 97.43%, 97.66%, 1.03, and 0.98, respectively, confirming the structured NN model's strong performance. The efficiency metrics derived from the NN model are displayed in Table 15.1, while the number of stages taken to structure the NN model is shown in Figure 15.8. The best NN model, acquired from MATLAB, is then incorporated in the PIC μC for real-time NCS parameter estimation. The program is created in μC using the MikroC Pro for PIC C compiler (Version 6.4.0). The application has the same floating-point precision as MATLAB and is 9.84 kilobytes in size, taking up 45% of RAM and 57% of ROM. The sampling rate for NCS data is one kilohertz. The diagnostic outcome predicted by the classifier is displayed on an LCD panel (Figure 15.2).

The embedded μC-based decision-making platform processes the real-time signals collected from the signal conditioning module and estimates the NCS parameter values upon which the overall decision on normal or abnormal conditions of the subjects are assessed. Real-time experimentation on various subjects and subsequent repeated trials further reveal the efficacy of the developed framework. Notably, the optimal NN paradigm incorporated in the μC module is suitably trained for the normal and abnormal data classes using best-suited settings while tuning the NN model. This is evident from the high PPV value obtained from the NN model, which explicitly denotes the detection of positive cases. Thus, the overall performance of each sub-module of the proposed design, along with the μC module integrated with an intelligent NN algorithm derived using MATLAB simulation using the NCS_{GNRC} dataset, infers high-level detection accuracy of anomalies while assessing the unhealthy subjects.

TABLE 15.1

Comparison of Performance Parameters of the Modelled NN Structure.

NN/Number of Layers	Epoch [Iteration]	Computational Time [s]	MSE [× 10^{-10}]	Activation Function	Learning Model
BPNN/3	87	6.19	1.988	Logsigmoid	GDA
BPNN/4	112	7.12	1.107	Logsigmoid	GDA

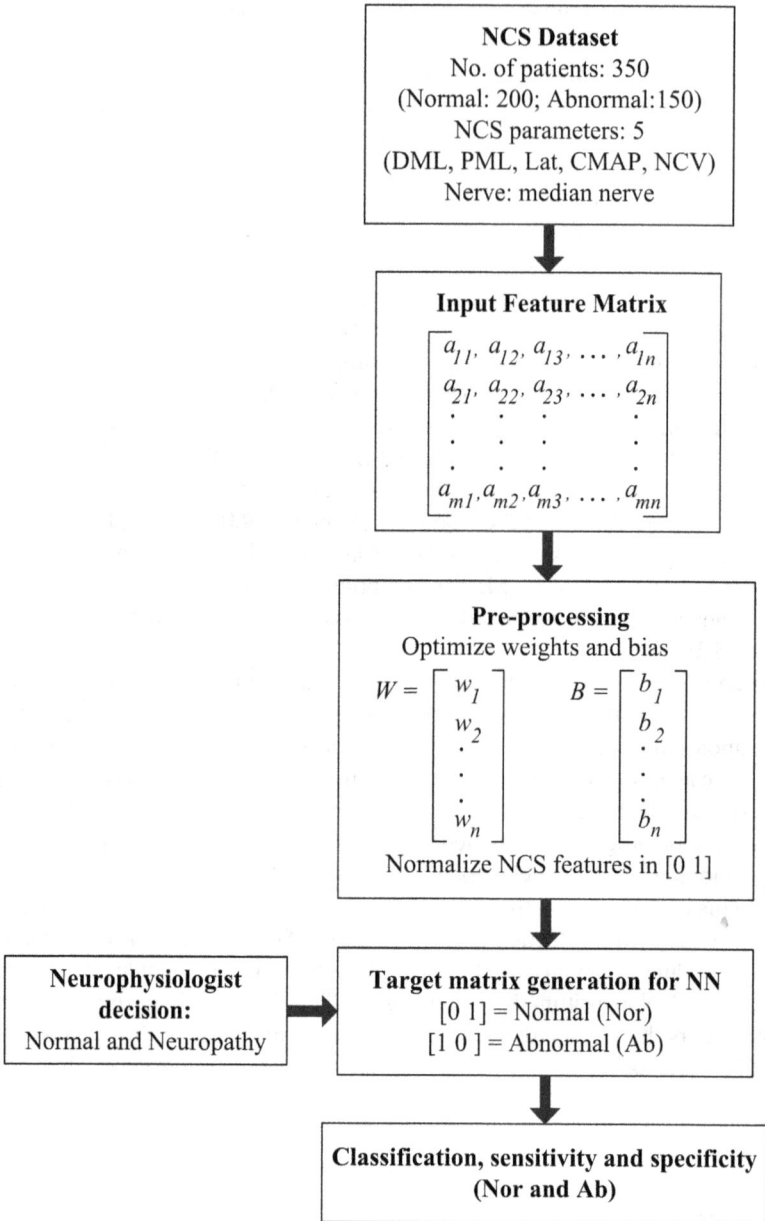

FIGURE 15.8   Different steps involved in finding the optimized NN model.

15.2.7 µC-BASED NCS PARAMETER ESTIMATION
AND DECISION-MAKING MODULE

Accurate analysis of NCS parameters, viz. DML, PML, Lat, CMAP, and MNCV, play a crucial role in diagnosing DN [62–64]. For that, a µC-based NCS parameter estimation and decision-making platform capable of performing automatic diagnosis on the signal extracted from the nerve under examination is employed, which forms the core of the embedded design platform. As a result, creating a high-performance µC-based platform having instant decision-making capability requires the integration of an ideal intuitive algorithm.

In this regard, many embedded design systems consider NN a suitable and effectively used algorithm for real-time application due to its compatibility and reliability [65]. Nonetheless, the NN complexity largely depends upon neuron arrangement, the number of layers, and the number of neurons [20, 65]. To achieve the best performance in the case of a non-linear problem scenario, a three-layered feed-forward backpropagation is derived from the MATLAB simulation using an offline NCS_{GNRC} dataset, and network performance parameters are derived, as mentioned earlier. The technique is then developed in the µC module for real-time NCS estimate and detection, which will ultimately provide inference on the severity class of the disease for efficient diagnosis. Figure 15.9 represents the step-by-step process flow of the µC-based NCS parameter estimation and decision-making scheme. Table 15.2 provides the reference range for NCS parameters for the median nerve.

Sequences of laboratory experiments are carried out to guarantee the refinement of the proposed design platform. Moreover, proper care has been taken to ensure the appropriate setting of the laboratory environment. All the readings have been taken at room temperature with a relative humidity of approximately 60%. Ten participants take part in the experiment: six men (S1–S6) and four women (S7–S10), ranging in age from 25 to 40 (mean: 29.2 ± 1.6 years), height from 5.1 to 5.11 feet (mean: 5.4 ± 0.14 feet), and weight from 51 to 90 kilograms (mean: 68.4 ± 10.4 kilograms). All participants are asked for their agreement and informed of the NCS recording technique in order to ensure the essential cooperation and efficient gathering of NCS signals. Moreover, before experimenting, the subjects are made aware of mild discomfort due to necessary electrical stimulation. The skin of the subjects is cleaned with alcohol to remove sticking dirt and is then applied with the electrode gel to achieve minimum resistivity at the skin-electrode interface for proper recording of NCS signals. The signal acquisition process starts with applying very low stimulating voltages to the nerve under examination, which gradually increases until SS attains SR. The occurrence of SR is further asserted from the LabVIEW software panel, which is integrated with a data acquisition card that enables visual investigation of the morphology of the recorded NCS signal at different stimulating voltages for better analysis. The voltage applied from the neurostimulator for stimulating different subjects lies in the range of 35–60 volts. Importantly, it is intriguing to see that the signal shape begins to deform beyond the SS, where the best CMAP, i.e., the SR, is attained. In addition, all of the SS factors were considered when deciding how to

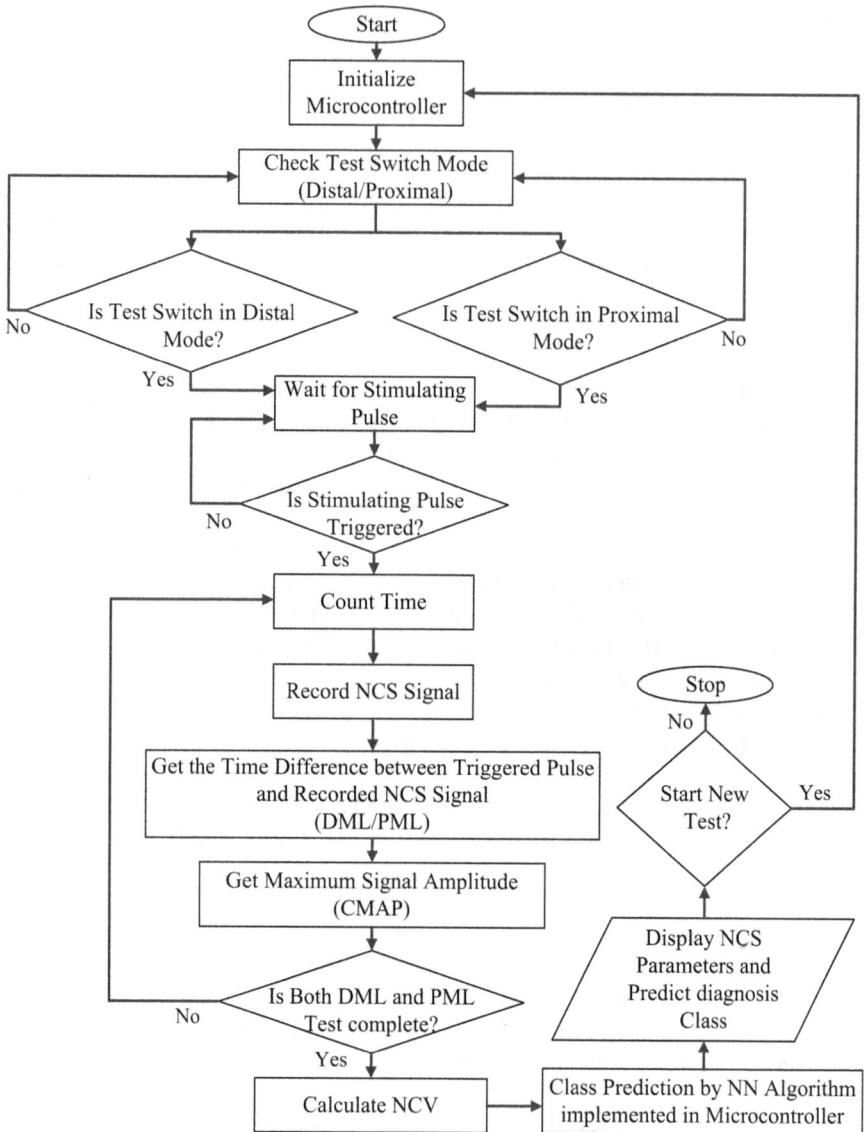

FIGURE 15.9 Step-by-step schematic flow of the μC-based parameter estimation and diagnosis decision algorithm.

evaluate the participants with neurological problems. Five real-time recorded NCS measurements at SS for ten patients (S1–S10) are shown in Table 15.3, along with the matching diagnosis for DN. Table 15.4 provides a comparison of the reported design methodologies with the proposed design setup in terms of various characteristic features.

TABLE 15.2

Reference Range of Electrophysiological NCS Parameters (Features) for Median Motor Nerve [73].

NCS Parameters	Normal Range (Nor)	Abnormal Range (Ab)
DML (in milliseconds)	$1.5 \leq DML < 3.2$	$3.2 < DML \leq 13.88$
PML (in milliseconds)	$6.25 \leq PML \leq 9.0$	$3.2 < DML \leq 13.88$
CMAP (in millivolts)	$6.25 \leq PML \leq 9.0$	$0.5 < CMAP \leq 12.60$
NCV (in meter/second (m/s))	$56.7 < MNCV \leq 84.94$	$23.33 < MNCV \leq 56.7$

15.3 SIGNIFICANCE OF NCS MEASUREMENT

The significance of NCS measurement lies in evaluating NCS data and extracting meaningful features from underlying nerves under examination to determine the physiological state of the patient's health. However, the clinical interpretation of NCS depends on measuring the individual's data with a reference range of various NCS parameters extracted from healthy subjects [73] (Table 15.2). These reference ranges are attributed to determine normal ranges of the NCS parameters, above and below which a given nerve parameter is considered abnormal and indicates DN. The NCS reference ranges generally depend on the data acquisition systems setting; therefore, different laboratories have different reference ranges of NCS parameters. Moreover, the placement of electrodes also affects the NCS recordings and can vary parameter values [73].

Various NCS parameters obtained and estimated by the proposed μC-based IHMD has a significant physiological definition and explanation. As such, the recorded CMAP indicates the action potential collectively generated by the stimulated neurons in the region of electrical stimulation [74]. This can further be explained as a measure of efficient neuromuscular transmission and the combined action potential collectively generated by the recorded muscles. The latencies recorded by stimulating the distal and proximal stimulation sites, i.e., DML and PML, are one of the prominent components of NCS. Both latencies measure the time elapsed during the signal propagation from the stimulation site to the recorded site [75]. The conduction velocity of the nerve, or MNCV, amidst two points of stimulation along the nerve segment, is also calculated using the total delay determined from the PML and DML (Figure 15.1). It is worth noting that impairment of axons results in lower CMAP amplitudes [73, 74]. On the other hand, demyelination of the nerve membrane causes longer NCS signal propagation delay, the consequence of which is prolonged DML, PML, and slow conduction velocity (MNCV) [76].

15.4 CONCLUSION AND DISCUSSION

This study demonstrated the potential application of a μC-based data acquisition system embedded with an advanced NN algorithm for the evaluation of DN. The

TABLE 15.3

Estimation of NCS Parameters for 10 Subjects and Their Corresponding Diagnosis Decision on DN Using the Proposed µC-based Design Setup [d = 240 millimetres for Male and Female Subjects].

Subject	DML (ms)	Mean DML (ms)	PML (ms)	Mean PML (ms)	Lat (PML-DML) (ms)	Mean Lat (ms)	CMAP (mV)	Mean CMAP (mV)	MNCV (m/s)	Mean MNCV (ms)	Diagnosis Situation
S1	3.20	3.24	7.20	7.22	4.00	3.98	21.05	21.05	60.00	60.30	Nor
	3.25		7.22		3.97		21.07		60.45		
	3.26		7.23		3.97		21.04		60.45		
S2	3.08	3.07	6.52	6.52	3.44	3.44	26.77	26.76	69.76	69.62	Nor
	3.07		6.53		3.46		26.76		69.36		
	3.06		6.50		3.44		26.75		69.76		
S3	3.10	3.10	6.21	6.20	3.11	3.11	28.25	28.23	77.17	77.25	Nor
	3.09		6.20		3.11		28.24		77.17		
	3.10		6.20		3.10		28.23		77.41		
S4	2.88	2.87	6.65	6.65	3.77	3.78	24.77	24.76	63.66	63.54	Nor
	2.87		6.65		3.78		24.75		63.49		
	2.86		6.64		3.78		24.77		63.49		
S5	3.27	3.26	6.92	6.92	3.65	3.65	25.56	25.56	65.75	65.69	Nor
	3.26		6.92		3.66		25.54		65.57		
	3.26		6.91		3.65		25.56		65.75		
S6	2.65	2.65	6.38	6.38	3.73	3.73	19.87	19.86	64.34	64.34	Nor
	2.64		6.37		3.73		19.86		64.34		
	2.65		6.38		3.73		19.86		64.34		
S7	2.25	2.25	6.10	6.10	3.85	3.85	23.12	23.12	62.37	62.34	Nor
	2.26		6.09		3.83		23.12		62.66		
	2.24		6.11		3.87		23.12		62.01		

(Continued)

TABLE 15.3
(Continued)

Subject	DML (ms)	Mean DML (ms)	PML (ms)	Mean PML	Lat (PML-DML) (ms)	Mean Lat (ms)	CMAP (mV)	Mean CMAP (mV)	MNCV (m/s)	Mean MNCV (ms)	Diagnosis Situation
S8	2.12	2.10	6.19	6.19	4.07	4.07	21.78	21.78	58.96	58.81	Nor
	2.10		6.19		4.09		21.77		58.67		
	2.10		6.18		4.08		21.78		58.82		
S9	2.97	2.97	6.75	6.74	3.78	3.77	24.47	24.47	63.49	63.65	Nor
	2.97		6.74		3.77		24.46		63.66		
	2.97		6.74		3.77		24.47		63.82		
S10	2.42	2.42	6.44	6.44	4.02	4.02	29.91	29.91	59.70	59.70	Nor
	2.41		6.43		4.02		29.92		59.70		
	2.42		6.44		4.02		29.91		59.70		

TABLE 15.4

Comparative Analysis of Reported Design Methodologies with Proposed Design Setup with Regard to Various Characteristic Features. Here, SP: Specialized Personnel, SE: Surface Electrode, MP: Monophasic.

Feature	[66]	[67]	[68]	[69]	[70]	[71]	[72]	Proposed Work
Working	Req SP	Not req SP	Not req SP	--	--	Not req SP	--	Not req SP
Nerve	Sural	Median	Median, Ulnar	Median, Ulnar	Median	Ulnar	Sciatic	Median motor
Sensor	SE³	SE	Pad/ring	SE	SE	SE	Cuff	Ag/AgCl disc SE
Sensor position	Fixed	Fixed	Fixed	Fixed	--	Fixed	Fixed	Adjustable
Stimulus duration	[50-100] μs	< 1 ms	0.2 ms	--	< 1 ms	1 ms	[50-200] μs	~ 62 ms
Decision on neuropathy	Not instant	Instant	Not instant	Not instant	Not instant	--	--	Instant
Trigger pulse	--	--	--	--	--	MP	MP	MP

efficiency of the NN has been validated by studying various per-performance measures, which represent NN as the best method to study the possibility of early and reliable diagnosis decisions on DN.

A μC-based data acquisition system is proposed for online NCS parameter estimation and to provide diagnosis decisions on DN. The system includes a designed voltage control neurostimulator for stimulating the nerve under examination in order to record NCS signals for disease diagnosis. The proposed setup works on a battery-based power supply with two nine-volt lithium-ion batteries which can work up to 12 hours continuously. The signal conditioning module employs a Butterworth filter (fourth-order) with a roll-off factor of $\pm$ 24 decibels per octave to acquire and process the recorded NCS signal. The signal conditioning module is tested using a real-time NCS signal achieving 95.7% SNR. Next, an optimal NN algorithm is developed using a three-fold cross-validation scheme using an offline NCS_{GNRC} dataset. The implementation of NN models has been validated as one of the best-suited methods for detecting DN, thus offering an early and reliable decision on the diagnosis of DN. The choice of cut-off utilized at the output is a crucial component in assessing the discrimination capacity of ANNs. In the case of DN prediction, NN is advantageous for diagnosis sensitivity because it produces a relatively small number of false unhealthy cases and no false healthy cases; therefore, the diagnosis specificity would deteriorate. Moreover, the NN algorithm can automatically decide a cut-off through a hard limit function at the output node, which can drive the output to either zero or one, i.e., Abnormal (Ab) or Normal (Nor). Thus, the derived NN algorithm is implemented in μC for real-time NCS parameter estimation and decisions on nerve disorders. Obtained experimental evidence of the proposed system by performing real-time laboratory testing on healthy subjects ensures the reliability and applicability of the setup in and outside the laboratory environment for critical examination of patients with DN for early diagnosis.

COMPETING INTERESTS

None of the authors have any competing interests to report.

GRANT INFORMATION

This research work is funded by the Department of Science and Technology, Government of India (Fund Sanction Order No. DST/INSPIRE Fellowship/2018/ IF180845).

ACKNOWLEDGEMENT

The authors would like to acknowledge the Department of Neurophysiology, Guwahati Neurological Research Centre (GNRC), Assam, India, for providing a nerve diagnosis dataset for carrying out this research work.

REFERENCES

1. Wild, S.; Roglic, G.; Green, A.; Sicree, R.; King, H. Global prevalence of diabetes: Estimates for the year 2000 and projections for 2030. *Diabetes Care* 2004, 27(5), 1047–1053.
2. Roglic, G. WHO global report on diabetes: A summary. *Int. J. Noncomm Dis.* 2016, 1(1), 3.
3. Centers for Disease Control and Prevention. *National Diabetes Statistics Report: Estimates of Diabetes and Its Burden in the United States, 2014.* US Department of Health and Human Services, 2014.
4. Beets, G. EU demographics: Living longer and reproducing less. *Pharm. Policy Law* 2007, 9(1/2), 29–40.
5. You, Y.; Liu, Z.; Chen, Y.; Xu, Y.; Qin, J.; Guo, S.; Huang, J.; Tao, J. The prevalence of mild cognitive impairment in type 2 diabetes mellitus patients: A systematic review and meta-analysis. *Acta Diabetol.* 2021, 58(6), 671–685.
6. Abbott, C.A.; Malik, R.A.; Van Ross, E.R.; Kulkarni, J.; Boulton, A.J. Prevalence and characteristics of painful diabetic neuropathy in a large community-based diabetic population in the UK. *Diabetes Care* 2011, 34(10), 2220–2224.
7. Callaghan, B.C.; Cheng, H.T.; Stables, C.L.; Smith, A.L.; Feldman, E.L. Diabetic neuropathy: Clinical manifestations and current treatments. *Lancet Neurol.* 2012, 11(6), 521–534.
8. Dyck, P.J.; Kratz, K.M.; Karnes, J.L.; Litchy, W.J.; Klein, R.; Pach, J.M.; Wilson, D.M.; O'Brien, P.C.; Melton, L. The prevalence by staged severity of various types of diabetic neuropathy, retinopathy, and nephropathy in a population-based cohort: The Rochester Diabetic Neuropathy Study. *Neurology* 1993, 43(4), 817–817.
9. Partanen, J.; Niskanen, L.; Lehtinen, J.; Mervaala, E.; Siitonen, O.; Uusitupa, M. Natural history of peripheral neuropathy in patients with non-insulin-dependent diabetes mellitus. *N. Engl. J. Med.* 1995, 333(2), 89–94.
10. Kong, X.; Schoenfeld, D.A.; Lesser, E.A.; Gozani, S.N. Implementation and evaluation of a statistical framework for nerve conduction study reference range calculation. *Comput. Methods Programs Biomed.* 2010, 97(1), 1–10.
11. Talukdar, C.; Hazarika, A.; Singh, A.; Das, N.; Bhuyan, M. A biofeedback based auto-controlled neurostimulator design for proper NCS signal acquisition and measurement. *Int. J. Eng. Adv. Technol. (IJEAT)* 2020, 9(3), 2249–8958.
12. Peckham, P.H.; Knutson, J.S. Functional electrical stimulation for neuromuscular applications. *Annu. Rev. Biomed. Eng.* 2005, 7, 327–360.
13. Kong, X.; Lesser, E.A.; Gozani, S.N. Nerve conduction studies: Clinical challenges and engineering solutions. *IEEE Eng. Med. Biol. Mag.* 2010, 29(2), 26–36.
14. Barthakur, M.; Hazarika, A.; Bhuyan, M. Rule based fuzzy approach for peripheral motor neuropathy (PMN) diagnosis based on NCS data. In *International Conference on Recent Advances and Innovations in Engineering (ICRAIE-2014)*, Jaipur, India, May 2014, 1–9. IEEE.
15. Singh, A.; Hazarika, A.; Talukdar, C.; Bhuyan, M.; Dutta, L.; Barthakur, M.; Chakraborty, K. Microcontroller-based online nerve parameter estimation for diagnosis of healthy subject using real-time nerve conduction study signal acquired using voltage controlled neurostimulator. *IEEE Trans. Industr. Inform.* 2021, 17(11), 7546–7553.
16. Talukdar, C.; Hazarika, A.; Singh, A.; Barthakur, M.; Bhuyan, M. Voltage controlled stimulator for nerve conduction study. In *2019 2nd International Conference on Innovations in Electronics, Signal Processing and Communication (IESC)*, Shillong, India, March 2019, 13–17. IEEE.

17. Meesad, P.; Yen, G.G. Combined numerical and linguistic knowledge representation and its application to medical diagnosis. *IEEE Trans. Syst. Man Cybern. A Syst. Hum.* 2003, 33(2), 206–222.
18. Kazemi, M.; Moghimbeigi, A.; Kiani, J.; Mahjub, H.; Faradmal, J. Diabetic peripheral neuropathy class prediction by multicategory support vector machine model: A cross-sectional study. *Epidemiol. Health* 2016, 38, 1–7.
19. Fioretti, S.; Scocco, M.; Ladislao, L.; Ghetti, G.; Rabini, R.A. Identification of peripheral neuropathy in type-2 diabetic subjects by static posturography and linear discriminant analysis. *Gait Posture* 2010, 32(3), 317–320.
20. Dutta, L.; Talukdar, C.; Hazarika, A.; Bhuyan, M. A novel low-cost hand-held tea flavor estimation system. *IEEE Trans. Ind. Electron.* 2017, 65(6), 4983–4990.
21. Shoeb, A.; Carlson, D.; Panken, E.; Denison, T. A micropower support vector machine based seizure detection architecture for embedded medical devices. In *2009 Annual International Conference of the IEEE Engineering in Medicine and Biology Society*, Minneapolis, USA, September 2009, 4202–4205. IEEE.
22. Cui, S.; Wang, D.; Wang, Y.; Yu, P.W.; Jin, Y. An improved support vector machine-based diabetic readmission prediction. *Comput. Methods Programs Biomed.* 2018, 166, 123–135.
23. Heymann, A.D.; Azuri, J.; Kokia, E.; Monnickendam, S.M.; Shapiro, M.; Shalev, G. Systemic Inventive Thinking: A new tool for the analysis of complex problems in medical management. *IMAJ-RAMAT GAN* 2004, 6(2), 67–69.
24. Khosrow-Pour, M., ed. *Inventive Approaches for Technology Integration and Information Resources Management*. IGI Global, 2014.
25. Leong, J.; Hjorth, L.; Choi, J.H.J. Inventive approaches to data tracking in more-than-human worlds. In *The Routledge Companion to Mobile Media Art*, Routledge, 2020, 259–269.
26. Oaklander, A.L.; Nolano, M. Scientific advances in and clinical approaches to small-fiber polyneuropathy: A review. *JAMA Neurol.* 2019, 76(10), 1240–1251.
27. Hansson, P. Neuropathic pain: Clinical characteristics and diagnostic workup. *Eur. J. Pain* 2002, 6, 47–50.
28. Telleman, J.A.; Herraets, I.J.; Goedee, H.S.; van Asseldonk, J.T.; Visser, L.H. Ultrasound scanning in the diagnosis of peripheral neuropathies. *Pract. Neurol.* 2021, 21(3), 186–195.
29. Pantelopoulos, A.; Bourbakis, N.G. Prognosis—A wearable health-monitoring system for people at risk: Methodology and modeling. *IEEE Trans. Inf. Technol. Biomed.* 2010, 14(3), 613–621.
30. Bourbakis, N.; Gallagher, J. A synergistic co-operative framework of health diagnostic systems for people with disabilities and the elderly: A case study. In *Proceedings of the 12th WSEAS International Conference on Computers*, Heraklion, Greece, July 2008, 730–735.
31. Van Lerberghe, W. *The World Health Report 2008: Primary Health Care: Now More Than Ever*. World Health Organization, 2008.
32. Cheng, B.; Wu, P. Recycled iontronic from discarded chewed gum for personalized healthcare monitoring and intelligent information encryption. *ACS Appl. Mater. Interfaces* 2021, 13(5), 6731–6738.
33. Kim, N.; Wei, J.L.J.; Ying, J.; Zhang, H.; Moon, S.K.; Choi, J. December. A customized smart medical mask for healthcare personnel. In *2020 IEEE International Conference on Industrial Engineering and Engineering Management (IEEM)*, Singapore, December 2020, 581–585. IEEE.

34. Mustafa, T.; Varol, A. Review of the internet of things for healthcare monitoring. In *2020 8th International Symposium on Digital Forensics and Security (ISDFS)*, Chattanooga, USA, June 2020, 1–6. IEEE.

35. Lmberis, A.; Dittmar, A. Advanced wearable health systems and applications-research and development efforts in the European Union. *IEEE Eng. Med. Biol. Mag.* 2007, 26(3), 29–33.

36. Gatzoulis, L.; Iakovidis, I. Wearable and portable ehealth systems. *IEEE Eng. Med. Biol. Mag.* 2007, 26(5), 51–56.

37. Andreu-Perez, J.; Leff, D.R.; Ip, H.M.; Yang, G.Z. From wearable sensors to smart implants--Toward pervasive and personalized healthcare. *IEEE Trans. Bio Med. Eng.* 2015, 62(12), 2750–2762.

38. Lanagan, J.; Caulfield, B.; Smeaton, A.F. Utilising wearable and environmental sensors to identify the context of gait performance in the home, Dublin, Ireland, June 2011.

39. Tsai, T.H.; Tsai, H.C.; Wu, T.K. A CMOS micromachined capacitive tactile sensor with integrated readout circuits and compensation of process variations. *IEEE Trans. Biomed. Circuits Syst.* 2014, 8(5), 608–616.

40. Romero, L.E.; Chatterjee, P.; Armentano, R.L. An IoT approach for integration of computational intelligence and wearable sensors for Parkinson's disease diagnosis and monitoring. *Health Technol.* 2016, 6(3), 167–172.

41. Nayyar, A.; Puri, V.; Nguyen, N.G. BioSenHealth 1.0: A novel internet of medical things (IoMT)-based patient health monitoring system. In *International Conference on Innovative Computing and Communications: Proceedings of ICICC 2018*, 2019, 1, 155–164. Springer Singapore.

42. Yang, S.; Zhou, P.; Duan, K.; Hossain, M.S.; Alhamid, M.F. emHealth: Towards emotion health through depression prediction and intelligent health recommender system. *Mob. Netw. Appl.* 2018, 23(2), 216–226.

43. Elouni, J.; Ellouzi, H.; Ltifi, H.; Ayed, M.B. Intelligent health monitoring system modeling based on machine learning and agent technology. *Multiagent Grid Syst.* 2020, 16(2), 207–226.

44. Tamilselvi, V.; Sribalaji, S.; Vigneshwaran, P.; Vinu, P.; GeethaRamani, J. IoT based health monitoring system. In *2020 6th International Conference on Advanced Computing and Communication Systems (ICACCS)*, March 2020, 386–389.

45. Gahlot, S.; Reddy, S.R.N.; Kumar, D. Review of smart health monitoring approaches with survey analysis and proposed framework. *IEEE Internet Things J.* 2018, 6(2), 2116–2127.

46. Sung, M.; Marci, C.; Pentland, A. Wearable feedback systems for rehabilitation. *J. Neuroeng. Rehabil.* 2005, 2, 1–12.

47. Lin, B.S.; Chou, N.K.; Chong, F.C.; Chen, S.J. RTWPMS: A real-time wireless physiological monitoring system. *IEEE Trans. Inf. Technol. Biomed.* 2006, 10(4), 647–656.

48. Mundt, C.W.; Montgomery, K.N.; Udoh, U.E.; Barker, V.N.; Thonier, G.C.; Tellier, A.M.; Ricks, R.D.; Darling, R.B.; Cagle, Y.D.; Cabrol, N.A.; Ruoss, S.J. A multiparameter wearable physiologic monitoring system for space and terrestrial applications. *IEEE Trans. Inf. Technol. Biomed.* 2005, 9(3), 382–391.

49. Chien, J.R.C.; Tai, C.C. A new wireless-type physiological signal measuring system using a PDA and the Bluetooth technology. *Biomed. Eng. Appl. Basis Commun.* 2005, 17(05), 229–235.

50. Tura, A.; Badanai, M.; Longo, D.; Quareni, L. A medical wearable device with wireless Bluetooth-based data transmission. *Meas. Sci. Rev.* 2003, 3(2), 1–4.

51. Pantelopoulos, A.; Bourbakis, N.G. A survey on wearable sensor-based systems for health monitoring and prognosis. *IEEE Trans. Syst. Man Cybern.* 2009, 40(1), 1–12.

52. Whelan, R.; Soose, R.J. Implantable neurostimulation for treatment of Sleep Apnea: Present and future. *Otolaryngol. Clin. North Am.* 2020, 53(3), 445–457.

53. Strand, N.H.; D'Souza, R.; Wie, C.; Covington, S.; Maita, M.; Freeman, J.; Maloney, J. Mechanism of action of peripheral nerve stimulation. *Curr. Pain Headache Rep.* 2021, 25(7), 1–9.

54. Oldroyd, P.; Malliaras, G.G. Achieving long-term stability of thin-film electrodes for neurostimulation. *Acta Biomater.* 2022, 139, 65–81.

55. Gayakwad, R.A. *Op-Amps and Linear Integrated Circuit Technology.* Prentice Hall, 1983.

56. Misra, U.K.; Kalita, J. *Clinical Neurophysiology: Nerve Conduction, Electromyography, Evoked Potentials.* Elsevier Health Sciences, 2019.

57. Ward, T.E. *Sensor Signal Conditioning for Biomedical Instrumentation,* Taylor & Francis Group, LLC, *2016.*

58. Abeyratne, U.R.; Kinouchi, Y.; Oki, H.; Okada, J.; Shichijo, F.; Matsumoto, K. Artificial neural networks for source localization in the human brain. *Brain Topogr.* 1991, 4(1), 3–21.

59. Basheer, I.A.; Hajmeer, M. Artificial neural networks: Fundamentals, computing, design, and application. *J. Microbiol. Methods* 2000, 43(1), 3–31.

60. Jain, A.K.; Mao, J.; Mohiuddin, K.M. Artificial neural networks: A tutorial. *Computer* 1996, 29(3), 31–44.

61. Yu, C.C.; Liu, B.D. A backpropagation algorithm with adaptive learning rate and momentum coefficient. In *Proceedings of the 2002 International Joint Conference on Neural Networks. IJCNN'02 (Cat. No. 02CH37290),* May 2002, 2, 1218–1223.

62. Zhang, Y.; Li, J.; Wang, T.; Wang, J. Amplitude of sensory nerve action potential in early stage diabetic peripheral neuropathy: An analysis of 500 cases. *Neural Regen. Res.* 2014, 9(14), 1389.

63. Thaisetthawatkul, P.; Logigian, E.L.; Herrmann, D.N. Dispersion of the distal compound muscle action potential as a diagnostic criterion for chronic inflammatory demyelinating polyneuropathy. *Neurology* 2002, 59(10), 1526–1532.

64. Herrmann, D.N.; Ferguson, M.L.; Logigian, E.L. Conduction slowing in diabetic distal polyneuropathy. *Muscle Nerve* 2002, 26(2), 232–237.

65. Hazarika, A.; Barman, P.; Talukdar, C.; Dutta, L.; Subasi, A.; Bhuyan, M. Real-time implementation of a multidomain feature fusion model using inherently available large sensor data. *IEEE Trans. Ind. Inform.* 2019, 15(12), 6231–6239.

66. Boettcher, B.; Cryan, M.; Gozani, S.N.; Herb, G.; Kong, X.; Williams, M.; Fendrock, C.; NeuroMetrix Inc. Apparatus and method for the automated measurement of sural nerve conduction velocity and amplitude. 2015 U.S. Patent 9,173,581.

67. Gozani, S.N.; NeuroMetrix Inc. Apparatus and methods for assessment of neuromuscular function. 1998 U.S. Patent 5,851,191.

68. Tolonen, U.; Kallio, M.; Ryhänen, J.; Raatikainen, T.; Honkala, V.; Lesonen, V.; Study Group. A handheld nerve conduction measuring device in carpal tunnel syndrome. *Acta Neurol. Scand.* 2007, 115(6), 390–397.

69. Armstrong, T.N.; Dale, A.M.; Al-Lozi, M.T.; Franzblau, A.; Evanoff, B.A. Median and ulnar nerve conduction studies at the wrist: Criterion validity of the NC-stat automated device. *J. Occup. Environ. Med.* 2008, 50(7), 758–764.

70. Rosier, R.N. Digital electroneurometer. 1989 US Patent No. 4807643.

71. Cossul, S.; Rettore Andreis, F.; Favretto, M.A.; de Castro Antonio Jr, A.; Marques, J.L.B. Portable microcontroller-based electrostimulation system for nerve conduction studies. *IET Sci. Meas. Technol.* 2020, 14(6), 695–703.

72. Hernandez-Reynoso, A.G.; Nandam, S.; O'Brien, J.M.; Kanneganti, A.; Cogan, S.F.; Freeman, D.K.; Romero-Ortega, M.I. Miniature electroparticle-cuff for wireless peripheral neuromodulation. *J. Neural Eng.* 2019, 16(4), 046002.

73. Barthakur, M.; Hazarika, A.; Bhuyan, M. Classification of peripheral neuropathy by using ANN based nerve conduction study (NCS) protocol. *Int. J. Commun. Syst.* 2014, 5(1), 31.

74. Isose, S.; Kuwabara, S.; Kokubun, N.; Sato, Y.; Mori, M.; Shibuya, K.; Sekiguchi, Y.; Nasu, S.; Fujimaki, Y.; Noto, Y.; Sawai, S. Utility of the distal compound muscle action potential duration for diagnosis of demyelinating neuropathies. *J. Peripher. Nerv. Syst.* 2009, 14(3), 151–158.

75. Cohn, T.G.; Wertsch, J.J.; Pasupuleti, D.V.; Lofsgaarden, J.D. Nerve conduction studies: Orthodromic vs antidromic latencies. *Arch. Phys. Med. Rehabil.* 1990, 71(8), 579–582.

76. Barthakur, M.; Hazarika, A.; Bhuyan, M. A computer-assisted technique for nerve conduction study in early detection of peripheral neuropathy using ANN. *Int. J. Electron. Commun. Eng. Tech.* 2013, 4(5), 47–65.

16 Critical Analysis of Current Healthcare Applications for Diagnosis of Diseases
Pitfalls and Future

*Tumul Vikram Singh, Qazi Amanur Rahman Hashmi,
Nitu Dogra, Ankur Saxena,
Deepshikha Pande Katare, and
Ruchi Jakhmola Mani*

16.1 INTRODUCTION

Digital health is an umbrella term that includes mHealth and other newly developing technological topics. The delivery of health services and healthcare-related information via smartphone technology is referred to as "mobile health", also known as mHealth, and is a subset of electronic health (eHealth) (World Health Organisation, 2019). eHealth is a term used to describe the secure and cost-effective use of information and communication technology in the field of medicine (such as healthcare services and health monitoring). Digital health is a further subset of eHealth. Even though digital health is a subset of eHealth, it has far more diverse and varying applications than eHealth alone (Wang et al., 2021). Digital health emulates and progresses the concept of eHealth to more intelligent and interconnected devices for digital consumers by implementing digital transformation in the healthcare industry and by adapting software, hardware, and services to meet specific needs (Bernstein, 2021). Several digital technologies, including the Internet of Things and artificial intelligence (AI), are widely used in the healthcare industry. Telecare, telehealth, telemedicine, mHealth, digital health, and eHealth services are examples of technology-enabled care, which combines medical technology, digital media, and mobile communications (Deserno & Jakob, 2020). It focuses on the citizen as the centre, collects health data from the user, and tracks their social interactions in real time, then performs sophisticated analysis to learn from the data in order to model and improvise as many social and economic activities as possible (Lupton, 2014).

DOI: 10.1201/9781003363361-16

In 2019, similar terms, such as medical information technology, mobile health, digital medical, and mobile medicine, were amalgamated by the World Health Organization (WHO) into the term "digital health" (Bernstein, 2021). Stakeholders involved in the digital healthcare field include patients, healthcare professionals, researchers, application developers, medical device manufacturers, and distributors. Today's healthcare system is becoming increasingly reliant on digital technology.

Artificial intelligence (AI), the Internet of Things (IoT), big data analysis, and distributed computing services such as cloud computing are all crucial to the advancement of digital health. These technologies are integrated and used cohesively during the preparation and implementation process. The Internet of Things is the network that connects all simple objects capable of performing autonomous tasks, using a variety of information-detecting devices. The medical industry has a lot of potential for IoT applications (Gharote et al., 2015). The Internet of Things can be used by hospitals to collect and distribute medical data on ongoing drugs and medications prescribed to patients, as well as to implement adaptable and intelligent management systems (Ahmadi et al., 2019). The drug identification system, implemented by utilizing novel IoT approaches, has the potential to reduce medication errors caused by humans while also increasing medical staff productivity (Gutierrez et al., 2017). Human intelligence may be augmented and improved by implementing artificial intelligence, which will help in simulating human decision-making and reasoning processes with machine learning (Haenlein & Kaplan, 2019). AI utilizes several disciplines, such as cognitive science, neurophysiology, mathematics, and information theory, and combines them with computational techniques, such as expert systems, machine learning, natural language processing, autonomous planning, image processing, and other technologies (Nadarzynski et al., 2019). AI may use massive amounts of data to automatically learn, gain expertise, and make correct predictions. By providing auxiliary diagnosis and therapy, AI may reduce the effort required of medical professionals, increasing their job productivity and quality of care (Liu et al., 2020).

Cloud computing is a model for delivering computing resources and a medium for distributing computing technology. It virtualizes computer resources and makes them available as services across the network by integrating multiple servers, processes and applications, data, and other resources. Cloud computing services enable users to gain access to the mainframe and process information at any time and from any location (Kuo, 2011). Cloud computing is useful for medical research and can improve medical services (Narayan et al., 2010). Big data is a term used to describe a collection of data that is extremely huge in size and cannot be analyzed in a short amount of time using traditional human methods, due to its size and variability. Healthcare is one of the commercial sectors with the greatest potential for big data applications (Priya et al., 2020). Since the advent of the big data era, clinical data has grown exponentially, demonstrating the constant increase in medical data volume (Moharana et al., 2020). Big data technologies efficiently regulate hospital management and the resulting improvement in hospital medical quality. Furthermore, the technologies involved in big data-processing technologies may provide precise and scientifically significant information to medical professionals to aid in diagnosis and treatment while decreasing the rate of incorrect diagnoses.

The global market for digital health is estimated to be valued at US$211 billion in 2022, with a compound annual growth rate (CAGR) of 18.6% in the time period of 2023 to 2030. Rising smartphone adoption, improved internet connectivity brought about by the rollout of 4G and 5G technologies, advancements in the infrastructure of healthcare, the increasing demands to moderate healthcare costs, an increase in the prevalence of chronic diseases, and increased accessibility to virtual care are some of the key factors driving market growth. Furthermore, major corporations are emphasizing the delivery of cutting-edge apps to improve user experience, such as Microsoft's Solo platform in collaboration with Teladoc Health. The goal of this platform is to improve clinician and patient access across the virtual healthcare arena (Bernstein et al., 2021).

16.2   WHAT IS MHEALTH?

The Global Observatory for eHealth (GOe), an initiative launched by the World Health Organization, defines mHealth as the use of mobile devices in the practice of medicine and public health (Kay et al., 2011). As of December 2022, 2.5 billion people worldwide own a mobile phone, which gives rise to a significant opportunity for mHealth to provide unparalleled access to specialized clinical diagnostics and treatment recommendations. The number of smartphone users worldwide is expected to reach seven billion by the end of 2025. Furthermore, many users own multiple devices, which makes it so that there are more mobile devices than users. Over 18.2 billion mobile devices are expected to be in use worldwide by the end of 2025 (Bernstein, 2021).

According to a recent systematic review, interactive symptom checkers are the most commonly explored type of diagnostic software, with an estimated 50 million app-based self-triage users worldwide. However, only 34% of non-emergent patients received adequate triage assistance, and diagnoses were only 55% accurate. Apps for diagnosing specific symptoms, such as hand or knee pain, have been shown to frequently provide incorrect recommendations. Symptom checker applications, according to studies, frequently take a risk-averse approach, which may result in unnecessary consultations in non-emergency situations (Millenson et al., 2018).

The other major class of diagnostic applications examines images or data from integrated sensors in smartphones using algorithms. A systematic review published in 2017 found 30 publications examining 35 applications, the majority of which were designed to screen images for melanoma or identify tremors using movement analysis (Buechi et al., 2017). However, the available data does not support the notion that photo-screening applications could serve as a clinical consultation (The Lancet Oncology, 2018).

According to 63% of respondents to the recent "Global mHealth Developer Survey", smartphone adoption is the primary driver of mHealth, while the biggest barrier to mHealth is the lack of standardization (50%), regulations (49%), and market transparency (49%). Remote information transmission, data collection and illness outbreak surveillance, diagnostic therapy and assistance, and medication adherence and remote monitoring are the four distinct uses of mHealth for global development (Blynn et al., 2021).

In the aftermath of the COVID-19 pandemic, the potential of mHealth applications has garnered huge interest, in both the public and private sectors. As of December 2022, the average number of new cases is still over 500,000 (Bernstein, 2021). At the onset of the pandemic, a glaring need for an easy-to-access healthcare service was evident. People were afraid to break lockdown restrictions to visit hospitals. The large influx of cases also stressed healthcare facilities (Karan & Wadhera, 2021). There were mass shortages of triage medications and masks worldwide. Their increasing demands put a huge financial burden on the healthcare sector. There was an average 7.4% reduction in GDP in Europe in 2020 (Conte et al., 2020). This effect on the global economy was also reflected in shortages in healthcare budgets. Many patients were unable to visit the hospital and get treatment for complications, due to the medical systems being already overloaded while dealing with COVID cases. mHealth services could enable healthcare professionals to detect and monitor minor illnesses remotely, without the need for physical intervention and contact.

16.3   HEALTHCARE APPLICATIONS

In this chapter, the different healthcare apps (symptom checker apps) are explored. Symptom checker applications utilize numerous artificial intelligence and machine learning algorithms, such as natural language processing (NLP), Bayesian networks, decision trees, rule-based systems, deep learning, etc. to generate results. The exact integration and working of these algorithms are not shared in the public domain, probably to safeguard intellectual property. Nevertheless, natural language processing is usually used to identify patterns and relationships in user inputs. The user inputs their symptoms into the app, typically in the form of selecting predetermined options. The apps often use NLP algorithms to analyze the user's text and identify relevant keywords and phrases. The apps then use these keywords and phrases to generate a list of potential medical conditions that match the user's symptoms. They may also ask the user additional questions to gather more information about their symptoms or medical history, which can help to refine the list of potential conditions. Finally, the user is provided with information about the potential conditions, including symptoms, causes, and treatment options. Some apps may also provide a recommendation to seek medical help if the user's symptoms are severe or persistent. Symptom checker apps can also use Bayesian networks to provide a more accurate and reliable diagnosis for the user. A Bayesian network is a type of probabilistic graphical model that represents a set of variables and their conditional dependencies using a directed acyclic graph. Bayesian networks are used to construct a probabilistic network that represents the relationships between the symptoms and medical conditions, which are used to calculate the probability of different medical conditions. Bayesian networks can be particularly useful in healthcare applications because they allow for the integration of prior knowledge and data into the diagnosis process. This can help to account for the complexity and uncertainty of medical conditions and can lead to a more accurate and personalized diagnosis for the user. The apps have a knowledge base that consists of medical data. Specific keywords entered by the user are recognized and the knowledge base is utilized to generate a result. However, as specified above, the specifics of the internal workings and algorithms of the apps are copyrighted and licensed and are not available for public use.

The objective of this work was to elucidate whether all the healthcare apps are working in sync or not, i.e., if they are capable of predicting similar diseases/disorders for a patient profile. Prior to the analysis of the apps, many profiles involving multiple symptoms were analyzed, and it was later realized that, to maintain a common baseline for the different apps used, the simplest symptoms must be selected. The medical knowledge base of each app is different, along with their working algorithms, which gives rise to a huge number of different combinations of questions asked and diagnoses recommended. Therefore, two virtual profiles were created with minimal symptoms, i.e., hypertension, diabetes, and headache (Figure 16.1).

Therefore, in order to follow a similar workflow, headache was selected as the only immediate symptom (Stovner et al., 2022). Patient 1 is a 40-year-old male with a history of hypertension and diabetes. Patient 2 is also a 40-year-old male and has no prior history of any prevalent illnesses (Figure 16.1)

Furthermore, the workflows for providing input into the app were created (for example, Figure 16.4 represents the workflow of Ada). The workflows were analyzed and a comparative analysis of their procedures and results was conducted. The functionality of the apps was elaborated and their utility was assessed based on their results. The five apps that were assessed were selected on the basis of market availability, platform of usage, and ease of use. The results of the trial have been provided

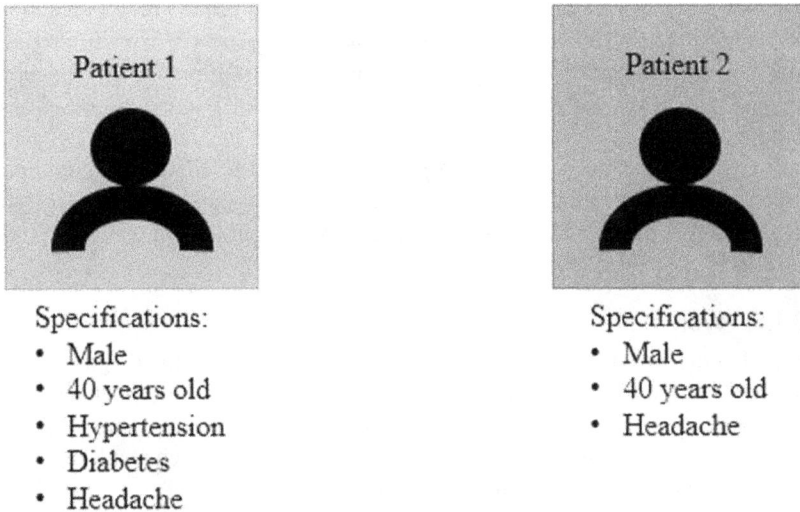

Patient 1

Specifications:
- Male
- 40 years old
- Hypertension
- Diabetes
- Headache

Patient 2

Specifications:
- Male
- 40 years old
- Headache

FIGURE 16.1 Illustrating the hypothetical patient profiles created for the two-patient trial strategy, which is utilized for all apps. The same profile was selected to limit the variability in workflows and diagnoses of the different apps.

along with the comparative analysis. The variability in the results of the different apps for the same symptoms was accentuated. Lastly, the possible future improvements and modifications to the working of these apps were also discussed.

16.3.1   ADA

Ada is a Berlin-based health firm that has developed and manages a user-based self-assessment web tool. It was developed by Claire Novorol, Daniel Nathrath, and Martin Hirsch. The app began as a tool for doctors, before being modified in 2016 to adapt the presentation of medical information in a way that patients could understand. The app compares user-described symptoms to symptoms of individuals of a similar age and gender, and then calculates the probability that the patient has a certain ailment. The Ada app is presently accessible in English, German, Spanish, Portuguese, Swahili, Romanian, and French. By September 2020, the Ada app had been downloaded ten million times and 20 million symptom evaluations had been performed.

ADA is a CE (Conformité Européenne) Class 1 medical device which is HIPAA (Health Insurance Portability and Accountabilty Act) and GDPR (General Data Protection Regulation) compliant. The CE Class 2a certification process for the app is currently underway. Ada Health's medical knowledge base covers around 30,000 ICD-10 codes, which are the alphanumeric codes used by doctors to represent different diagnoses. It is one of the most diverse and largest knowledge bases of any such system in the market space. Ada Health, in addition to placing its symptom assessment app in the hands of patients, offers a suite of corporate solutions in which partners pay to embed and thoroughly integrate its triage technology into their websites and digital services. That means businesses may utilize it to provide an entrance point for their customers, directing them to the appropriate service and providing administrative assistance by equipping physicians with health information supplied by patients via the Ada interface (as well as the AI's own evaluation) ahead of the appointment.

In a study conducted, it was discovered that around 97.8% of the participants submitted that it was "very or quite easy" to use Ada, around 88% of the participants agreed that they would use Ada again, and 85% would recommend it to others (Figure 16.2).

16.3.1.1   Working

The app begins working with the basic information and starts the diagnostic questionnaire. The app has a clean and simple interface with easy-to-understand questions (Figure 16.3). To reduce the complexity and maintain the same diagnostic criteria across all apps, we have opted to select the answers which result in the least number of possible questions asked to the individual.

Referencing the workflow of the app (Figure 16.4), Ada prioritizes smoking, the presence of high blood pressure, and diabetes as the basic diagnostic markers. Then, we are asked to enter the symptom that is troubling us the most. Any such entry gives multiple pre-defined symptoms to choose from, which helps in clarifying any

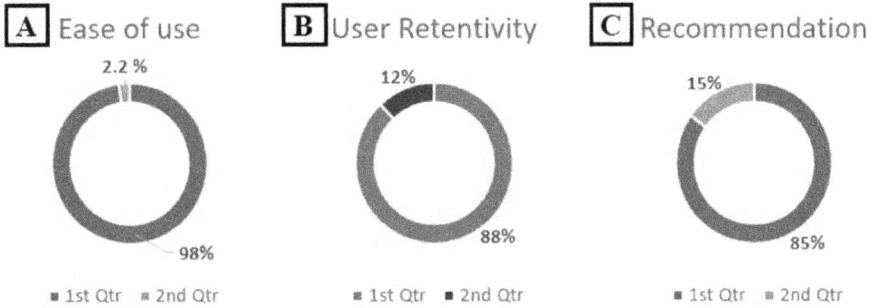

FIGURE 16.2 Demonstrating the descriptive statistics of Ada usage, namely (A) the ease of use, (B) user retentivity and (C) recommendation by users to other people.

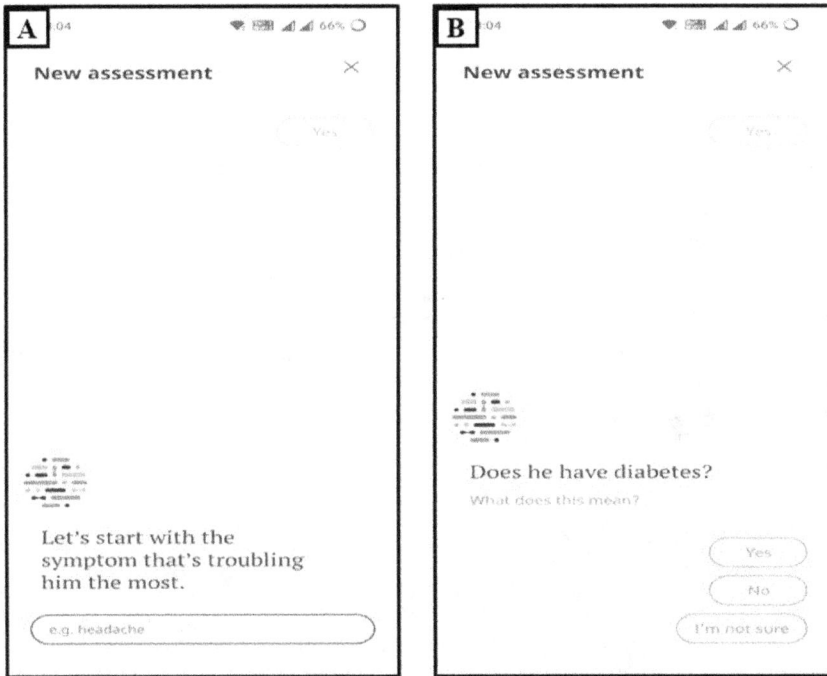

FIGURE 16.3 (A) Depicting the interface of the Ada app (B) Depicting the app's clean and simple interface and easy-to-understand questions.

doubts about the condition that the user might have. It also provides a small definition of the selected symptom, which is extremely helpful in making the selection. After entering the symptoms, the app asks further questions to predict the condition more accurately. It starts by inquiring about the location, duration, and type of pain experienced by the individual. The type of pain is extremely important because it is

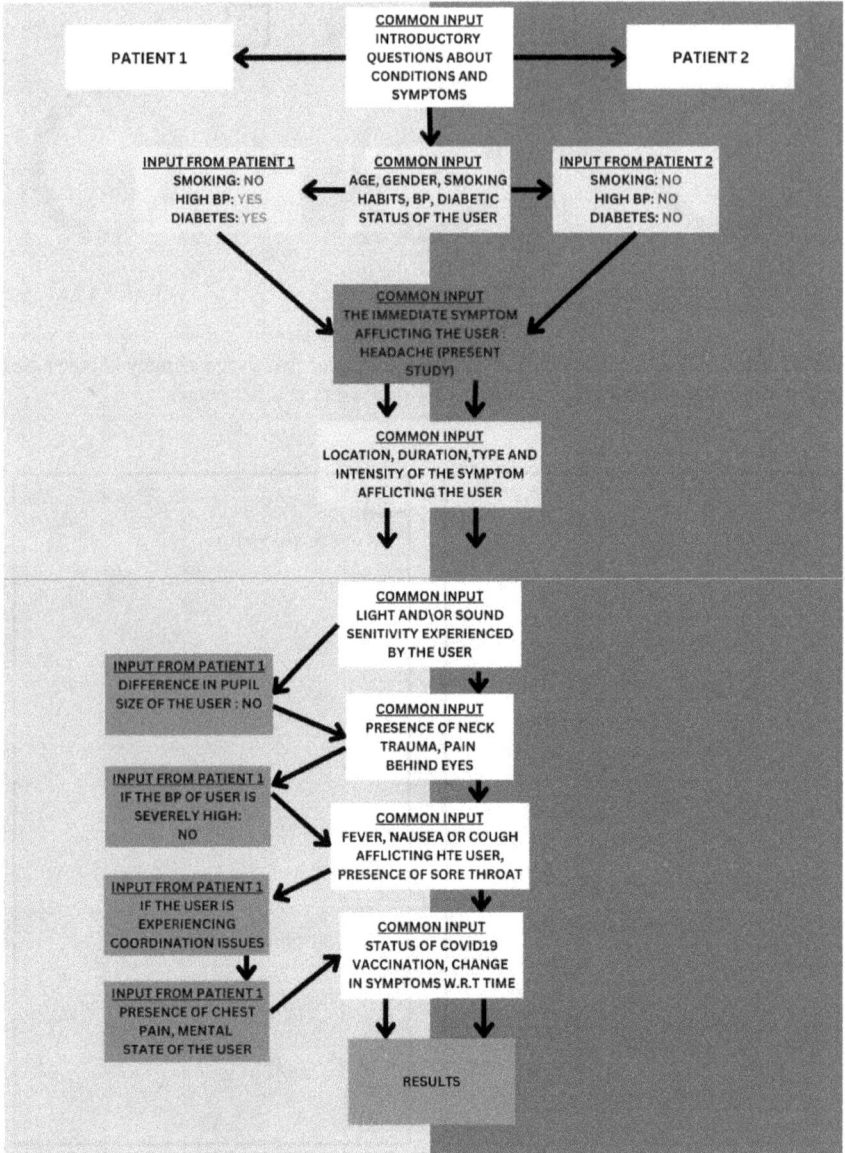

FIGURE 16.4 Depicting the workflow of the Ada app. The demarcation between the questions asked of Patient 1 and Patient 2 is represented. Patient 1 (located on the left side) was asked more specific questions about certain conditions (highlighted in blue), possibly due to the presence of pre-existing conditions. The red box indicates the entry of the common symptom, while the green box denotes the results.

a major biological marker. For example, migraines generally result in a pounding, pulsating headache accompanied by nausea, while tension headaches are described as a squeezing headache.

The app then once again asks for any other symptoms experienced by the individual. As stated above, we have opted to create the most fundamental diagnostic trial by selecting only one afflicting condition. After entering "no" to a question asking whether there are any further conditions, the diagnostic questions become more specific. The app further asks about any hypersensitivity to sound or light or accompanying nausea, to rule out underlying medical complications. It also asks if the individual noticed any difference in pupil size while the headache was present, which is a classical indication of tension or migraine headaches. The app then asks generalized questions such as recent head or neck trauma, fever, cough, generalized muscle weakness, etc. A striking question asked is whether the individual has had the COVID-19 vaccine administered in the past three weeks. Any delayed headache occurring after the vaccine can be an indicator of vaccine induced cerebral vascular thrombosis (Hanse et al., 2022).

The final question asked by the app is if the symptoms have gradually worsened, gotten better, or stayed the same with time. Then, the app presents a detailed report about the different conditions the individual might have, along with the likelihood of them occurring. The questions asked and the answers given are displayed in the Table 16.1. The results have also been provided for a comparative study.

In testing, the app was discovered to be extremely user-friendly. The interface is clean and smooth and does not overwhelm the user with excessive medical information. The questions asked are framed in an extremely easy-to-understand manner and the options provided are sufficient to cover most possible answers. The average time to provide a diagnosis is five minutes, however, it can vary, depending on the user's comprehension and understanding of their condition.

Ada has one of the most versatile and adaptive algorithms and presents the results in the most descriptive manner (Figure 16.5).

16.3.2 Mediktor

Mediktor is the most advanced and accurate artificial intelligence-based solution for triage, pre-diagnosis, and decision assistance. The contact with users begins by asking them to record their symptoms or just how they feel in an open text box using their own words. From there, considering data such as gender, age, risk factors, and vital signs, Mediktor employs AI and intuition to generate hypotheses about the circumstances that users may be experiencing. It then iterates to select the appropriate question to confirm or reject the various hypotheses. Patients might be asked a variety of questions. Images are used to demonstrate and enhance comprehension when a question is difficult to grasp.

Mediktor safeguards users' data in compliance with the European Union's and the European Economic Area's General Data Protection Regulation (GDPR). In the United States, Mediktor conforms with the Health Insurance Portability and Accountability Act (HIPAA).

TABLE 16.1

Depicting the differences and similarities in the working of the different apps assessed in the study. A clear contrast in the number of questions asked and the time required for diagnosis between the different apps can be observed.

App	Platform Availability	Introductory Questions	Number of Questions Asked	Time Required for Use	Diagnosis Representation	Links
Ada	IOS, Android, and web-based tool	• Gender • Age • Smoking • Hypertension • Diabetes	Around 25	Around five minutes	Probability based on patient history	https://ada.com/, httos://play.google.com/store/apps/details?id=com.adn.ada.app&hl=en IN&gl=US
Mediktor	IOS, Android, and web-based tool	• Gender • Age	Around 30	Around five minutes	Symptomatic evidence-based	https://www.mediktor.com/en-us,https://play.google.com/store/a_pos/details?id=com.teckelmedical.mediktorghl=en IN&girLIS
5ymotomate	IOS, Android, and web-based tool	• Age • Gender • Weight • Hypertension • Smoking - Injury • Cholesterol	Around 30	Around five minutes	Symptomatic evidence-based	https://symptomate.com/,https://play.gooele.com/store/aoos/details?id=com.5vmotomate.mobile&h1=en IN&gl=US
MayaMD	IOS and Android	• Age • Gender	Around ten	Around two minutes	Symptomatic evidence-based	httos://www.mayantclAii,httos://olay.google.com/store/apos/details?id=ai.mavamd.mayamd&hl=en IN&gl=US
WebMD	IOS, Android and, web-based tool	• Gender • Age • Medication	Around five	Less than a minute	Direct symptom-matching	https://www.webmd.com/httos://play.gooele.com/store/apps/details?id=com.webmd.android&hi=en IN&gl=US

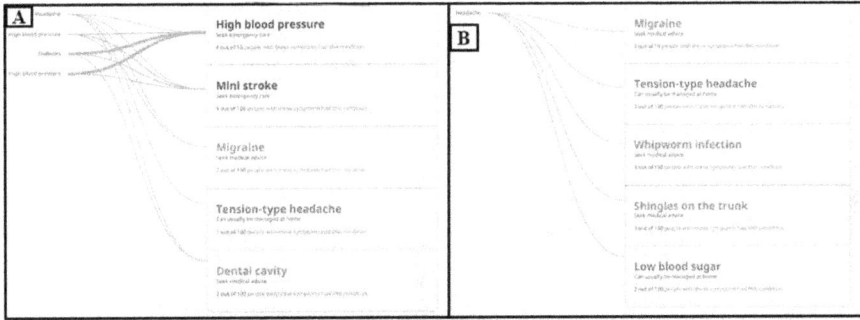

FIGURE 16.5 The results for the Ada app are displayed. (A) The results for Patient 1 are specific to conditions tying headaches to pre-existing conditions, while (B) displays the results for Patient 2, which include common conditions that can cause headaches.

16.3.2.1 Working

The app functions like a chatroom window, by asking about the most debilitating condition (Figure 16.6). After that, the app asks general questions about the person taking the assessment. The app then proceeds to ask about the location of the patient. Then, the app presents the patient with a list of further symptoms, which increase according to the options selected. The list of symptoms changes according to the combination of symptoms selected.

A striking feature of this app is that there are no questions asked about the pre-existing conditions or comorbidities of the patient. This further simplifies the use of the app, but the diagnosis might not be as accurate as other apps. As observed, we cannot distinguish between the results by having different pre-existing conditions. The app has one of the simplest and easiest-to-understand workflows (Figure 16.7). There are not many diverging paths that can be selected, and users should not have any trouble entering their details and symptoms and getting a diagnosis.

The app enquires about the most debilitating symptom first. It then follows up by asking about the age, gender, and geographical location of the user. The location is used to correlate to any local disease or endemics prevalent in the region. Furthermore, the app asks the user to input additional information pertaining to the symptom, such as the onset of the symptom, the duration, the type of pain perceived, and specific questions such as sensitivity to light and sound, dizziness, etc. The app tries to cover all the diagnostic questions that are related to the disease. It then presents the diagnosis in a symptomatic evidence-based manner (Figure 16.8).

16.3.3 SYMPTOMATE

Symptomate was developed in 2012 as a smart tool for symptom-checking. They employ an AI-based engine linked to a thorough database of medical knowledge. Over ten million people use it worldwide and it is available in 20 languages. Symptomate

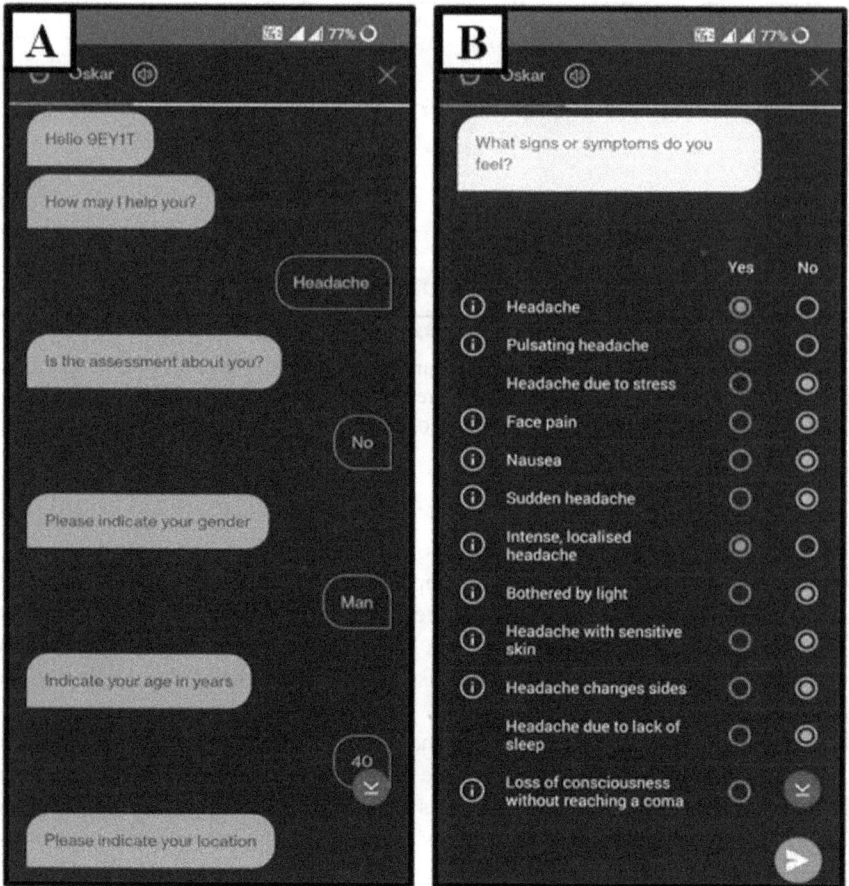

FIGURE 16.6 Depicting the interface of the Mediktor app. (A) The app works in a fairly-simple and easy-to-understand manner. (B) The additional symptoms are provided with a yes/no option.

is part of Infermedica. They developed it based on best practices applied by their excellent team of specialists, who want to increase everyone's access to primary care. Leading healthcare organizations around the world employ Infermedica's early symptom assessment and digital triage solutions.

Symptomate is renowned for its precise outcomes and user-friendly user interface (UI) (Figure 16.9). In addition to having a mobile app for iOS and Google Play, Symptomate has now created a website for PC users. It has been downloaded over 100,000 times and has a 4.2-star rating on Google Play. According to the developers, it can evaluate more than 740 conditions in three minutes, and reviews posted online show that consumers have repeatedly found it to be correct. Symptomate has a global rank of over 1500 in the health and fitness category (according to Google Apps statistics), including Canada, the United Kingdom, Germany, France, etc. Recent

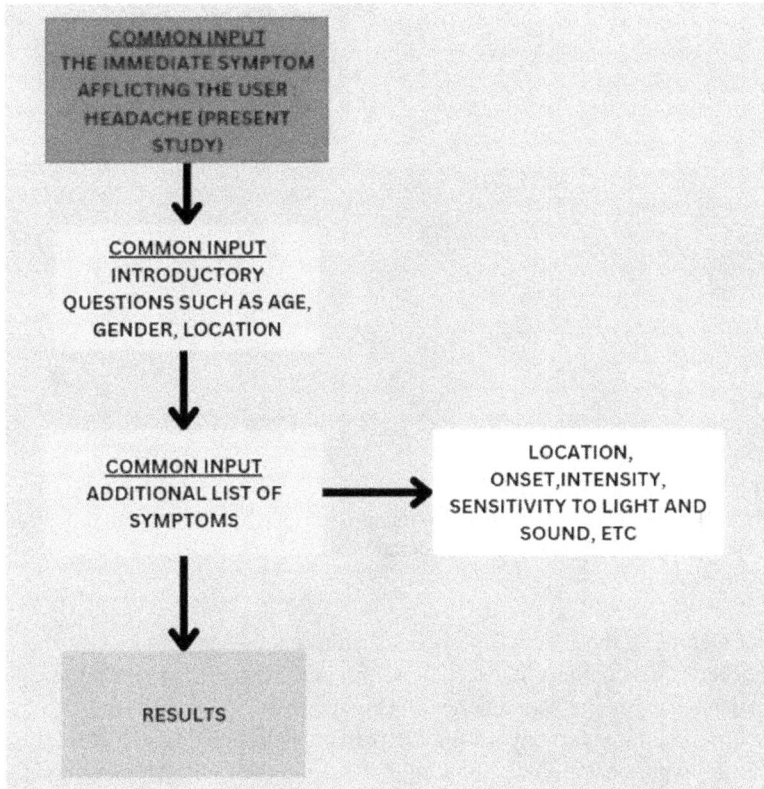

FIGURE 16.7 Depicting the workflow of the Mediktor app. The workflow is fairly simple without too many diverging paths. The red box denotes the entry of the symptom afflicting the user, while the green box denotes the results. As we can see, there is no distinction between the workflows for Patient 1 and Patient 2, because Mediktor does not take preexisting conditions into account before asking about the most immediate symptom.

statistics show that the rating of the application has drastically decreased over the past few months. The majority of Symptomate's traffic comes from individual user searches on the Google Play store and app recommendations.

16.3.3.1 Working

Symptomate is easy to use (Figure 16.10). Patients share the symptoms that are bothering them. Then, much like with a real doctor, they respond to a series of questions in order to better understand their condition. A list of the most likely conditions, along with an explanation, description, and recommendation on the level of care that would be most appropriate, is given to the patient at the conclusion of each checkup. As stated above, we have predetermined two hypothetical patients as the subjects for the diagnostic trial. The same patients will be taken into consideration across all the apps we are testing, so as to maintain a standard, and to compare each application's results afterwards. The base symptom for our diagnostic is headache.

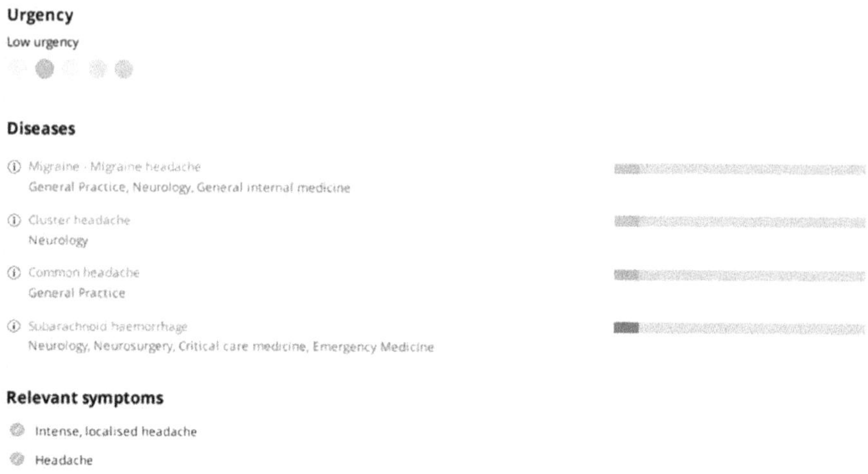

Urgency

Low urgency

Diseases

ⓘ Migraine · Migraine headache
General Practice, Neurology, General internal medicine

ⓘ Cluster headache
Neurology

ⓘ Common headache
General Practice

ⓘ Subarachnoid haemorrhage
Neurology, Neurosurgery, Critical care medicine, Emergency Medicine

Relevant symptoms

🟢 Intense, localised headache

🟢 Headache

FIGURE 16.8 The result from the Mediktor app is displayed. As observed, Mediktor does not take pre-existing conditions into consideration, which exempts us from adopting the two-patient trial strategy.

After feeding in the general questions, such as name, age, and gender, the symptom checker's questionnaire starts. A flowchart of the questions in the application for both patients has been attached herewith (Figure 16.9).

The questionnaire starts by asking the patient about their weight, if they are suffering from hypertension, their smoking habits, and their cholesterol content. After these general questions, the Symptomate asks for the main symptom which is causing the patient the most trouble. Headache is the base symptom for Patient 1 and Patient 2. For Patient 1, we also added diabetes as a symptom. After adding diabetes and headache for Patient 1, it asked for the blood glucose level and went on to ask for the geographic location, which was common for both patients.

Furthermore, it asked the patient how often the headaches occur, since when the headaches have been happening, how long they occur for, and the intensity of the headaches. Just like a doctor asks for other questions unrelated to the main symptom, Ada asked whether the patient has a sore throat, or is having trouble hearing any sounds, if they have a runny nose, or if are they grinding their teeth. All of these questions have some relation to the root problem, headache. The grinding of teeth signifies that the patients may have bruxism, runny nose, and sore throat, all of which are general symptoms of the common cold, which can also cause headaches.

Moreover, it asks for the specific location of the headache, which is a very important question for the identification of the root problem. Usually, headaches at the back of the head and near the temples are tension headaches, headaches behind the eyes and forehead are migraines, behind one eye are cluster headaches, and behind an ear can be caused by an ear infection. For Patient 1, it asked how much their BP (blood pressure) was, then went back to the common question, which was whether the patient's jaw was frozen, and whether they had pain behind their eyes. A frozen

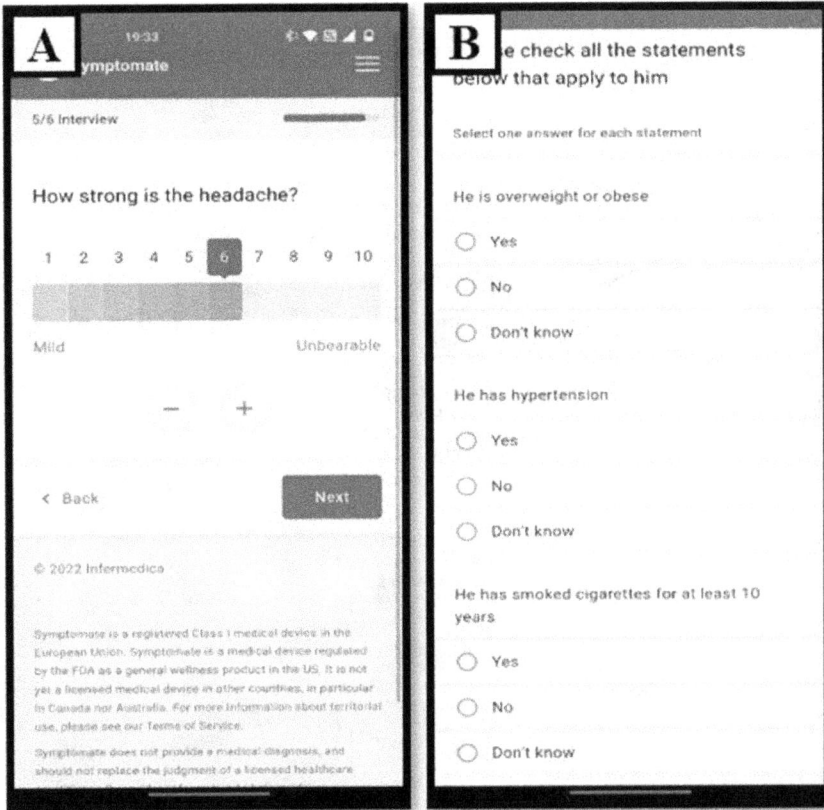

FIGURE 16.9 Depicting the interface of Symptomate app. (A) For specifying the intensity of the symptom. (B) List of additional symptoms.

jaw alongside a headache is an indicator of Temporomandibular joint dysfunction or TMJ syndrome. For Patient 1, this was the last and final question, and it started processing the results which will be compared in the results section of this chapter.

However, for Patient 2, there was one more question remaining. It asked whether the headaches worsen in the morning, whether the headaches occur when the patient is stressed, whether they occur during physical activity, and whether the intensity of the headaches increases when bending down. After this, the results for Patient 2 were processed.

The results of Symptomate are attached (Figure 16.11) in the following Diagnoses section.

16.3.4 MayaMD

MayaMD, an innovative AI healthcare startup formed in 2019, has developed a cutting-edge patient interaction platform that empowers both patients and physicians.

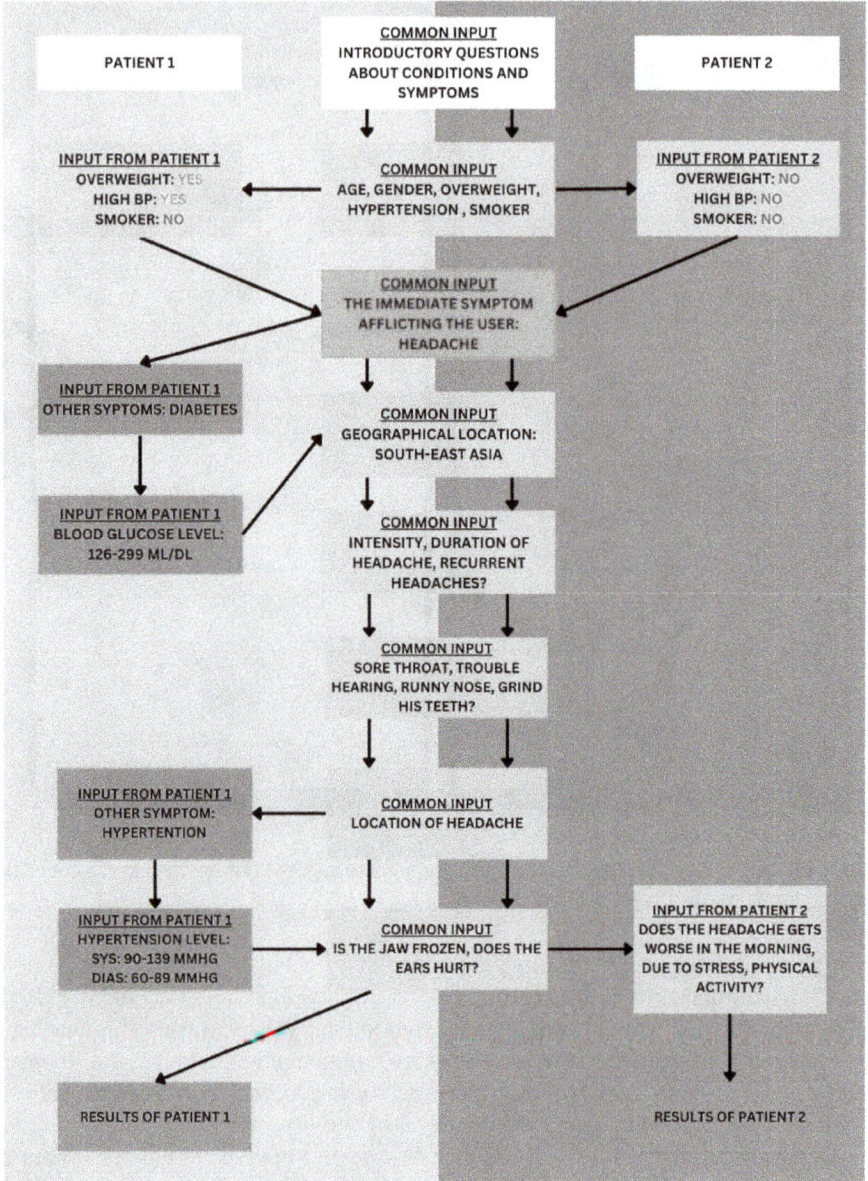

FIGURE 16.10 Depicting the workflow of the Symptomate app. It takes the geographical location of the user along with the pre-existing conditions to recommend a diagnosis. The blue box depicts the questions asked specifically to Patient 1. The red box denotes the input for the symptom (Headache), while the green box denotes the results.

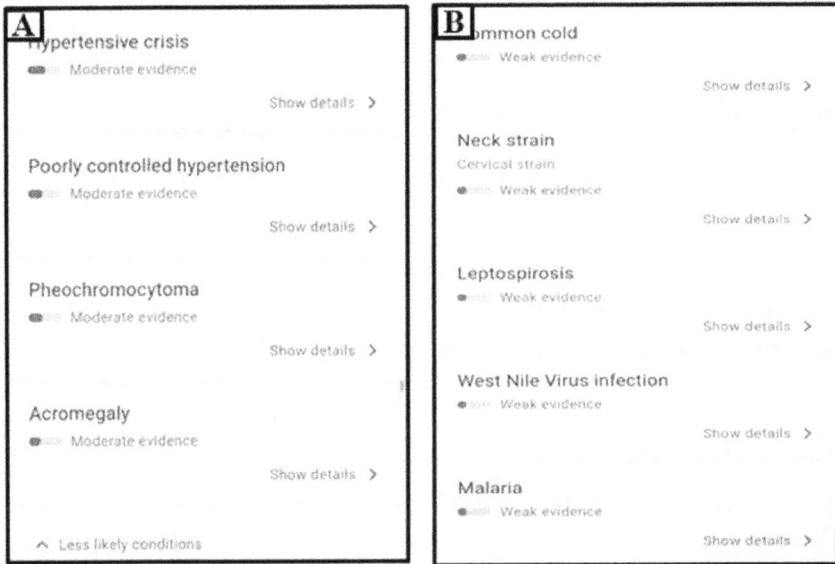

FIGURE 16.11 The results for the two patients are displayed for the Symptomate app. (A) Result for Patient 1. As we can see, the results are focused on pre-existing conditions. (B) The result for Patient 2, are extremely varied, covering all the common causes for headaches.

They are made to improve collaboration and communication between doctors and patients, resulting in the best possible patient experience. They offer services for telemedicine platforms, remote patient monitoring, clinical decision support tools, and AI patient engagement or symptom checkers. They seek to cut the cost of care by directing patients toward less-expensive care options, providing patient education tools for improved health literacy, increasing patient satisfaction, using conversational interfaces for better engagement, reducing readmissions and medical errors, and providing instantaneous medical answers.

MayaMD is a robust symptom checker and virtual health assistant that uses AI to give unrivalled access to medical information and knowledge (Figure 16.12). MayaMD can process any number and combination of symptoms, physical indicators, lab results, medications, and past medical history to produce a patient note at the clinician level. MayaMD leverages AI and the critical-thinking techniques of top doctors to deliver insightful information in less than 90 seconds. It is among the quickest and most potent health assistants on the market. MayaMD is accessible both on iOS and Google Play. With 170 reviews and more than 100,000 downloads, it has a Google Play rating of 4.2 out of 5 stars. MayaMD claims to be able to assess more than 10,000 symptoms and diseases, with a triage accuracy rate of 94% in less than 90 seconds. According to the official website (https://www.mayamd.ai/) , the application has been downloaded more than 400,000 times in more than 170 nations. Although detailed statistics about MayaMD are not yet accessible, it can be inferred from recent trends that the apps popularity has been rising in recent years. MayaMD

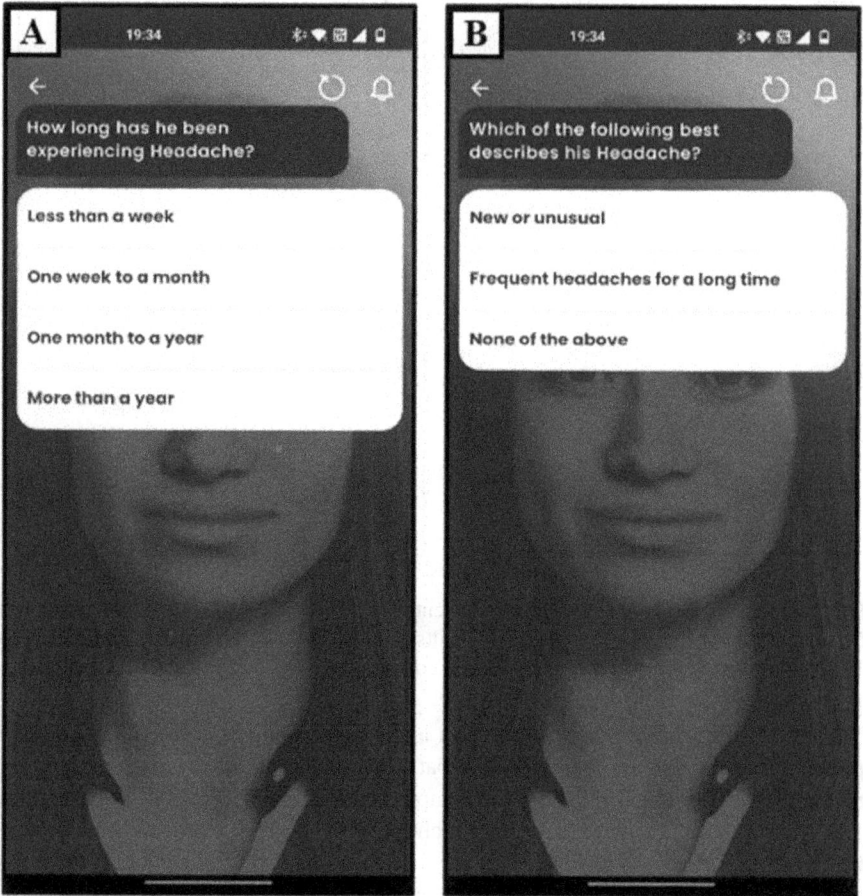

FIGURE 16.12 Illustrating the interface of the WebMD app. (A) Question inquiring about the onset of the headache. (B) Question inquiring about the nature of the headache.

is currently ranked about 7000 in the health and fitness area in the United States (according to Google Apps statistics).

16.3.4.1 Working

The flow of questions in MayaMD is straightforward. After answering general questions, such as name, age, and gender, the symptom checker's questionnaire starts (Figure 16.13).

You feed it a symptom, and it asks questions related to the symptom, then moves on to ask about the next symptom. This process is repeated until the patient enters "no" in the "Other symptoms?" question, after which it generates a result. The base symptom for our study of all these apps is headache, which was entered after the application asked for basic information like gender and age. After "headache" was

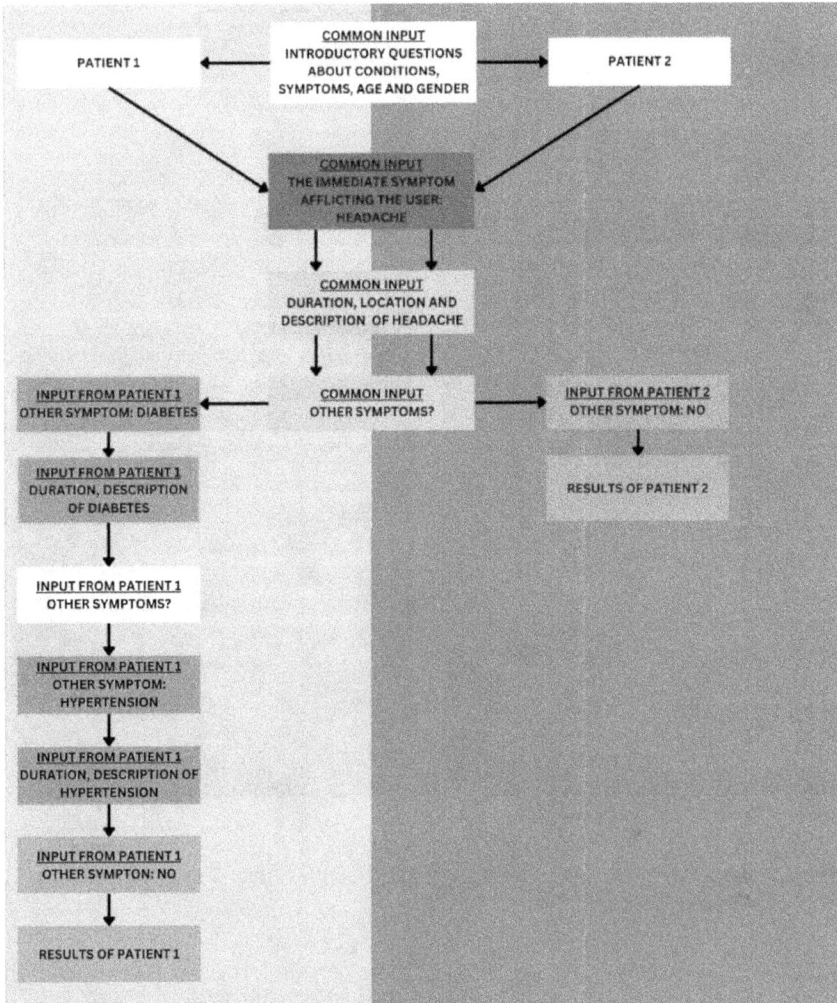

FIGURE 16.13 Depicting the workflow of the MayaMD app. It has a relatively less complex workflow, with the app only focusing on the immediate symptoms and pre-existing conditions.

entered, the app asked since when had the headache been happening, and for a description of the headache, whether it was new or unusual, or if headaches were frequent, and what part of the brain was most affected by the headache. Since this was the only symptom for Patient 2, it generated a result for them.

As Patient 1 had more pre-existing complications like diabetes, the app asked since when the patient has had diabetes, and asked the same about hypertension. After that, it generated a result for Patient 1, which will be compared with the results

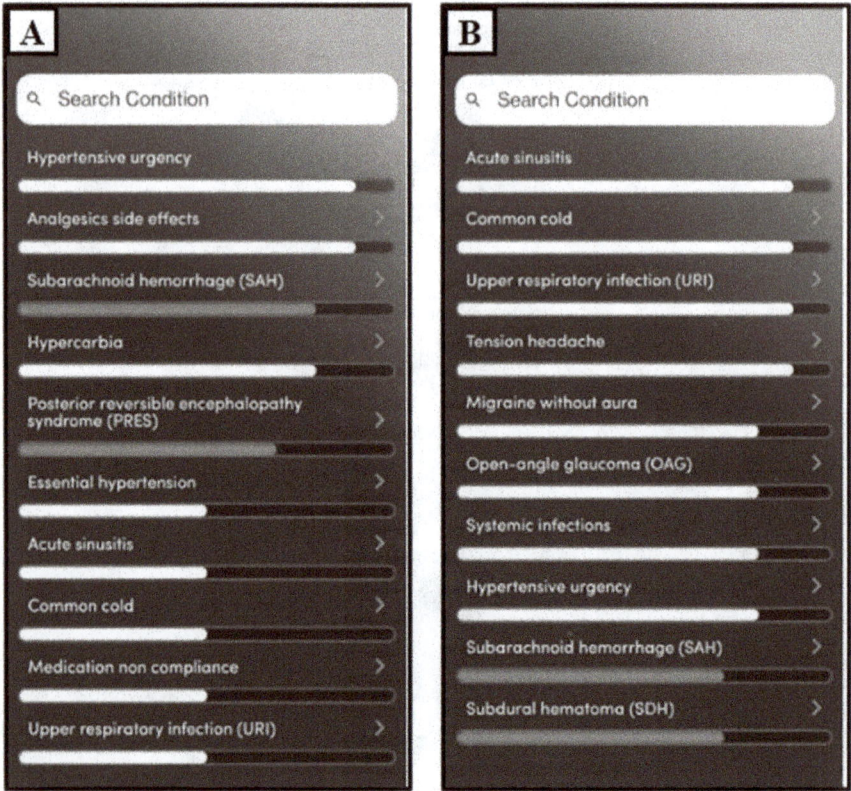

FIGURE 16.14 As observed, the results are varied, possibly due to the different pre-existing conditions of the patients. The results are more complicated for Patient 1 and simpler, in terms of diagnostic criteria, for Patient 2.

for both patients from all the applications. The app's interface is pretty basic, the questionnaire is very straightforward, and it provides results in 90 seconds.

The results of MayaMD are attached (Figure 16.14) in the Diagnoses section.

16.3.5 WebMD

The WebMD app has many integrated features integrated. It provides users with multiple services, such as symptom checker, medicine reminders, drug interactions database, allergy tracker, and pill identifier. It also includes up-to-date articles about the most recent innovations in the medical field. On selecting the symptom checker option, we are presented with a rather simple interface, which asks about the age and gender of the user (Figure 16.15). After that, it provides a body-map of sorts to assist in entering symptoms. It then shows the results in the next step. It has one of the simplest workflows, which does not require a pictorial depiction for its analysis.

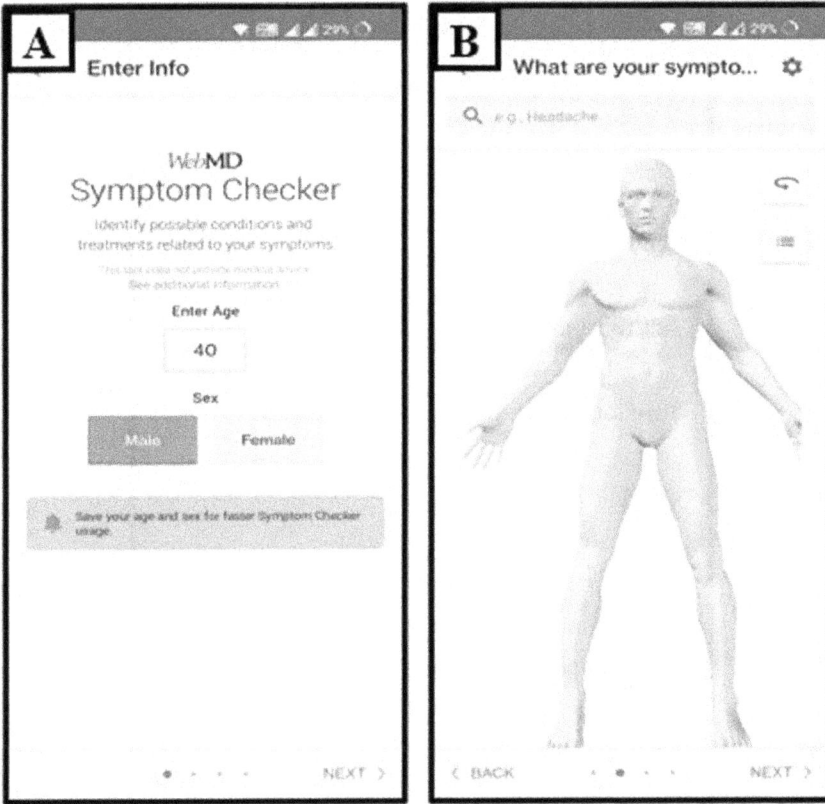

FIGURE 16.15   Illustrating the interface of WebMD app. (A) Window for inputting the age and gender of the user. (B) Window for entering the symptom afflicting the user. A figure is also provided, on which the user can select the part of the body affected, which will provide them with multiple options of symptoms to choose from.

16.3.5.1   Working

WebMD has the most straightforward procedure and result interface. It displays the strength of the results and their likelihood. Since WebMD does not take pre-existing conditions into consideration while dealing with the immediate symptom, the two-patient trial strategy to understand the functioning of this app is not viable here. Only one patient with the headache symptom is selected for the trial (Figure 16.16).

16.4   COMPARISON OF OUTPUTS FROM HEALTHCARE APPS

In this section, the results of the different apps that were evaluated are depicted in a cumulated manner. There is a huge difference in the way the results are displayed by each app. There are varying degrees of explanation and statistics provided by each app. As a common theme, the possible diagnosis is displayed as the probability

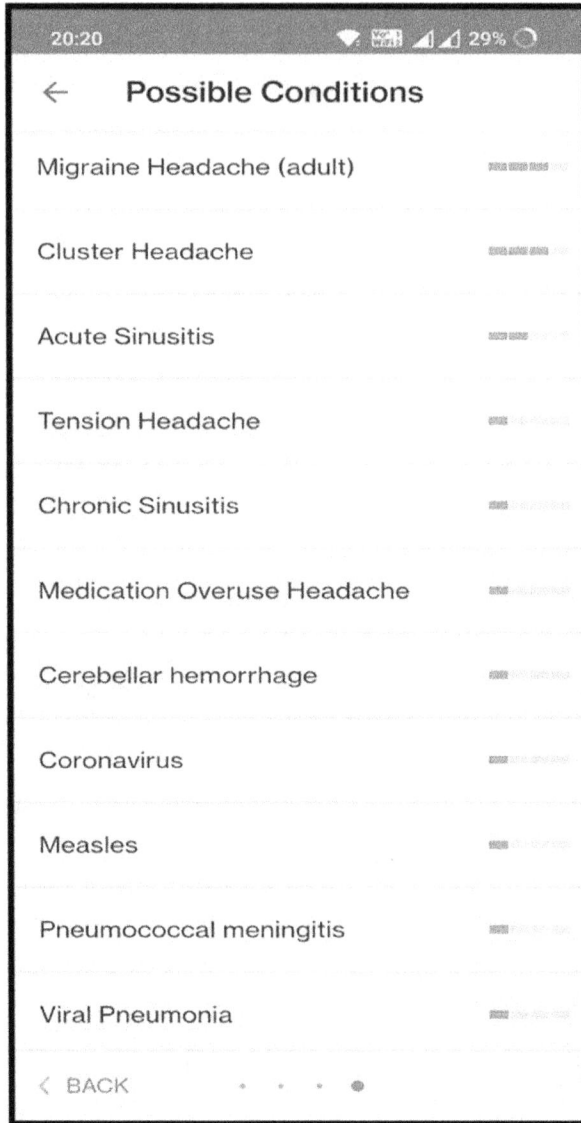

FIGURE 16.16 The results for WebMD are displayed. Due to the lack of input of pre-existing conditions, the diagnoses are extremely varied, ranging from common conditions.

of whether the patient has that condition. A basic comparison of the apps is presented in Table 16.1. The difference in the workflows of the apps can be elucidated by the variability in their introductory questions, the number of questions asked, and the representation of the diagnoses recommended. As observed from the consensus workflow (Figure 16.17), each app broadly follows a common path. The objective is

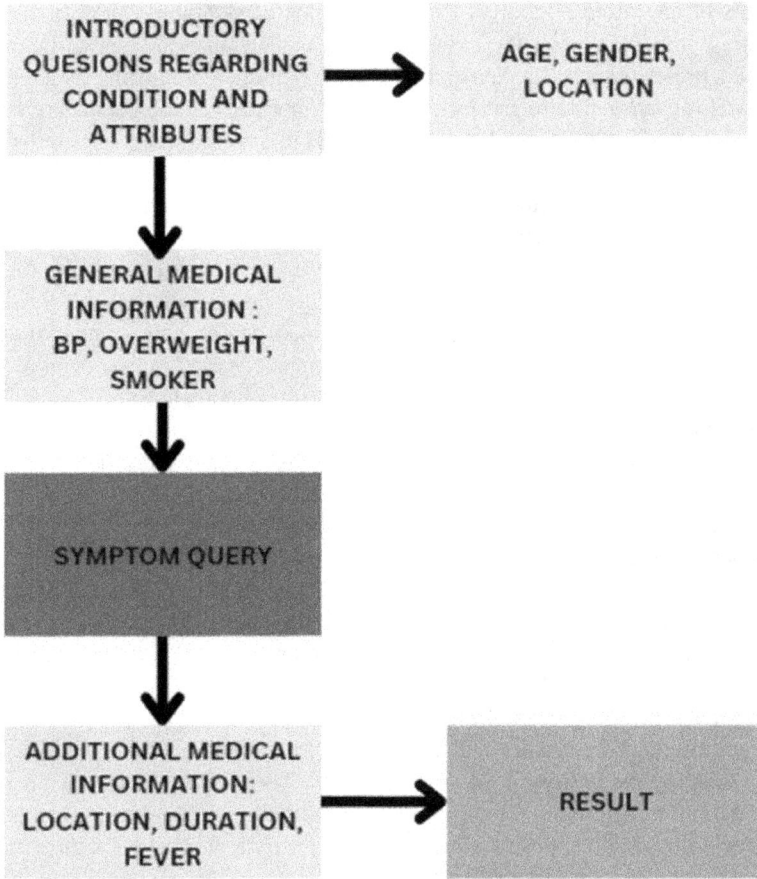

FIGURE 16.17 A consensus workflow is depicted. There is a high degree of similarity in the workflows of the apps. The immediate symptoms along with pre-existing conditions are entered to create a symptomatic profile of the patient. The red box denotes the entry of the most debilitating symptom, while the green box denotes the results.

to ascertain the diagnostic profile of the user, based on the input which contains the afflicting symptom and pre-existing condition.

16.5 CONCLUSION

Digital health is an umbrella term that covers many eHealth aspects. mHealth is a subset of digital health which refers to the utilization of mobile devices for improving public health. mHealth along with various other fields, such as telehealth, telemedicine, digital health, etc., makes up technology-enabled care. It is defined as the integration of technological techniques into healthcare to meet the needs of the people.

Diagnosis of any disease involves the identification of symptoms by an individual, performing clinical tests on the individual, the verification of disease afflicting the individual, prescribing medication and treatment plans, and monitoring for any future changes. However, due to recent lockdowns and shortages in the healthcare field, it was extremely difficult for people to visit hospitals to undergo treatment for diseases. The integration of digital healthcare in the medical field can help tackle this problem. Medical professionals can augment their diagnosis by utilizing digital health devices. A person can perform a diagnostic test of their symptom at their home using mHealth applications, without visiting a diagnostician and limiting their exposure to the contaminants present in the hospital. However, there are many challenges that the digital health industry needs to overcome. The need for high-quality data is one of the main technical obstacles in the creation of healthcare apps powered by AI. A lot of high-quality data is needed to train AI algorithms. This information must be representative of various patient populations and include information on a wide range of illnesses, symptoms, and treatments. It can be difficult to create AI algorithms that are accurate and inclusive, though, because medical data is frequently fragmented, siloed, and hard to access. The requirement to make the algorithms transparent and understandable presents another technical challenge. Understanding how a particular diagnosis or treatment recommendation is reached by an AI algorithm is essential in the healthcare industry. This is crucial to ensure the algorithms are trustworthy and safe, as well as to foster trust among patients, healthcare professionals, and the creators of AI-based healthcare apps. Explainable AI is a topic that is still being researched, but it is a difficult one that needs to be developed further.

The requirement for privacy and security in the creation of healthcare apps powered by AI presents another technical challenge. These apps frequently deal with private patient information, which needs to be shielded from unauthorized access. This necessitates the creation of effective data security and encryption measures, as well as adherence to laws like HIPAA and GDPR.

Another technical issue that requires attention is interoperability. With various data standards and communication protocols, healthcare systems are frequently complicated and fragmented. AI-based healthcare apps must be able to communicate effectively with healthcare providers and be able to work with current healthcare systems in order to be effective.

Last, but not least, creating healthcare apps based on AI necessitates a multidisciplinary strategy that involves experts in medicine, data science, computer science, and engineering. It can be difficult to effectively collaborate and communicate between various teams, but this is necessary.

There has been a huge surge in the number of healthcare apps produced and used by people, possibly due to the COVID-19 pandemic. The large volume of apps available makes it confusing for people to decide which app to select for their needs. As we can see from the above sections, there is a huge variability in the workflows and results of each app. We can create a consensus workflow for easier analysis and interpretation. The basis of all symptom-checking apps is working on textual data provided by the users. The app correlates the textual with the medical knowledge base present in the app. This leads to a huge variability in results, as seen above.

The questions asked by the apps were framed extremely differently to obtain medical data, and this ambiguous nature of the questioning leads to a difference in the understanding of the condition.

In the current work, it was observed that Ada is one of the most sophisticated and user-friendly apps. It provided the greatest number of diagnoses and has one of the most diverse medical knowledge bases supporting the application. Symptomate and Mediktor have the added benefit of asking the user to input their geographical location to account for regional diseases and endemics. WebMD has one of the fastest computation times and least complex workflows. However, further development in this field is possible by assimilating clinical test values as input and integrating more detailed patient history into the healthcare app algorithms.

16.6   DISCUSSION

In the current work, the functioning of different symptom-checking apps was analyzed and recorded. There is a high degree of variability in the diagnoses provided by the apps which is apparent due to differences in their functioning and knowledge bases. The chosen apps reported different outcomes on patient profiles, which will cause confusion for the user. The apps utilize text-based data entered by the user, combined with the pre-defined options available on their portal. The user selects the options provided on the interface of the mobile app in the form of a question. This questionnaire is based on the knowledge base of the app and the algorithm used in its functioning. These apps can take a further take by assimilating new features like accepting clinical values from the user, i.e., their bioassay references (LFTs, KFTs, etc.). and adding them to the pre-existing algorithm to optimize them further for individual cases. These values will help in selecting a more specific and accurate diagnosis for the symptoms provided by the user. Providing the user with options containing multiple ranges of values, instead of asking for exact clinical values, will also be beneficial.

Furthermore, a centralization of the database of these apps will help in increasing their usability and utility. For example, a feature called 'Health-locker' can be created, which will help the user in keeping their clinical test reports and hospital visit prescriptions in a single place. A similar initiative has been launched by Ayushman Bharat Digital India, a digital health initiative launched under the Ayushman Bharat program, in conjunction with DigiLocker. As part of the second level of the initiative to integrate Ayushman Bharat and DigiLocker, vaccination records, doctor prescriptions, lab results, hospital discharge summaries, and other health records can now be stored and accessed on the safe cloud-based storage platform of DigiLocker.

The utility of such a repository lies in creating a health record and a customized symptom checker for the user. This will help in keeping track of the comorbidities of the user and help in avoiding conditions such as the Long COVID syndrome (Raveendran et al., 2021), chronic diabetes, hypertension, etc.

Additionally, research and development can be performed on this data by designing guidelines that protect the privacy of the user and the ethicality of using the data. This will help in providing the research community with detailed and specific diagnostic data, which can be used for future clinical studies.

REFERENCES

Ahmadi, H., Arji, G., Shahmoradi, L., Safdari, R., Nilashi, M., & Alizadeh, M. (2019). The application of internet of things in healthcare: A systematic literature review and classification. *Universal Access in the Information Society, 18*(4), 837–869.

Bernstein, C. (2021, March 11). *What is Digital Health (Digital Healthcare) and why is it important?* Health IT. Retrieved December 15, 2022, from https://www.techtarget.com /searchhealthit/definition/digital-health-digital-healthcare.

Blynn, E., & Aubuchon, J. (2009). *Piloting mHealth: A research scan.* Knowledge Exchange Management Sciences for Health.

Buechi, R., Faes, L., Bachmann, L. M., Thiel, M. A., Bodmer, N. S., Schmid, M. K., Job, O., & Lienhard, K. R. (2017). Evidence assessing the diagnostic performance of medical smartphone apps: A systematic review and exploratory meta-analysis. *BMJ Open, 7*(12), e018280.

Conte, A., Lecca, P., Sakkas, S., & Salotti, S. (2020). *The territorial economic impact of COVID-19 in the EU: A RHOMOLO analysis* (No. JRC121261). Joint Research Centre (Seville site).

Deserno, T. M., & Jakob, R. (2020, October). Accident & emergency informatics: Terminologies and standards are needed for digital health in the early rescue chain. In *2020 IEEE 14th international conference on application of information and communication technologies (AICT)* (pp. 1–5). IEEE.

Esteban-Cartelle, H., Gutierrez, R. V., & Fernández-Ferreiro, A. (2017). Technology and telemedicine in hospital pharmacy, it has come to stay.

García-Azorín, D., Do, T. P., Gantenbein, A. R., Hansen, J. M., Souza, M. N. P., Obermann, M., Pohl, H., Schankin, C. J., Schytz, H. W., Sinclair, A., Schoonman, G. G., & Kristoffersen, E. S. (2021). Delayed headache after COVID-19 vaccination: A red flag for vaccine induced cerebral venous thrombosis. *The Journal of Headache and Pain, 22*(1), 1–5.

Gharote, M. S., Sodani, A., Palshikar, G. K., Tibrewala, P. A., Saproo, K., & Bendre, A. (2015). *Efficient vaccine distribution planning using IoT.* TATA Consultancy Services.

Haenlein, M., & Kaplan, A. (2019). A brief history of artificial intelligence: On the past, present, and future of artificial intelligence. *California Management Review, 61*(4), 5–14.

Karan, A., & Wadhera, R. K. (2021). Healthcare system stress due to Covid-19: Evading an evolving crisis. *Journal of Hospital Medicine, 16*(2), 127. https://doi.org/10.12788/jhm .3583.

Kay, M., Santos, J., & Takane, M. (2011). mHealth: New horizons for health through mobile technologies. *World Health Organization, 64*(7), 66–71.

Kuo, M. H. (2011). Opportunities and challenges of cloud computing to improve health care services. *Journal of Medical Internet Research, 13*(3), e1867.

Liu, R., Rong, Y., & Peng, Z. (2020). A review of medical artificial intelligence. *Global Health Journal, 4*(2), 42–45.

Lupton, D. (2014). Critical perspectives on digital health technologies. *Sociology Compass, 8*(12), 1344–1359.

Millenson, M. L., Baldwin, J. L., Zipperer, L., & Singh, H. (2018). Beyond dr. Google: The evidence on consumer-facing digital tools for diagnosis. *Diagnosis, 5*(3), 95–105.

Moharana, M., Pandey, M., & Routaray, S. S. (2020). Why big data, and what it is: Basics to advanced big data journey for the medical industry. In Edited by Valentina Emilia Balas, *Handbook of data science approaches for biomedical engineering* (pp. 221–249). Academic Press.

Nadarzynski, T., Miles, O., Cowie, A., & Ridge, D. (2019). Acceptability of artificial intelligence (AI)-led chatbot services in healthcare: A mixed-methods study. *Digital Health, 5*, 2055207619871808.

Narayan, S., Gagné, M., & Safavi-Naini, R. (2010, October). Privacy preserving EHR system using attribute-based infrastructure. In *Proceedings of the 2010 ACM workshop on cloud computing security workshop* (pp. 47–52).

Raveendran, A. V., Jayadevan, R., & Sashidharan, S. (2021). Long COVID: An overview. *Diabetes and Metabolic Syndrome: Clinical Research and Reviews*, *15*(3), 869–875.

Stovner, L. J., Hagen, K., Linde, M., & Steiner, T. J. (2022). The global prevalence of headache: An update, with analysis of the influences of methodological factors on prevalence estimates. *The Journal of Headache and Pain*, *23*(1), 1–17.

The Lancet Oncology. (2018). Digital oncology apps: Revolution or evolution? *The Lancet Oncology*, *19*(8), 999. https://doi.org/10.1016/S1470-2045(18)30542-4.

Vidhyalakshmi, A., & Priya, C. (2020). Medical big data mining and processing in e-health care. In Edited by Min Chen, *An industrial IoT approach for pharmaceutical industry growth* (pp. 1–30). Academic Press.

Wang, Q., Su, M., Zhang, M., & Li, R. (2021). Integrating digital technologies and public health to fight Covid-19 pandemic: Key technologies, applications, challenges and outlook of digital healthcare. *International Journal of Environmental Research and Public Health*, *18*(11), 6053.

World Health Organization. (2019). *WHO guideline: Recommendations on digital interventions for health system strengthening: Web supplement 2: Summary of findings and GRADE tables* (No. WHO/RHR/19.7). World Health Organization.

17 Machine Learning-Based Decision Support System for Optimal Treatment of Acute Inflammation Response with Specific Patient Conditions

Selami Beyhan and Meriç Çetin

17.1 INTRODUCTION

Mathematical modelling has been recently addressed for many diseases with non-linear time-varying dynamics and multiple-equilibrium points. These mathematical models of diseases can be used to predict the future dynamics of the diseases as well as to design a model-based controller. Therefore, control-theoretic approaches have been recently applied for the drug dosage regulation of serious diseases to achieve a desired treatment period including diabetes, tuberculosis, HIV, COVID-19, etc. [1].

It is known that inflammation is a pathological cause of many diseases [2, 3]. The cause of a pathogenic bacterial infection is invading bacteria and secreted inflammatory mediators [4]. Serious diseases, such as COVID-19, autoimmune diseases, arthritis, chronic respiratory disease, inflammatory bowel, psoriasis, coronary heart diseases, psychological disorders, neurological diseases, or cancer etc., are examined and treated on the basis of inflammation [5, 6]. The response of the immune system to such a pathogenic infection occurs as inflammation [7, 8]. Inflammation control becomes more important [9], especially in critical diseases, as inflammation damages the infected tissues. According to the response of the autoimmune system, the inflammation that damages the tissues can be eliminated with the infusion of anti-inflammatory drugs [10]. Delayed therapy may reduce the patient's chances of survival [11]. Therefore, it is necessary to optimize the treatment for critical conditions. Anti-inflammatory control based on drug infusion is important in terms of providing less costly and more effective pharmaceutical treatments [12]. In the literature, there are several studies on the solution of the inflammation control problem.

DOI: 10.1201/9781003363361-17

Day et al. designed a non-linear model predictive controller [4] to specify appropriate treatments for *in silico* patients with inflammatory disease]. Bara et al. presented an optimal controller [13] for anti-inflammatory treatment. Rigatos et al. developed state estimation [14] for a non-linear acute inflammatory model using the particle filter.]. Hogg et al. presented a non-linear controller [12] for acute inflammation that describes the reaction to bacterial infection.

Reinforcement learning (RL) is a machine learning method that constructs human-like decision-makers without the need for system information, so that actions, rewards, and states are enough to build a reinforcement agent [15]. It solves the dynamic programming problem with a different learning mechanism which designs its actions based on reactions from the environment, receives a reward value based on its interaction with the environment to perform the learning process, and finds the best behaviour to maximize it [16]. Due to its sophisticated learning mechanism, reinforcement learning-based strategies have been utilized for accurate treatments of diseases. In addition, the treatment processes can be planned for different goals, such as minimizing the total amount of drugs to reduce the damage caused by serious side effects or effectively increasing the number of healthy cells. Martín-Guerrero et al. used a reinforcement learning approach [17] for personalized anemia management with a chronic renal failure. A patient-specific anaesthesia problem was solved in [18] and an optimal insulin injection policy has been proposed for the control of blood glucose with type one diabetes in [19]. Liu et al. have proposed deep learning models [20] that detect lung cancer. Recently, a comprehensive review of the reinforcement learning treatment of diabetic control and anaemia has been presented in [21]. An intelligent system based on reinforcement learning that can provide automatic assistance to patients whose treatment process needs to be followed at home was presented in [22].

Following that, the main goal of this chapter is to improve the learning capability of reinforcement agents by the design of experiments and particular reward functions for the stabilization of AIR in septic and aseptic cases. The reinforcement agents are rewarded based on the recovered tissue, such that they learn how to produce the drug dosages under the limits of inflammation dynamics. Dynamic Q-learning and radial basis function-based value approximation agents are designed to learn and face some important patient-specific cases. First, reinforcement agents are learned with different initial values of states, some parameters are randomly assigned in the learning phase, and disturbances are added to be uncertainties. Second, some of the treatment dosages are assumed to be zero, to be considered as randomly forgotten treatment times or ineffective drug dosages. These two design scenarios cover many different treatment conditions for the inflammation response. By doing that, it is aimed that the reinforcement agents can robustly learn the treatment behaviour in a general sense under severe conditions. For the learning capability of the agents, novel reward-value functions are proposed under unknown disturbances and ineffective treatment periods for optimal treatments. Drug dosage levels are generated in discrete levels for practical application in medicine. In computational results, the treatment results of aseptic and septic death cases are shown, where the proposed reward-value functions are compared for the effectiveness of agents in terms of root-mean-squared performances of state stabilization, applied drug dosage amounts, and maximum value of the states.

17.2 MATHEMATICAL MODELLING OF ACUTE INFLAMMATORY RESPONSE

The mathematical model of acute inflammatory response (AIR) [8] – inflammation caused by various pathogenic factors – is as follows.

$$
\begin{aligned}
\dot{P} &= k_{pg}P\left(1-\frac{P}{P_\infty}\right)-\frac{k_{pm}s_m P}{\mu_m+k_{mp}P}-k_{pn}f\left(N^*\right)P,\\
\dot{N^*} &= \frac{s_{nr}R}{\mu_{nr}+R}-\mu_n N^*+u_p(t),\\
\dot{D} &= k_{dn}\frac{f^6\left(N^*\right)}{x_{dn}^6+f^6\left(N^*\right)}-\mu_d D,
\end{aligned}
\tag{17.1}
$$

$$
\dot{C_A}=s_c+k_{cn}\frac{f\left(N^*+k_{cnd}D\right)}{1+f\left(N^*+k_{cnd}D\right)}-\mu_c C_a+u_a(t),
\tag{17.2}
$$

with

$$
R=f\left(k_{np}P+k_{nn}N^*+k_{nd}D\right),
\tag{17.3}
$$

and

$$
f(x)=\frac{x}{1+(\frac{C_A}{C_\infty})^2}
\tag{17.4}
$$

where P stands for the pathogen population responsible for causing inflammation, N^* relates to the activated phagocytes that manage inflammation and the early pro-inflammatory mediators produced by N^*, D symbolizes the tissue damage, while C_A represents anti-inflammatory mediators (such as cortisol and interleukin-10) [23]. The production of the anti-inflammatory mediator directly alleviates inflammation by preventing excessive tissue damage caused by severe inflammation. The input values u_a and u_p are used for anti-inflammatory and pro-inflammatory therapy, respectively. The term $f(x)$ in (4) represents the influence of activated phagocytes on the development of damaged tissue. Parameters of the AIR model are given in [8]. There are three stable equilibrium points in the AIR model: a healthy case, an aseptic case, and a septic case [23]. In the healthy scenario, P,N^*,D are equal to zero and C_A is at the background level. In the aseptic case, N^*,C_A,D mediators are elevated and pathogen P has been eliminated. In the septic case, all mediators $\left(N^*, C_A, D\right)$ with pathogen P are at high levels.

17.3   REINFORCEMENT LEARNING-BASED TREATMENT

Reinforcement learning is an approximate solution to the dynamic programming problem. Dynamic programming is concerned with predicting what will happen in the process before making the next decision when deciding about any state. In these changes, decisions cannot be evaluated independently, and a balance is considered between the current cost and the total cost. For the stochastic problem that aims to improve long-term performance by sacrificing short-term performance, an agent's decision-making mechanism is modelled by the Markov decision process (MDP) [16]. In RL, the agent designs its actions based on the reactions from the environment. The environment is often modelled as an MDP defined by a series of states, actions, transition probabilities, and expected values. The policy function learns the dynamics based on the environmental rewards of the corresponding actions. After enough trials and learning, the agent selects the best action to maximize the reward for optimal decision-making. According to these definitions, a finite MDP is expressed in a group of mathematical terms $\left(S, A, P, R\right)$, as follows.

1. Set of states: $S = s_1, s_2, \ldots, s_N$ where $s \in S$,
2. Action set: $A = a_1, a_2, \ldots, a_n$ where $a \in A$,
3. State transition probabilities (action to be taken in s state): $P_{sa}\left(.\right) \in \{0,1\}$

where $P: S \times A \times S \rightarrow \left[0,1\right]$, discount factor: $\gamma \in \left[0,1\right)$,

4. Reward function (limited by absolute r_{max}.): where $R: S \times A \rightarrow \mathbb{R}$.

The main elements of MDP are the policy, the reward function, the value function, and the model of the environment [16]. In Figure 17.1, the general schematic representation of the MDP is depicted.

In MDP, the agent based on one of the states $(s_t \in S)$ takes one of the actions $(a_t \in A)$ for every t discrete time. The environment rewards the agent who switched to s_{t+1} because of the selected action a_t with r_t.

$$
\begin{aligned}
r_t &= r\left(s_t, a_t\right), \\
s_{t+1} &= \delta\left(s_t, a_t\right).
\end{aligned}
\tag{17.5}
$$

It can be assumed that the functions $r\left(.\right)$ and $\delta\left(.\right)$ are initially deterministic and a part of the environment. The agent does not need to know these functions. The solution of the MDP or the strategy that the agent should achieve its process-related policy $\pi: S \rightarrow A$. The policy is represented by a lookup table or a function that can be stochastic or deterministic [16]. The task of this policy is to ensure that the next-most appropriate action is selected, depending on the current observed state, i.e., $\pi\left(s_t\right) = a_t$. The most important question is how the agent will learn this plan. One of

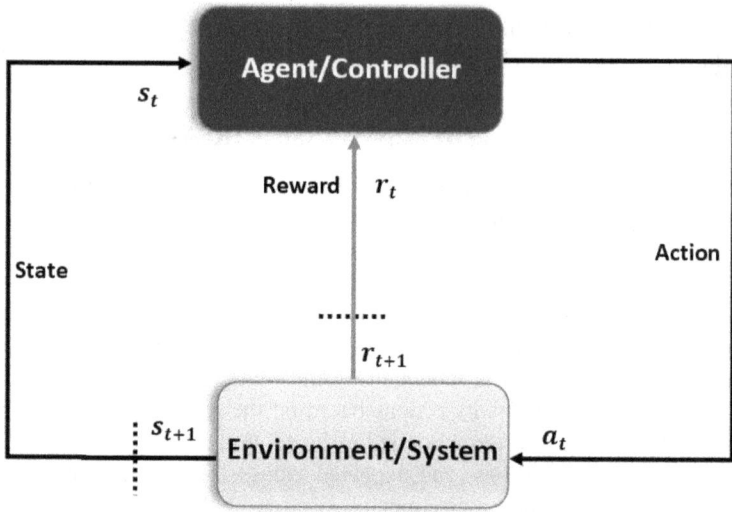

FIGURE 17.1   The general block diagram of the MDP.

the solutions to the decision-making problem in the MDP is the selection of the policy that constitutes the biggest cumulative reward. The cumulative reward value obtained with the π of the system starting at s_t is defined as $G(s_t) = r_t + \gamma r_{t+1} + \gamma^2 r_{t+2} + \ldots$, where $0 \le \gamma \le 1$ is the discount factor. The value function calculates how the agent will be good in each state. Two functions – state value ($V^\pi(s)$) and action value ($Q^\pi(s,a)$) – are utilized to predict the future reward. According to [16], the state-value function is preferred when one has knowledge of the environment/system model, and the action-value function is preferred when it is a model-free concept. $V^\pi(s)$ is defined under policy π as

$$V^\pi(s_t) = \sum_{i=0}^{\infty} \gamma^i r_{t+i}. \tag{17.6}$$

The optimal policy (π^*) that must be obtained because of learning is the policy that maximizes the cumulative reward. $V^*(s)$ that is an optimal state-value function can be expressed as

$$V^*(s) = \max_{\pi} \; V^\pi(s), \tag{17.7}$$

$$\forall s \in S.$$

In addition, the optimal action-value function is

$$Q^*(s,a) = \max_{\pi} \; Q^\pi(s,a), \tag{17.8}$$

$$\forall s \in S, \quad \forall a \in A.$$

Regardless of the initial state and decision, according to Bellman's optimality criterion in dynamic programming, all decisions must be an optimal policy. The Bellman optimality equation is expressed as

$$V^*(s) = \max_{\pi}\left(r(s_t, a_t) + \gamma V^*\left(\delta(s_t, a_t)\right)\right). \tag{17.9}$$

When the Markov decision process is exactly modelled, which means that the transition possibilities and rewards are known, Bellman's optimality approach is expected to produce a general solution. In real-time applications, due to the MDP not being modelled exactly, this solution cannot be applicable. Instead, it is preferable to develop a method through policy iteration and value iteration while trial-and-error continues randomly online. Q-learning is an off-policy Temporal difference (TD) learning method [24]. TD optimizes control through the experiences gained from episodes, in which the agent moves from an initial state to a target state by making stochastic decisions. In RL, when the number of states, actions, and transitions are known, then, for a certain number of episodes, the reward function is assumed to be able to sweep almost all the space with random trials from a starting point. As a result of these trials, a lookup table or value function containing the optimal plan to be followed is created according to the obtained experience.

Tabular reinforcement learning techniques are designed for scenarios where there is a limited number of states and actions, allowing the value function to be represented as a lookup table where each state corresponds to an input. The value-update rule for $TD(\lambda)$ is written as

$$V(s_t) \leftarrow V(s_t) + \alpha \sum_{k=t}^{\infty} \lambda^{k-t}\left[r_{t+1} + \gamma V(s_{t+1}) - V(s_t)\right], \tag{17.10}$$

$$\lambda < 1, \quad 0 < \alpha < 1.$$

α is the learning rate and the term $r_{t+1} + \gamma V(s_{t+1}) - V(s_t)$ is the temporal-difference error. In $TD(\lambda)$ learning, the reward update is performed with Equation 17.10, while the action selection is randomly advanced and is the basis for direct-approximation methods. Then, Q-learning has been proposed by improving the policy update.

$$Q(s_t, a_t) \leftarrow Q(s_t, a_t) + \alpha\left[r_{t+1} + \gamma \max_{a_{t+1}} Q(s_{t+1}, a_{t+1}) - Q(s_t, a_t)\right]. \tag{17.11}$$

Q-learning greedily develops the policy regarding action values by maximum operator and the agent does not need to know any δ or r functions of the MDP. Function approximation-based methods are utilized to solve the curse of dimensionality when infinite states or actions exist. Continuous state-based discrete-action RL is most suitable for the treatment of AIR. Based on TD learning, radial functions-based value approximations are designed for ten levels of dosages. In RL that relies on value approximation, the experiences are utilized to refine a value function that provides an approximate evaluation of the optimal policy [25]. Tabular methods may not generalize problems involving very large states and/or actions, and value approximation-based RL can be preferred for problems that require fast convergence. The value function is commonly approximated as a set of basis functions:

$$\phi(s_t) = \left[\phi_1(s_t) \quad \phi_2(s_t)\ldots \quad \phi_n(s_t) \right] \tag{17.12}$$

where $\phi_i : S \to \mathbb{R}$ are the basis functions. In radial basis function representation, $\phi_i(s) = e^{-\frac{\|c_i - s\|^2}{2\sigma^2}}$. c_i and σ are the centre and width of the radial basis functions, respectively. Radial basis functions are suitable to represent value functions that may have discontinuities as they generalize locally [26]. Using a linear combination of features, value functions are approximated as

$$\hat{V}(s_t, w) = \phi^T(s_t) w = \sum_{j=1}^{n} \phi_j(s) w_j \tag{17.13}$$

where $w = \begin{bmatrix} w_1 & w_2 \ldots w_m \end{bmatrix}$ are known as the tunable weights of the function approximator that are updated with optimization techniques. Update rules such as gradient descent are used in function approximation. In order to minimize the objective function, the negative direction of the gradient vector $\left(J(w) = \left[\dfrac{\partial F(w)}{\partial w_1} \quad \dfrac{\partial F(w)}{\partial w_2} \ldots \dfrac{\partial F(w)}{\partial w_n} \right] \right)$ is chosen as the search direction. An update step is calculated as " $w = -\dfrac{1}{2} \alpha J(w)$. Function approximators can be used for state-action values such that $\hat{Q}(s_t, a_t, w) \approx Q(s_t, a_t)$. Then, policy evaluation is performed by using $\hat{Q}(s_t, a_t, w)$. The objective function is defined as

$$F(w) = \mathbb{E} \left[Q(s_t, a_t) - \hat{Q}(s_t, a_t, w)^2 \right]. \tag{17.14}$$

Finally, the target is formulated by the maximum TD target as

$$" w = \alpha \left[r_{t+1} + \gamma \max_{a_{t+1}} \hat{Q}(s_{t+1}, a_{t+1}, w) - \hat{Q}(s_t, a_t, w) \right] \nabla_w \hat{Q}(s_t, a_t, w). \tag{17.15}$$

17.3.1 Proposed Reward Value Functions

Remember that when the large state-action space and a high number of unknowns make it impossible to find the exact solution of MDP, reinforcement learning is used by assuming equal transition probabilities and particularly chosen reward values. In the literature, different constant values are used to reward the reinforcement models; however, there is no detailed discussion and comparison for the management of treatments.

It is known that reward values directly affect the learning behaviour of the reinforcement models. In general, reward values are defined as discrete pairs of zero and one for planning and strategical applications. For continuous problems, reward

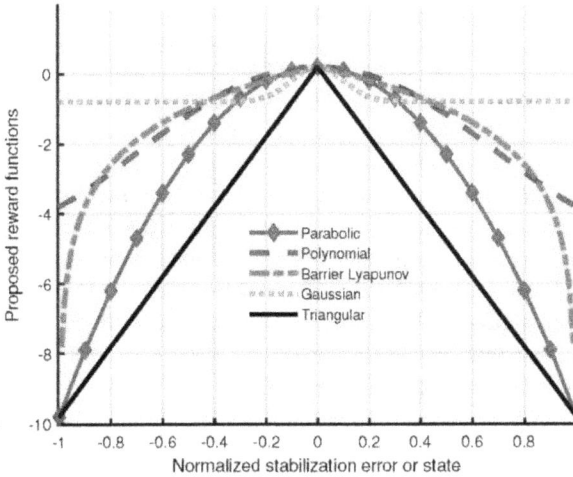

FIGURE 17.2 Proposed reward functions for stabilization. (a) Random disturbance. (b) Ineffective or forgotten drug times.

values are based on the function of the states. In this chapter, the reinforcement learning models are being taught the treatment of the AIR by the following reward value functions. The proposed reward functions for stabilization are illustrated in Figure 17.2. The maximum reward function values are designed as 0.2 when it is close to zero, to improve convergence behaviour.

Case 1: Parabolic function

$$r(e) = -10e^2 + 0.2,$$ (17.16)

Case 2: Polynomial function

$$r(e) = 2e^4 - 6e^2 + 0.2,$$ (17.17)

Case 3: Barrier Lyapunov function

$$r(e) = 0.2 - log(\rho / (\rho - |e|)^2),$$ (17.18)

Case 4: Gaussian function

$$r(e) = exp(-0.5(e / \sigma)^2) - 0.8,$$ (17.19)

Case 5: Triangular function

$$r(e) = \begin{cases} 0.2 + 10e & \text{if} \quad e < 0, \\ 0.2 - 10e & \text{if} \quad e \geq 0 \end{cases}$$ (17.20)

17.4 COMPUTATIONAL RESULTS

In this section, treatment results with and without disturbance conditions have been investigated respectively for the septic and aseptic death cases. A one-hour sampling time is chosen to be clinically feasible and the initial conditions and parameters vary, corresponding to the septic and aseptic cases. k_{pg} makes it challenging for conventional control methods to manage septic situations. However, the proposed controllers here control both cases efficiently, even under disturbances and ineffective treatment periods. Ineffective treatment samples and disturbances have also been taken into consideration to represent ineffective and forgotten drug uptake, to make a therapy plan compatible with the clinical data which are illustrated in Figure 17.3.

For the reinforcement learning models, $\alpha = 0.9$, $\gamma = 1$, $\epsilon = 0.3$, the simulation period is 240 hours and the number of episodes is selected as 1000. The state vector of the tabular reinforcement model is defined in two-dimensional vector as $\left[N^*, C_A \right]$ where the discrete state-space is constructed linearly spaced in $\left[0,2 \right]$ with ten discrete levels. The action vector, i.e., drug dosage level, is defined linearly spaced in $\left[0,1 \right]$ with five discrete levels. In all simulations, the anti-inflammatory drug is ended around 50th hour, since the pathogen is already minimized and the inflammation is therefore left to the autonomous form. In addition, the limits of the states are thought of in the reinforcement learning models as $\left[0,2 \right]$ when this limit is exceeded, and a specific reward value function is activated. This means that they are not good actions to be selected in future. For the value approximation-based reinforcement model, RBF functions of ten actions are selected with centres linearly spaced in $\left[0,1 \right]$.

The pathogen growth rate (k_{pg}) in AIR dynamics is an important parameter for inflammation control. The smaller values of the k_{pg} correspond to the aseptic case in AIR, while larger values of k_{pg} represent the septic case. In the septic case, where the pathogen level exceeds the threshold value, inflammation control becomes difficult and a treatment with a strong pro-inflammatory component is required to prevent

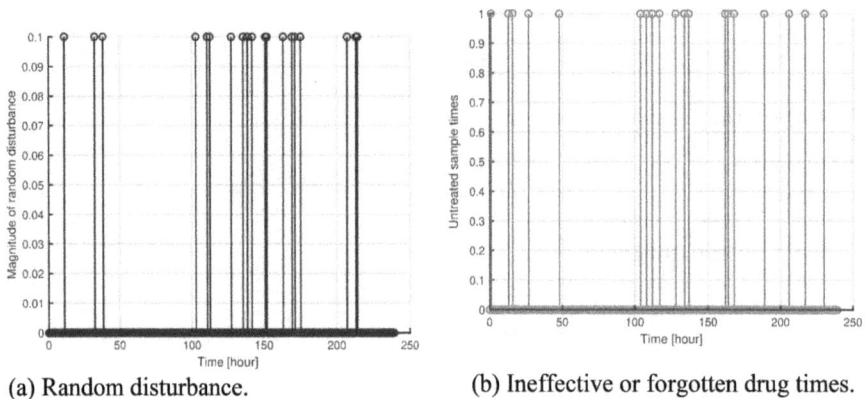

(a) Random disturbance.   (b) Ineffective or forgotten drug times.

FIGURE 17.3 The random disturbances and ineffective treatment samples used for aseptic and septic death cases.

septic consequences. Therefore, in this chapter, dynamic Q-learning for the aseptic case and value approximation-based reinforcement learning for the septic case were designed.

17.4.1 ASEPTIC DEATH CASE: DYNAMIC Q-LEARNING-BASED TREATMENTS

In simulations for the AIR model, the measured output states and the applied control dosages are assumed in discrete levels. If the inflammation dynamics exceed their limits, it is crucial to restore the patient to a healthy case using optimal treatment, or the immune system will be unable to counteract the increased pathogen attack. The initial conditions of these variables are taken as $P = 1.5, N^* = 0, D = 0, C_A = 0.125$, and $k_{pg} = 0.3$, respectively. The numerical values related to dynamic Q-learning-based inflammation control for an aseptic case without disturbance and ineffective treatment samples have been illustrated in Figure 17.4. Figure 17.4a and Figure 17.4b show stabilized variables of the AIR for the aseptic scenario. u_a and u_p therapy

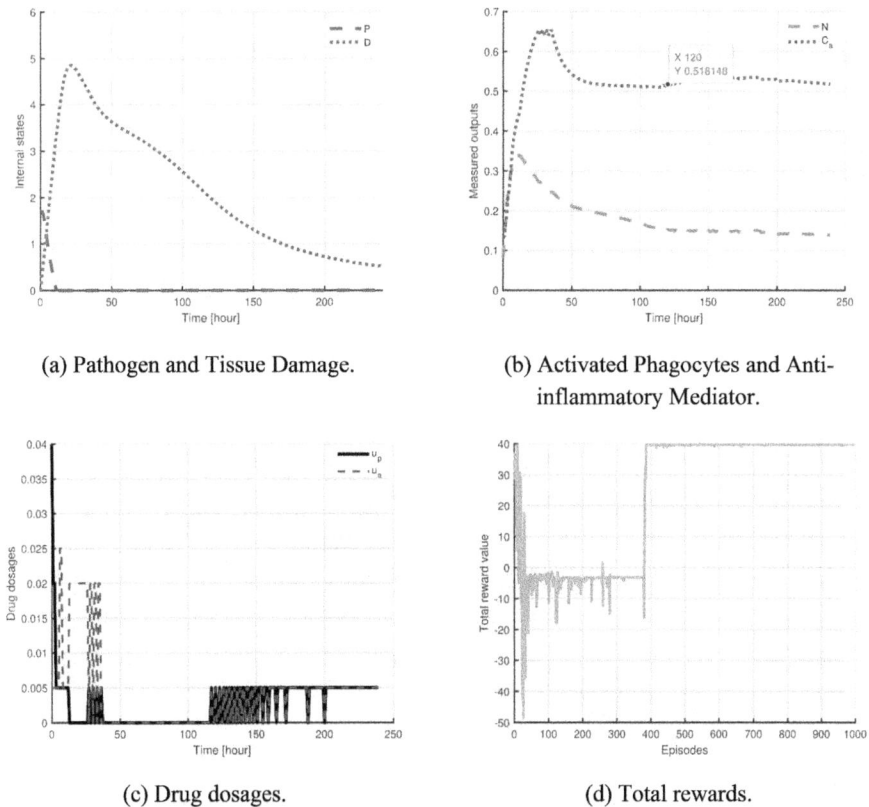

(a) Pathogen and Tissue Damage.

(b) Activated Phagocytes and Anti-inflammatory Mediator.

(c) Drug dosages.

(d) Total rewards.

FIGURE 17.4 Aseptic death case without disturbance and ineffective treatment samples: dynamic Q-learning control.

signals obtained with no disturbance are shown in Figure 17.4c. The stabilization results for aseptic cases with disturbance and ineffective treatment samples have been illustrated in Figure 17.5. The stabilized dynamics of AIR have been given in Figure 17.5a and Figure 17.5b, respectively. Drug dosage inputs are illustrated in Figure 17.5c. Total reward values for the aseptic death case are given in Figure 17.4d and Figure 17.5d, respectively.

17.4.2 SEPTIC DEATH CASE: RBF VALUE APPROXIMATION-BASED TREATMENTS

Value approximation-based RL is preferred when there are infinite states of continuous time systems. When the inflammation dynamics exceed their limits in the septic case, value approximation-based RL aims to minimize P and D levels by using the lowest drug doses. The initial conditions are chosen as $P = 1, N^* = 0, D = 0, C_A = 0.125$, $k_{pg} = 0.6$ for the septic scenario parameters of the AIR model. The value approximation-based reinforcement learning inflammation control results for the septic

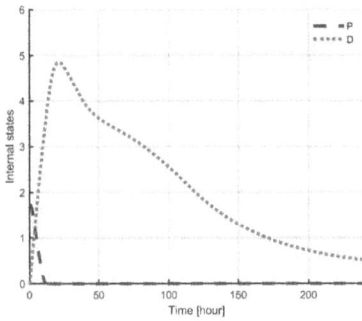

(a) Pathogen and Tissue Damage.

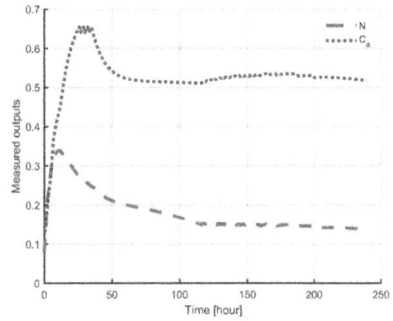

(b) Activated Phagocytes and Anti-inflammatory Mediator.

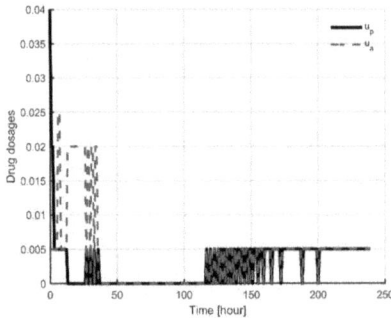

(c) Drug dosages.

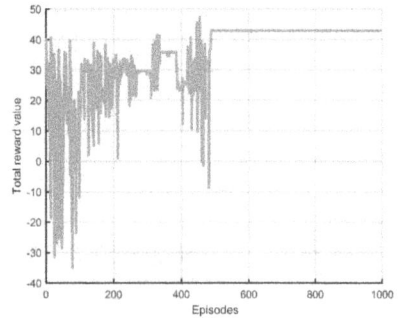

(d) Total rewards.

FIGURE 17.5 Aseptic death case with disturbance and ineffective treatment samples: dynamic Q-learning control.

case without disturbance and ineffective treatment samples have been illustrated in Figure 17.6. For the septic case, the dynamics of the AIR obtained are illustrated in Figure 17.6a and Figure 17.6b, respectively. u_a and u_p therapy signals obtained with no disturbance in value approximation-based control are shown in Figure 17.6c. Like the tabular reinforcement learning approach, disturbances were taken into account for a therapy plan compatible with clinical data in value approximation-based reinforcement learning control. The simulation results for the septic case with disturbance and ineffective treatment samples have been illustrated in Figure 17.7. The dynamics of the AIR have been given in Figure 17.7a and Figure 17.7b, respectively. Anti-inflammatory and pro-inflammatory therapy signals are shown in Figure 17.7c. The aim here is to ensure that the P and D disappear as quickly as possible by using these therapies. Total reward values for the septic death case are given in Figure 17.6d and Figure 17.7d.

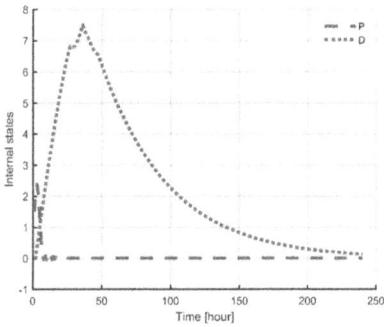

(a) Pathogen and Tissue Damage.

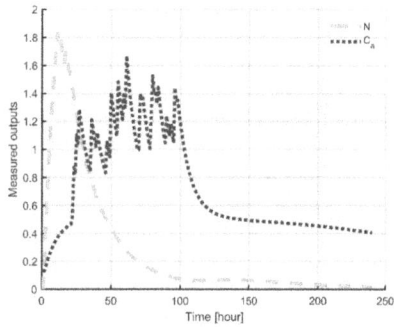

(b) Activated Phagocytes and Antiinflammatory Mediator.

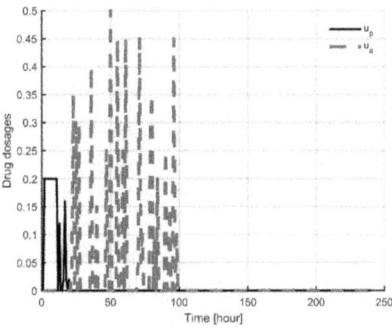

(c) Drug dosages.

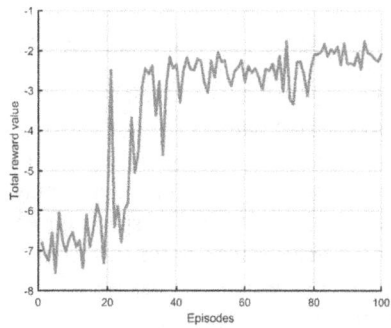

(d) Total rewards.

FIGURE 17.6   Septic death case without disturbance and ineffective treatment samples: RBF value approximation control.

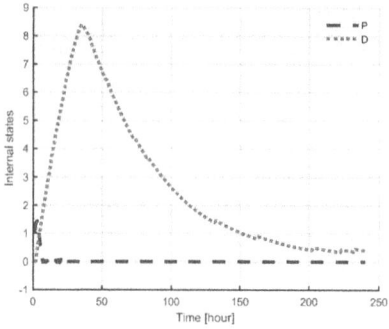

(a) Pathogen and Tissue Damage.

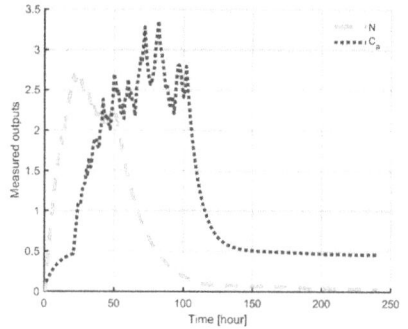

(b) Activated Phagocytes and Anti-inflammatory Mediator.

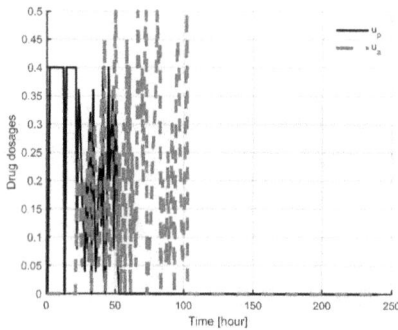

(c) Drug dosages.

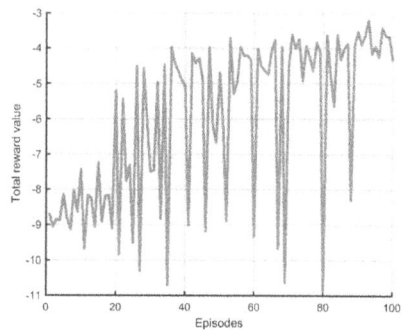

(d) Total rewards.

FIGURE 17.7   Septic death case with disturbance and ineffective treatment samples: RBF value approximation control.

17.5   DISCUSSION AND COMPARISON

The immune response to pathogenic infection or trauma both attempts to eliminate the invasive pathogen threat and promote tissue repair. It is very important to plan patient-specific treatment for rapidly progressing medical conditions such as acute inflammation, as mortality rates may increase when treatment with broad-spectrum drugs is used instead of specific treatment. In this chapter, reinforcement learning-based treatment of acute inflammatory conditions under external disturbances and ineffective treatments has been performed to calculate the optimum drug dose and timing of the treatment, which will strengthen the immune system to prevent possible damage to tissues and lead the patient to a healthy case. The pro-inflammatory mediator and anti-inflammatory mediator reference points are assumed to be around zero for healthy patients. Computational results can be evaluated as follows: it was observed that a large N^* value destroys the pathogen level faster by causing tissue damage. This result activates the anti-inflammatory response (C_A) while reducing the value of N^*. The anti-inflammatory mediator directly abates inflammation by preventing tissue damage produced by inflammation. In this process, the anti-inflammatory therapy signal (u_a) can increase the C_A value and minimize tissue damage while causing pathogen growth. On the other hand, if the pro-inflammatory therapy signal (u_p) rapidly decreases the pathogen while increasing the N^* value, irreparable risks to the organs can occur.

Remember that the rewarding functions are constructed based on the negative power of the stabilization errors for designed reinforcement learning models. In the learning period, maximization of the reward value implies the minimization of the inflammation states or stabilization error. If the reinforcement models are compared in terms of stabilization speed, value approximation models are found to be much faster than the tabular reinforcement models, even though septic dynamics are stabilized. When the disturbance and ineffective treatment periods are added to the damaged state and anti-inflammatory drug dosage, respectively, then the total rewards of both reinforcement models oscillate, since the manifolds corresponding to disturbed states change unexpectedly and new state-action pairs are rewarded, which means that the reinforcement models can sweep larger state-action spaces so that they are ready to make better decisions in large spaces for future patients.

In the stabilization dynamics, the drugs $(u_a$ and $u_p)$ are applied to the N^* and C_A states to compensate the P and D dynamics. Therefore, it is assured that the N^* and C_A converge to zero, but that does not mean that the N^* and C_A stabilized; true control dosages must be chosen. In the results, the P and D states are specially checked for stability. According to Table 17.1, the reward value functions are compared for the maximum state values of the AIR model. The polynomial and Gaussian reward functions provided smaller P and D values, which is important for sensitive patients. For the mean return values of the treatments, the root-mean-squared values of the states and control dosages are shown in Table 17.2.

For the lower amounts of drug dosages, parabolic reward values are suitable for treatment. The triangular reward value is preferable for the smaller stabilization error. Note that these results are to emphasize the details when different dosages are applied and the consequences obtained from sensitive patients. In a general sense, it

TABLE 17.1
Maximum Values of States

Reward Value Functions	P	N^*	D	C_A
Parabolic	1.6853	0.5097	3.9420	0.7533
Polynomial	1.8529	0.8896	5.7766	0.8034
Barrier Lyapunov	1.6853	0.3470	5.3475	0.6613
Gaussian	1.6853	0.4357	3.7150	0.7523
Triangular	1.6853	0.4561	3.9830	0.7533

TABLE 17.2

RMS Values of Stabilization

Reward Value Functions	N^*	C_A	u_a	u_p
Parabolic	0.1059	0.6120	0.0018	0.0220
Polynomial	0.1106	0.5558	0.0028	0.0202
Barrier Lyapunov	0.1220	0.6460	0.0044	0.0283
Gaussian	0.1612	0.6236	0.0074	0.0281
Triangular	0.1095	0.5555	0.0027	0.0202

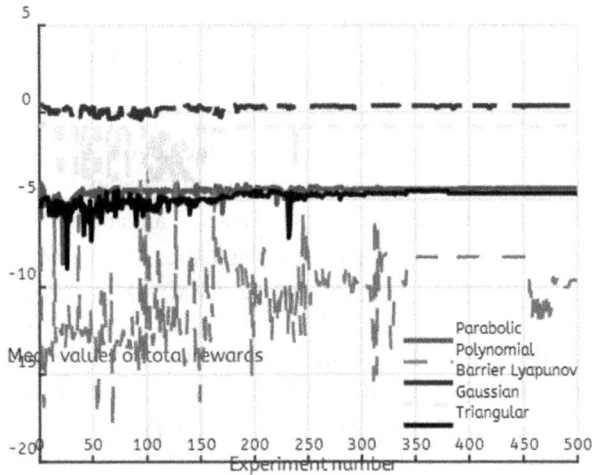

FIGURE 17.8　Mean return values of 500 experiments.

is seen that the convergence of the triangular and parabolic reward-value functions-based reinforcement learning models is fast and more robust compared to the other reinforcement agents. The mean total return values of the treatments corresponding to the mean of the 500 episodes are shown in Figure 17.8. This means that each learning phase is performed by 500 episodes, then, after each learning phase, the results are recorded. The mean return values after 100 epochs are given in the table. To be a fair comparison, the results in the tables are obtained with the same random disturbances and random ineffective treatments.

17.6　CONCLUSIONS

Reinforcement models with novel reward functions were designed to stabilize the inflammatory response dynamics under specific conditions. Computational results based on the proposed treatment models provide a satisfactory level of stabilization performance for possible applications in future. Designed reward-value functions have resulted in different stabilization results that are important for specific patients' conditions. In the future, actor-critic reinforcement models with deep neural network approximations can be designed for policy and value approximations to provide improved treatments for specific conditions of patients.

REFERENCES LIST

1. Cherruault Y. *Mathematical Modelling in Biomedicine: Optimal Control of Biomedical Systems* (Vol. 23). Berlin: Springer Science and Business Media, 2012.
2. Kumar R, Gilles C, Yoram V, Carson CC. "The dynamics of acute inflammation". *Journal of Theoretical Biology*, 230(2), 145–155, 2004.
3. Parker RS, Gilles C. "Systems engineering medicine: Engineering the inflammation response to infectious and traumatic challenges". *Journal of the Royal Society. Interface / The Royal Society*, 7(48), 989–1013, 2010.
4. Day J, Jonathan R, Gilles C. "Using nonlinear model predictive control to find optimal therapeutic strategies to modulate inflammation". *Mathematical Biosciences and Engineering*, 7(4), 739, 2010.
5. Huang Z, Shuang L, Li-li L, Jiao-yang C, Fen L, Wen-cheng Q, Da-ming S, Hans G. "Predicting the morbidity of chronic obstructive pulmonary disease based on multiple locally weighted linear regression model with k-Means clustering". *International Journal of Medical Informatics*, 139, 104141, 2020.
6. Araujo DC, Adriano AV, Karina BGB, Maria GC. "Prognosing the risk of COVID-19 death through a machine learning-based routine blood panel: A retrospective study in Brazil". *International Journal of Medical Informatics*, 165, 104835, 2022.
7. Day J, Chase C, Rami N, Ruben Z, Gary A, Yoram V. "Inflammation and disease: Modelling and modulation of the inflammatory response to alleviate critical illness". *Current Opinion in Systems Biology*, 12, 22–29, 2018.
8. Reynolds A, Jonathan R, Gilles C, Judy D, Yoram V, Bard E. "A reduced mathematical model of the acute inflammatory response: I. derivation of model and analysis of anti-inflammation". *Journal of Theoretical Biology*, 242(1), 220–236, 2006.
9. Bara O, Djouadi SM, Day J, Lenhart S. "Immune therapeutic strategies using optimal controls with L1 and L2 type objectives". *Mathematical Biosciences*, 290, 9–21, 2017.
10. Ramirez-Zuniga I, Jonathan ER, David S, Gilles C. "Mathematical modeling of energy consumption in the acute inflammatory response". *Journal of Theoretical Biology*, 460, 101–114, 2019.
11. Radosavljević V, Kosta R, Zoran O. "A data mining approach for optimization of acute inflammation therapy". *IEEE International Conference on Bioinformatics and Biomedicine*, Philadelphia, October 4–7, 2012.
12. Rigatos G, Krishna B, Abbaszadeh M. "Nonlinear optimal control of the acute inflammatory response". *Biomedical Signal Processing and Control*, 55, 101631, 2020.
13. Bara O, Day J, Djouadi SM. "Optimal control of an inflammatory immune response model". *54th IEEE Conference on Decision and Control*, Osaka, December 15–18, 2015.
14. Hogg JS, Gilles C, Robert SP. "Acute inflammation treatment via particle filter state estimation and mpc". *IFAC Proceedings Volumes*, 43(5), 272–277, 2010.

15. Funk N, Dominik B, Vincent B, Sebastian T. "Learning event-triggered control from data through joint optimization". *IFAC Journal of Systems and Control*, 16, 100144, 2021.
16. Sutton RS, Andrew GB. *Reinforcement Learning: An Introduction*. London: MIT Press, 1998.
17. Martín-Guerrero JD, Faustino G, Emilio SO, Jürgen S, Mónica CM, Víctor JT. "A reinforcement learning approach for individualizing erythropoietin dosages in hemodialysis patients". *Expert Systems with Applications*, 36(6), 9737–9742, 2009.
18. Moore BL, Larry DP, Vivekanand K, Periklis P, Kevin P, Anthony GD. "Reinforcement learning for closed-loop propofol anesthesia: A study in human volunteers". *The Journal of Machine Learning Research*, 15(1), 655–696, 2014.
19. Ngo PD, Susan W, Anna H, Jan M, Fred G. "Reinforcement learning optimal control for type-1 diabetes". *IEEE EMBS International Conference on Biomedical & Health Informatics*, Las Vegas, Nevada, March 4–7, 2018.
20. Liu Z, Chenhui Y, Hang Y, Taihua W. "Deep reinforcement learning with its application for lung cancer detection in medical internet of things". *Future Generation Computer Systems*, 97, 1–9, 2019.
21. Tejedor M, Ashenafi ZW, Fred G. "Reinforcement learning application in diabetes blood glucose control: A systematic review". *Artificial Intelligence in Medicine*, 104, 101836, 2020.
22. Naeem M, Giovanni P, Antonio C. "A reinforcement learning and deep learning based intelligent system for the support of impaired patients in home treatment". *Expert Systems with Applications*, 168, 114285, 2020.
23. Bara O, Michel F, Cédric J, Judy D, Seddik MD. "Toward a model-free feedback control synthesis for treating acute inflammation". *Journal of Theoretical Biology*, 448, 26–37, 2018.
24. Watkins CJCH. "Learning from delayed rewards". PhD thesis, King's College, Cambridge, 1989.
25. Hasselt HV. "Reinforcement learning in continuous state and action spaces". In *Reinforcement Learning*, 207–51, Berlin, Heidelberg: Springer, 2012.
26. Konidaris G, Sarah O, Philip T. "Value function approximation in reinforcement learning using the Fourier basis". *Twenty-Fifth AAAI Conference on Artificial Intelligence*, San Francisco, August 7–11, 2011.

18 Digital Histopathology
Paving Future Directions Towards Predicting Diagnosis of Disease Via Image Analysis

Rishita Singh, Nitu Dogra, Ravina Yadav,
Angamba Meetei Potshangbam,
Deepshikha Pande Katare, and
Ruchi Jakhmola Mani

18.1 INTRODUCTION

Human health is a concept that has continued to be studied for decades to understand the impact or effect of disease at the cellular level and how it affects the body and its immunity. Nowadays, disease is a commonly used word and is referred to as the anomalous condition which negatively affects the structure or function of normal cells and eventually affects the entire organism. It manifests in the body at specific structural and functional levels and has a known cause which develops from genetic or environmental exposure. Depending on certain features, diseases are categorized as acute, in which the start of the disease is abrupt, for a short time span, or chronic, in which a patient may experience months or years of disease-related symptoms (Tizard and Musser, 2022).

Pathology is a fundamental medical discipline that mainly focuses on the visualization of diseased tissues and cells. It is the field that studies the causes and effects of a disease at a cellular level, which is essential for disease diagnosis. From the beginning, the examination of such pathological slides starts with sampling, i.e., collecting samples either during surgery or autopsy, after which the tissue is observed under a microscope. The introduction of digital scanning technologies in bioimaging has been evolving, as there has been a need for more computational methods to analyze a pathological slide, as the microscopic evaluation of cells is still the gold-standard method for classification, especially in tumour pathology. Automatic image analysis and decision making in histopathology is a challenging but promising area of research (Adiga and Chaudhuri, 2000; Meijering, Meijering, 2020). Pathology is now moving towards digitization, which makes computer-based image analysis

DOI: 10.1201/9781003363361-18

tools more accessible and capable of producing objective, quantitative slide evaluations. Digital pathology (DP) is a field-emerged technique used for handling large-magnification images of pathologic slides (Ibrahim et al., 2020). Histopathology is the study of diseased cells that foretells the symptoms which might occur after that stage and hence correlate with the disease. As imaging technology advances quickly, there is a growing need to evaluate stained tissue sections. This procedure is made feasible by DP, which includes automatically taking images (scanning slides) and interpreting and visualizing markers with the aid of software (Kuczkiewicz-Siemion et al., 2022). Artificial intelligence (AI) and machine learning (ML) concepts have been extensively useful for pathologic image analysis, which has provided essential support for medical study and clinical practice. DP is an arrangement of procedures that adds diagnostic value through information technology (IT)-assisted analysis of image data (van der Laak et al., 2021; Jahn et al., 2020).

In this chapter, the importance of histopathology in disease diagnosis at the cellular level is discussed. Digital images can be obtained by digitizing complete histopathological whole slide images (WSIs) using a high-resolution scanner. Different software for image analysis like ImageJ, Fiji, Qu Path, Orbit, etc. enable us to perform the analysis quickly and accurately and are discussed in detail. ML algorithms for feature extraction and segmentation and image-based convolutional neural networks (CNN) are commonly used for image analysis in the upcoming or latest software. Understanding the importance of the exchange of image data among the software and the need for software to be interoperable can benefit pathologists and clinicians in the exchange of patients' data, which is also discussed in this chapter.

18.2   IMPORTANCE OF HISTOPATHOLOGY FOR CLINICIANS

An important branch of biology called histology examines the microscopic structure of the cell anatomy of an organism, which is essential for diagnosis. Alternatively, histopathology is the study of a diseased cell, where certain changes or physical or functional variations causing disease are recorded. Images from histology and histopathology are crucial in diagnosis, since they can be used to assess the condition of a specific biological structure, support the diagnosis of diseases like cancer, or examine the anatomy of cells and tissues. These images are an important source that decides the state of the cell (Arevalo and Cruz-Roa, 2014). Based on reports, diagnosis can be made by studying a small piece of tissue, called a biopsy, which can be from the liver, skin, or other organs. This field of study is crucial, as it enables histopathologists to understand the disease at the molecular level. They are responsible for cell diagnosis, providing a report containing all descriptions of the cell, like the shape, size, and findings about the cell or the tissue. It is challenging but essential for clinicians to interpret it and make a decision for treatment.

Therefore, cooperation between histopathologists and clinicians is useful for making a clear diagnosis and determining the severity of the disease. Histological studies of biological samples often lead to a structure-function relationship. Understanding the normal structure and function of various tissues is essential for interpreting the changes that occur during disease. For example, the cells or tissues undergo certain changes like shrinking or enlargement of certain areas, either in the membrane, cytoplasm, or any organelle. Changes in cell structure indicate that the cell is not working properly, and, hence, will lead to disease. These histology images help clinicians guide the treatment modalities.

With the development of the microscope, pathologists can analyze and classify specimens under various magnifications, enabling them to see details that would otherwise be invisible to the naked eye. In modern healthcare biomedical imaging, "a world without imaging is not imaginable" (Meijering, 2020). Analysis techniques and automatic image representations are being successfully used in the area of medical imaging. For instance, several computational techniques make use of the growing number of sizable open-access biological image databases. The process of converting histopathological slides into digital imaginings utilizing a whole slide scanner, and then analyzing these images, is known as DP. Fresh fields of research like bioimage informatics and DP are progressively developing (Arevalo and Cruz-Roa., 2014; Jahn et al., 2020).

18.3 DISEASE BIOLOGY

Disease can develop when an external stimulus changes the cell's environment, which prevents the cell from sustaining homeostasis. In some situations, disease represents spontaneous variations in the cell's capacity to multiply or function naturally. Every disease has certain distinguishing symptoms, through which we can recognize the type of disease. An abnormal condition of a cell or tissue which negatively affects the structure or function of an organism is termed a disease

Why is it important to understand what a disease is? Modern medicine has unprecedented capabilities. New ethical responsibilities come with the potential to conduct effective, successful interventions in people's health. Knowing information about a disease helps physicians to diagnose and treat it. For instance, if we want to make sure that limited healthcare resources are efficiently distributed, we need to have a clear understanding firstly of what a disease is, and secondly which diseases are most worth spending time and money to treat (Scully, 2004).

18.3.1 MANIFESTATION OF DISEASE AT THE CELLULAR LEVEL

A cell is a structural and functional unit that is enclosed by a membrane. Cells are the smallest animate units from which diseases originate (Peterson, 2021). Any changes or disturbances can cause functional variation at the cellular level, leading to structural change. For example, see Figure 18.1, in which a normal cell has a large cytoplasm, a single nucleolus, and a spherical nucleus shape, whereas a cancer cell has a small cytoplasm, multiple nucleoli, and an irregular nucleus shape.

Some diseases originate due to spontaneous variations in the cell's ability to multiply and function normally, while others are caused by external stimuli that cause changes in the cell's environment, and which prevent the cell from maintaining homeostasis. Cells need to adapt to such new surroundings. Hyperplasia (i.e., growth in the number of cells), hypertrophy (i.e., increase in cell size), atrophy (i.e.,

NORMAL CELLS and CANCER CELLS

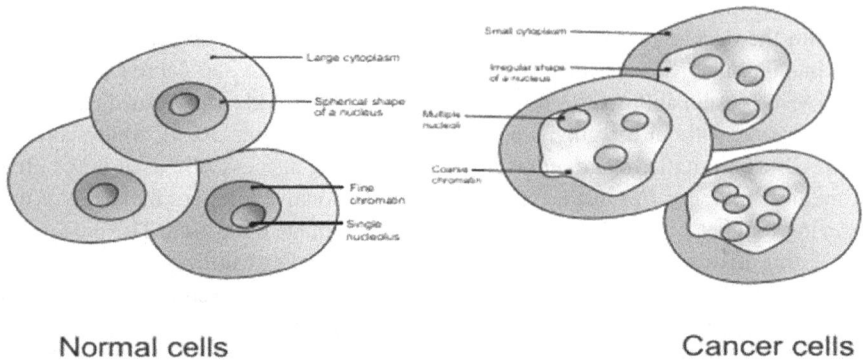

Normal cells   Cancer cells

FIGURE 18.1   Morphological differences between normal and diseased cells

reduction in cell size), or metaplasia (i.e., transformation of one cell type to another) are instances of such adaptations that could be physiological or pathological depending on whether a stimulus is normal or abnormal. The cell can adjust up to a certain limit, but if the stimulus remains beyond that limit, the cell and organ may fail. Death can occur if they are unable to adapt to the pathologic stimulus (Kemp et al., 2008).

Red blood cells are normally rounded and disc-shaped. In sickle cell anaemia, some red blood cells become deformed and resemble a sickle shape. These unusually formed cells are where the disease gets its name. Some cell changes could result in cell death, which could be due to having an excessive chemical environment or external forces like extreme pressure, temperature, etc. causing accidental death, resulting in necrosis or apoptosis, which could be recognized by the shrinking of the cytoplasm later due to condensation of the nucleus (DeBerardinis and Thompson, 2012).

18.3.2 Disease Diagnosis

Identifying the cause of illness or disease is considered a diagnosis. To diagnose is to find the cause of a disease to establish a diagnosis and for the health practitioner to use a combination of treatment methods. Treatment of a disease requires the power of observation and an understanding of human anatomy and physiology. A medical diagnosis is evaluated by observing the patient's symptoms and examining the patient's area of concern (Wexler, 2013). It has important implications for patient care and research. It is considered a process that is categorized by the medical profession to designate a particular condition. If the diagnosis is accurate and timely, the patient has the best opportunity to get the best treatment, leading to a positive change in the body (Balogh et al., 2015).

18.3.3 DIAGNOSTIC PROCESS

The process of identification of the disease by determining its cause through the evaluation of symptoms, physical examination, medical history, or reports is known as a diagnosis. The diagnostic process is how a medical professional identifies a disease by looking into a person's symptoms. Early indications which appear during the disease are often undifferentiated, which makes it challenging for the physician to make an accurate diagnosis.

The primary step is to get the medical history of the patient. This involves the clinicians getting previous medical records of the patient's health, and collecting information regarding any past or current signs and symptoms, any family history of disease, or information about any medications taken. Health practitioners often think that a patient's medical history is the key to diagnosis. For instance, a review of physiological symptoms such as cardiovascular, gastrointestinal (GI) digestive disorders, and neurologic disorders are included in the medical history, through which symptoms of the disease are experienced. Physical examination is the thorough observation of the patient's temperature, blood pressure, weight, and height, and further inspection of any marks or rash on the skin or other body parts. A physical examination can help the clinician understand the next step to be taken in the diagnosis and prevent any unnecessary testing (Wexler, 2013; Balogh et al., 2015).

18.3.4 DIAGNOSTIC TESTING

As the medical history and physical examination are taken, it is necessary to take a diagnostic test to confirm the diagnosis, which is to know the main cause of the disease. Testing can identify or classify a condition that is physically visible. Which kind of test is to be taken entirely depends on the symptoms and assumed diagnosis. For example, coronary artery disease (CAD), is a disease that could be identified by an image, by studying the blockage in an artery, even without the presence of symptoms. There are a few procedures that help the physician recognize the origin of the disease, which helps them further understand the disease and the treatment.

18.3.5 BLOOD TEST

A blood test is a laboratory examination that is performed on a blood sample. It is the most-commonly used test done as a routine check-up. Multiple tests could be done, such as tests for blood sugar levels in diabetes, and tests for malaria, dengue, and typhoid. A blood test provides a complete blood count, consisting of white blood cells (WBCs), basophils, monocytes, plasma content, and serum content.

18.3.6 ULTRASOUND

Images of the internal organs are captured using high-frequency sound waves, also known as sonography. This is used to diagnose tumours and examine gallbladder diseases, and can also provide a view of the uterus and kidneys. For example, the doctor advises an ultrasound if the patient is having pain or swelling, which requires an internal view of the organs. The images produced by ultrasound are not as precise as images obtained through methods like magnetic resonance imaging (MRI) and computed tomography (CT) scans.

18.3.7 MRI

Magnetic resonance imaging (MRI) is a non-invasive imaging technology that provides a three-dimensional detailed anatomical image. An MRI scanner has a "transmitting" coil that produces a magnetic field and a "receiver" coil, which obtains the current which goes to a computer to give the image, created by the position and intensity of the signals (Bulas and Egloff, 2013). MRI technology has been playing an increasingly significant role in biomedical research and clinical diagnosis. Mainly, MRI scans are performed on the brain, spine, and musculoskeletal system. It is a diagnostic tool to study bodily functions and dysfunction (Dong et al., 2015; van Beek et al., 2019).

18.3.8 CT Scan

Computed Tomography (CT) has transformed diagnostic decisions to become more precise. It has many advantages over other methods, as it can be completed in minutes, and it is widely used by physicians to approve or exclude a diagnosis. CT scans are often used to examine circulatory system diseases and diagnose cancer conditions, inflammatory diseases, and head or internal organ injuries (Balogh et al., 2015). The rapid utilization of CT scans has led to a concern about evidence that ionizing radiation delivered during scanning causes the development of solid organ cancer and leukaemia. It is becoming a more appealing imaging modality due to its advanced 3D resolution along with shorter scanning time (Power et al., 2016).

Medical imaging is commonly utilized almost in all fields of medicine and plays a crucial part in forming diagnoses. For a varied range of conditions, imaging technology advancements have improved clinicians' ability to recognize and identify treatment options and permit the patient to avoid more invasive procedures. Developing measurement systems that accurately reflect the data provided by diagnostic imaging is a current challenge for diagnostic imaging systems. The non-invasive imaging tests mentioned above are widely acknowledged to have resulted in a significant decrease in invasive testing. Medical imaging, like other types of diagnostic testing, has limitations (Balogh et al., 2015). The reliability, validity, and specificity of a diagnostic test are taken into consideration when deciding whether to perform it or not, as are the test's duration and its financial expense, along with any possible risks to the patient (Wexler, 2013).

18.3.9 Role of Histopathology in Diagnosis

Viewing the diagnosis from a different perspective can tell us not only the changes occurring at the tissue level but also the actual condition of the tissue. Pathology plays a vital role in providing patients with quality care treatments, but it does not get the deserved recognition (Fischer et al., 2021). Histopathology provides an understanding or knowledge of the disease, resulting in effective treatment. Additionally, new infections which were discovered in histopathology have been directed towards new diagnostic problems and challenges. The standardization and reliability of histopathological diagnoses have steadily increased, largely due to audits, external quality assurance, reporting, and growing specialization. New infections that emerged later in the 20th century, such as HIV, AIDS, and the coronavirus, among others, had an impact on histopathology as well (Underwood, 2017). People were mainly unaware that samples removed by biopsies, screening tests, and surgical removals are analyzed by pathologists (Fischer et al., 2021). The addition of digital cameras to microscopes has been one of the most significant changes in pathology in recent ages. Histological images were initially captured digitally as a still image or a film of the microscopic field of vision.

18.3.10 HISTOPATHOLOGY PRACTICE

The last ten years have seen a rapid evolution in the field of histopathology, with advancements in DP and now well-established developments in molecular diagnosis (Rakovic et al., 2022). The histological findings of pathological diagnoses that conflict with the clinical and radiological impression can all be explained in part by pathologists (Fischer et al., 2021). With digitization, advances have also been made in image analysis.

The term "histopathology" denotes the study of prepared tissue using a microscope. Histopathology's basic techniques first appeared in the 19th century, and they remain largely unchanged today. They focus on the use of light microscopy to examine stained tissue sections that have been formalin-fixed and paraffin-embedded (Rakovic et al., 2022). For a long time, histopathologists used standard hematoxylin and eosin (H&E) and specific-stained slides to examine their pathological diagnostic reports of the tissue growth forms and morphology of cells. The most frequently used is eosin dye, which is an acidic colouring substance that stains basic, negatively charged tissues like the cytoplasm. The nucleus of the cell, which is acidic, receives colour from the other companion colour, hematoxylin, which is basic. Even though special tissue staining is no longer used, even if available, the results would not have been suitable. Only a small number of private sectors claim to be manufacturing high-quality slides, but techniques still need to be standardized. If a slide is created following the standard usage of advanced nations, there is a range of technically skilled individuals who are available and can accurately interpret the slide (Horai et al., 2019). Modern facilities and tools must be available, as well as qualified personnel who can collect the samples, prepare them, stain them, and read the slides. As there is improvement in the field of IT, there is tremendous improvement in medical imaging and image processing as well (Sikandar, 2018). This methodology also includes the proper collection and processing of tissues along with their comparison and assessment with clinical pathology (Elmore, 2012).

With the implementation of AI approaches, it is critical to comprehend the level of detail the public wants to know about these developments, their role in diagnostic procedures, the likelihood that the public will accept these changes, as well as how we will communicate these developments. With the implementation of DP over the past ten years, there have been more advancements. Instead of using a microscope, DP scans the glass slide and examines the complete slide image digitally on a computer screen (Rakovic et al., 2022).

18.4   IMAGE ANALYSIS: DIGITAL IMAGE TECHNIQUE

Tissue slides are examined under a microscope by the pathologist at several magnifying stages such as 10×, 20×, 40×, and so on, to view various cells, nuclei, and glands and detect similarities between the structures of a normal versus a diseased slide. As the disease is detected, a classifying procedure is carried out to deal with the spread of infected cells over the slide of tissue. The prediction and consequent treatment for each patient are further planned based on the grade or level of disease. A measurable evaluation of these images is critical for a fair diagnosis. One well-known interface like Fiji or QuPath can be used for a variety of tasks when a deep learning technique is incorporated into a versatile toolkit (Meijering, 2020). Furthermore, the advancement of digital scanners now offers digital image information or data for computer-assisted image analysis using digital image processing algorithms for pathological image acquisition. Therefore, it acts as a crucial topic of research, mainly in histopathological imaging, in addition to diagnostics, where numerous image processing techniques can be used for the analysis of images for disease analysis (diagnosis) and prediction. Histology offers a clinical basis for medical study, education, or practice (Belsare and Mushraf, 2012). Furthermore, diagnosis or detection by the histopathology image is the "gold standard" in identifying or diagnosing a wide range of diseases, inclusive of nearly all kinds of cancer. Meanwhile, the structure of the images provides a huge amount of information, which again introduces a new challenge for automated or computerized image analysis (Gurcan et al., 2009).

Numerous methods of automatic image analysis and classification have been developed, since the manual examination of microscopic pictures take time and relies on a human expert (Nedzved et al., 2007).

A DP image is analyzed through feature extraction, segmentation, and classification algorithms, which input images and segment the nuclei into small regions see Figure 18.2. Techniques such as edge, region, and structural-based are used to segment the nuclei (Rani and Amsini, 2018).

1. **Segmentation:** Diagnosis of diseases for histopathologic images deals with the identification of histologic features like cell nuclei, glands, etc. The morphologic presence of such structures (i.e., size, shape, and colour intensity) is an important indicator of disease. For examining these indicators, histopathology images must first be separated or segmented. There are different magnification levels for segmentation approaches; for nucleus separation magnification is at 40× and for cell identification it's at 20×.

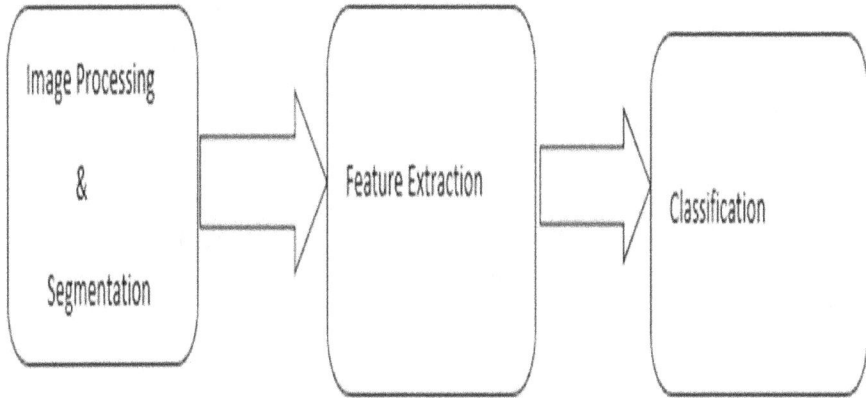

FIGURE 18.2 Flow chart depicting the common process of image analysis in digital histopathology applications

Histology images are stained with different proportions, which is critical to eliminate the consequence of variation. Image segmentation is an important step in automatic medical diagnosis based on microscopic images after preprocessing. It distinguishes between objects of interest and the background (Belsare and Mushraf, 2012). Mostly, histopathology cancer images are taken for the research field. They are used in disease analysis to find the presence of cancer cells. Various computerized algorithms are used to detect nuclei. Pathologists analyze the valuable information and form microscopic colour images (Rani and Amsini, 2018).

2. **Feature Extraction:** After segmentation and following division, characteristics are extracted from the image and features are observed at a cellular level to assess the morphologic features of abnormalities or categorize the image for various diseases. Cellular level characteristics concentrate on calculating the individual cells' features without taking their spatial dependence into account. The structural, textural, or intensity-based features can be retrieved from a single cell. The size and shape of the nucleus serve as the foundation for features like object-level (Belsare and Mushraf, 2012; Rani and Amsini, 2018).

3. **Classification:** After feature extraction and segmentation, the images are classified through classifier techniques. These are used to classify a huge number of datasets. The pathology images are classified via ML algorithms such as neural networks, Bayesian classifiers, support vector machines (SVM), etc. The choice of classifier is crucial for dealing with huge, dense datasets for histopathology images. Various classifiers are used to classify images to diagnose abnormality in images after segmentation and feature extraction. For example, a cell is given to one of the classes and later classified by the grade of malignancy, such as in tumours. Many ML algorithms are used for histopathological image classification, such as logistic

regression, k-nearest neighbours, neural networks, etc. Those are used to differentiate between cancer-affected cells and others from images and to identify the particular location (Belsare and Mushraf, 2012; Rani and Amsini, 2018).

However, dimensional analysis of histopathology imagery has lately become the backbone of most computerized histopathological image analysis practices, leading to digital histopathology (DH). Despite the advancements made thus far, there are still many studies to be done in this area, because of the range of imaging techniques and disease-specific traits (Gurcan et al., 2009).

18.5 SOFTWARE USED IN IMAGE ANALYSIS

Algorithms for image analysis have been implemented for object classification (like types of cells), object counting (like nucleus counting), region segmentation (such as tumour delineation), or image quality control, known as image analysis packages (e.g., detection of artifacts). All of these are mostly built upon the foundational libraries such as Tensorflow, OpenSlide, Keras, PyTorch, or scikit-learn, for deep learning (DL) and (computer vision) OpenCV (Marée, 2019). Image segmentation and image classification are the general steps of image analysis by DH. In this task of classification, the algorithm takes the whole histopathology image slide as the input and gives as the output the label of the input image (Xu et al., 2017). The workflow of contemporary pathology is becoming increasingly digital, culminating in the use of computer screens to view scanned histology slides (Aeffner et al., 2019).

Traditionally, the bioimage software frameworks were mostly created in C/C++ or Java, but in the past ten years, Python has quickly gained popularity in the scientific community. C/C++ is still the language of choice for computer graphics since it can provide good performance. CNN in DL is the algorithm that is used the most in image analysis software like CellProfiler and HistoClean. Some applications, like Fiji and QuPath, are in Java, which makes them easily portable and multi-platform, meaning they can run on Windows, Mac, and Linux (Levet et al., 2021). There are certain software or applications for image analysis of histopathological images, such as ImageJ/Fiji, Qu Path, CellProfiler, Icy, and Cytomine, some of which are explained here.

18.5.1 IMAGEJ/FIJI

ImageJ (https://imagej.nih.gov/ij/) is Java-built image analysis software widely used in the biological sciences and other fields. It is a potent image processing platform that is open source and was created at National Institutes of Health (NIH) by Wayne Rasband. Since its original release in 1997, ImageJ has excelled in various scientific endeavours and projects, specifically in life sciences. ImageJ's development directions presently tend to focus on solving bioimaging-related issues. However, the majority of image processing processes or algorithms are commonly useful (Rueden et al., 2017).

ImageJ's abilities vary from simple tasks like opening images in different formats, annotating or marking, image processing, and running basic workflows on images, to advanced projects like visualizing and analyzing large amounts of image data by applying ML algorithms. WSIs can be used by adding plugins. ImageJ can be extended and customized by using macros and scripting. ImageJ allows users to section or segment, track particles, and record datasets. Segmentation, also known as object delineation, allows biologists to computationally segment or separate specific regions in images (Schroeder et al., 2021).

Image datasets have become increasingly huge, typically spanning multiple gigabytes and frequently exceeding terabytes. This type of data is challenging to open and difficult to view, mark, or quantify utilizing ImageJ's typical image screen or window. Fiji (https://fiji.sc/) enables biological image analysis that is more intensive and widespread than ImageJ. It enables quick processing of image prototyping methods. It involves current software engineering practices, which combine robust software libraries along with a varied range of scripting languages. ImageJ is a tool that has been used for a long time and has been an open-source option for bioimage analysis. It is known for users to section or segment, track particles, and record datasets, useful in image preprocessing. ImageJ as well as Fiji which is a plugin included-distribution is used for deep image investigations and ideally suitable for single-image processing. The driving idea of design in ImageJ was to keep things simple, particularly in the interface, which is minimalist and has maintained its original design to the present day. Behind the built of the software it conceals extensibility and its actual power. Unlike a centralized development paradigm, it was easily expanded by the developer community. Plugins are more sophisticated, modular software components that increase the product's capability.

In Fiji, the image is opened by clicking the File option the image can be adjusted by changing the image type (eight-bit, 16-bit, etc.), and can also be cropped. Adjusting the brightness, colour contrast, and subtracting the background are some steps that are performed, by using "Image>Adjust>Threshold", the image's threshold can be set automatically or manually for image preprocessing for cellular and single-image analysis.

In the Analyze tab, clicking "Analyze Particles" can be used for image analysis, along with using plugins like Trackmate and TissueAnalyzer. The data can be summarized or plots can be formed for visualization. Figure 18.3 shows the Fiji image analysis for two types of cells: one liver cell and one brain cell sample taken from laboratory work (Jakhmola-Mani et al., 2020). The results of the analysis are given in Table 18.1.

Fiji makes it easy to apply new algorithms into ImageJ plugins that can be shared with end-users via updates. It offers a robust and reliable distribution system that guarantees new algorithms are made available to its large user base. Because of ImageJ's extensive use, wide implementation, and extensible plugin architecture, scientists from many different fields like it as a tool. However, primarily, ImageJ was created by biologists for other biologists, and as a result, its development and architecture do not adhere to contemporary principles of software engineering. As a result, it becomes less appealing to deliver new solutions using the platform. To solve

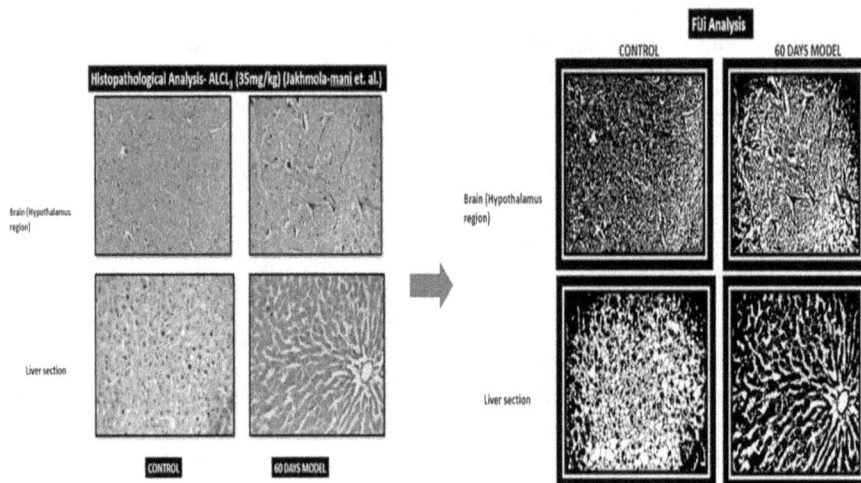

FIGURE 18.3　Fiji analysis of brain (hypothalamus region) and liver section

TABLE 18.1
Analysis Results of Images by Fiji Software

	Cell Count	Total Area	Avg Size	Area (%)
Brain (hypothalamus region) of control sample	3968	93908	23.666	31.166
Liver section of control sample	1175	155025	131.936	49.841
Brain (hypothalamus region) of 60-days model	2049	120469	58.792	43.177
Liver section of 60-days model	949	88441	93.194	30.405

this limitation in ImageJ, a brand-new open-source software venture called Fiji. Fiji improves ImageJ's fundamental architecture, while letting researchers concentrate on creating new, cutting-edge approaches to biological image analysis. Fiji adds new core capabilities while maintaining ImageJ's compatibility (Schindelin et al., 2012). The Figure 18.4 showing threshold image after converting the RGB in eight or 16 bits from the File tab using the analyze particles option to identify count of cells. The summary shows the details of image such as count total, area, mean etc., the plot of area to mean of count of the cells can be visualized.

18.5.2　CLIJ

CLIJ is a graphical processing unit (GPU) accelerated image processing library in ImageJ/Fiji. The majority of routine image processing activities can be completed by

(A)

(B)

(C)

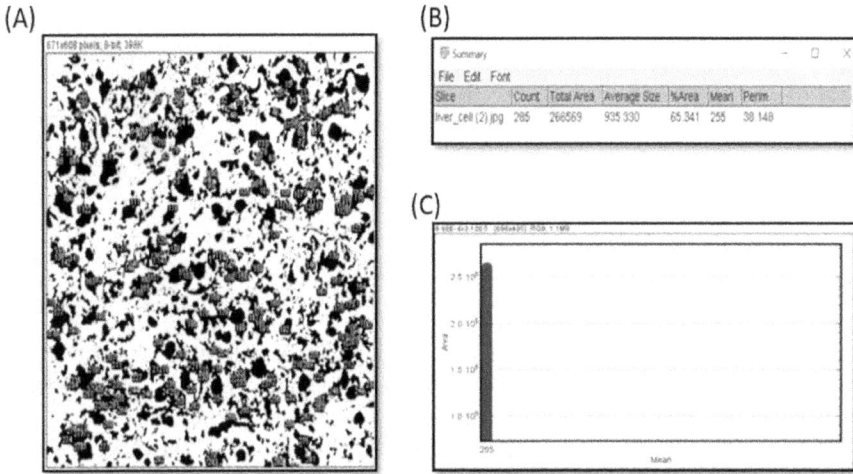

FIGURE 18.4 Fiji software (A) threshold image, (B) summary or details of measurement, (C) plot of area mean

creating flexible workflows using only basic operations in tools like ImageJ and Fiji. However, most of these procedures were developed at a time when general-purpose processing on GPUs was not very widespread.

As a result, GPUs are not utilized in normal workflows composed of fundamental ImageJ functions. CLIJ was created as an adaptable and reusable GPU acceleration framework in Fiji to solve this problem. It also adds modified versions of fundamental ImageJ operations that utilized the open computer language (OpenCL) framework, which runs on GPUs, in which it implements a variety of image processing features (Haase et al., 2019). It can perform various operations faster by having more processing cores and faster memory. It comes along with various operations for filtering, binarizing, filtering, mathematical operations for images, and transformations (https://github.com/clij/clij2).

It can be installed in different software. To install it in Fiji/ImageJ, we can follow certain steps: by clicking Help > Update, clicking on "Manage Update Sites", and selecting the CLIJ/CLIJ2 update sites. After the update restarts the software, if it is updated successfully, it will be shown in the toolbar (see Figure 18.5).

18.5.3 QuPath

An open-source bioimage analysis programme called QuPath (https://qupath.github .io/) was built to respond to the growing demand for an extensible, easy-to-use, and open-source resolution for both DP and WSIs. QuPath is an innovative cross-platform Java programme for quantitative pathology and bioimage analysis. The user interface was created using JavaFX and the underlying software was developed using Java 8. QuPath offers researchers a wide range of tools for the identification of

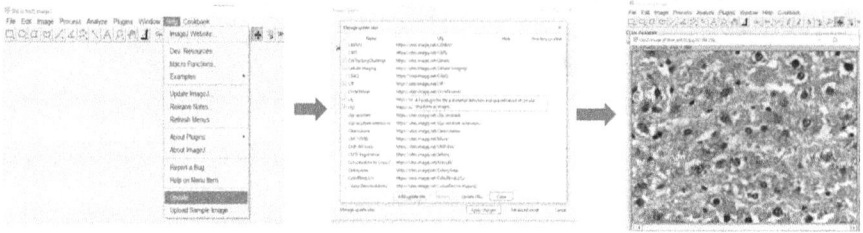

FIGURE 18.5   Installation of Clij in Fiji

tumours and biomarker evaluation in high-throughput, as well as strong batch processing and scripting capabilities, with an expandable platform for the creation and exchange of new algorithms for the analysis of complicated tissue images.

The new QuPath software upgrade improves the diagnostic abilities of the pathologist by allowing image analysis to be run on areas of any shape and size, in contrast to earlier software versions, where the area of analysis was restricted to either the entire field of view or a squared-off selection. Its hierarchical, object-based data architecture is a key component of QuPath's capability and a significant technical differentiator between QuPath and other bioimaging analysis applications. An image's structure or region is referred to here as an "object", which can be generated or altered using either interactive drawing tools such as those used to mark a particular region of interest (ROI) or automatic separation instructions (for example, "identify specific cell/nuclei"). The object can take on various types, such as detection or annotation, and is equipped to handle classifications and measurements. In addition, it designates ROI while also featuring a 'cell detection' capability. Lastly, QuPath permits developers to implement extensions to address their novel problems and applications, as well as to share data with other programmes, like ImageJ and MATLAB, that would otherwise only handle partial slides. In QuPath, an object plays a crucial role; a cell, artery, gland, tumourous region, or biopsy can all be regarded as an object in an image. This item captures the shape as well as some of its characteristics (Bankhead et al., 2017).

It typically allows quantitative analysis of the image, including detecting cells or identifying cells, based on markers classifying cells, and measuring different features, such as size, shape, distance, or area. If the built-in capabilities are not insufficient for analysis, there's the option to exchange data seamlessly with QuPath and Fiji (where a huge number of plugins are available), meaning that there can be an easy exchange of data between software, which can enhance the quality and accuracy of analysis, covering the broad range of requirements in bioimage analysis see Figure 18.6 (Dobson et al., 2021).

There is a Workflow tab in the QuPath software, where all the commands that were run on the image can be seen. Generally, the first command is the "Set image type" command, where the type of image can be set, such as "Brightfield or Fluorescence" or "Brightfield(H&E)". To automate this step, click the Run menu. A new dialog box will allow for the selection of images. Finally, press "OK", which will apply the

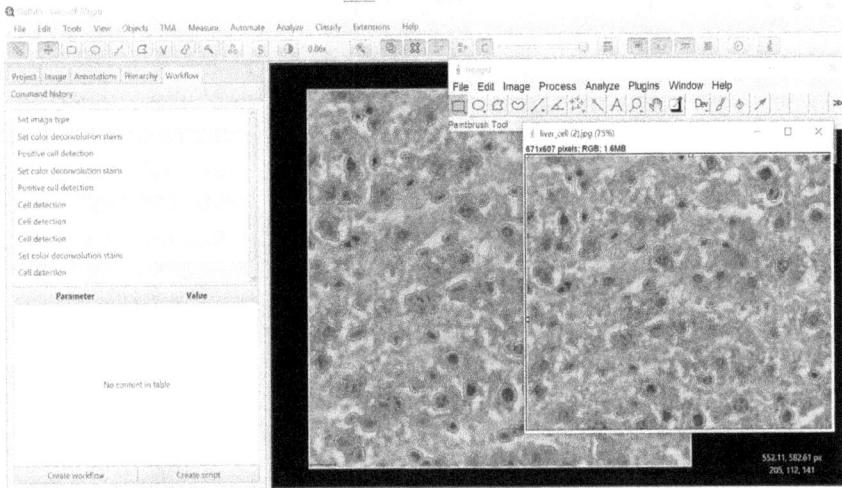

FIGURE 18.6 Image data exchange between QuPath and ImageJ shows interoperability feature (here, positive cell count from QuPath is send to ImageJ)

script to the selected image. Complex workflows in QuPath can be completed with little scripting. QuPath has its own script editor that can be selected in the Automate tab (Burri, 2022).

Histological study of a tissue or cell section has been challenging for pathologists, due to the time required, along with the risk of partial explanation (Aeffner et al., 2019). But this software enables whole slide image analysis, helping save time. The nucleus/cell area ratio is a particularly helpful parameter for tumour cell identification. Because tumour nuclei are typically larger and more tightly packed than non-tumour nuclei, this value is typically higher for tumour cells. Both of these properties are included in the nucleus/cell area ratio measurement. The measurement is somewhat "noisy", which contributes to the nucleus/cell area ratio's limited use (Bankhead et al., 2017). Here, as seen in Figure 18.7, the nucleus/cell ratio is 0.082. As observed, there is significant variation on a cell-by-cell basis, but, overall, tumour cells exhibit higher values (i.e., more yellow/white colour in tumour areas).

18.5.4 CELLPROFILER

CellProfiler (https://cellprofiler.org/releases) is a free and open-source software designed to help biologists with no prior experience in computer vision or programming to automatically calculate characteristics from hundreds of images. Advanced image analysis techniques and algorithms are available as separate modules that can be connected sequentially to create a pipeline. The "pipeline" is utilized to recognize and quantify biological objects and characteristics in images. The CellProfiler biological image analysis tool is widely used to gather a comprehensive set of morphologic, structural, and textural information about cells and organisms on the screen.

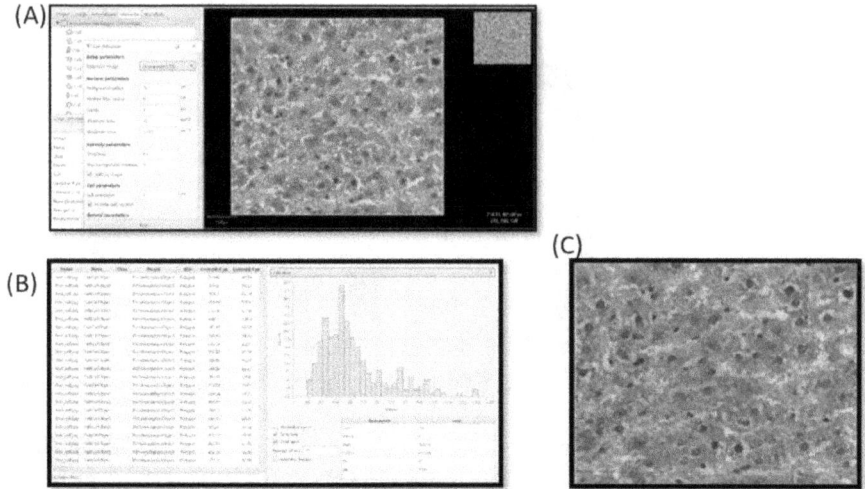

FIGURE 18.7 QuPath (A) cell detection in QuPath showing cell nuclei and cell wall, (B) showing all the detections measurement, (C) density map showing region where a higher number of cells is present

Additionally, it has the linked or flexible cell-tracing abilities of time-lapse tests, like the linear assignment problem (LAP) approach, that offer reliable tracking by bridging sequential openings and catching object unions and splits (Bray and Carpenter, 2015). Originally created in MATLAB, CellProfiler was rewritten in Python 2 in 2010, reaching its official end-of-life in 2020. Several changes have been made to the CellProfiler user interface in response to comments from biologists, with the aim of making the application more approachable and user-friendly.

A more feature-rich 3D viewer that allows users to analyze any plane in a volume has now taken the place of the simple 3D viewer first offered in CellProfiler 3.0, and several previous modules have also been improved. The threshold model was completely redesigned to enable adaptive use of all previously developed threshold algorithms, offering users more options in images with significantly changeable backgrounds. "MeasureObjectSizeShape" may record up to 60 new shape measures for each item, including bounding box positions, image moments, and inertia tensors, which are now available in scikit-image. Tissue segment analysis stands out as a possible area for development. As system memory is frequently insufficient to load the complete image at once, the huge file sizes associated with tissue specimens present a difficulty for image analysis. CellProfiler evaluates a wide range of properties, including area, intensity, shape, and texture, identifying cellular and sub-cellular parts in the image. It features pipelines where various image analysis modules can be applied.

It can answer a variety of biological questions, such as cell size, shape, or sub-cellular patterns of DNA. Furthermore, it has advanced algorithms for the analysis of images, which correctly differentiate swarmed cells and non-mammalian cells.

is optimized for the analysis of two-dimensional (2D) images, as the software operates on a modular pipeline concept. Each module within the software is specifically designed for image processing, contributing to the creation of a structured pipeline. This pipeline facilitates the application of various image analysis modules for tasks such as evaluating cellular properties, including size, shape, and sub-cellular patterns. Each module is designed to be placed in a specific order for images, contributing to the formation of a pipeline that leads to image processing see Figure 18.8. Currently, there are over 50 modules available for use. Measurements are available using its built-in viewing with tools for data plotting. It can be accessible in Microsoft Excel (as CSV) or OpenOffice Calc (Carpenter et al., 2006) .

In CellProfiler, there is "IdentifyPrimaryObject", module aids in the identification of objects like nuclei. Comparable to Fiji, this process involves several steps, including Gaussian Blur, Thresholding, Fill Holes, and the declumping of objects using Watershed, followed by Analyze Particles. This sequence highlights the software's interoperability. In Fiji, the process involves several steps, whereas in CellProfiler, these same steps are encapsulated in a module, providing easy accessibility for analysis. It has a feature for building a pipeline: first, the image can be loaded by opening or dragging and dropping, then select the image type (RGB, Gray), then on the left-hand side double-click the window to add modules, like ColourToGray > IdentifyPrimaryObjects > IdentifySecondaryObjects (see Figure 18.8). The results can be exported as a CSV file (Ward et al., 2022).

As an open-source platform, CellProfiler is for image analysis. It is used to create reproducible analysis pipelines, modular for larger-scale studies. The modules present in the software can be arranged to form the pipeline in different orders according to specific needs for the analysis of images (Flach et al., 2022). It is the better option of the software available for large-scale pipelines for image analysis (see Figure 18.9).

18.5.5   ICY

Icy is free, open-source, and available at http://icy.bioimageanalysis.org/. Icy is a platform for collaborative bioimage informatics that combines software with a high-end visual programming framework for the smooth creation of sophisticated imaging workflows, as well as a community website for sharing tools and resources. By promoting and supporting the reusability, modularity, standardization, and management of algorithms and protocols, Icy expands the principles of reproducible research. The BioImage Analysis Lab at the Institute Pasteur developed Icy in 2011. It was created with the intention of addressing the broadest range of biological applications, facilitating simple access to cutting-edge image analysis methods, and promoting reproducibility research (de Chaumont et al., 2012). Icy provides a platform for sharing and publishing collaborative algorithm developments, encourages code sharing and reusability to speed up the creation of new algorithms, and streamlines user feedback and support via a community website (de Chaumont et al., 2013).

Icy is a Java-based desktop application that is supplemented with a website, which acts as a central location for the contribution and exchange of protocols, scripts, and

(A)

(B)

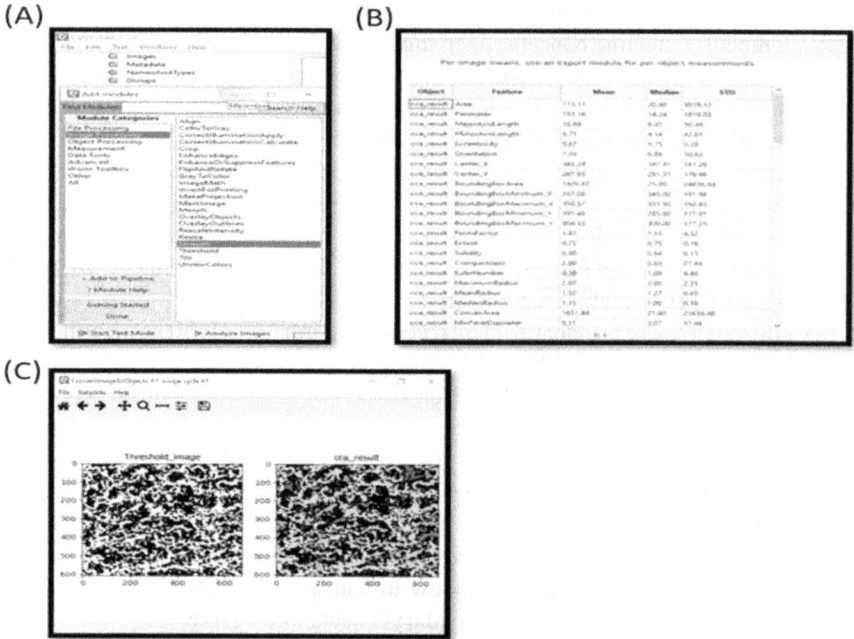

(C)

FIGURE 18.8 CellProfiler software (A) adding module to pipeline, (B) thresholding image (ConvertImageToObject), (C) object measurements

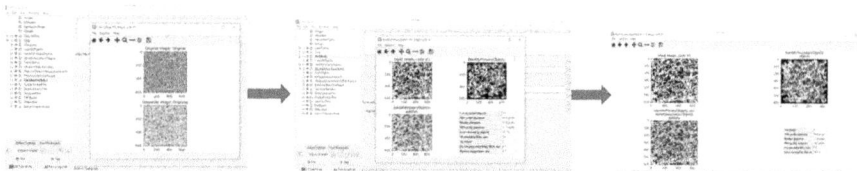

FIGURE 18.9 Shows the modular pipeline i.e., adding modules to the image from the left tab and showing the changes in images

plugins. The interface features a ribbon-style toolbar that is very reminiscent of one such tool found in Microsoft's Office Suite, which makes it extremely simple to use. Icy also incorporates bio-formats to read images for loading WSIs, but it is not able to support the organization of multi-resolution pyramids, which creates a memory management issue when reading very high-resolution images. Icy can be combined with Cytomine as a plugin called Icytomine. To use Icy analysis tools in WSIs, this plugin creates a bridge between the two applications (Gonzalez Obando et al., 2019).

Icy has certain features like spot detection, feature extraction, and best thresholder, which chooses the best auto-thresholding technique. It also has an Active Cells plugin, which implements fast active contours for image segmentation (see Figure 18.10). Icy has "protocols" which refers to bioimage analysis workflows and

(A)

(B)

(C)

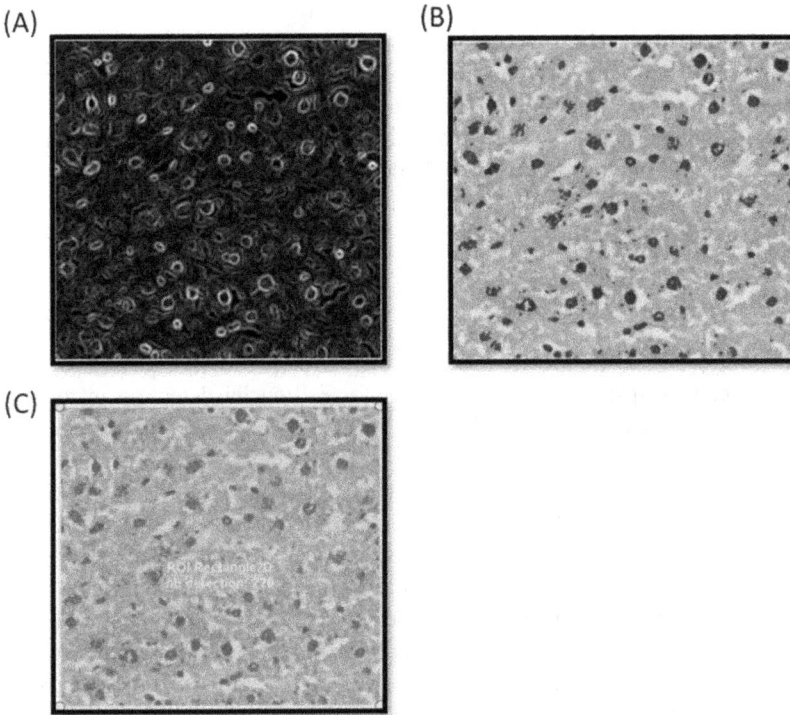

FIGURE 18.10 Icy software (A) feature detector, (B) best threshold (MaxEntropy), (C) number of detections using spot detector

automating many images (batch processing) that is constructed using a graphical programming language. Protocols can be shared or reused directly from the Icy website.

18.5.6 HALO

HALO (v2.2.1870.17, Indica Labs, Albuquerque, NM, USA) is an image analysis software. It allows the study of tissue segmentation using AI. It is commercial software, unlike ImageJ and Fiji. It quantifies various histopathological images which can be used. It simplifies finding the changes that take place. With the increase in the development of information technology there is increased development in DP. There has been a boom in the use of ML and AI to analyze and diagnose pathological tissues. In the HALO software, histopathological features are analyzed and quantified. There is a tissue classifier module that uses a random forest algorithm, which is among the methods in ML. Random Forest is a classification algorithm that consists of multiple classifiers to solve a complex problem and improves the performance of the model. It contains numerous decision trees, which compute the average to enhance predictive accuracy. The tissue classifier module is trained to learn the morphological features, separating them into different classes, and the region of interest is quantified. After separation, each cell is analyzed in detail by other modules, such as vacuoles or cytonuclear modules. Moreover, combinations of various modules can analyze some other findings or features as well. It is hard to use more detailed features in images, whereas, by using DL with CNN, it could be possible to recognize the morphological features of a detailed tissue structure, including single-cell death or inflammatory cells. Setting the parameters of HALO is simple, which makes it easy-to-use for those who lack experience in image analysis.

18.5.7 CYTOMINE

Cytomine app (http://www.cytomine.be/), was developed by the ULiège Cytomine Research team (https://uliege.cytomine.org) for cell/nuclei detection in regions of interest (ROIs), encapsulating the Stardist Python code (https://github.com/stardist/stardist).

DH has been used more frequently in research as well as in the clinical field. Equally, modern tissue/cell imaging techniques, such as imaging mass-spectrometry, are thought to be a very promising avenue for improving molecular or cellular pathology diagnosis. Due to the lack of collaborative software for sharing associated data for multimodal analysis (i.e., simultaneous examination and integration of data from multiple modes or types of imaging), new data sources are still frequently underutilized. The Cytomine software, operating in adherence to the open-science paradigm, is supported by new features that are specifically developed to enhance multimodal analysis (see Figure 18.11). The new version of Cytomine is a web-first, free tool which makes it possible to share data by molecular imaging or traditional

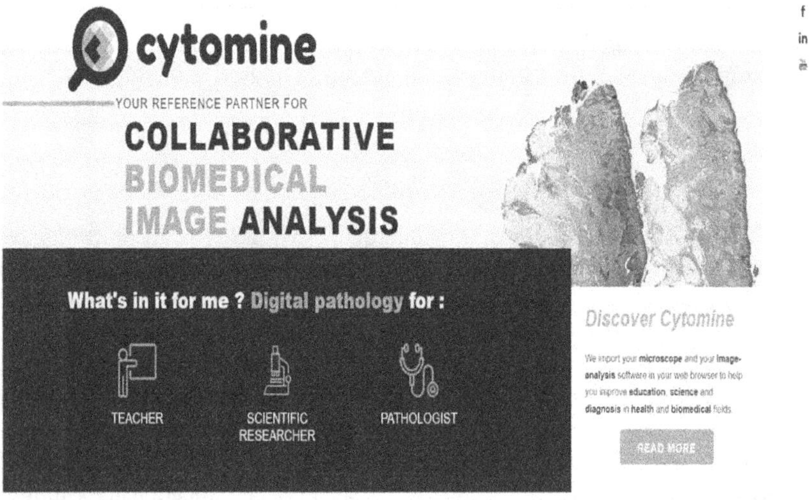

FIGURE 18.11   Homepage of Cytomine

histology. It enables highly collaborative analysis of multi-gigapixel imaging data, made possible by a rich web environment. The developers had the following goals in mind when creating this tool: to provide guidelines for remote and collaborative work, to rely on data models that make it simple to standardize, organize, and semantically annotate imaging datasets, and to effectively support multi-gigapixel high-resolution images (Rubens et al., 2019; Marée et al., 2016).

18.5.8   HistoClean

HistoClean is an open-source software which can be downloaded from GitHub (https://github.com/HistoCleanQUB/HistoClean). It is a preprocessing programme/application for use in DP in DL projects. It is a GUI which combines many image processing components into a single, user-friendly toolset. Python 3.8 and Anaconda3 were used to develop HistoClean. The Tkinter toolbox (v8.6) was used to create the GUI. The goal of HistoClean is to close the knowledge gap that exists between biomedical scientists, pathologists, and computer scientists by offering a clear-picture preprocessing and augmentation method that can be used without any past coding experience. We used HistoClean to improve the model's accuracy at the tile, ROI, and patient level (McCombe et al., 2021) by preprocessing the image for a simple CNN used for the identification of stromal growth, showing that HistoClean may be utilized to enhance a typical DL system using conventional picture augmentation and preprocessing approaches. These software frameworks enable the advancement of digital image analysis (DIA) algorithms through the usage of ML from predetermined features. This makes it possible for histopathologists who serve as consultants and bioimage analyzers to respond to challenging research problems in human tissue. It intends to complete the ecosystem of DP frameworks and other open-source tools for bioimage analysis. According to the computational techniques often utilized in histologic image preprocessing, HistoClean is an image processing toolkit which is divided into five functional modules: image patching, image normalization, whitespace thresholding, dataset balancing, and augmentation (see Figure 18.12).

Computer scientists, biomedical experts, and pathologists all are working together to develop DL models in histopathological analysis. To train basic CNN to predict stromal maturity, HistoClean can optimize the input pictures. We evaluate these models to show the value of a very simple CNN foundation. HistoClean is the software that easily implements and evaluates histopathological image pre-processing and augmentation procedures. CNN is a DL algorithm designed especially for images and videos. It takes images as input, extracts the features and later classifies them. It is inspired by the workings of the human brain's visual cortex. It has various different layers, and each one has its own function. It allows us to learn hierarchical representations of local image features from data (Abbas et al., 2020). CNN has various filters, and each filter extracts some of the information and then identifies images by combining all the features.

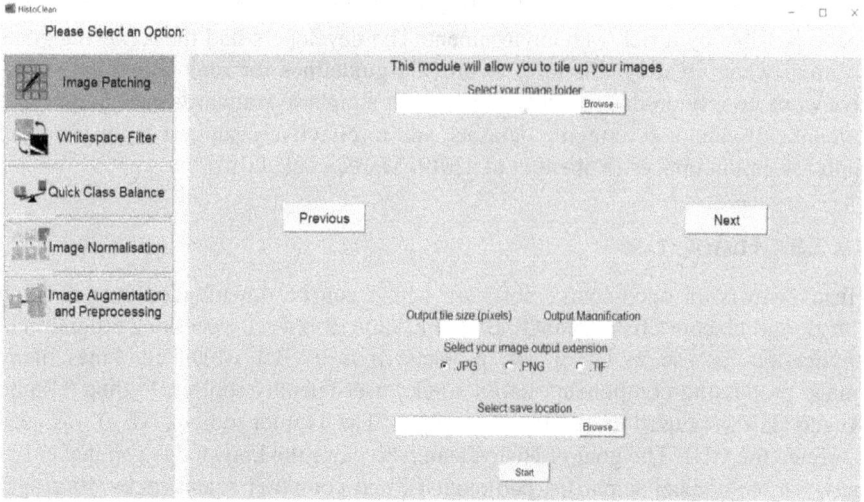

FIGURE 18.12   User interface of HistoClean

18.5.9 ORBIT

Orbit (http://www.orbit.bio/) is a whole slide image analysis programme available for free (Figure 18.13). It was created in Java and works on Linux, Mac, and
Windows operating systems. Swing is used to implement its user interface, although
it can alternatively be run headlessly from the command line. Utilizing a tile-based
map reduce implementation framework, Orbit's flexible tile-processing engine

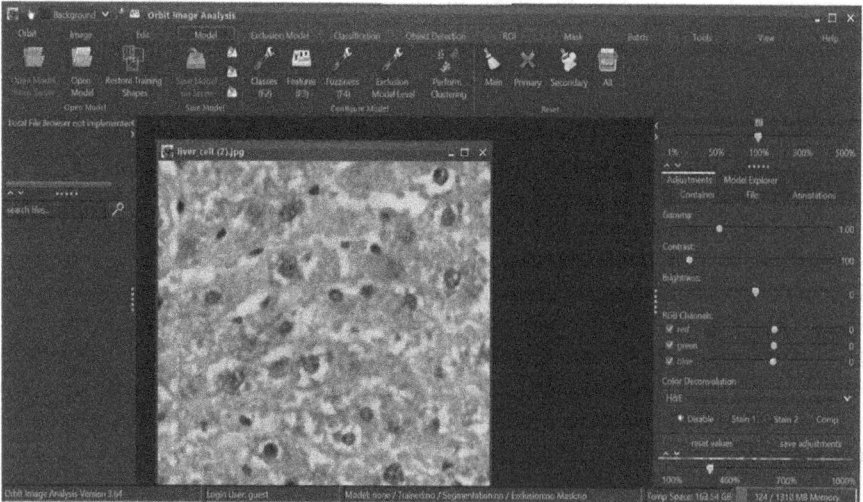

FIGURE 18.13   Orbit software interface for Orbit image analysis

enables the execution of various analysis algorithms provided by Orbit and other platforms. Orbit can be used to link an OMERO image server or run locally as a standalone application. It allows the reading of WSIs using bio-formats. It puts an emphasis on pixel and object classification and object separation. It uses ML tools like SVM. New algorithms can be added using plugins like Groovy script editor or external software. It can work in a collaborative environment (Stritt et al., 2020; Allan et al., 2012).

18.5.10   INTEROPERABILITY AND LICENCING

As a result, of digital imaging bioimage analysis has emerged as a key step in incorporating data science methodologies into the life sciences. Building an extension or plugin for already-existing software is a middle-ground position. Software such as Fiji, CellProfiler, ImageJ, and ImageJ extensibility has been crucial to their success, leading to the development of numerous cutting-edge algorithms as plugins for these systems. Using the CLIJ library as an instance, you can add several advanced image processing algorithms implemented as plugins for software like Fiji and Icy. The term "interoperability" refers to the capability of several software to work together in a coordinated manner or workflow, or their ability to replace each other. Interoperability can be likely to be attained via two methods: (i) external interoperability, through the usage of common file libraries and formats, and (ii) via a plugin mechanism for internal interoperability.

It is a critical issue to be addressed, as it will allow software packages to work together seamlessly and efficiently by their ability to exchange data and algorithms. To achieve interoperability between bioimage software, the standardization of data formats or protocols is required. Many software tools use different formats like JPEG, JPG, PNG, TIFF, and OME-TIFF, which allows users to exchange image data between platforms. In Figure 18.6, the image data exchange between ImageJ and QuPath is shown. In addition, several initiatives have been developed to promote interoperability between bioimage software, such as the Bio-Formats library, which provides a common interface for reading and writing image data in a variety of formats. Software can be regarded as interoperable with other applications that handle similar data if it stores processing data in standard file formats like CSV, TXT, or common picture file formats. Software that offers unique, closed-source file formats for handling data is incompatible with other programmes and acts as a barrier. For example, in CellProfiler, after completing the image analysis pipeline, the output data can be exported in CSV format by using the "ExportToSpreadsheet" module. This module allows users to select which measurements to export and in which format, including CSV. The exported CSV file can be easily opened and analyzed in other software tools, such as Microsoft Excel or R. In addition to standardized file formats, interoperability can be achieved by using common programming languages and application programming interfaces (APIs). Interoperability between bioimage software is critical for the efficient and effective analysis of large and complex image datasets.

Similarly, in QuPath, the analysis results can be exported in CSV format by using the "Export measurements" command, which exports the measurements of the selected objects in a tabular format. Users can choose which measurements to include in the output file and how to organize the columns. Internal interoperability can be performed at a higher level through plugin methods, which make it possible for modules with different origins to interact with one another within a given software programme. In the field of image data science, programmes like ImageJ/Fiji, Icy, or CellProfiler are well-known as platforms that can be extended utilizing plugin architectures.

Despite its significance, licencing is a feature of open-source software which developers sometimes neglect. The licence should be specified from the beginning; however, this is not always the case once the source code is released. As it specifies how others may utilize the source code for a particular project, licencing is crucial. OpenSource.org is an Open Source Initiative (OSI) and is a helpful resource which keeps track of the accepted open-source licences used for choosing the license. Mostly, software are freely available and accessing the license is not always required. For example, QuPath is open-source and freely available, licensed under the GNU General Public License v3.0.

Platforms like Cytomine enable remote collaboration so that specialists in several locations can work simultaneously on the same slide. In contrast to other platforms, QuPath offers a wide range of tools for tissue microarray investigation (Escobar Díaz Guerrero et al., 2022).

Each software has its own features for instance, in Fiji auto-threshold is currently supported in RGB only for eight- to 16-bit image sizes. Furthermore, annotation can be added to classify the cells on the basis of the intensity of the cell. Similarly, QuPath classification could easily be done, as there is hierarchical cell detection, positive cell detection, and tissue micro analysis (TMA). It could provide better results if the region of interest is small, but if it is bigger, image calculation might be affected. New features are constantly added to Fiji, as an open-source image processing software that is constantly being updated with new features and improvements by the developers over time, such as the plugin system in Fiji 2.0, which allows users to easily install and use new plugins that add new features like image processing algorithms, data visualization, three-dimensional (3D) image analysis, etc. Another instance is the addition of the Bio-Formats image reader to Fiji. Bio-Formats is a library that allows Fiji to read a wide variety of image formats that are commonly used in biological research. In QuPath, classification of objects (ex. cells) could be annotated as a tumour cells, positive cells, or negative cells more easily than in ImageJ/Fiji (Escobar Díaz Guerrero et al., 2022). The comparison between the software is shown in Table 18.2 and Table 18.3.

CellProfiler has a pipeline in which modules are added according to requirements. It has ML tools, whereas ImageJ has ML tools with plugins. HistoClean GUI is simple and does have more required information on the image analysis documentation than QuPath. Cytomine has integrative collaborative tools, whereas QuPath has partially collaborative tools and Orbit does not.

TABLE 18.2

Comparison of the Software listed for Image Analysis

Software / Application	Type of Platform	Main Programming Language	Common Features	Major Features	WSI (Whole Slide Imaging)	Release Year
ImageJ/Fiji	Desktop	Java	Image processing, covers most areas of biological analysis	With plugins	Using SlideJ	1997
Cell Profiler	Desktop	MATLAB later python	Image preprocessing such as cell density, track cells, colonization	Ease of use, continuous improvement, versatility using pipelines	External Software e.g. Orbit	2005
Cytomine	Web-based	Groovy/Java	Annotation, image management tool, viewing multiple images	Organize, explore, and analyze multi-gigapixel imaging data over the internet, images stored in cloud, object classification, pixel segmentation	Bio-formats, OpenSlide (yes)	2016
Qu Path	Desktop	Java	Smart Annotation tools, analyze whole slide image, cell detection and classification	Allow exchange of files with ImageJ and MATLAB, object-based classification, density maps, tools for TMA	Bio-formats and OpenSlide (yes)	2016
Orbit	Desktop with certain web-based properties	Java	Object classification, pixel classification	Compatible with ImageJ, advanced whole slide image viewer	Bio-formats (yes)	2016
Icy	Desktop	Java	Annotate, quantify bioimaging data	Covers a wide range of biological applications, collaborative Adobe Photoshop for image analysis, GUI ribbon-style, resembles Microsoft Office Suite	Using plugin or external software (yes)	2011

TABLE 18.3

Comparison of Software Based on Cell Features (Number of Detections of Cells, Mean Area of Cells, Mean Perimeter of Cells)

Tools/Software	Number of Detections of Cells	Mean Area (Average Size) of Cells (px²)	Mean Perimeter of Cells (px)
Fiji	285	935.33	38.14
Qu Path	258	428.51	76.6
Icy	220	Individual area size is available (μm^2)	Individual perimeter is available (μm)
CellProfiler	278	715.11	151.16

Thus, the current work emphasizes the efficacy and utility of these applications in predicting the diagnosis of disease at a cellular level.

18.6 CONCLUSION

Pathologists can now use digital image analysis on tissue sections, due to the digitization of glass slides and the creation of specialized software tools, which can now recognize and quantify events that were previously observed through a microscope. With a focus on the software's key strengths and drawbacks, this chapter sought to present a comprehensive list of computational tools that can be used by computer scientists and pathologists. It also discussed the various difficulties that could arise in DP. One of these difficulties is in reading WSIs, because of their varied and complex formats. Although many of them can be read using libraries like OpenSlide or Bio-Formats, none of the libraries currently support all of the market-available formats. Combining them as a whole turns out to be a feasible and preferable solution. Other common bioimaging software boost performance by using extra plugins and external software. However, using platforms created especially for DP offers easier understanding for WSIs than using standard tools of bioimaging. The use of the software varies for user's differing needs for analysis; some require single-image processing, for which Fiji/ImageJ is considered the better choice, and some require multiple images for batch processing and building pipelines, for which CellProfiler and QuPath are tools available.

As we study different histopathological image analysis software, we learn about their different features, such as their ability to detect objects in images, calculate cell area and perimeter, work with whole slide images (WSIs) and Bio-Format images, and provide all the required information. Working together seamlessly with software, either by transfer of image data or protocols integrating different image analysis tools into a single workflow, makes interoperability between software effective for large image data. Different software showed certain differences in each of their detections as we got the result for the image, which could be seen from Figures 18.3 to 18.10. To achieve the comparative scenario, multiple software was used for the same image, showing different results. A cell that undergoes various changes due to the occurrence of a disease is important for clinicians to observe and understand to achieve a diagnosis, but it would be easier if it could be done digitally as it would save time and provide quick and efficient results. In comparison to the traditional method, bioimaging tools use ML and DP algorithms, which can be helpful in accurately analyzing the results for the diagnosis. The aim is to have more intuitive software paving a new way in DH: software which is easy, user-friendly, and robust, and in which annotations or detections could be understood by experts. However, there is no such perfect software or tool on which we can be fully dependent, and we must choose among available software according to different user needs.

There are different algorithms that are used in software in DP like ML. Digital image analysis is important in observation or detection; generally k-nearest neighbours, neural networks, etc. are used. AI and ML algorithms are being developed to diagnose diseases using software image processing, which would be promising in healthcare. Bioimage software is striving to integrate AI and ML to improve and automate medical imaging practice and quantitative image analysis.

18.7 DISCUSSION

With advancing technology, the field of medicine, or the healthcare sector, is advancing rapidly. There is a need for advancement in medical diagnosis, such as in imaging techniques. AI or ML tools have a great impact on the diagnosis and treatment of diseases. Pathologists make use of image analysis by obtaining DH to help them diagnose cancer subtypes and tumours, as well as minimize their workload. Clinicians say that ML and DL could help in tracing tumours and lesions. The software which is used in this analysis is a tool that can be improved and used effectively. In histopathology, where the diseased cell is studied, identification and correct prediction are very important. Common traditional methods have been found to be time- and resource-consuming. Interoperability is important because it enables researchers and healthcare providers to use the tools that are best suited for their needs and to easily exchange data and results between different systems. This can improve efficiency and enhance the accuracy of bioimage analysis (Levet et al., 2021). DH is widely used to get quick results in a short time with accurate disease prediction in certain areas of research and diagnosis.

As per the result of the study of certain tools and software, we observed that a combination of these tools, having multiple ML and DL technologies, improved the computational power and accuracy of analyses. For instance, cell detection could be combined with detecting changes that take place in the cells, indicating the changes at every stage of the cell, which could be helpful for clinicians. These tools should have more user-friendly interfaces or GUI and the documentation should be well-explained for the end-users or for beginners, as it is very difficult to understand the correct usage of software without any proper clarification on the steps to perform image analysis (i.e., it should be less complex). Robust and effective algorithms for tissue analysis and diagnosis should be included and the description of its diagnostic approach should be improved (i.e., there should be constant additions of new updates with different algorithms for cell detection or diseased cell prediction cell). The combined feedback by the pathologist, histopathologist, and clinicians is important for improving the development of software for the timely diagnosis of a disease. Moreover, collaborative tools could be improved for easy exchange of data or images, allowing improvement in the results (Escobar Díaz Guerrero et al., 2022). The ability of different software programmes to work together, exchange data, and use the same standards and protocols make the software interoperable, which is important in the field of bioimage analysis.

REFERENCES

Abbas, A., Abdelsamea, M. M., and Gaber, M. M. (2020). DeTrac: Transfer learning of class decomposed medical images in convolutional neural networks. *IEEE Access*, 8, 74901–74913. https://doi.org/10.1109/access.2020.2989273

Adiga, P. U., and Chaudhuri, B. B. (2000). Region based techniques for segmentation of volumetric histo-pathological images. *Computer Methods and Programs in Biomedicine*, 61(1), 23–47. https://doi.org/10.1016/S0169-2607(99)00026-7

Aeffner, F., Zarella, M. D., Buchbinder, N., Bui, M. M., Goodman, M. R., Hartman, D. J., Lujan, G. M., Molani, M. A., Parwani, A. V., Lillard, K., Turner, O. C., Vemuri, V. N. P., Yuil-Valdes, A. G., and Bowman, D. (2019). Introduction to digital image analysis in whole-slide imaging: A white paper from the digital pathology association. *Journal of Pathology Informatics*, 10(1), 9. https://doi.org/10.4103/jpi.jpi_82_18

Allan, C., Burel, J. M., Moore, J., Blackburn, C., Linkert, M., Loynton, S., Macdonald, D., Moore, W. J., Neves, C., Patterson, A., Porter, M., Tarkowska, A., Loranger, B., Avondo, J., Lagerstedt, I., Lianas, L., Leo, S., Hands, K., Hay, R. T., Patwardhan, A., Best, C., Kleywegt, G. J., Zanetti, G., and Swedlow, J. R. (2012). OMERO: Flexible, model-driven data management for experimental biology. *Nature Methods*, 9(3), 245–253. https://doi.org/10.1038/nmeth.1896

Arevalo, J., and Cruz-Roa, A. (2014). Histopathology image representation for automatic analysis: A state-of-the-art review. *Revista de Medicina*, 22(2), 79–91.

Balogh, E., Miller, B. T., and Ball, J. (2015). *Improving Diagnosis in Health Care*. The National Academies Press.

Bankhead, P., Loughrey, M. B., Fernández, J. A., Dombrowski, Y., McArt, D. G., Dunne, P. D., McQuaid, S., Gray, R. T., Murray, L. J., Coleman, H. G., James, J. A., Salto-Tellez, M., and Hamilton, P. W. (2017). QuPath: Open source software for digital pathology image analysis. *Scientific Reports*, 7(1), 1–7. https://doi.org/10.1038/s41598-017-17204-5

Belsare, A. D., and Mushrif, M. M. (2012). Histopathological image analysis using image processing techniques: An overview. *Signal and Image Processing*, 3(4), 23. https://doi.org/10.5121/sipij.2012.3403

Bray, M. A., and Carpenter, A. E. (2015). CellProfiler Tracer: Exploring and validating high-throughput, time-lapse microscopy image data. *BMC Bioinformatics*, 16(1), 1–7. https://doi.org/10.1186/s12859-015-0759-x

Bulas, D., and Egloff, A. (2013). Benefits and risks of MRI in pregnancy. *Seminars in Perinatology*, 37(5), 301–304. https://doi.org/10.1053/j.semperi.2013.06.005

Burri, O. (2022, October 17). QuPath: Taking full control through workflows, scripting, and extensions. Retrieved February 10, 2023, from https://analyticalscience.wiley.com/do/10.1002/was.0004000312

Carpenter, A. E., Jones, T. R., Lamprecht, M. R., Clarke, C., Kang, I. H., Friman, O., Guertin, D. A., Chang, J. H., Lindquist, R. A., Moffat, J., Golland, P., and Sabatini, D. M. (2006). CellProfiler: Image analysis software for identifying and quantifying cell phenotypes. *Genome Biology*, 7(10), 1–11. https://doi.org/10.1186/gb-2006-7-10-r100

De Chaumont, F., Dallongeville, S., Chenouard, N., Hervé, N., Pop, S., Provoost, T., Meas-Yedid, V., Pankajakshan, P., Lecomte, T., Le Montagner, Y., Lagache, T., Dufour, A., and Olivo-Marin, J. C. (2012). Icy: An open BioImage informatics platform for extended reproducible research. *Nature Methods*, 9(7), 690–696. https://doi.org/10.1038/nmeth.2075

De Chaumont, F., Dallongeville, S., Provoost, T., Lecomte, T., Dufour, A., and Olivo-Marin, J. C. (2013, September). Icy: A user-friendly environment for algorithm development and deployment. In *21st European Signal Processing Conference (EUSIPCO 2013)* (pp. 1–5). IEEE.

DeBerardinis, R. J., and Thompson, C. B. (2012). Cellular metabolism and disease: What do metabolic outliers teach us? *Cell*, 148(6), 1132–1144. https://doi.org/10.1016/j.cell.2012.02.032

Dobson, E. T. A., Cimini, B., Klemm, A. H., Wählby, C., Carpenter, A. E., and Eliceiri, K. W. (2021). ImageJ and CellProfiler: Complements in open-source BioImage analysis. *Current Protocols*, 1(5), e89. https://doi.org/10.1002/cpz1.89

Dong, Z., Andrews, T., Xie, C., and Yokoo, T. (2015). Advances in MRI techniques and applications. *BioMed Research International*, 2015, 1–2. https://doi.org/10.1155/2015/139043

Elmore, S. A. (2012). Enhanced histopathology of the immune system: A review and update. *Toxicologic Pathology*, 40(2), 148–156. https://doi.org/10.1177/0192623311427571

Escobar Díaz Guerrero, R., Carvalho, L., Bocklitz, T., Popp, J., and Oliveira, J. L. (2022). Software tools and platforms in Digital Pathology: A review for clinicians and computer scientists. *Journal of Pathology Informatics*, 13, 100103. https://doi.org/10.1016/j.jpi.2022.100103

Fischer, G., Anderson, L., Ranson, M., Sellen, D., and McArthur, E. (2021). Public perceptions on pathology: A fundamental change is required. *Journal of Clinical Pathology*, 74(12), 812–815. https://doi.org/10.1136/jclinpath-2020-206873

Flach, R. N., Fransen, N. L., Sonnen, A. F. P., Nguyen, T. Q., Breimer, G. E., Veta, M., Stathonikos, N., van Dooijeweert, C., and van Diest, P. J. (2022). Implementation of artificial intelligence in diagnostic practice as a next step after going digital: The UMC Utrecht perspective. *Diagnostics (Basel, Switzerland)*, 12(5), 1042. https://doi.org/10.3390/diagnostics12051042

Gonzalez Obando, D. F., Mandache, D., Olivo-Marin, J. C., and Meas-Yedid, V. (2019, April). Icytomine: A user-friendly tool for integrating workflows on whole slide images. In *European Congress on Digital Pathology* (pp. 181–189). Cham: Springer. https://doi.org/10.1007/978-3-030-23937-4_21

Gurcan, M. N., Boucheron, L. E., Can, A., Madabhushi, A., Rajpoot, N. M., and Yener, B. (2009). Histopathological image analysis: A review. *IEEE Reviews in Biomedical Engineering*, 2, 147–171. https://doi.org/10.1109/RBME.2009.2034865

Haase, R., Royer, L. A., Steinbach, P., Schmidt, D., Dibrov, A., Schmidt, U., Weigert, M., Maghelli, N., Tomancak, P., Jug, F., and Myers, E. W. (2019). Clij: GPU-accelerated image processing for everyone. *Nature Methods*, 17(1), 5–6. https://doi.org/10.1038/s41592-019-0650-1

Horai, Y., Mizukawa, M., Nishina, H., Nishikawa, S., Ono, Y., Takemoto, K., and Baba, N. (2019). Quantification of histopathological findings using a novel image analysis platform. *Journal of Toxicologic Pathology*, 32(4), 319–327. https://doi.org/10.1293/tox.2019-0022

Ibrahim, A., Gamble, P., Jaroensri, R., Abdelsamea, M. M., Mermel, C. H., Chen, P. C., and Rakha, E. A. (2020). Artificial intelligence in digital breast pathology: Techniques and applications. *Breast (Edinburgh, Scotland)*, 49, 267–273. https://doi.org/10.1016/j.breast.2019.12.007

Jahn, S. W., Plass, M., and Moinfar, F. (2020). Digital pathology: Advantages, limitations and emerging perspectives. *Journal of Clinical Medicine*, 9(11), 3697. https://doi.org/10.3390/jcm9113697

Jakhmola-Mani, R., Mittal, K., and Pande Katare, D. (2020). Alarm test: A novel chemical-free behavioural assessment tool for zebrafish. *Zebrafish in Biomedical Research*. https://doi.org/10.5772/intechopen.91181

Kemp, W. L., Burns, D. K., and Brown, T. G. (Eds.). (2008). Chapter 1. Cellular pathology. *Pathology: The Big Picture*. McGraw Hill. https://accessmedicine.mhmedical.com/content.aspx?bookid=499andsectionid=41568284

Kuczkiewicz-Siemion, O., Sokół, K., Puton, B., Borkowska, A., and Szumera-Ciećkiewicz, A. (2022). The role of pathology-based methods in qualitative and quantitative approaches to cancer immunotherapy. *Cancers*, 14(15), 3833. https://doi.org/10.3390/cancers14153833

Levet, F., Carpenter, A. E., Eliceiri, K. W., Kreshuk, A., Bankhead, P., and Haase, R. (2021). Developing open-source software for bioimage analysis: Opportunities and challenges. *F1000Research*, 10, 302. https://doi.org/10.12688/f1000research.52531.1

Marée, R. (2019). Open practices and resources for collaborative digital pathology. *Frontiers in Medicine*, 6, 255. https://doi.org/10.3389/fmed.2019.00255

Marée, R., Rollus, L., Stévens, B., Hoyoux, R., Louppe, G., Vandaele, R., Begon, J. M., Kainz, P., Geurts, P., and Wehenkel, L. (2016). Collaborative analysis of multi-gigapixel imaging data using Cytomine. *Bioinformatics*, 32(9), 1395–1401. https://doi.org/10.1093/bioinformatics/btw013

McCombe, K. D., Craig, S. G., Pulsawatdi, A. V., Quezada-Marín, J. I., Hagan, M., Rajendran, S., Humphries, M. P., Bingham, V., Salto-Tellez, M., Gault, R., and James, J. A. (2021). HistoClean: Open-source software for histological image preprocessing and augmentation to improve development of robust convolutional neural networks. *Computational and Structural Biotechnology Journal*, 19, 4840–4853. https://doi.org/10.1016/j.csbj.2021.08.033

Meijering, E. (2020). A bird's-eye view of deep learning in BioImage analysis. *Computational and Structural Biotechnology Journal*, 18, 2312–2325. https://doi.org/10.1016/j.csbj.2020.08.003

Nedzved, A., Belotserkovsky, A., Lehmann, T. M., and Ablameyko, S. (2007, February). Morphometrical feature extraction on colour histological images for oncological diagnostics. In *5th International Conference on Biomedical Engineering*, ACTA Press, 379 - 384).

Power, S. P., Moloney, F., Twomey, M., James, K., O'Connor, O. J., and Maher, M. M. (2016). Computed tomography and patient risk: Facts, perceptions and uncertainties. *World Journal of Radiology*, 8(12), 902–915. https://doi.org/10.4329/wjr.v8.i12.902

Rakovic, K., Colling, R., Browning, L., Dolton, M., Horton, M. R., Protheroe, A., Lamb, A. D., Bryant, R. J., Scheffer, R., Crofts, J., Stanislaus, E., and Verrill, C. (2022). The use of digital pathology and artificial intelligence in histopathological diagnostic assessment of prostate cancer: A survey of Prostate Cancer UK supporters. *Diagnostics*, 12(5), 1225. https://doi.org/10.3390/diagnostics12051225

Rani, U., and Amsini, A. (2018). Image processing techniques used in digital pathology imaging: An overview. *International Journal of Engineering Research in Computer Science and Engineering (IJERCSE)*, 5(1)

Rubens, U., Hoyoux, R., Vanosmael, L., Ouras, M., Tasset, M., Hamilton, C., Longuespée, R., and Marée, R. (2019). Cytomine: Toward an open and collaborative software platform for digital pathology bridged to molecular investigations. *Proteomics: Clinical, Applications*, 13(1), e1800057. https://doi.org/10.1002/prca.201800057

Rueden, C. T., Schindelin, J., Hiner, M. C., DeZonia, B. E., Walter, A. E., Arena, E. T., and Eliceiri, K. W. (2017). ImageJ2: ImageJ for the next generation of scientific image data. *BMC Bioinformatics*, 18(1), 1–26. https://doi.org/10.1186/s12859-017-1934-z

Schindelin, J., Arganda-Carreras, I., Frise, E., Kaynig, V., Longair, M., Pietzsch, T., Preibisch, S., Rueden, C., Saalfeld, S., Schmid, B., Tinevez, J. Y., White, D. J., Hartenstein, V., Eliceiri, K., Tomancak, P., and Cardona, A. (2012). Fiji: An open-source platform for biological-image analysis. *Nature Methods*, 9(7), 676–682. https://doi.org/10.1038/nmeth.2019

Schroeder, A. B., Dobson, E. T., Rueden, C. T., Tomancak, P., Jug, F., and Eliceiri, K. W. (2021). The ImageJ ecosystem: Open-source software for image visualization, processing, and analysis. *Protein Science*, 30(1), 234–249. https://doi.org/10.1002/pro.3993

Scully, J. L. (2004). What is a disease? *EMBO Reports*, 5(7), 650–653. https://doi.org/10.1038/sj.embor.7400195

Sikandar, A. (2018). Histopathology: An old yet important technique in modern science. In *Histopathology - an Update*. IntechOpen. https://doi.org/10.5772/intechopen.76908

Stritt, M., Stalder, A. K., and Vezzali, E. (2020). Orbit image analysis: An open-source whole slide image analysis tool. *PLOS Computational Biology*, 16(2), e1007313. https://doi.org/10.1371/journal.pcbi.1007313

Tizard, I. R., and Musser, J. M. B. (2022). Infectious diseases and their causes. *Great American Diseases*, 1–17. https://doi.org/10.1016/b978-0-323-98925-1.00005-2

Underwood, J. C. (2017). More than meets the eye: The changing face of histopathology. *Histopathology*, 70(1), 4–9. https://doi.org/10.1111/his.13047

van Beek, E. J., Kuhl, C., Anzai, Y., Desmond, P., Ehman, R. L., Gong, Q., Gold, G., Gulani, V., Hall-Craggs, M., Leiner, T., Lim, C. C. T., Pipe, J. G., Reeder, S., Reinhold, C., Smits, M., Sodickson, D. K., Tempany, C., Vargas, H. A., and Wang, M. (2019). Value of MRI in medicine: More than just another test? *Journal of Magnetic Resonance Imaging*, 49(7), e14–e25. https://doi.org/10.1002/jmri.26211

van der Laak, J., Litjens, G., and Ciompi, F. (2021). Deep learning in histopathology: The path to the clinic. *Nature Medicine*, 27(5), 775–784. https://doi.org/10.1038/s41591-021-01343-4

Ward, A. O., Janbandhu, V., Chapman, G., Dunwoodie, S. L., and Harvey, R. P. (2022). An image analysis protocol using CellProfiler for automated quantification of post-ischemic cardiac parameters. *Star Protocols*, 3(1), 101097. https://doi.org/10.1016/j.xpro.2021.101097

Wexler, B. (2013). *Health and Wellness: Illness Among Americans*. Gale, Cengage Learning.

Xu, Y., Jia, Z., Wang, L. B., Ai, Y., Zhang, F., Lai, M., and Chang, E. I. (2017). Large scale tissue histopathology image classification, segmentation, and visualization via deep convolutional activation features. *BMC Bioinformatics*, 18(1), 1–17. https://doi.org/10.1186/s12859-017-1685-x

19 Artificial Intelligence Techniques to Design Epitope-Mapped Vaccines and Diagnostics for Emerging Pathogens

Hina Bansal and Navya Aggarwal

19.1 INTRODUCTION

Since the dawn of the first vaccines, healthcare systems have appropriately developed a technique that can manipulate our bodies to fight pathogens by priming our innate immunity against that specific pathogen. These vaccines are conventionally prepared by using live or attenuated pathogens as a whole or by using their subunits. These substances are recognized by our bodies as foreign and thus attacked by cellular and humoral immunity. However, these traditional vaccines have some major drawbacks in today's scenario. Traditional methods to make vaccines can take up to 15 years, at a huge expense (Parvizpour et al. 2020). These vaccines also pose risks, as they can have adverse effects and induce disorders, the disease itself, and in extreme cases, death (Soria-Guerra et al., 2015). Such a long and costly process is undesirable both to the industry and to the health of the general populace. This leads to the development of epitope vaccines using immunoinformatic techniques in the fields of genomics and proteomics. These vaccines have the capacity to have both preventative and curative impacts. The computational method is not only affordable but also prompts a focused, protracted immune response and, most significantly, it saves time. The vaccines are also considered to be safer, as there is no risk of pathogen revival. The fundamental idea behind an epitope vaccine is that immunity acquired by adaptation is regulated by lymphocytes (B-cells and T-cells). These cells are not capable of identifying pathogens wholly, but they detect the molecular components called antigens by permitting a fit between antibody cell-surface structures (paratopes) with antigen surface epitopes. This recognition happens on the surface of the cells. These antigens have a defined group of amino acids called epitopes, which are capable of activating the receptors (Raoufi et al., 2020). These regions may span an area of 600 to 1000 Angstrom in loops and 15–25 residues in length (Potocnakova

DOI: 10.1201/9781003363361-19

et al. 2016). A design with multiple epitopes is predicted to have better antigenicity and immune response, as a close-to-perfect vaccine must be a single molecule that is able to adequately elicit a response from both B- and T-cells in the majority of the population (multitarget), with a deficit of non-protective epitopes, target-conserved epitopic sequences in variably mutating pathogens, and, thus, should be highly effective and efficient (Gershoni et al., 2007; Almeida et al., 2012; Iurescia et al., 2012).

Major steps involved in epitope vaccine development were earlier performed *in vivo*, however, seeing how costly and time-consuming they were, *in silico* tools were developed. These tools involve creating algorithms for the analysis of prospective B-cell epitopes and T-cell epitopes. Another major goal is to determine the binding affinities of potential peptides to antibodies. These methods involve various tools that depend on artificial intelligence technology. Artificial intelligence is a technology, or rather a subfield of computational science, which deals with problem-solving on robust datasets while mimicking decision-making capabilities and essentially learning and deciphering patterns and answers in a manner similar to the human mind (Mohammad, 2020; Kundu and Mondal, 2022). In this chapter, we will throw light on different artificial intelligence tools used for epitope prediction, also focusing on various techniques used in the given tools. Artificial intelligence (AI) and machine learning (ML) provide a close-to-perfect alternative to finding vaccine epitopes that have the ability to stimulate specific immune responses. These are formulations of small sequences of proteins (peptides), in contrast to conventional vaccines, which usually contain dead or attenuated pathogens. AI and ML techniques help in data analysis and prediction. Essentially, they help in the analysis of multiple genomes, peptides, structures, and their various properties, then shortlist the epitopes which produce the best response, are the safest, and give the most population coverage.

19.2 LYMPHOCYTES (B-CELLS AND T-CELLS)

Lymphocyte cells are a type of white blood cell responsible for providing an organism with its only means to recognize and fight a specific pathogen or foreign substance – an antigenic epitope for instance – thus being responsible for antigen-specific immunity. There are two types of lymphocytes present in the human body: B-cells, which are deployed to provide humoral immunity, and T-cells, which are linked to cell-mediated immunity (Cano and Lopera, 2013; Calder et al., 2022).

19.2.1 B-Cells

They are Y-shaped proteins that are capable of recognizing antigens exposed to solvent through its receptors (Figure 19.1 (a,b)). These B-cell receptor proteins consist of immunoglobulins which are membrane-bound. After stimulation, these cells divide and secrete antibodies (specialized proteins called immunoglobulins). B-cells can have a different impact depending on the antigen, such as neutralization of toxins and pathogens, or flagging them for apoptosis (Wild 2013).

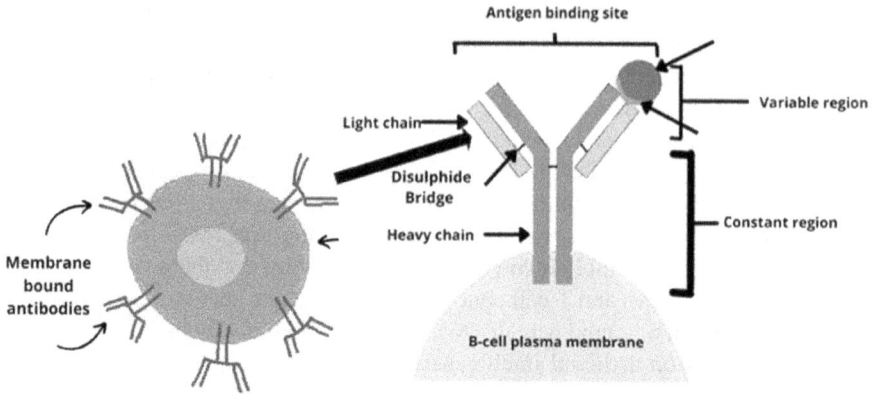

FIGURE 19.1 (a) B-cell lymphocytes (b) Antigen-antibody complex

19.2.2 T-Cells

T-cells are mainly of two types: helper T-cells, which activate B-cells by producing cytokines, and killer T-cells, which kill the infected cells by use of toxins (Duru et al., 2022). They comprise a specific receptor on their surface that allows the identification of antigens, which are displayed on the cells presenting antigens attached to major histocompatibility complex (MHC) molecules. T-cells can be represented as class one MHC molecules, which are identified by CD8 T-cell subset, and class two MHC molecules, which are recognized by CD4 T-cell subset. Because of this, there are two types of T-cell epitopes (Figure 19.2).

CD8 T-cells are labelled as cytotoxic T lymphocytes (CTL), whereas CD4 T-cells are considered regulatory (Treg) or helper (Th) T-cells [12]. T-helper cells magnify the response of the immune system, and three types exist: Th1 leads to the cell-mediated

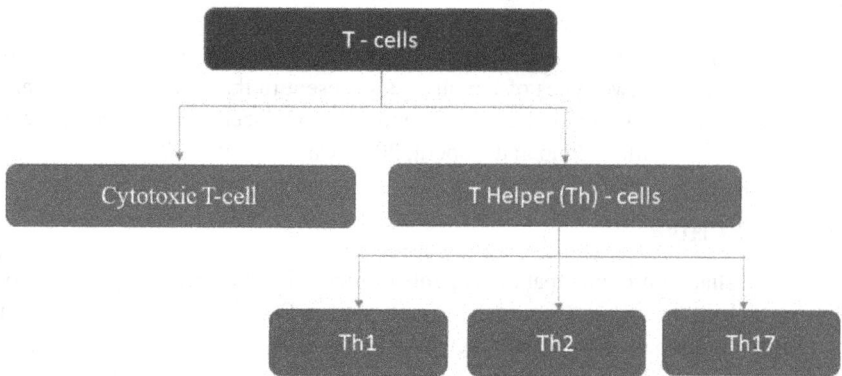

FIGURE 19.2 Types and subtypes of T-lymphocyte cells in humans

response by the use of macrophages and cytotoxic killer T-cells; Th2 provides a humoral immune response by triggering antibodies; and Th17 leads to apoptosis of viruses and other pathogens and an increased inflammatory response by creating a link between adaptive and innate immunity (Gagliani and Huber, 2017; Sagu et al., 2022).

19.3 ARTIFICIAL INTELLIGENCE TECHNIQUES

The following are some of the most prevalent artificial intelligence techniques that may be applied for epitope prediction.

19.3.1 MACHINE LEARNING

Machine learning methods have lately been in the spotlight due to their techniques which prevent error-prone calculations from occurring during the estimation of the protein-ligand interaction. This is usually worked upon in terms of entropic changes and ligand solvation (Raza et al., 2020). There are two major methods to perform the learning process: unsupervised learning and supervised learning. The technique of supervised learning consists of labelled data, with the aim to predict the result from the input provided, while unsupervised learning has unlabelled input, where the machine itself finds the hidden patterns in the input and output datasets supplied (Love, 2002; Napolitano et al., 2013). The majority of drug discovery, epitope prediction, and cheminformatic tools are based on a supervised approach.

19.3.2 ARTIFICIAL NEURAL NETWORKS

This approach is employed to parameterize the quantitative structure-activity relationship (QSAR) model in a nonlinear sense. This model is inspired by the human brain and, thus, is made up of layers of nodes connecting like biological neurons. The biological neuron has dendrites (which receive information), cell bodies (for processing), and axons (which carry processed information outward). This is mimicked by the artificial neural networks (ANN) model, which strives to draw conclusions from limited data provided like a human brain (Dobchev and Karelson, 2016). It has three major layers: an input information layer, a hidden layer, and an output generation layer. Here, hidden layers are multiple in number and connected by a weighted relationship, which is estimated by backpropagation (Buciński et al., 2009; Brusic and Flower, 2004). ANN has several benefits, such as being able to identify both linear and nonlinear patterns in input data, being able to self-improve, being able to handle erroneous data, and being based on a higher-order model that is able to decipher complex relationships in the dataset. They need preprocessed data, such as peptide alignment, before presentation (Brusic and Flower, 2004).

19.4 DEEP LEARNING

Deep neural networks (DNNs) are based on the deep learning technique, an extension of artificial neural networks. They are extensively applied in the processing of unstructured high dimensional learning for machine vision (learning which involves analysis of data by relying on patterns and inference) (Coley et al., 2018) and natural language processing (a technique used for voice recognition by computers much like humans do) (Najafabadi et al., 2015; Chowdhary, 2020). DNN has been observed to outperform other machine learning approaches in specific pharmaceutical arenas such as predicting biological activity, toxicity, and absorption, distribution, metabolism, excretion, and toxicity (ADMET) properties. DNN consists of multiple layers of neurons to achieve a high level of abstraction of data. It aims to reduce the overfitting issue. To solve the data extraction of features and dimensions, reduction mechanisms are also incorporated. Convolutional neural networks (CNNs) are used to determine the scores for protein-ligand interaction, by applying the 3D-CNN approach, where proteins are visualized as 3D images (Najafabadi et al., 2015; Schneider et al., 2019; Raza et al., 2020). Recurrent neural networks (RNNs) are also employed for predictions. Protein structure prediction is also a major use of DNN.

19.4.1 Autoencoder-Based Approach

An autoencoder is a neural network model used for the extraction of features from the unsupervised method. It is a feed-forward network, where input and output are the same. It consists of three components: an encoder, a decoder, and a distance function (code). The encoder takes high-dimensional input and compresses it into a lower-dimensional code several orders smaller, which is then injected into the machine, while the decoder reconstructs the original input by learning (Blaschke et al., 2017; Jordan, 2018; Michelucci, 2022). A bottleneck is provided so that the network learns and doesn't just memorize input values (Dertat, 2017). The distance function measures the deviations and differences between the processed output and the original input. This method is used to create identical characteristics in the output layer and the input layer. It helps in transforming raw data into an internal characteristic used for classification and identification purposes.

19.4.2 Text Mining

Text mining, also called text analytics, is an artificial intelligence-centred approach that makes use of natural language processing to convert unstructured and unorganized text data, such as the data provided by databases and documents, into more appropriate and manageable structured data, which is then suitable for further analysis, to use in machine learning algorithms, or for further predictive work (Linguamatics, 2019). Existing data present in the plethora of biomedical and pharmaceutical literature and works and detailed and versatile datasets at our disposal are potential sources of an information bank regarding drugs, diseases, proteins, epitopes, antigens, toxicity, genetic data, pathogens, and their features (Dash et al., 2019; Raza et al., 2020).

19.4.3 Hidden Markov Model

The hidden Markov model is a statistical high-order method used in artificial intelligence algorithms capable of recognizing complex relationships in data. These algorithms do not require the preprocessing of proteins before their training (Brusic and

Flower, 2004). They allow predictions of sequences of unidentified variables from a set of known and observed variables. The model can determine the probabilistic feature of any random process (Roy and Hasan, 2021). It is found to be most suitable for the prediction of peptides of MHC molecules and to characterize motifs with an inherent structure arrangement (Raoufi et al., 2020). This model was reported to be a high-accuracy predictor of peptides binding to MHC molecules (Mamitsuka, 1998).

19.4.4 SUPPORT VECTOR MACHINE

Support vector machine belongs to the class of supervised learning algorithms that aims at creating the best line that divides n-dimensional space (where n gives the number of features) into separate classes, so that the new data point can be added to the right category (Suthaharan, 2016). The boundary of the best decision is also called a hyperplane. Extreme points called support vectors are chosen to make the hyperplane (Wang, 2022). This method majorly helps in the classification of training data, along with the advantage of being able to train on small peptide datasets (Brusic and Flower, 2004).

19.4.5 QUANTITATIVE STRUCTURE-ACTIVITY RELATIONSHIP

This is a mathematical computational method that portrays relationships between the chemical structural properties and biological activity (such as metabolism, toxicity, absorption, and excretion) of the molecules (Kwon et al., 2019). Different properties lead to the different biological activities of the peptides. Using statistical methods, it relates the measured activity of a molecule with regard to the biological response to its physiochemical structure. The most prevalent approach is random forest. The input data is usually molecular descriptors, from which molecular property is predicted (Ivanciuc, 2009).

19.5 *IN SILICO* VACCINE DESIGN

Currently, only a small number of infectious diseases have vaccines, so there is a serious need for quick vaccine design for many lethal and emerging pathogens. Several reports have already been published that emphasize the importance of *in silico* techniques for vaccine design and outline the steps of AI and computational techniques that can be utilized for vaccine design and assessment of drugs (Bhakta et al., 2021; Thomas et al., 2022). An AI-based model can be a comprehensive way to design novel vaccine candidates in an extensive molecular space. AI employs algorithm structures to explore and discover the characteristics of the incoming data and to generate autonomous decisions to achieve particular goals. Additionally, it can quickly inspect drug targets, find hit and lead compounds, and optimize drug structure design (Lv et al., 2021).

An artificial intelligence-based approach reduces the time it takes to sort extensive data and thus provides the most relevant information. The steps involved in

Biological Data Extraction

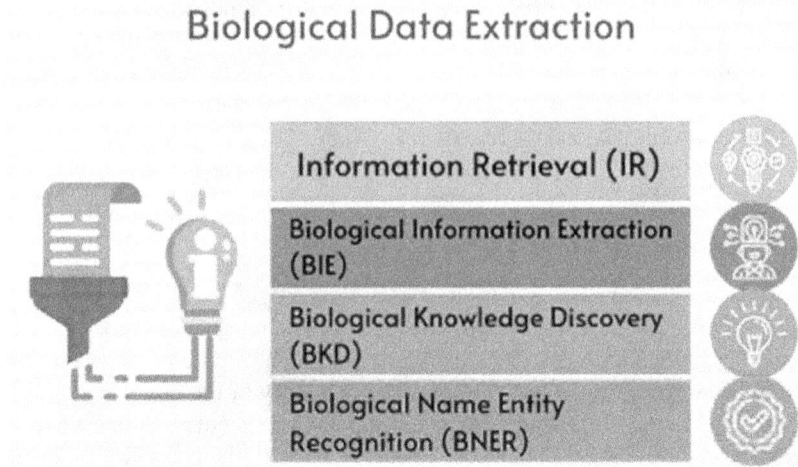

FIGURE 19.3 Steps for biological data extraction

biological data extraction are the retrieval of information (IR), followed by biological information extraction (BIE), biological knowledge discovery (BKD), and, finally, biological name entity recognition (BNER) (Figure 19.3).

Malone et al. in 2020 employed an artificial intelligence technique to outline the process of designing a vaccine against SARS-CoV-2 that has a suitably wide range of T-cell epitopes able to serve worldwide. They utilized the national electrical code (NEC) Immune Profiler suite to generate epitope maps. Then, the Monte Carlo simulation model was used to check the significance level of epitope maps. They explored around 3400 virus sequences to find a pattern suggesting that the viral infection is less likely to be presented by infected host cells and subsequently recognized by the host immune system. After that, epitope hotspots that appeared in less-conserved parts of the viral proteome were eliminated through a sequence conservation study, and, lastly, a digital twin simulation model was used to simulate various hotspot combinations (Malone et al., 2020).

Mazzocco et al. in 2021 applied a machine learning model to investigate the immunogenicity of epitopes. The data from viral epitope experimental T-cell immunogenicity were used to train the model. They made use of publicly available immunogenicity data for coronavirus for modal validation. Additionally, they also carried out analyses of epitope conservation among various strains and the hazard of immunotoxicity (Mazzocco et al., 2021).

Yang et al. in 2021 proposed DeepVacPred, a cutting-edge AI-based tool for multi-epitope vaccine design. They used a deep neural network algorithm for predictions and validation of the model. The model determines the potency of the input peptide sequence to be a vaccine candidate or not. First, the model allows for the initial reduction of the number of potential vaccine subunits to around 30, followed by additional evaluation and vaccine design (Yang et al., 2021).

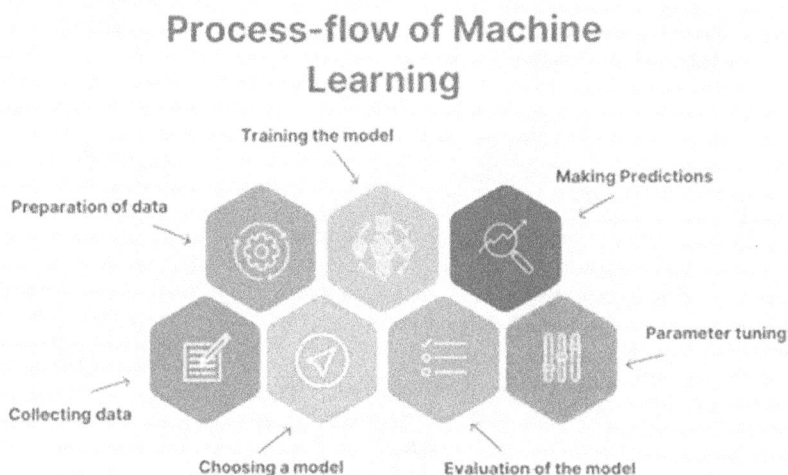

FIGURE 19.4   Seven stages in machine learning process flow

Additionally, molecular docking is one of the most extensively applied approaches for drug and vaccine discovery projects. It can identify binding orientations between molecules and help deduce drug-protein interactions such as epitope-paratope interaction (Raza et al., 2020). This method quantifies the binding affinity and strength of ligands with receptors using two main components: a search algorithm and a scoring function (Meng et al., 2011). All possible conformation and the orientations of the ligand in the active site of its receptor are predicted, along with the free energy involved. Monte Carlo, systematic search, genetic algorithm, simulated annealing, and various other algorithms are utilized for this search algorithm development. This is converted into a mathematic function by the scoring method. Scoring can be based on physical, empirical (experimental), or knowledge-based information available on ligand and receptor interactions (Sliwoski et al., 2013).

The process flow of machine learning for drug design consists of seven stages: collection of data, preparation of data, choosing a model, training it, evaluation of the model, parameter tuning, and, finally, making predictions (Brzić et al., 2022). Numerous algorithms used in this approach are random forest (RF), deep neural network (DNN), deep learning (DL), and support vector machines (SVM) (Figure 19.4). The accuracy of the model relies on the quality and quantity of data used in training the algorithm, along with the validation process for the ready model.

19.6   DATABASES FOR EPITOPES

For the computational research process and the study of epitope prediction, data to train artificial intelligence is needed. This data may be served by databases that have been curated over the years to provide all the information regarding the immunological peptides and their physiochemical properties that are needed. The names and links of major databases for epitopes of lymphocytes are listed in Table 19.1.

TABLE 19.1
List of Databases for Epitopes of Lymphocytes

Database Name	Description	Type	Reference
AntiJen	Quantitative kinetic, diffusion coefficient, thermodynamic binding, and cellular data for peptide interactions including T-cell epitopes, B-cell epitopes, major histocompatibility complexes (MHCs), TAP transporters, lymphocyte receptors, and immunological interaction. Downloading of data is not allowed.	Both	Mazzocco et al. (2021), McSparron et al. (2003)
BciPep	Contains experimentally approved linear (continuous) B-cell epitopes obtained from public databases as well as available literature. The database contains data from PubMed, Swiss-Prot, MHCBN, and Protein DataBank. Epitopes are categorized into immunogenic, immunodominant, and null-immunogenic.	B-cells	Meng et al. (2011)
IEDB-3D	IEDB (Immune Epitope Database) is a highly detailed data resource cataloging experimentally defined B- and T-cell epitopes, along with MHC ligand binding belonging to a variety of organisms. It contains data on different epitopes such as source antigen, structure and sequence of epitopes, obtained from public databases, peer-reviewed literature, submissions done directly, and patent applications. It has a fully embedded application called EpitopeViewer, which permits visualization of the antigen structure. It has several tools attached to it for various processes such as the calculation of intermolecular contacts.	Both	Michelucci, (2022), Mixter (1999)
Epitome	It gives access to a number of antibody–antigen complexes, comprising visualization and annotation of residues, along with structural properties of binding areas. Data entry is collected from Protein DataBank.	Both	Mohammad, (2020)
SDAP	SDAP (or Structural Database of Allergenic Proteins) includes structures, sequences, and epitopes of allergenic antigens. It also allows the matching of allergen and peptide and the cross reactivity.	Both	Najafabadi et al. (2015)

(Continued)

**TABLE 19.1
(Continued)**

Database Name	Description	Type	Reference
AntigenDB	Data about T-cell epitopes, MHC binding peptides, their characteristics, expression of genes, and post-translational modifications (PTMs). Provides external links to other databases and also includes binding affinity of MHC proteins, TAP binders, cleavage sites connected PTMs, and T-cell epitopes.	T-cells	Napolitano et al. (2013)
Cancer Immunity Peptide Database	Contains tumor T-cell antigens for cancer immunity collected experimentally.	Both	Parvizpour et al. (2020)
CrossTope	CrossTope contains 3D structures of MHC I complexes. These immunogenic peptides contained are obtained from experiments and literature. These complexes are termed pMHC-I.	T-cells	Peters et al. (2005)
HIV Molecular Immunology Database	It contains information about experimentally found B-cell and T-cell epitopes. Also containing information such as escape mutations, overlapping functional domains in epitopes, and cross-reactivity.	Both	Ponomarenko et al. 2010
SEDB	Data about T-cell epitopes, MHC-binding peptides, their characteristics, expression of genes, and post-translational modifications (PTMs). Provides external links to other databases and also includes binding affinity of MHC proteins, TAP binders, cleavage sites connected PTMs, and T-cell epitopes.	Both	Potocnakova et al. (2016)
IEDB binding	Artificial neural network with SMM-align algorithm Is used. It is a comprehensive and multipurpose database with the largest co of human immune epitopes. It contains hyperlinks to other databases and includes T-cell assay and MHC-binding assays collected from literature and experimental data. It also provides 3D database (IEDB 3D) and tools for the prediction of TAP binding, MHC binding, and proteasome cleavage.	T-cells	Raoufi et al. (2020), Raza et al. (2020)
IMGT/ 3Dstructure-DB	It contains information and 3D configurations of TCR–peptide–MHC and peptide–MHC complexes with annotation with IMGT-ONTOLOGY classification concepts including domain information. Non-peptide epitopes and precalculated contact residue are also available.	T-cells	Reynisson et al. (2021)

(Continued)

TABLE 19.1
(Continued)

Database Name	Description	Type	Reference
JENPEP	It contains MHC-I, plus MHC-II and TAP-binding peptides' data, along with other T-cell epitopes. It can also help in quantitative prediction, and it is the predecessor of AntiJen.	T-cells	Roy and Hasan (2021)
MHCBN	An inclusive catalogue curated for MHC peptides (binding and non-binding) which are assayed, including TAP and T-cell epitopes. It contains hyperlinks for significant databases, and epitope mapping and creating datasets is also available.	T-cells	Rubinstein et al. (2009)
MHCPEP	It is a database that contains peptide sequences with information such as MHC specificity, binding affinity, activity, identification of T-cell epitope, anchor positions, etc. Data has been curated from published literature and experimentally collected data. Predefined classification of responses and binding affinity helps in the building of classifiers and studying correlations.	T-cells	Sagu et al. (2022)
MPID-T2	It contains crystal structures of peptide–MHC complexes coupled with TCR–peptide–MHC. Precalculated intermolecular parameters such as hydrogen bonding, gap index, gap volume, docking angles, and binding angles, among others.	T-cells	Saha et al. (2005)

19.7 COMPUTATIONAL TOOLS FOR EPITOPE PREDICTION

Different tools apply various methods in order to predict and formulate B-cell and T-cell epitopes in the most accurate fashion. These tools provide us with means for prediction through a number of features and properties of both the antigen and the antibody.

19.7.1 B-CELL EPITOPE PREDICTION TOOLS

B-cell lymphocyte epitopes are mainly divided into two major types that are linear and conformational, as explained before. Hence, the tools themselves have been made to cater to particular needs, enumerated in Table 19.2.

19.7.2 T-CELL EPITOPE PREDICTION TOOLS

Prediction for T-cell epitopes depends on major histocompatibility complexes, to which they bind, which are of two types: MHC-I and MHC-II. Thus, on that basis, the tools and their application differ, as described in Table 19.3.

TABLE 19.2
Prediction Tools for B-Cell Epitopes

Type	Name	Description	Reference
Prediction Tools for Linear B-cell Epitopes	ABCPred	Method: Artificial (Recurring) Neural Network by using fixed length pattern together with the prediction of short peptide sequences. Remarks: Trained on random peptides for negative datasets. The first server employed at prediction of continuous epitopes.	Saha and Raghava (2006)
	BCPREDS	Method: Support Vector Machine (using string kernel). Remarks: Supports ABCPred, BCPred, BayesB, and AAP methods to predict short peptide sequences.	Sanchez-Trincado et al. (2017)
	Bcepred	Method: Works on kernel-based Support Vector Machine approach. Remarks: Physiochemical properties like flexibility, hydrophilicity, polarity, and surfaces exposed are studied on a non-redundant database. Allows choosing of methods between BCPred, FBCPred, and amino acids pair scaling approach (AAP).	Schlessinger et al. (2006)
	Bepipred	Method: Hidden Markov Model (HMM) with a propensity scale approach. Based on the random forests approach for training. Remarks: Low sensitivity, it has a number of physicochemical propensities to scale comprising hydrobocity, solvent accessibility, antigenicity, hydrophilicity, and secondary structures.	Schneider et al. (2019)
	LBtope	Method: artificial neural network working on support vector machine. Remarks: It makes use of a machine learning approach using AAP, dipeptide composition, and binary profile of the antigen.	Sela-Culang et al. (2014)
	LEPS	Method: Support vector machine using physiochemical propensities and mathematical morphology.	Serdari et al. (2019)
	PEOPLE	Method: Propensity scale method using physicochemical propertiesRemarks: Employs a multiparametric algorithm working on hydrophilicity, secondary structure, and flexibility along with analysis of β-turns of the peptide chains and amino acids.	Sharma et al. (2012)
	SVMtrip	Method: support vector machine approach using tripeptide composition vectors. Remarks: Similarity and propensity of tripeptides are applied together for prediction.	Singh et al. (2013)
Prediction Tools for Conformational B-cell Epitopes	CBTOPE	Method: support vector machine method capable of working on an amino acid sequence for prediction. Remarks: Physiochemical and sequence-derived profiles are used to create binary vectors and to generate and predict epitope propensity.	Singh and Raghava (2001)
	EPITOPIA	Method: Naïve Bayes, a classifier of machine learning method. Remarks: Physiochemical properties along with structural geometry are used to create vectors with a sliding window of seven amino acid residues.	Sinigaglia et al. (2013)
	PEASE	Method: Machine learning model by scoring antigen and surface exposed residue. Remarks: It uses antigen and antibody attachment patterns, where relative composition and residue cooperativity improves the scoring method.	Sliwoski et al. (2013)

(Continued)

TABLE 19.2
(Continued)

Type	Name	Description	Reference
Prediction Tools which Support both Types of B-Cells	BayesB	Method: Support vector machine with Bayes feature extraction.	Soria-Guerra et al. (2015)
	COBEpro	Method: Support vector machine having Gaussian kernel, with solvent accessibility anticipated with ACCpro and secondary structure predicted using SSpro. Remarks: COBEpro can predict only a single peptide at a time. Another limitation of COBEpro is that it can only be applied for the prediction of chains of peptides smaller than 1,500 residues.	Suthaharan (2016)
	BEST	Method: Support vector machine-based tool working on sequence-derived chain of amino acid. Remarks: BEST performs better than several modern sequence-based B-cell epitope predicting tools such as ABCPred, COBEpro, BCPred, and CBTOPE. It uses a scoring system having sequence conservation, secondary structure prediction, relative solvent accessibility, and likeness to experimentally obtain B-cell epitopes.	Sweredoski and Baldi (2008)

TABLE 19.3
T-Cell MHC-I Type Prediction Tools

Type	Name	Description	Reference
T-cell MHC-II Type Prediction Tools	IL4pred	Method: Support vector machine classifier used. Remarks: Works with amino acid composition, amino acid propensity, dipeptide composition, and physiochemical properties as features.	Thomas et al. (2022)
	MHC2Pred	Method: Support vector machine algorithm is used. Remarks: It can be used for vaccine design, immunotherapy, diagnostics in immune systems, cellular immunology along with prediction.	Tieri et al. (2007)
	NetMHCII	Method: Artificial neural network. Remarks: Predicts MHC-II class supertypes.	Tong et al. (2007)
	NetMHCIIpan	Method: Artificial neural network. Remarks: Predicts MHC-II class supertypes.	Tong et al. (2007)
TAP binding and CTL Prediction Tools	TAP Pred	Method: Support vector machine is utilized to forecast binding peptide affinity. Remarks: It is indispensable for recognizing MHC-I T-cell epitopes which are restricted in nature.	Vahedi et al. (2022)
	CTLPred	Method: CTLPred is a prediction method that uses ANN, SVM, and Quantitative matrices in order to predict CTL epitopes. Remarks: It provides a choice for selecting a combined approach or a consensus of all three methodologies used and MHC alleles can be fixed and changed according to the user.	Wang et al. (2011)

(Continued)

TABLE 19.3
(Continued)

Type	Name	Description	Reference
T-cell MHC-I type Prediction Tools	NetCTL	Method: Artificial neural network (ANN) with regression. Remarks: It is capable of predicting binding affinity of MHC-I complexes, supertypes, TAP-binding efficiency and proteasomal cleavage at C-terminal of six vertebrates including humans.	Wang (2022)
	IEDB binding	Method: Artificial neural network with SMM – align algorithm is used. Remarks: IEDB – AR provides prediction tools for TAP binding, MHC binding, and proteasome cleavage to help with better prediction of T-cells.	Raoufi et al. (2020), Raza et al. (2020)
	KISS	Method: Kernel-based inter-allele peptide binding prediction SyStem (or KISS), runs on an SVM (support vector machine) algorithm which is multitasking kernel-based.	Almeida et al. (2012)
	NetMHC	Method: Artificial neural network-based tool. Remarks: It predicts binding affinity to different HLA (HLA-A2 and H-2Kk) alleles.	Wee et al. (2010)
	NetMHCpan	Method: Artificial neural network model which predicts binding affinity. Remarks: Prediction of the interaction of MHC-I class peptides, along with HLA-A as well as HLA-B supertypes for not only humans but even pigs, mice, chimpanzees, gorillas, cows, and macaques.	Wild (2013)
	nHLApred	Method: Artificial Neural Network with quantitative matrix technique. Remarks: Prediction of proteasomal cleavage. It also provides a choice between Compred and ANNPred, where Compred is a hybrid style of prediction.	Yang et al. (2021)
	WAPP	Method: Support vector machine with regression is applied. Remarks: A combination of TAP transport, proteasomal cleavage, and MHC-peptide binding for pathways of MHC-I antigen binding is applied. PCM (proteasomal cleavage matrices), SVMTAP (for TAP transport), and SVMHC (MHC binding) are used together for the most optimal predictions.	Yao et al. (2012)

19.8　SUMMARY AND CONCLUSION

Traditional vaccine development utilizes a lot of resources and is a laborious process. These resources can be saved by the use of artificial intelligence techniques to predict epitopes of both types of lymphocyte cells capable of generating an immune response. These techniques provide a close-to-perfect alternative for laboratory experimentation for smaller tasks and are an affordable choice. The addition of attenuated or dead pathogens can be avoided in the vaccine, and AI techniques have also provided insight into how Ag-Ab complexes are formed, biorecognition, and mapping of epitopes. Algorithms only get better as they get more and more data to work on, and the quality of the data increases, thus better predictions can be made with the regular use of these tools. The availability of a number of databases for both T-cells and B-cells leads to more work in the same paradigm. Possible epitopes which would have been ignored during experimentation can be obtained by the use of these tools. Medical issues such as immune intolerance, cytokine storm, or ineffectiveness can be also prevented. The presence of tools capable of predicting epitopes with the most possible accuracy helps reduce the time and resources spent on using an experimental approach to deduct and predict candidate epitopes. Artificial intelligence techniques are not only responsible for offering a time- and cost-saving option, but also a more accurate and desired immunogenic response with the fewest adverse effects possible. However, it is important to mention that such tools do not represent a substitute for the laboratory experiments necessary to verify and optimize the safety and efficacy of vaccines. Their role is to support the design of such experiments in order to reduce their number, the time needed, and the cost.

BIBLIOGRAPHY

Alix, A.J.P., 1999. Predictive estimation of protein linear epitopes by using the program people. *Vaccine*, 18(3–4), 311–314.

Almeida, R.R., Rosa, D.S., Ribeiro, S.P., Santana, V.C., Kallás, E.G., Sidney, J., Sette, A., Kalil, J., and Cunha-Neto, E., 2012. Broad and cross-clade CD4+ T-cell responses elicited by a DNA vaccine encoding highly conserved and promiscuous HIV-1 M-group consensus peptides. *PLOS ONE*, 7(9), e45267–e45267.

Ansari, H. and Raghava, G.P.S., 2010. Identification of conformational B-cell Epitopes in an antigen from its primary sequence. *Immunome Research*, 6(1), 6.

Ansari, H.R., Flower, D.R., and Raghava, G.P.S., 2009. AntigenDB: An immunoinformatics database of pathogen antigens. *Nucleic Acids Research*, 38(Suppl_1), D847–D853.

Bhakta, S., Paul, J., Bhattacharya, A., and Choudhury, S., 2021. Vaccine development through reverse vaccinology using artificial intelligence and machine learning approach. In *COVID-19: Tackling Global Pandemics through Scientific and Social Tools*(pp. 33–49). Academic Press.

Bhasin, M., Lata, S., and Raghava, G.P.S., 2007. TAPPred prediction of TAP-binding peptides in antigens. In Edited By Darren R. Flower *Methods in Molecular Biology*. Humana Press, 381–386.

Bhasin, M. and Raghava, G.P.S., 2007. A hybrid approach for predicting promiscuous MHC class I restricted T cell epitopes. *Journal of Biosciences*, 32(1), 31–42.

Blaschke, T., Olivecrona, M., Engkvist, O., Bajorath, J., and Chen, H., 2017. Application of generative autoencoder in De Novo Molecular design. *Molecular Informatics*, 37(1–2), 1700123.

Blythe, M.J., Doytchinova, I.A., and Flower, D.R., 2002. JenPep: A database of quantitative functional peptide data for immunology. *Bioinformatics*, 18(3), 434–439.

Brusic, V. and Flower, D.R., 2004. Bioinformatics tools for identifying T-cell epitopes. *Drug Discovery Today: BIOSILICO*, 2(1), 18–23.

Brzić, B., Botički, I., and Bagić Babac, M., 2022. Detecting deception using natural language processing and machine learning in datasets on COVID-19 and climate change. *SSRN Electronic Journal*, 16(5), 221.

Buciński, A., Wnuk, M., Goryński, K., Giza, A., Kochańczyk, J., Nowaczyk, A., Baczek, T., and Nasal, A., 2009. Artificial neural networks analysis used to evaluate the molecular interactions between selected drugs and human 1-acid glycoprotein. *Journal of Pharmaceutical and Biomedical Analysis*, 50(4), 591–596.

Calder, P.C., Berger, M.M., Gombart, A.F., McComsey, G.A., Martineau, A.R., and Eggersdorfer, M., 2022. Micronutrients to support vaccine immunogenicity and efficacy. *Vaccines*, 10(4), 568.

Cano, R.L.E. and Lopera, H.D.E., 2013. Introduction to T and B lymphocytes BT. In *Autoimmunity: From bench to bedside [Internet]*. El Rosario University Press.

Chowdhary, K.R., 2020. Natural language processing. In *Fundamentals of artificial intelligence*. Springer India, 603–649.

Coley, C.W., Green, W.H., and Jensen, K.F., 2018. Machine learning in computer-aided synthesis planning. *Accounts of Chemical Research*, 51(5), 1281–1289.

Dash, S., Shakyawar, S.K., Sharma, M., and Kaushik, S., 2019. Big data in healthcare: Management, analysis and future prospects. *Journal of Big Data*, 6(1), 1–25.

den Eynde, B.J. and van der Bruggen, P., 1997. T cell defined tumor antigens. *Current Opinion in Immunology*, 9(5), 684–693.

Dertat, A., 2017. Applied deep learning - Part 3: Autoencoders - Towards data science.

Dhanda, S.K., Malviya, J., and Gupta, S., 2022. Not all T cell epitopes are equally desired: A review of in silico tools for the prediction of cytokine-inducing potential of T-cell epitopes. *Briefings in Bioinformatics*, 23(5), bbac382.

Dobchev, D. and Karelson, M., 2016. Have artificial neural networks met expectations in drug discovery as implemented in QSAR framework? *Expert Opinion on Drug Discovery*, 11(7), 627–639.

Dönnes, P. and Kohlbacher, O., 2005. Integrated modeling of the major events in the MHC class I antigen processing pathway. *Protein Science*, 14(8), 2132–2140.

Duru, C., Ladeji-Osias, J., Wandji, K., Otily, T., and Kone, R., 2022. A review of human immune inspired algorithms for intrusion detection systems. In *2022 IEEE World AI IoT Congress, AIIoT 2022*.

Ehrenmann, F., Kaas, Q., and Lefranc, M.-P., 2009. IMGT/3Dstructure-DB and IMGT/DomainGapAlign: A database and a tool for immunoglobulins or antibodies, T cell receptors, MHC, IgSF and MhcSF. *Nucleic Acids Research*, 38(Suppl_1), D301–D307.

EL-Manzalawy, Y., Dobbs, D., and Honavar, V., 2008. Predicting linear B-cell epitopes using string kernels. *Journal of Molecular Recognition*, 21(4), 243–255.

Gagliani, N. and Huber, S., 2017. Basic aspects of T helper cell differentiation. In *Methods in Molecular Biology*, pp. 19–30.

Gao, J., Faraggi, E., Zhou, Y., Ruan, J., and Kurgan, L., 2012. BEST: Improved prediction of B-cell epitopes from antigen sequences. *PLOS ONE*, 7(6), e40104.

Gershoni, J.M., Roitburd-Berman, A., Siman-Tov, D.D., Tarnovitski Freund, N., and Weiss, Y., 2007. Epitope mapping: The first step in developing epitope-based vaccines. *BioDrugs : Clinical Immunotherapeutics, Biopharmaceuticals and Gene Therapy*, 21(3), 145–156.

Harris, L.J., Larson, S.B., Hasel, K.W., and McPherson, A., 1997. Refined structure of an intact IgG2a monoclonal antibody. *Biochemistry*, 36(7).

Iurescia, S., Fioretti, D., Fazio, V.M., and Rinaldi, M., 2012. Epitope-driven DNA vaccine design employing immunoinformatics against B-cell lymphoma: A biotech's challenge. *Biotechnology Advances*, 30(1), 372–383.

Ivanciuc, O., Schein, C.H., Braun, W., 2003. SDAP: Database and computational tools for allergenic proteins. *Nucleic Acids Research*, 31(1), 359–362.

Ivanciuc, O., 2009. Machine learning quantitative structure-activity relationships (QSAR) for peptides binding to the human Amphiphysin-1 SH3 domain. *Current Proteomics*, 6(4), 289–302.

Kim, Y., Ponomarenko, J., Zhu, Z., Tamang, D., Wang, P., Greenbaum, J., Lundegaard, C., Sette, A., Lund, O., Bourne, P.E., Nielsen, M., and Peters, B., 2012. Immune epitope database analysis resource. *Nucleic Acids Research*, 40(W1), W525–W530.

Kundu, S. and Mondal, P., 2022. A conceptual model for coeval time estimation of virtual reference service. *Internet Reference Services Quarterly*, 26(1), 31–55.

Kwon, S., Bae, H., Jo, J., and Yoon, S., 2019. Comprehensive ensemble in QSAR prediction for drug discovery. *BMC Bioinformatics*, 20(1), 1–12.

Larsen, J.E.P., Lund, O., and Nielsen, M., 2006. Improved method for predicting linear B-cell epitopes. *Immunome Research*, 2, 2.

Larsen, M.V., Lundegaard, C., Lamberth, K., Buus, S., Brunak, S., Lund, O., and Nielsen, M., 2005. An integrative approach to CTL epitope prediction: A combined algorithm integrating MHC class I binding, TAP transport efficiency, and proteasomal cleavage predictions. *European Journal of Immunology*, 35(8), 2295–2303.

Lata, S., Bhasin, M., and Raghava, G.P.S., 2009. MHCBN 4.0: A database of MHC/TAP binding peptides and T-cell epitopes. *BMC Research Notes*, 2(1), 61.

Love, B.C., 2002. Comparing supervised and unsupervised category learning. *Psychonomic Bulletin and Review*, 9(4), 829–835.

Lundegaard, C., Lamberth, K., Harndahl, M., Buus, S., Lund, O., and Nielsen, M., 2008. NetMHC-3.0: Accurate web accessible predictions of human, mouse and monkey MHC class I affinities for peptides of length 811. *Nucleic Acids Research*, 36(suppl_2), W509–W512.

Lv, H., Shi, L., Berkenpas, J.W., Dao, F.Y., Zulfiqar, H., Ding, H., Zhang, Y., Yang, L., and Cao, R., 2021. Application of artificial intelligence and machine learning for COVID-19 drug discovery and vaccine design. *Briefings in Bioinformatics*, 22(6), bbab320.

Malone, B., Simovski, B., Moliné, C., Cheng, J., Gheorghe, M., Fontenelle, H., Vardaxis, I., Tennøe, S., Malmberg, J.A., Stratford, R., and Clancy, T., 2020. Artificial intelligence predicts the immunogenic landscape of SARS-CoV-2 leading to universal blueprints for vaccine designs. *Scientific Reports*, 10(1), 22375.

Mamitsuka, H., 1998. Predicting peptides that bind to MHC molecules using supervised learning of hidden markov models. *Proteins: Structure, Function, and Genetics*, 33(4), 460–474.

Mazzocco, G., Niemiec, I., Myronov, A., Skoczylas, P., Kaczmarczyk, J., Sanecka-Duin, A., Gruba, K., Król, P., Drwal, M., Szczepanik, M., Pyrc, K., and Stępniak, P., 2021. AI aided design of epitope-based vaccine for the induction of cellular immune responses against SARS-CoV-2. *Frontiers in Genetics*, 12, 602196.

McSparron, H., Blythe, M.J., Zygouri, C., Doytchinova, I.A., and Flower, D.R., 2003. JenPep:0.167em A novel computational information resource for immunobiology and vaccinology. *Journal of Chemical Information and Computer Sciences*, 43(4), 1276–1287.

Meng, X.-Y., Zhang, H.-X., Mezei, M., and Cui, M., 2011. Molecular docking: A powerful approach for structure-based drug discovery. *Current Computer – Aided-Drug Design*, 7(2), 146–157.

Michelucci, U., 2022. Autoencoders. In *Applied Deep Learning with Tensorflow* 2, 257–283, Berkeley, CA: Apress.

Mixter, P.F., 1999. Fundamental immunology (4th edn) edited by W.E. Paul. *Immunology Today*, 20(12), 589.

Mohammad, S.M., 2020. Artificial intelligence in information technology. *SSRN Electronic Journal*. Available at SSRN 3625444.

Najafabadi, M.M., Villanustre, F., Khoshgoftaar, T.M., Seliya, N., Wald, R., and Muharemagic, E., 2015. Deep learning applications and challenges in big data analytics. *Journal of Big Data*, 2(1), 1–21.

Napolitano, F., Zhao, Y., Moreira, V.M., Tagliaferri, R., Kere, J., D'Amato, M., and Greco, D., 2013. Drug repositioning: A machine-learning approach through data integration. *Journal of Cheminformatics*, 5(1), 1–9.

Parvizpour, S., Pourseif, M.M., Razmara, J., Rafi, M.A., and Omidi, Y., 2020. Epitope-based vaccine design: A comprehensive overview of bioinformatics approaches. *Drug Discovery Today*, 25(6), 1034–1042.

Peters, B., Sidney, J., Bourne, P., Bui, H.-H., Buus, S., Doh, G., Fleri, W., Kronenberg, M., Kubo, R., Lund, O., Nemazee, D., Ponomarenko, J.V., Sathiamurthy, M., Schoenberger, S., Stewart, S., Surko, P., Way, S., Wilson, S., and Sette, A., 2005. The immune epitope database and analysis resource: From vision to blueprint. *PLOS Biology*, 3(3), e91.

Ponomarenko, J., Papangelopoulos, N., Zajonc, D.M., Peters, B., Sette, A., and Bourne, P.E., 2010. IEDB-3D: Structural data within the immune epitope database. *Nucleic Acids Research*, 39(Database), D1164–D1170.

Potocnakova, L., Bhide, M., and Pulzova, L.B., 2016. An introduction to B-cell epitope mapping and in silico epitope prediction. *Journal of Immunology Research*.

Raoufi, E., Hemmati, M., Eftekhari, S., Khaksaran, K., Mahmodi, Z., Farajollahi, M.M., and Mohsenzadegan, M., 2020. Epitope prediction by novel immunoinformatics approach: A state-of-the-art review. *International Journal of Peptide Research and Therapeutics*, 26(2), 1155–1163.

Raza, K., Maryam, and Qazi, S., 2020. An introduction to computational intelligence in COVID-19: Surveillance, prevention, prediction, and diagnosis. In *Studies in Computational Intelligence*. Springer Singapore, 3–18.

Reynisson, B., Alvarez, B., Paul, S., Peters, B., and Nielsen, M., 2021. NetMHCpan-4.1 and NetMHCIIpan-4.0: Improved predictions of MHC antigen presentation by concurrent motif deconvolution and integration of MS MHC eluted ligand data. *Nucleic Acids Research*, 48(W1), W449–W454.

Roy, K.C. and Hasan, S., 2021. Modeling the dynamics of hurricane evacuation decisions from twitter data: An input output hidden markov modeling approach. *Transportation Research Part C: Emerging Technologies*, 123, 102976.

Rubinstein, N.D., Mayrose, I., Martz, E., and Pupko, T., 2009. Epitopia: A web-server for predicting B-cell epitopes. *BMC Bioinformatics*, 10(1), 1–6.

Sagu, A., Gill, N.S., Gulia, P., Chatterjee, J.M., and Priyadarshini, I., 2022. A hybrid deep learning model with self-improved optimization algorithm for detection of security attacks in IoT environment. *Future Internet*, 14(10), 301.

Saha, S., Bhasin, M., and Raghava, G.P.S., 2005. Bcipep: A database of B-cell epitopes. *BMC Genomics*, 6(1), 1–7.

Saha, S. and Raghava, G.P.S., 2006. Prediction of continuous B-cell epitopes in an antigen using recurrent neural network. *Proteins: Structure, Function, and Bioinformatics*, 65(1), 40–48.

Sanchez-Trincado, J.L., Gomez-Perosanz, M., and Reche, P.A., 2017. Fundamentals and methods for T- and B-cell epitope prediction. *Journal of Immunology Research*, 2017, 1–14.

Schlessinger, A., Ofran, Y., Yachdav, G., Rost, B., 2006. Epitome: Database of structure-inferred antigenic epitopes. *Nucleic Acids Research*, 34(90001), D777–D780.

Schneider, P., Walters, W.P., Plowright, A.T., Sieroka, N., Listgarten, J., Goodnow, R.A., Fisher, J., Jansen, J.M., Duca, J.S., Rush, T.S., Zentgraf, M., Hill, J.E., Krutoholow, E., Kohler, M., Blaney, J., Funatsu, K., Luebkemann, C., and Schneider, G., 2019. Rethinking drug design in the artificial intelligence era. *Nature Reviews: Drug Discovery*, 19(5), 353–364.

Sela-Culang, I., Ashkenazi, S., Peters, B., and Ofran, Y., 2014. PEASE: Predicting B-cell epitopes utilizing antibody sequence. *Bioinformatics*, 31(8), 1313–1315.

Serdari, D., Kostaki, E.G., Paraskevis, D., Stamatakis, A., and Kapli, P., 2019. Automated, phylogeny-based genotype delimitation of the Hepatitis Viruses HBV and HCV. *PeerJ*, 2019(10), e7754.

Sharma, O.P., Das, A.A., R., K., M., S.K., and Mathur, P.P., 2012. Structural epitope database (SEDB): A web-based database for the epitope, and its intermolecular interaction along with the tertiary structure information. *Journal of Proteomics and Bioinformatics*, 5(3), 84–89.

Singh, H., Ansari, H.R., and Raghava, G.P.S., 2013. Improved method for linear B-cell epitope prediction using antigen's primary sequence. *PLOS ONE*, 8(5), e62216.

Singh, H. and Raghava, G.P.S., 2001. ProPred: Prediction of HLA-DR binding sites. *Bioinformatics*, 17(12), 1236–1237.

Sinigaglia, M., Antunes, D.A., Rigo, M.M., Chies, J.A.B., and Vieira, G.F., 2013. CrossTope: A curate repository of 3D structures of immunogenic peptide: MHC complexes. *Database*, 2013.

Sliwoski, G., Kothiwale, S., Meiler, J., and Lowe, E.W., 2013. Computational methods in drug discovery. *Pharmacological Reviews*, 66(1), 334–395.

Soria-Guerra, R.E., Nieto-Gomez, R., Govea-Alonso, D.O., and Rosales-Mendoza, S., 2015. An overview of bioinformatics tools for epitope prediction: Implications on vaccine development. *Journal of Biomedical Informatics*, 53, 405–414.

Suthaharan, S., 2016. Support vector machine. In *Machine Learning Models and Algorithms for Big Data Classification*. Springer US, 207–235.

Sweredoski, M.J. and Baldi, P., 2008. COBEpro: A novel system for predicting continuous B-cell epitopes. *Protein Engineering, Design and Selection*, 22(3), 113–120.

Thomas, S., Abraham, A., Baldwin, J., Piplani, S., and Petrovsky, N., 2022. Artificial intelligence in vaccine and drug design. *Methods in Molecular Biology*, 1, 131–146.

Tieri, P., Castellani, G.C., Remondini, D., Valensin, S., Loroni, J., Salvioli, S., and Franceschi, C., 2007. Capturing degeneracy in the immune system. *In Silico Immunology*, pp. 109–118.

Tong, J.C., Tan, T.W., and Ranganathan, S., 2007. Methods and protocols for prediction of immunogenic epitopes. *Briefings in Bioinformatics*, 8(2), 96–108.

Vahedi, F., Ghasemi, Y., Atapour, A., Zomorodian, K., Ranjbar, M., Monabati, A., Nezafat, N., and Savardashtaki, A., 2022. B-cell epitope mapping from eight antigens of Candida albicans to design a novel diagnostic kit: An immunoinformatics approach. *International Journal of Peptide Research and Therapeutics*, 28(4), 110.

Wang, H.-W., Lin, Y.-C., Pai, T.-W., and Chang, H.-T., 2011. Prediction of B-cell linear epitopes with a combination of support vector machine classification and amino acid propensity identification. *Journal of Biomedicine and Biotechnology*, 2011, 1–12.

Wang, Q., 2022. Support vector machine algorithm in machine learning. In *2022 IEEE Internationa l Conference on Artificial Intelligence and Computer Applications (ICAICA)*, pp. 750–756. IEEE.

Wee, L.J.K., Simarmata, D., Kam, Y.-W., Ng, L.F.P., and Tong, J.C., 2010. SVM-based prediction of linear B-cell epitopes using Bayes Feature Extraction. *BMC Genomics*, 11 (S4), 1–9.

Wild, D., 2013. The immunoassay handbook. In *Theory and Applications of Ligand Binding, ELISA and Related Techniques*, Newnes.

Yang, Z., Bogdan, P., and Nazarian, S., 2021. An in silico deep learning approach to multi-epitope vaccine design: A SARS-CoV-2 case study. *Scientific Reports*, 11(1), 3238.

Yao, B., Zhang, L., Liang, S., and Zhang, C., 2012. SVMTriP: A method to predict antigenic epitopes using support vector machine to integrate tri-peptide similarity and propensity. *PLOS ONE*, 7(9), e45152.

20 DN-Based DTI Model to Identify Potential Drug Molecules Against COVID-19

Santhosh Amilpur and Chandra Mohan Dasari

20.1 INTRODUCTION

The 2019 novel coronavirus which resulted in COVID-19 is one of the greatest medical challenges of the 21st century [12]. The majority of COVID-19 treatments were ineffective, and even after vaccination, there was still an increased risk of susceptibility. Since there is currently no effective treatment, it instilled a sense of urgency to develop potent therapeutic compounds through the study of drug discovery methods [53]. Two well-known approaches to the drug discovery process are small molecule development and antibody development. In the first, the molecules are created using computational approaches and serve as ligands to inhibit the target proteins, whereas in the latter, antibodies bind to the virus protein's surface to prevent it from attaching to the receptor of the host cell. Recent attempts to uncover prospective medications relied on drug repurposing of virtually tested, clinically authorized compounds, but these methods were found to be less effective [3]. In addition to these methods, drug repurposing through *de novo* molecular design using computational methods has demonstrated its dominance in the field of novel molecular generation and has produced significant contributions [40]. Deep generative models [20] have made considerable strides in a variety of areas, including bioinformatics [14] and the construction of realistic artworks [15].

Drug repurposing is a technique for finding new indications for medicines that have already received approval or that are still under research. Reusing existing drugs can deliver medications considerably faster and at a lower cost than generating new drugs because the safety of these drugs has previously been evaluated in clinical studies for other applications. For many years, academics and scientific researchers have promoted the idea that screening libraries of already-approved medications with a variety of tests could reveal new applications. Several well-known examples are Remdesivir [6] for the treatment of COVID-19, thalidomide for multiple myeloma,

DOI: 10.1201/9781003363361-20

and sildenafil citrate for erectile dysfunction. A potent remedy for developing disorders like COVID-19 is the medication repurposing technique.

The need for creating generative models to produce accurate and realistic compounds for *de novo* drug design has grown in the area of chemo-informatics. Simplified Molecular Input Line Entry Specification (SMILES) [47] strings that are formed from molecular graphs are typically used in this field to represent compounds. The enormous search space presents a significant obstacle to finding the appropriate therapeutic compounds during drug design. According to estimates, there are more than 10^{60} synthetically available drug-like compounds. From this collection of compounds, research experts choose and study molecules that firmly attach to biological targets and mimic the inhibitory mechanism of bacteria and viruses.

The virtual screening method examines a vast number of existing molecules in order to find suitable drug-like compounds using similarity-based measures, which has the effect of quantifying the relationship between molecules. On the other hand, in *de novo* drug design, the created unique compounds bind the biological targets. Generative models built on deep learning have succeeded in delivering cutting-edge solutions to a variety of issues, including text generation, image generation, and many others. This opens the door for the delivery of numerous potential candidate molecules, each of which has the necessary (drug-like) characteristics against a disease.

The likelihood of new diseases emerging has increased as a result of the COVID-19 outbreak. New drugs can be created to treat conditions that have been present for a long time but were previously incurable as disease pathology and metabolism are investigated. Furthermore, due to variations in metabolism, distinct drugs can be required to treat similar illnesses. One of the main reasons for the need to find new pharmaceuticals is the emergence of drug resistance brought on by the overuse of existing treatments. To maintain a healthy lifestyle, new medications must be created and tested. Deep learning and molecular docking are two computer methods for drug development that have received a lot of attention. Molecular docking works by employing a 3D simulation whereby drug molecules (ligands) locate their position within the target (protein) sites. Molecular docking analyzes how efficiently a drug molecule connects with biological targets. However, this method has two significant drawbacks: first, it is challenging to obtain the target protein's 3D structure; second, running massive simulations takes a lot of time and money. In order to find potential candidate compounds that are active against particular targets, computational *de novo* drug design approaches to aid in navigating through the huge chemical space of whole pharmaceuticals. Deep learning techniques automate the design and selection of potential compounds with particular desired features.

We propose the Deep-DTI model for *de novo* drug development conducive to the constraints of deep learning models generated at the molecular level. We use convolutional neural networks (CNN) for the discriminative method and generative adversarial networks (GAN) based on long short-term memory (LSTM) networks for this job. The model is rigorously trained using huge collections of molecules. In this method, we used reinforcement learning, which functions as a reward system by improving the generator depending on the validity of the sampled molecules, to update the weights of the generative model. As a result, the adversarial network, which comprises a generator and a discriminator, has acquired knowledge about the distribution of generalized compounds, enabling it to create new compounds that directly interact physiologically with viral proteins.

20.2 LITERATURE SURVEY

Deep generative neural networks have recently gained significant attention as a highly operational field, illuminating a potential new route for autonomous molecular production and optimization. The best choices for these representations are recurrent neural networks (RNNs); hence, RNN-based generation with one-hot encoding was widely used. Training these models straight away on visual representations has become a viable option in the field of neural network-based molecular graphs.

20.2.1 GENERATIVE NEURAL NETWORK ARCHITECTURES FOR MOLECULAR DESIGN

RNN, variational auto encoders (VAE), generative adversarial networks (GAN), and adversarial auto encoders (AAE) are examples of typical generative architectures for the creation of molecules. The two components of GAN are a generating model (G) that learns a map from a prior data distribution to sample new data points and a discriminative model (D) that learns to distinguish between samples that come from the real data distribution and from G. These two models were developed as deep neural networks using stochastic gradient descent. G and D can be thought of as two participants in a min-max game with distinct goals. AAE is presented as a conventional auto encoder- (AE-) regularized technique as a substitute for a Kullback-Leibler (KL) divergence [38], drawing inspiration from VAE and GAN. While in VAE a prior distribution is often imposed on the latent code using the KL regularization, in AAE the posterior distribution is matched to a preceding distribution using the KL regularization.

For deep generative models, there are often two different forms of molecular inputs: a 2D undirected molecular graph and a linear notation of SMILES [47]. The SMILES string is a preferred way of molecular representation in generative models that sample drug compounds. An RNN generative model for *de novo* molecule creation was initially created by Segler et al. [42]. The model architecture was built using three-tier LSTM layers. A broad generative model was trained on nearly 1.5 million molecules from the ChEMBL database [16]. They improved the general paradigm for developing new a formation with an appropriate job against a particular biological target based on the theory of transfer learning (TL). A similar LSTM model is used in conjunction with a sample temperature to rescale the probability distribution of output sequences, as proposed by Bjerrum et al. [7]. They trained nearly 2.7 million molecules taken from the ZINC database [19]. Between the created and trained molecules, the distributions of many molecular characteristics, including molar weight, projected logP, the number of hydrogen bonds, the number of rotatable bonds, and other chemical features, were compared. All of the estimated attributes had well-matched distributions, which indicated that the models only produced molecules close to the training set. Gupta et al. [18] built another comparable LSTM-based RNN model with various applications. With TL in mind, the pre-trained model was adjusted using three distinct ligand subsets: peroxisome proliferator-activated receptor (PPAR) inhibitors; trypsin inhibitors; and five structurally different TRPM8 blockers.

Reinforcement learning (RL) is often effective in resolving dynamic decision issues. By understanding an enforced episodic likelihood, taking into account both past probability and a specified reward function, a policy-based RL generative technique attempts to calibrate a pre-trained RNN generator to produce desired compounds. Using enhanced episodic probability RL, Olivecrona et al. [30] created REINVENT, for constructing novel molecules. To calibrate an RNN-based agent to produce molecules with specified desired features, they developed a policy-based RL. Popova et al. [34] developed ReLeaSE, an RL-based RNN model for producing novel chemical compounds with desired features. Unlike REINVENT, ReLeaSE integrates two deep neural networks: one a generator, the other a predictive network.

Gomez et al. [17] published the first *de novo* molecular generative model based on VAE, chemical VAE. ChemVAE's architecture comprises an encoder, a decoder, and a predictor. The encoder and decoder worked together to build the original VAE framework, and the VAE concept aimed to reduce model complexity during training. In VAE Grammar, proposed by Kusner et al. [25], a context-free grammar (CFG) was utilized to build a parse tree, which was then deconstructed into a series of production rules. They were supplied through a CNN encoder, followed by an RNN as a decoder to produce syntactically correct SMILES. These strings could be constructed iteratively by following production rules. Dai et al. [13] developed syntax-directed VAE (SDVAE) to account for both the syntax and semantics of SMILES.

AAE architecture was built on top of a regular AE, primarily by including an adversarial network to force the latent vector code to fit a certain target distribution. Kadurin et al. [21] created the first fingerprint-based AAE models, focusing on producing chemical fingerprints rather than actual molecules. Blaschke et al. [40] developed a SMILES-based AAE molecular generative model for *de novo* molecule design. Entangled conditional AAE (ECAAE) is a conditional AAE model that was recently presented by Polykovskiy et al. [34]. ECAAE incorporates predictive and joint disentanglement methodologies into supervised AAE to alleviate the problem of supervised AAE [38] being unable to handle disentanglement difficulties, which results in inconsistent conditional generation. ECAAE aims to increase the interpretability of latent space by combining it with the re-parameterization technique.

Deep learning algorithms have the potential to transform several procedures for discovering drugs [41]. Utilization of deep learning in drug development for novel coronaviruses is mainly concerned with therapeutic repurposing of the candidate medication compounds. Finding and forecasting new compounds for COVID-19, however, is a difficult challenge. In conjunction with this endeavour, Gordon et al. [32] discovered more than 60 human proteins that are connected to COVID-19. Li et al. [28] discovered 30 reformulated medications based on an examination of the coronavirus's major viral families' genomic sequences. A deep learning model was created by Beck et al. [5] based on using RNN and CNN to forecast the effectiveness of currently available, commercial antiviral medications against COVID-19. The creation of medical knowledge graphs is also a well-known method for medication repurposing. New drug-disease interactions can be accommodated in these graphs. Graphs are used most often in graph networks. Latent dimensional space edges and nodes are represented using embedding methods. The increased interest in developing graph models has resulted in a variety of graph representations. Concepts like the network medicine framework created by Gysi et al. [54] used graph representation to identify 81 potential repurposing candidates as part of a case study on COVID-19. Similarly, BenevolentAI [38] created an AI-powered knowledge network that forecasted a probable Baricitinib, a repurposed medication, used to treat COVID-19. A GAN and Generative auto encoder that utilizes crystalline ligands, protein structures, and other data has been suggested by Zhavoronkov et al. [23] to identify related proteins that recognize drug compounds for the primary coronavirus protease.

Reinforcement learning-based strategies for candidate drug development were developed by Tang et al. [45] to find molecules that bind to the novel coronavirus. Patankar [33] suggested an LSTM network that was used to train IC50 binding data, and compounds that might inhibit RNA-dependent RNA polymerase (RdRp) were screened in order to provide new molecules for attacking RdRp, which prevents viral RNA production. Using a variety of chemical datasets, Zhang et al. [51] described a deep learning method to identify drug-protein combinations for extensive virtual screening. A machine learning approach was presented by Kowaleswski et al. [24] to identify medicinal compounds. A deep generative LSTM-based model was recently presented by Amilpur et al. [2] to construct a targeted library of compounds and run docking simulations to discover prospective candidates. Although numerous methodologies for medication repurposing against SARS-CoV-2 have been developed using a variety of deep learning techniques, there are still few approaches that investigate treatment options in order to find novel drug-like molecules.

In this work, we present Deep-DTI, an adversarial model to develop *de novo* drug-like chemicals using reinforcement learning. Deep-DTI serves as a reward system to develop more reliable molecules and is conceptually comparable to existing active medications against coronavirus major protease. As an improved alternative to simulation-based docking techniques, we also present a unique drug-target interaction architecture to determine the binding affinity of the produced drugs against the target protein.

20.3 MATERIALS AND METHODS

This section provides a detailed explanation of Deep-DTI, which comprises new drug compounds and the structural information for drug-target interactions.

20.3.1 MOLECULAR REPRESENTATION

The simplified molecular input line entry system (SMILES) format, which is clearly specified on a set of syntactical norms, was proposed for the representation of molecules in a machine-readable manner [47] The SMILES representation of a molecule is based on conventions such as the depiction of atoms by their atomic symbol, the portrayal of metal atoms with their symbol in brackets, and the representation of single, double, and triple bonds with the symbols -, =, and #, respectively. The abstract characteristics and patterns that are crucial for identifying the qualities inside each sequence are recorded through deep learning techniques. Based on these characteristics, the generative model can comprehend the fundamental production rules of the SMILES language and produce legitimate molecules that adhere to those rules.

20.3.2 DATASETS COLLECTION

The molecular SMILES dataset for the generative model is put together by fusing two databanks, namely ChEMBL [16] and ZINC [43]. The databanks hold almost two million SMILES altogether. A chemoinformatics tool called RDKit [26] is used for the preparation of the data. It helps clean the data by applying normalization transforms to the functional groups and neutralizing the ionized acids and bases. Only SMILES with a length of between 32 and 128 characters are used to train the generative model. Following preprocessing, 1.3 million SMILES are filtered out and provided to the generative model for training. The suggested DTI model was trained using the BindingDB [29] dataset. BindingDB is a freely available dataset that contains binding affinities from protein-drug-like molecule interactions. The drug-target couples are chosen from among the several tests available based on the dissociation constant (Kd). The dataset contains 52,000 DTI pairings and their corresponding Kd scores. To maintain a steady training process, the Kd scores are changed to log-scale (P_{Kd}), as given in Equation 20.1.

$$P_{kd} = \log\left[K_d / 1e9\right]$$ (20.1)

20.3.3 NOVEL MOLECULES THROUGH THE GENERATIVE APPROACH

20.3.3.1 GANs

Models called generative adversarial networks [11] produce synthetic data that closely resembles the real data. RNN networks that can process sequential data include LSTMs and GRUs. By looking at the previously created tokens, these networks aim to optimize the log-likelihood of predicting the subsequent token in a given sequence. This method has exposure bias, which means that if one intermediate token is erroneous, the entire sequence produced from that time step will be impacted. It has been demonstrated that GANs can help to lessen the exposure bias issue [9]. It has been proven that the model surpassed all of its competitors in the job of generating sequences.

The adversarial approaches aim to reduce the difference between the synthetic data produced by a generative model and the real data that is provided. A discriminator (D) and generator (G) make up the GANs network. The fundamental concept is that G samples synthetic data (S) from a random distribution (Pr), including random noise given an initial distribution of actual data (Pt). Both the samples produced by Pt and Pr are used to train D. G attempts to select increasingly realistic data such that

D can no longer distinguish between created data (S in :Pr) and actual data (S in :Pt), based on how well D performs in categorizing the true and fake data.

As a result, the performance of the discriminator is used to optimize the generator's performance. Thus, the unsupervised problem, in which we only had real data, is changed into a supervised issue, in which we use a discriminator to discriminate between two classes of data. The entire setup has now been changed into a min-max issue, where a genuine sample must have a high likelihood of being drawn from the true distribution, which implies that the discriminator's predictions must be high. As a result, we want to increase the likelihood that the true sample is real. Similar to this, the discriminator seeks to categorize the fake sample as false with the lowest probability of prediction. The formulation of this is a cross-entropy loss, as in Equation 20.2.

$$min_G max_D E_{s \sim P_t} \log \left[D(S) \right] + E_{s \sim P_r} \left[\log \left(1 - D(G(S)) \right) \right] \qquad (20.2)$$

Two LSTM layers are stacked together to create the generator architecture, which may be used to produce sequences. θ serves as a generating parameter. Two convolutional layers that receive input from both Pt and $G(S_s$ in $P_r)$ and are parameterized by phi are stacked to create the discriminator model. These layers are then linked to a dense layer, and the cross-entropy provides the optimization function.

20.3.3.2 Reinforcement Approach for Updating the Generator's Weights

Since its conception, the GAN model has performed poorly when applied to sequential data. This is because the generator network is unable to control the creation of discrete outputs. We use reinforcement learning approaches to treat the creation of discrete tokens as a stochastic strategy [39] in order to get around the issue of generator differentiation. The following can be used to signify the SMILES sequence generated by the GAN approach. The SMILES sequence, given by $C = \{C_1, C_2, ..., C_N\}$, is produced by the θ parameterized generator indicated by G_θ (operating as an agent in reinforcement setting), where Ci corresponds to the character relevant to the SMILES vocabulary. If the concept is understood in terms of an RL setting, the current state (K) at time step(t) is the total amount of SMILES characters created for a sequence up until time t1, i.e., $K = \{C_1, C_2, ..., C_{t-1}\}$. Therefore, $G_\theta \left(\left(C_t | C_{1-(t-1)} \right) \right)$ is the formula for the stochastic policy model. Deterministic behaviour determines which character will be the next in the sequence. D_{phi} stands for the parameterized discriminator for phi. The sequences are checked to see whether they were produced from a generator (synthetic samples) or if they came from a genuine distribution by Dϕ, which is utilized to enhance the findings produced by the generator G_θ. Sequences from the generator are viewed as negative samples, whereas the original sequences from the dataset are treated as positive samples. As a result, the issue has been transformed into a supervised problem in which the discriminator is taught to distinguish between positive and negative inputs. The action value [44] is symbolized by Q[K, C], which represents the anticipated reward for creating a SMILES character at state K by applying policy G_θ, which is provided by Equation 20.3, where Rt[C] represents the overall reward for the whole series of characters that was created.

$$Q(K,C_t) = Q(K = C_{1:(t-1)}, C_t) = R_t(C) \tag{20.3}$$

To determine the optimum action at intermediate phases, or to maximize the predicted long-term reward, we must take into account the total expected benefit when the entire sequence is created. The validity function Rt(C) rewards the generator based on the generated SMILES when a full SMILES sequence is produced. Equation 20.4 provides the stochastic policy's predicted long-term reward (value function).

$$J(\theta) = E[R_t|K,\theta] = \sum_{C_i \in C} G_\theta(C_i|K).Q(K,C_i) \tag{20.4}$$

We employ the Monte Carlo search [49] to obtain the full sequence in advance of computing the reward function. For a given partial sequence, this creates the subsequent set of characters at an intermediate stage. The characters representing future states are stochastically sampled from state [k + 1] to N, completing the supplied sequence. The subsequent set of actions (choosing the best character for a larger reward) is determined by the future reward applied at each step. Figure 20.1 depicts the entire generative architecture. For our studies, the validity metric V(C) (using the RDKit library), as well as the discriminator's classification, are used as the total reward to update the generator's weights throughout the first generator training

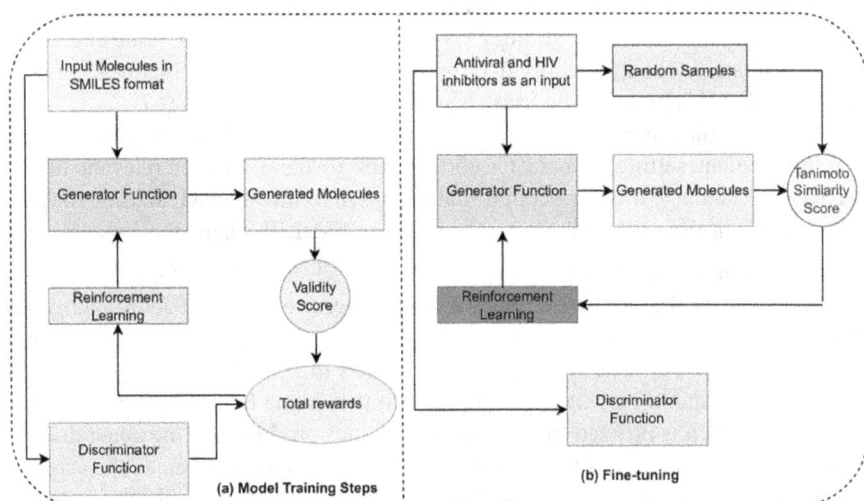

FIGURE 20.1   (a) Process for finding new drugs in which the reward is determined by the correctness of produced sequences and the discriminator's prediction. (b) The rewards from the Tanimoto Similarity Metric, which arbitrarily selects a sequence from the dataset and creates molecules to calculate comparable attributes, are used in the fine-tuning procedure.

procedure. Equation 20.5 illustrates the total reward R(C) for the action value as the sum of the validity score and the discriminator's prediction.

$$R(C) = \frac{1}{2} D_\varnothing(C) + \frac{1}{2} (V(C))$$
(20.5)

We fine-tune the generator on selected molecules once it samples more and more valid compounds. The goal is to transfer expertise in producing legitimate compounds to the area of developing molecules that particularly bond with the new coronavirus's major protease (3CLpro). The DTI model was then developed to determine the binding affinity scores of the produced compounds with the major protease.

20.3.4 DTI MODEL

Figure 20.2 depicts the suggested framework for binding affinity prediction. The raw protein sequences and the matching drug compounds in SMILES format are fed into the architecture. To begin, each SMILE character in the sequence is encoded as a number {A: 1, B:2, ... }. The encoded sequences are then sent into the proposed deep learning pipeline as inputs. Sequences, 1D convolution, and LSTM networks [10] are used as inputs because they are best suited for the analysis of sequence-based data.

20.3.4.1 D Convolutional Neural Network

Multiplication and addition are all that is involved in convolution. In 1D convolution, which is used for sequences, we move a filter through the encoded sequence. With random values, the filter is first filled. We specify the size of the filter at each convolution layer, which establishes the quantity of values from the sequence to be convolved. Convolution modifies the input sequence in accordance with the filter; hence, the values of the filter may also be learned. These filters take the input sequences and extract various patterns. The pooling layer receives the output of the convolutional layer and downsamples the inputs. Reducing the size of the feature maps, which in turn decreases the total number of learnable parameters, aids in the compact representation of the input-encoded sequence and speeds up learning.

20.3.4.2 Long Short-Term Memory (LSTM) Network

A kind of RNN called the LSTM can manage long-term dependencies without experiencing the vanishing gradient problem. This issue has been resolved by LSTM units, which extend the functionality of the conventional RNN unit by adding new gates, such as input and forget gates. A self-loop memory cell in the LSTM enables gradients to flow over lengthy sequences. The memory cell is in charge of managing how data moves between cells. The LSTM stores the input tokens from a specific phrase as continuous values in a distributed representation. Cell state C_i and hidden state h_i are additional states that may be discovered in LSTM cells. The memory cell is made up of three units: the forget unit F_i, the input unit I_i, and the output unit O_i, together with the weights assigned to each unit. These components limit the quantity of information flow while still allowing the LSTM cell to convey data from one time step to the next.

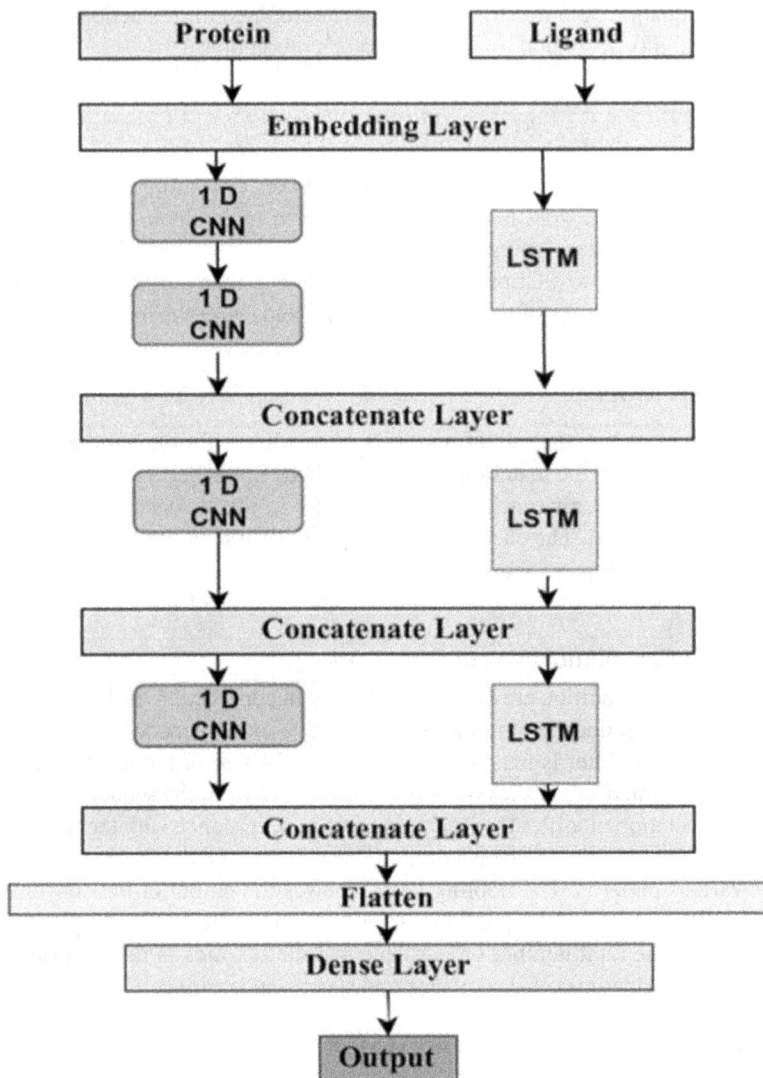

FIGURE 20.2   The architecture of the proposed DTI model.

20.3.4.3   DTI Architecture

Proteins and drug molecules are the two inputs used in the design for each data type. We fixed the length of the input proteins at 1024 characters, and we fixed the length of the drug molecules at 128 characters. Both forms of input are sent to an embedding layer once the input sequences have been encoded. For both inputs, the embedding layers' dimensionality is set at 32. As seen in Figure 20.2, a stack of two convolutional layers receives the embedded vectors corresponding to the protein as its initial input. In between each convolutional layer, maxpooling is utilized. An LSTM layer is passed through with the embedded vectors corresponding to the drug molecules. In each of the first stacked convolutional layers, the total number of feature mappings is 128. The pooling size is four in the first max-pooling layer. The input-embedded protein sequence's dimensions are changed from 1024×32 to 256×128 as a result. The pool size is two for the second maximum tier. By further reducing the protein representation's dimension from 256×128 to 128×128, the input protein sequences are given a compact form. The LSTM layer's total number of hidden units is set at 128. The dimensions of the input drug molecules are changed from 128×32 to 128×128. These dimensions allow the outputs of the stacked convolutional layers and the LSTM layer to be concatenated. To extract underlying characteristics from protein sequences, stacked 1D convolutional layers are used, whereas an LSTM layer is used to extract features from pharmacological compounds.

The characteristics derived from the stacked convolutional layers of protein sequences and drug compounds are then transferred via a concatenate layer. The concatenate layer merges two vector representations of the same form into a single vector representation. We feed this concatenated representation into both the convolutional layer and the LSTM, which both have the same number of feature mappings and hidden units, resulting in a multi-view learning paradigm [52]. This method allows both LSTM and convolutional layers to extract underlying information and apply the best of both. We repeat this method by concatenating the outputs of these layers and passing the concatenated representation to both the LSTM and the convolutional layer. The final concatenated version reflects the combination of both the protein and its associated molecule representation in a simplified manner. This representation is then processed further to create a flat layer and then a dense layer. The prediction of the dissociation constant (Kd), which represents the interaction between the protein and the ligand, is seen as a regression issue.

20.3.4.4 Implementation Details

Using Python's TensorFlow library as a backend, the drug creation and interaction prediction models were trained [v3.7]. The models have been trained on a Tesla P100 GPU. Using a chemo-informatics molecular modelling tool package called RDKit [26], all the preprocessing procedures needed for validating, cleaning, and computing the physiochemical characteristics on SMILES strings are completed.

20.4 RESULTS AND DISCUSSION

In this work, we focus on three different issues. The first is the generation of a sizable collection of molecules through adversarial training. The second is passing on the expertise inproducing reliable compounds and perfecting the generator to screen for powerful pharmacological molecules that block the 3CLpro protease of COVID-19 utilizing the Tanimoto similarity between pre-existing inhibitors as a reinforcement technique. The final objective is to use the created DTI prediction model to determine the binding affinity of the synthesized compounds.

20.4.1 GENERATOR QUALITY METRICS

After training the model, we took a sample of around 10,000 compounds and evaluated their quality, which is important for drug design. Validity, uniqueness, and novelty are the three quality criteria utilized to assess the created compounds. The following is a description of these quality indicators. Let S represent the total number of drug molecules that were sampled from the generator, V represent the total number of chemically sound molecules, and N represent the total number of training samples.

(1) Validity [QM_{Valid}]: This measures the total number of valid molecules out of all the generated molecules, as shown in Equation 20.6.

$$QM_{Valid} = \frac{|V|}{S} \tag{20.6}$$

For calculating the reward of the generated sequence by the RL model, the validity metric is used.

(2) Uniqueness [QM_{Unique}]: This lists the total number of unique molecules out of all valid molecules. The equation for uniqueness is shown below in Equation 20.7.

$$QM_{Unique} = \frac{set(V)}{|V|} \tag{20.7}$$

1. Novelty [QM_{Novel}]: This indicates the total number of molecules generated that do not appear in the training set, as shown in Equation 20.8.

$$QM_{Novel} = 1 - \frac{|set(V) \cap N|}{|set(V)|} \tag{20.8}$$

20.4.2 EVALUATION METRICS FOR DRUG-TARGET INTERACTION

We used two assessment measures to assess the effectiveness of the DTI model: the Concordance index [CI] and the root-mean-squared error [RMSE]. Let y_i represent the actual result of the ith sample, $\hat{y}_i$ represent the projected result of the ith sample, and N represent the total number of samples. The RMSE value is then determined as indicated in Equation 20.9. The RMSE calculates the difference between expected and actual values.

$$RSME(y_i, \hat{y}_i) = \sqrt{\frac{1}{N} \sum_{i=1}^{N} (y_i - \hat{y}_i)^2} \tag{20.9}$$

Let b_i denote the prediction value of larger affinity δ_i and b_j denote the prediction value for smaller affinity δ_j, then the concordance index is given by Equation 20.10.

$$CI = \frac{1}{Z} \sum_{\delta_i > \delta_j} h\left(b_i - b_j\right) \tag{20.10}$$

where Z is a normalization constant and h[x] denotes a step function:

$$\left(x\right) = \begin{cases} 1, & if \ x > 0 \\ 0.5, & if \ x = 0 \\ 0, & if \ x < 0 \end{cases} \tag{20.11}$$

This statistic compares two randomly selected drug-target pairings' expected binding affinities to their actual affinities in the same order.

20.4.3　NOVEL MOLECULE GENERATION

The early stopping mechanism ended the training process after 15 epochs of training the generator since the validity of the generator's samples had not improved. Following training, we took 10,000 or so molecules from the generator for sampling. The model was able to create valid SMILES at a rate of 93.12%; of these legitimately generated sequences, 94.23% are unique, and the novelty of molecules is 100%. In addition, as a baseline for the suggested strategy, we trained an LSTM-based generative model. This model is made up of three stacked LSTM layers coupled to a single fully connected later with 128 units with softmax activation. Based on hyper-parameter tweaking, the number of hidden units at each layer is set at 256. THE LSTM-based generator created valid SMILES at a rate of 72.15%, and 97.38% of these validly generated sequences are unique, and the novelty of molecules is 90.12%. We modify the generator's measure from validity to Tanimoto similarity to sample compounds that particularly bind to 3CL protease [4]. The model is then run again on a new dataset of widely viable antiviral medicines and a few HIV inhibitors. Figure 20.3 shows a few representative molecules from the suggested generator model, together with their IDs.

As indicated in Table 20.1, we also included a few existing models and made distinctions between the proposed generative model and the baseline models, based on a number of different factors. Although several generative models are used to generate unique molecules, each of them has been tuned for a distinct goal. For instance, ReLeaSE produced a comparable reinforcement learning strategy for the goal of suppressing JAK2 kinase, and Bjerrum et al. developed their model for the task of creating a retrosynthetic pathway of groups, among other models, as indicated in Table 20.1. The proposed model was adjusted to work against the primary coronavirus protease and has produced respectable outcomes, as reported in the next subsection. We feel the proposed model has offered a potential avenue for the identification of new therapeutic compounds in light of the findings shown in Table 20.1.

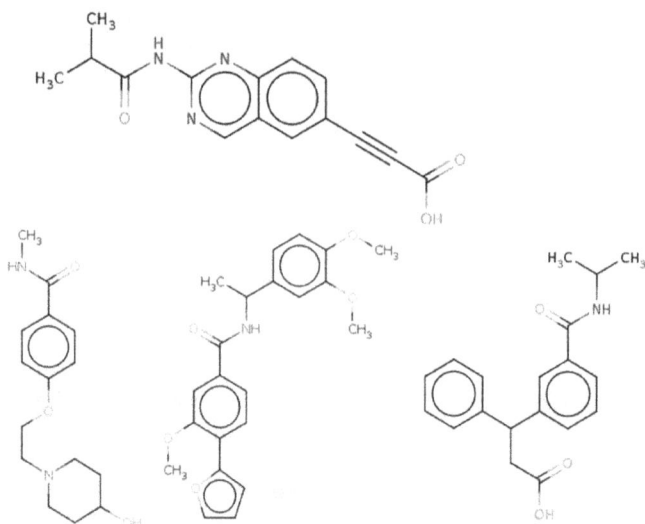

FIGURE 20.3   Potential sampled molecules that bind 3CL proof the novel coronavirus with their molecular IDs.

20.4.4   ADDITIONAL TRAINING OF THE GENERATOR FOR SAMPLING DRUG MOLECULES ACTIVE AGAINST 3CLPRO PROTEASE OF COVID-19

Following training on the available databanks, the generator produced legitimate compounds, and the model was well-versed in developing unique and acceptable drug-like molecules that differed from the training set. The goal of our investigations is to transfer knowledge of producing realistic molecules and tweak the model to develop realistic therapeutic molecules that can specifically bind to coronavirus's primary protease. We gathered a few current antiviral medicines, HIV inhibitors, and prescription drugs that were effective against SARS-CoV to create a new training set for this purpose. The generator was then trained on this set using the Tanimoto similarity index as the reward function. If a created molecule has a Tanimoto similarity with the training set between 0.5 and 0.7, the policy generates a positive reward, modifying the weights of the generator to develop molecules close to the existing inhibitors that might potentially block 3CL protease. We selected 10,000 molecules from the trained model, of which 96.17% were acceptable SMILE sequences. Out of the compounds that were authentically generated, 86.23% and 99.12% were unique andnovel molecules, respectively. We also created the DTI model, and using it, we determined the equilibrium dissociation constant (K_d) of the compounds produced against the SARS-CoV-2 protease.

TABLE 20.1
Comparison of the Generator's Quality Metrics of the Proposed Generative Model with Other Baseline Architectures

Architecture Type	Model Name	Dataset used	Size of Molecule	No. of Trained Molecules	No. of Generated Molecules	Generator Quality Metrics	Task
RNN- and AE-Based Architectures	Grammar VAE [25]	ZINC	< 39 heavy atoms	250,000	100,000	7.2% (V)	Penalized logP
	SD VAE [13]	ZINC	< 39 heavy atoms	250,000	100,000	43.5% (V)	Penalized logP
	AAE [8]	ChEMBL	< 121 characters	1.3 million	No data	77.4% (V)	Drug analogue generation
	ECAAE [34]	ZINC	< 58 characters	1.8 million	10,000	No data	Structural analogue
RNN-Based Architecture with RL	REINVENT [30]	ChEMBL	10–50 heavy atoms	1.5 million	12,800	94%(V), 90% (N)	Drug analogue generation
	ReLeaSE [35]	ChEMBL	No data	1.5 million	1 million	95%(V), 95.3% (N)	Inhibitor of JAK2
	ChemTS [48]	ZINC	No data	250,000	No data	No data	Penalized logP
RNN-Based Architecture	Segler et al. [42]	ChEMBL	No data	1.4 million	976,327	97.7%(V), 89.4% (N)	Plasmodium falciparum,5 - HT2A
	Bjerrum et al. [7]	ZINC	No data	1,611,889	50,000	98%(V), 63% (N)	Retrosynthetic route
	Gupta et al. [18]	ChEMBL	34–74 heavy atoms	541,555	30,107	93%(V), 92% (N)	PPARs, Trypsin
	Amilpur et al. [2]	ChEMBL, ZINC	34–128 characters	290,000	10,000	70.5% (V), 98.99% (N), 99.83% (U)	CLPro protease

(Continued)

TABLE 20.1

Comparison of the Generator's Quality Metrics of the Proposed Generative Model with Other Baseline Architectures (Continued)

Architecture Type	Model Name	Dataset used	Size of Molecule	No. of Trained Molecules	No. of Generated Molecules	Generator Quality Metrics	Task
GNN- and RNN-Based Architecture	ATNC [37]	ChemDiv	< 91 characters	15000	157,986	72%(V), 77% (N)	No. of unique heterocycles
	RANC [36]	ChemDiv	< 91 characters	15000	896,000	58%(V), 48% (N)	No. of unique heterocycles
	Deep-DTI	ChEMBL, ZINC	48–132 characters	2.9 million	10,000	93.12% (V)	3CLpro main protease of COVID-19

QM_{valid}, QM_{Unique}, QM_{Novel} are represented as V, U, N, respectively.

20.4.5 Evaluating newly created compounds that bind 3CL protease

Due to its role in the viral replication process, the primary protease or chymotrypsin-like protease (3CLpro) of the new coronavirus is being investigated as a crucial target for drug interactions. Since this protease is involved in the production of non-structural proteins (Nsp), which are crucial to the replication process, we selected 3CLpro as the site for the pharmacological target. We gathered the 3CL protease's FASTA format and encoded it as an integer sequence. All of the unique compounds created following training on antiviral inhibitors were utilized to predict against the protease. For the DTI model to predict K_d against the 3CL protease, these produced molecules were encoded into integer form. We created a deep learning-based DTI model because it produces more accurate findings than molecular docking techniques. The main shortcoming of such techniques is that they are overly reliant on scoring algorithms to predict precise binding energies. This is owing to flaws in the prediction of intermolecular interaction terms, such as entropy change [50] and solvation impact, as well as the fact that only a few intermolecular interactions that are potentially significant are included. Additionally, the docking technologies' usage of X-ray crystal structures of ligands results in errors when identifying the water molecules that serve as a link between the binding molecule and the ligand. Due to these drawbacks, we suggest a deep learning-based solution that not only overcomes the aforementioned issues but also performs better while quickly processing millions of compounds.

20.4.5.1 Comparison of the proposed model with other baseline models

Since the majority of the baseline models have demonstrated their ability to determine the measure of inhibition of a process indicated by Ki. We initially trained our model with Ki as the goal value to demonstrate a valid comparison to other current models. The performance of various models in terms of RMSE and concordance index (CI) to predict affinity on the BindingDB dataset is reported in Table 20.2. GanDTI [46] reported the best RMSE from the baseline models, which is 0.721, in which both drugs and proteins were represented as embedded sequences, which

TABLE 20.2
Comparison of proposed DTI model with existing models on BindingDB dataset

Model	RMSE	CI
GanDTI [46]	0.721	–
DeepAffinity[a] [22]	0.740	
DeepDTA[a] [31]	0.782	0.812[b]
MONNa [27]	0.764	–
DeepCDA [1]	0.899	0.822
Deep-DTI	**0.698**	**0.852**

[a]Results are taken from [46], [b]reported from [1].

is equivalent to our technique. As opposed to the stated baseline models, proposed model for drug-target interaction had a higher RMSE. The proposed DTI displayed an overall RMSE score of about 0.698. In terms of CI measure, the proposed model reported a CIscore of about 0.852, which is an improvement over the two previous models by Ozturetal [31], which had a CI score of about 0.812, and by Abbas et al. [1] with a CI score of about 0.822. Moreover, we experimented with removing the intermediate concatenation layers and just keeping the final concatenation layer in order to assess the performance gain achieved by merging features generated by CNN and LSTM networks. We obtained RMSE scores of 0.718 and CI scores of around 0.812 without the use of intermediary concatenation layers. Although K_i also displays the dissociate constant, its focus is largely on the inhibitor's binding to the enzyme. Therefore, since K_i is broader and calculates the equilibrium between dissociated components and ligand-protein complex, we utilize it to describe the binding affinity of newly created therapeutic compounds against 3CLpro of the novel coronavirus.

20.4.5.2   An evaluation of the binding affinity of the top ten produced potential drug molecules

We tested proposed DTI model against the COVID-19 primary protease using drug compounds from the generative model. In addition to the compounds created, we have included several commercially available antiviral drugs [5] in canonical SMILES style taken from PubChem. Table 20.3 shows the binding affinities of the created molecules and existing drugs. We kept all generated molecules in ascending order of their binding affinities and the top ten molecules are named M001...M010. With a projected binding affinity of 15.37 nanomolars (nM), which is much higher than Remdesevir's (1557.35 nM), as predicted by the model, M001 has emerged as the leading contender among other produced compounds. Abacavir and Atazanavir, which had binding affinity ratings of 43.51 nM and 48.68 nM, respectively, have displayed the best results among HIV medications. Molecular IDs from M001 to M003 have demonstrated the greatest outcomes when compared to currently available prospective antiviral medications that have been utilized to treat SARS-CoV-2. The prospective medications may now be examined *in vitro* and *in vivo* based on these findings.

20.5   CONCLUSION

We present a generative adversarial network-based reinforcement learning technique using molecular metrics as targets in this research. The model is well-versed in molecular grammar and has produced legitimate compounds. We further adjusted the model to produce substances that selectively bind to the primary coronavirus protease. We put forth a cutting-edge drug-target interaction model based on deep learning to illustrate the binding affinity of the created compounds. On the BindingDB dataset, the proposed DTI model outperformed other existing models in predicting equilibrium constant [Ki] values. Our model was then trained to predict dissociation constant (Kd) scores. We expected the effects of produced pharmacological

TABLE 20.3

Binding Affinity Score Comparison of Generated and Existing Drugs Predicted by ReGen-DTI

ID	SMILE	K_d (nM)
M001	CNC(=O)c1ccc(OCCN2CCC(O)CC2)cc1	**15.37**
M002	COc1cc(C(=O)NC(C)c2ccc(OC)c(OC)c2)ccc1c1ccco1	33.13
M003	COc1cc(C=Cc2ccc(C(=O)NC3CC3)cc2)cc(OC)c1OC	40.92
M004	CC(C)C(=O)Nc1nc2ccc(C#CC(=O)O)cc2cn1	46.32
M005	CC(C)NC(=O)c1cccc(C(CC(=O)O)c2ccccc2)c1	50.78
M006	Cc1ccc(C(=O)Nc2ccc(F)c(C3(C)C=C(N)C3)n2)cc1N(C)C	75.73
M007	COC(=O)c1ccc2nc(N3CCN(C(=O)C(C)CC3)[nH]c2c1	78.01
M008	O=C(O)C1=C(C2CCN(CCc3ncc4ncncc4n3)CC2)C1=O	102.08
M009	CC(C)C(=O)NC(Cc1ccccc1)C(O)CNCCc1ccccc1	168.75
M010	CC1(C)OC(=O)C(CCCC2CCCCC2)Cc2ccccc21	225.46
Dolutegravir	CC1CCOC2N1C(=O)C3=C(C(=O)C(=CN3C2)C(=O)NCC4=C(C=C(C=C4)F)F)O	2458.33
Ritonavir*	CC(C)C1=NC(=CS1)CN(C)C(=O)NC(C(O)C)(C(=O)NC(CC2=CC=CC=C) CC(C)(CC3=CC=CC=C3)NC(=O)OCC4=CN=CS4)O	2247.78
Entecavir	C=C1C(CC(C1CO)O)N2C=NC3=C2N=C(NC3=O)N	2215.04
Remdesivir	CCC(CC)COC(=O)C(C)NP(=O)(OCC1C(C(C(O1)(C#N)2=CC=C3N2N=CN=C3N)O)O)OC4=CC4	1557.35
Efavirenz	C1CC1C#CC2(C3=C(C=CC=C3)Cl)NC(=O)O2)C(F)(F)F	1507.03
Atazanavir*	CC(C)(C)OC(C(=O)NC(CC1=CC=CC=C1)C(CN(CC2=CC=CC=C(C=C2)C3=CC=CC=C2)3)NC(=O)OC(C)(C)C)NC(=O)OC)O)NC(=O)OC	48.68
Abacavir*	C1CC1NC2=C3C(=NC(=N2)N)N(C=N3)C4CC(C=C4)CO	43.51

*Indicates HIV drugs.

compounds on 3CLpro main protease of coronavirus based on this. When compared to known antiviral medications such as Remdesevir, the generated drug molecules bound well with the major protease with the least binding affinity.

REFERENCES

1. Karim Abbasi, Parvin Razzaghi, Antti Poso, Massoud Amanlou, Jahan B Ghasemi, and Ali Masoudi-Nejad. Deepcda: Deep cross-domain compound–protein affinity prediction through LSTM and convolutional neural networks. *Bioinformatics*, 36(17):4633–4642, 2020.
2. Santhosh Amilpur and Raju Bhukya. Predicting novel drug candidates against COVID-19 using generative deep neural networks. *Journal of Molecular Graphics and Modelling*, 110:108045, 2022.
3. Heba Askr, Enas Elgeldawi, Heba Aboul Ella, Yaseen AMM Elshaier, Mamdouh M Gomaa, and Aboul Ella Hassanien. Deep learning in drug discovery: An integrative review and future challenges. *Artificial Intelligence 56: Review*:1–63, 2022.
4. Dávid Bajusz, Anita Rácz, and Károly Héberger. Why is tanimoto index an appropriate choice for fingerprint-based similarity calculations?*Journal of Cheminformatics*, 7(1):1–13, 2015.
5. Bo Ram Beck, Bonggun Shin, Yoonjung Choi, Sungsoo Park, and Keunsoo Kang. Predicting commercially available antiviral drugs that may act on the novel coronavirus [SARS-COV-2] through a drug-target interaction deep learning model. *Computational and Structural Biotechnology Journal*, 18:784–790, 2020.
6. John H Beigel, Kay M Tomashek, and Lori E Dodd. Remdesivir for the treatment of COVID-19-preliminary report reply. *The New England Journal of Medicine*, 383(10):994–994, 2020.
7. Esben Jannik Bjerrum and Richard Threlfall. Molecular generation with recurrent neural networks [RNNS]. *arXiv Preprint ArXiv:1705.04612*, 2017.
8. Thomas Blaschke, Marcus Olivecrona, Ola Engkvist, Jürgen Bajorath, and HongmingChen. Application of generative autoencoder in de novo molecular design. *Molecular Informatics*, 37(1–2):1700123, 2018.
9. Tong Che, Yanran Li, Ruixiang Zhang, R Devon Hjelm, Wenjie Li, Yangqiu Song, and YoshuaBengio. Maximum-likelihood augmented discrete generative adversarial networks. *arXiv Preprint ArXiv:1702.07983*, 2017.
10. Francois Chollet. *Deep Learning with Python*. Simon and Schuster, 2021.
11. Antonia Creswell, Tom White, Vincent Dumoulin, Kai Arulkumaran, Biswa Sengupta, and Anil ABharath. Generative adversarial networks: An overview. *IEEE Signal Processing Magazine*, 35(1):53–65, 2018.
12. David Cyranoski. Profile of a killer: The complex biology powering the coronavirus pandemic. *Nature*, 581(7806):22–27, 2020.
13. Hanjun Dai, Yingtao Tian, Bo Dai, Steven Skiena, and Le Song. Syntax-directed variational autoencoder for structured data. *arXiv Preprint ArXiv:1802.08786*, 2018.
14. Chandra Mohan Dasari, Santhosh Amilpur, and Raju Bhukya. Exploring variable-length features [motifs] for predicting binding sites through interpretable deep neural networks. *Engineering Applications of Artificial Intelligence*, 106:104485, 2021.
15. Ahmed Elgammal, Bingchen Liu, Mohamed Elhoseiny, and Marian Mazzone. Can: Creative adversarial networks, generating "art" by learning about styles and deviating from style norms. *arXiv Preprint ArXiv:1706.07068*, 2017.

16. Anna Gaulton, Louisa J Bellis, A Patricia Bento, Jon Chambers, Mark Davies, Anne Hersey, Yvonne Light, Shaun McGlinchey, David Michalovich, Bissan Al-Lazikani, John POverington. ChEMBL: A large-scale bioactivity database for drug discovery. *Nucleic Acids Research*, 40(D1):D1100–D1107, 2012.

17. Rafael Gómez-Bombarelli, Jennifer N Wei, David Duvenaud, José Miguel Hernández-Lobato, Benjamín Sánchez-Lengeling, Dennis Sheberla, Jorge Aguilera-Iparraguirre, Timothy D Hirzel, Ryan P Adams, and Alán Aspuru-Guzik. Automatic chemical design using a data-driven continuous representation of molecules. *ACS Central Science*, 4(2):268–276, 2018.

18. Anvita Gupta, Alex T Müller, Berend JH Huisman, Jens A Fuchs, Petra Schneider, and Gisbert Schneider. Generative recurrent networks for de novo drug design. *Molecular Informatics*, 37(1–2):1700111, 2018.

19. John J Irwin, Teague Sterling, Michael M Mysinger, Erin S Bolstad, and Ryan G Coleman. Zinc: A free tool to discover chemistry for biology. *Journal of Chemical Information and Modeling*, 52(7):1757–1768, 2012.

20. Natasha Jaques, Shixiang Gu, Dzmitry Bahdanau, José Miguel Hernández-Lobato, Richard E Turner, and Douglas Eck. Sequence tutor: Conservative fine-tuning of sequence generation models with kl-control. In *International Conference on Machine Learning*, 1645–1654. PMLR, 2017.

21. Artur Kadurin, Alexander Aliper, Andrey Kazennov, Polina Mamoshina, Quentin Van-haelen, Kuzma Khrabrov, and Alex Zhavoronkov. The cornucopia of meaningful leads: Applying deep adversarial autoencoders for new molecule development in oncology. *Oncotarget*, 8(7):10883, 2017.

22. Mostafa Karimi, Zhangyang Wang Di Wu, Yang Shen. Deepaffinity: Interpretable deep learning of compound–protein affinity through unified recurrent and convolutional neural networks. *Bioinformatics*, 35(18):3329–3338, 2019.

23. Aman Chandra Kaushik and Utkarsh Raj. Ai-driven drug discovery: A boon against COVID-19?*AI Open*, 1:1–4, 2020.

24. Joel Kowalewski and Anandasankar Ray. Predicting novel drugs for SARS-COV-2 using machine learning from a >10 million chemical space. *Heliyon*, 6(8):e04639, 2020.

25. Matt J Kusner, Brooks Paige, and José Miguel Hernández-Lobato. Grammar variational autoencoder. In *International Conference on Machine Learning*, 1945–1954. PMLR, 2017.

26. Greg Landrum. RDKit: A software suite for cheminformatics, computational chemistry, and predictive modeling. *Greg Landrum*, 8, 2013.

27. Shuya Li, Fangping Wan, Hantao Shu, Tao Jiang, Dan Zhao, and Jianyang Zeng. Monn: A multi-objective neural network for predicting compound-protein interactions and affinities. *Cell Systems*, 10(4):308–322, 2020.

28. Xu Li, Yu Jinchao, Zhiming Zhang, Jing Ren, Alex E Peluffo, Wen Zhang, Yujie Zhao, Jiawei Wu, Kaijing Yan, Daniel Cohen, W Wang. Network bioinformatics analysis provides insight into drug repurposing for COVID-19. *Medicine in Drug Discovery*, 10:100090, 2021.

29. Tiqing Liu, Yuhmei Lin, Xin Wen, Robert N Jorissen, and Michael K Gilson. Bindingdb: A web-accessible database of experimentally determined protein–ligand binding affinities. *Nucleic Acids Research*, 35(suppl 1):D198–D201, 2007.

30. Thomas Marcus Olivecrona, Ola Engkvist, and Hongming Chen. Molecular de- novo design through deep reinforcement learning. *Journal of Cheminformatics*, 9(1):1–14, 2017.

31. Hakime Öztürk, Arzucan Özgür, and Elif Ozkirimli. Deepdta: Deep drug–target binding affinity prediction. *Bioinformatics*, 34(17):i821–i829, 2018.

32. Matthew J O'Meara, Jeffrey Z Guo, Danielle L Swaney, Tia A Tummino, and Ruth Hüttenhain. A SARS-COV-2-human protein-protein interaction map reveals drug targets and potential drug-repurposing. *BioRxiv*, 2020.

33. Sayalee Patankar. Deep learning-based computational drug discovery to inhibit the RNA dependent RNA polymerase: Application to SARS-COV and COVID-19, 2020.

34. Daniil Polykovskiy, Alexander Zhebrak, Dmitry Vetrov, Yan Ivanenkov, Vladimir Aladinskiy, Polina Mamoshina, Marine Bozdaganyan, Alexander Aliper, Alex Zhavoronkov, and Artur Kadurin. Entangled conditional adversarial autoencoder for de novo drug discovery. *Molecular Pharmaceutics*, 15(10):4398–4405, 2018.

35. Mariya Popova, Olexandr Isayev, and Alexander Tropsha. Deep reinforcement learning for de novo drug design. *Science Advances*, 4(7):eaap7885, 2018.

36. Evgeny Putin, Arip Asadulaev, Yan Ivanenkov, Vladimir Aladinskiy, Benjamin Sanchez-Lengeling, Alán Aspuru-Guzik, and Alex Zhavoronkov. Reinforced adversarial neural computer for de novo molecular design. *Journal of Chemical Information and Modeling*, 58(6):1194–1204, 2018.

37. Evgeny Putin, Arip Asadulaev, Quentin Vanhaelen, Yan Ivanenkov, Anastasia V Aladinskaia, Alex Aliper, and Alex Zhavoronkov. Adversarial threshold neural computer for molecular de novo design. *Molecular Pharmaceutics*, 15(10):4386–4397, 2018.

38. Peter Richardson, Ivan Griffin, Catherine Tucker, Dan Smith, Olly Oechsle, Anne Phelan, Michael Rawling, Edward Savory, and Justin Stebbing. Baricitinib as potential treatment for 2019-ncov acute respiratory disease. *Lancet*, 395(10223):e30, 2020.

39. Benjamin Sanchez-Lengeling, Carlos Outeiral, Gabriel L Guimaraes, and Alan Aspuru-Guzik. Optimizing distributions over molecular space. An Objective-Reinforced Generative Adversarial Network for Inverse-Design Chemistry [Organic], 2017.

40. Luana Carine Schünke, Blanda Mello, Cristiano André da Costa, Rodolfo Stoffel Antunes, Sandro José Rigo, Gabriel de Oliveira Ramos, Rodrigo da Rosa Righi, Juliana Nichterwitz Scherer, and Bruna Donida. A rapid review of machine learning approaches for telemedicine in the scope of COVID-19. *Artificial Intelligence in Medicine*:102312, 2022.

41. Dalton Schutte, Jake Vasilakes, Anu Bompelli, Yuqi Zhou, Marcelo Fiszman, Hua Xu, Halil Kilicoglu, Jeffrey R Bishop, Terrence Adam, and Rui Zhang. Discovering novel drug-supplement interactions using SuppKG generated from the biomedical literature. *Journal of Biomedical Informatics*, 131:104120, 2022.

42. Marwin HS Segler, Thierry Kogej, Christian Tyrchan, and Mark P Waller. Generating focused molecule libraries for drug discovery with recurrent neural networks. *ACS Central Science*, 4(1):120–131, 2018.

43. Teague Sterling and John J Irwin. Zinc 15–ligand discovery for everyone. *Journal of Chemical Information and Modeling*, 55(11):2324–2337, 2015.

44. Richard S Sutton and Andrew G Barto. *Reinforcement Learning: An Introduction.* MIT Press, 2018.

45. Bowen Tang, Fengming He, Dongpeng Liu, Fei He, Tong Wu, Meijuan Fang, Zhangming Niu, Zhen Wu, and Dong Xu. Ai-aided design of novel targeted covalent inhibitors against SARS-COV-2. *Biomolecules*, 12(6):746, 2022.

46. Shuyu Wang, Peng Shan, Yuliang Zhao, and Lei Zuo. Gandti: A multi-task neural network for drug-target interaction prediction. *Computational Biology and Chemistry*, 92:107476, 2021.

47. David Weininger. SMILES, a chemical language and information system. 1. Introduction to methodology and encoding rules. *Journal of Chemical Information and Computer Sciences*, 28(1):31–36, 1988.

48. Xiufeng Yang, Jinzhe Zhang, Kazuki Yoshizoe, Kei Terayama, and Koji Tsuda. Chemts: An efficient python library for de novo molecular generation. *Science and Technology of Advanced Materials*, 18(1):972–976, 2017.

49. Yu Lantao, Weinan Zhang, Jun Wang, and Yong Yu Seqgan. Sequence generative adversarial nets with policy gradient. In *Proceedings of the AAAI Conference on Artificial Intelligence*, Vol. 31(1), 2017.

50. Elizabeth Yuriev, Mark Agostino, and Paul A Ramsland. Challenges and advances in computational docking: 2009 in review. *Journal of Molecular Recognition*, 24(2):149–164, 2011.

51. Haiping Zhang, Konda Mani Saravanan, Yang Yang, MD Hossain, Junxin Li, Xiaohu Ren, Yi Pan, and Yanjie Wei. Deep learning based drug screening for novel coronavirus 2019-nCov. *Interdisciplinary Sciences: Computational Life Sciences*, 12(3):368–376, 2020.

52. Jing Zhao, Xijiong Xie, Xin Xu, and Shiliang Sun. Multi-view learning overview: Recent progress and new challenges. *Information Fusion*, 38:43–54, 2017.

53. A Zhavoronkov, V Aladinskiy, A Zhebrak, et al. *Potential COVID-2019 3c-Like Protease Inhibitors Designed Using Generative Deep Learning Approaches*, vol. 2, 2020.

54. Yadi Zhou, Fei Wang, Jian Tang, Ruth Nussinov, and Feixiong Cheng. Artificial intelligence in COVID-19 drug repurposing. *The Lancet Digital Health*, 2(12):e667–e676, 2020.

21 Deep Learning-Based Chatbots for Patient Queries

Priya Vijay, K. Jayashree, R. Babu, and K. Vijay

21.1 INTRODUCTION

Artificial intelligence (AI) is bringing a revolution and transformation in healthcare, driven by the expansion of analytics tools and the accessibility of healthcare data. Artificial intelligence in health care can be broadly classified into two categories based on the data (Jiang et al., 2017). The first category works with structured data like health reports, scan reports, and images, applying machine learning (ML) algorithms. The second category applies natural language processing to the reports and text to detect the disease and to provide suggestions and solutions based on analysis.

The expert system (Athota et al., 2020) not only diagnoses the disease based on input, but can also answer queries raised by the user. An expert system application can educate and counsel patients with the integration of hardware, software, and specialized data through reasoning and analysis. One such expert system is the chatbot. In recent years, doctor consultation has become a difficult task, due to the pandemic situation or due to economic rise. So, an automatic answering system can help the medical field give consultation and suggestions to patients. Chatbots can provide answers for all sorts of structured data records, using machine learning (ML) as well as natural language processing (NLP) techniques.

This chapter flows in the direction of explaining chatbot components, types of chatbots, how deep learning chatbots can be built, describing deep learning algorithms to analyze reports and images and make suggestions based on reports, security, ethics and statutory rules about chatbot use. The chapter ends with future research directions that can be carried out further in developing chatbots for healthcare.

21.1.1 COMPONENTS OF CHATBOTS

Smart chatbots are made up of natural language understanding (NLU), natural language generation (NLG), and machine learning layers (Bhirud et al., 2019). The architecture of artificial intelligence-based chatbots is shown in Figure 21.1.

The structure of chatbots (Bhattad and Atkar, 2021) used for answering FAQs normally comprises three components: NLU to categorize the user's intent, dialogue

DOI: 10.1201/9781003363361-21

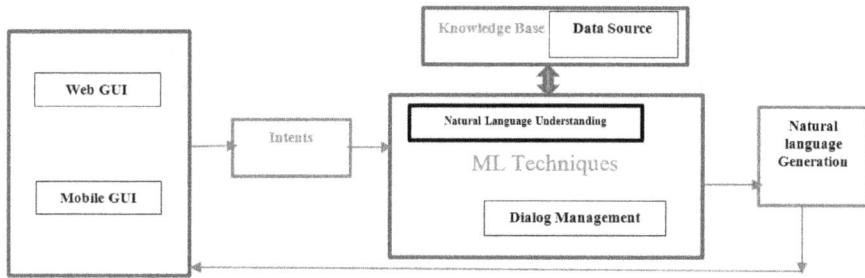

FIGURE 21.1 Architecture of chatbot system

management (DM) to determine the user's intent, and NLG to generate a response in natural language.

The main objective of a chatbot is language recognition since it needs to understand the queries raised by users on web or mobile graphical user interface (GUI) (Karri, 2020). The cornerstone for language recognition is natural language processing. The unstructured text received from the user is converted to a structured format by extracting relevant terms and patterns from the user content using NLU algorithms. The NLU system needs to comprehend each word of a sentence in order to comprehend the sentence as a whole. The first objective is to separate the phrases into their component words, which is what it signifies. The algorithm then has to grasp the grammar of the sentence in order to understand the words. This is accomplished by understanding the parts of speech of each word in the sentence.

The "brain" of the chatbot engine is its knowledge base (Chuan and Morgan, 2020), which typically contains key phrases and the responses related to them. The knowledge base is the source of data the chatbot uses to generate responses throughout the dialogue management stage. The majority of extant chatbots now use structured texts to construct their knowledge bases, because they provide labelled utterance-response (or Q-R) pairs that the chatbot engine can store. The knowledge base might be open domain or closed-domain (restricted domain). A conversational agent, a chatbot with an open domain knowledge base, can reply to a range of user inputs.

The dialogue management stage categorizes the inquiry type and selects the pertinent category of responses the chatbot can use in response. After the chatbot has chosen a response, the dialogue manager (DM) must decide on a variety of communication techniques, employ linguistic gimmicks to make it look human, and then deliver the message. The user, the system, or both may be in charge of the dialogue, depending on the interaction method chosen during the creation of the DM system. When user-directed initiative is used, the user opens the dialogue, and the system responds. The issue with this strategy is that the user could give vague inputs, to which the system may not know how to react. When using system-directed initiative, the system controls the conversation and the user responds to questions. This greatly minimizes the number of ambiguous responses from the user, but it also reduces the system's flexibility and restricts the user's behaviour. In diverse circumstances, the mixed-initiative technique enables the user and system to take the lead in the conversation. The second step is to select an error handling and confirmation mechanism.

The reverse task of NLU is performed by NLG. It is the process of transforming the system's output into understandable representations in natural language for the user. NLG is the process of creating text/speech from patterns generated by the system. The system produces results in a structured way so that it can process and understand them quickly. The system knowledge base is represented by NLG in a natural or conversational language representation that the user may easily understand.

21.1.2 TYPES OF CHATBOT

A variety of criteria can be used to categorize chatbots (Bhattad and Atkar, 2021; Adamopoulou and Moussiades, 2020), including knowledge domain, service offered, goals, input and response method, human assistance, and construction approach. The types of chatbots are shown in Figure 21.2.

The knowledge a chatbot can access or the volume of data it is educated on are taken into account in classification based on the knowledge domain. Chatbots with open domains can converse about general subjects and respond correctly, but chatbots with closed domains are concentrated in a single knowledge domain and may not be able to answer questions from other users.

The emotional closeness of the chatbot to the user, the level of intimate connection, and the function the chatbot performs are all taken into account when classifying the chatbot based on the service offered. Interpersonal chatbots fall under the category of communication. They don't accompany the user, but they do gather information and give it to them. Intrapersonal chatbots reside within the user's personal domain. They are companions to the user and understand the user in the same way that humans do. Inter-agent chatbots become ubiquitous when all chatbots require some inter-chatbot communication capabilities. Protocols are already required for inter-chatbot communication.

Goal-based classification takes into account the main objective that chatbots try to accomplish. The goal of informative chatbots, like FAQ chatbots, is to give the user access to information that has been pre-stored or is readily available from a fixed source. The aim of chat-based or conversational chatbots is to correctly answer the statement that is supplied to them by talking to the user in a human-like manner. Chatbots that are task-based carry out a single activity, such as making a flight reservation or offering assistance. These chatbots are sophisticated when it comes to requesting information and comprehending the user's input.

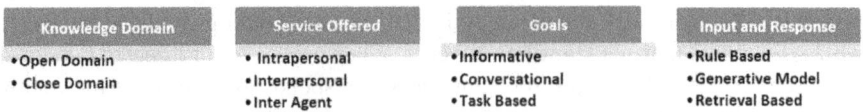

Knowledge Domain	Service Offered	Goals	Input and Response
• Open Domain	• Intrapersonal	• Informative	• Rule Based
• Close Domain	• Interpersonal	• Conversational	• Generative Model
	• Inter Agent	• Task Based	• Retrieval Based

FIGURE 21.2 Classification of chatbots

The way of processing inputs and producing replies is taken into account in classification based on the input processing and response generation approach. Three models are employed to generate acceptable responses: generative models, rule-based models, and retrieval-based models. The majority of the initial chatbots, including many internet chatbots, were constructed using rule-based model architecture. They select the system's response in accordance with a set of fixed, established rules, based on lexical analysis of the input text, without producing any new text responses. The retrieval-based paradigm, which differs just slightly from the rule-based model in that it uses application programming interface (API) to query and evaluate available resources, offers additional flexibility. Before using the matching method to pick responses, a retrieval-based chatbot retrieves some response candidates from an index. The generative model, which is based on the most recent and past user messages, produces replies more effectively than the other models. These chatbots use deep learning and machine learning techniques to make them more human-like.

The development of deep learning chatbots for the healthcare industry is best served by generative, conversational, inter-agent, and open domain chatbots since these types of chatbots must be able to analyze reports and photos and have a broad range of domain knowledge.

21.2   DEEP LEARNING CHATBOTS FOR HEALTHCARE

The medical chatbots (Fadhil and Schiavo, 2019) can be of three types, namely informative chatbots, conversational chatbots, and prescriptive chatbots. The least intrusive method is provided by informative chatbots, which gradually introduce the patient to the world of medical knowledge. These chatbots use the most basic AI algorithms to disseminate information through preprogrammed responses. Conversational chatbots can answer particular queries, making them better able to handle the patient's issues. The degree of their intelligence can, however, differ: some can only respond to questions that have been asked in a clear and concise manner, whereas others can spot patterns and deduce broader meanings. NLP is a subtype of machine learning that is used by complex conversational bots. They must receive training before being released, in order to efficiently process speech. Prescriptive chatbots provide actual medical advice based on the information provided by the user, in addition to responding to the patient's inquiries. The prescriptive chatbots use deep learning algorithms along with NLP techniques.

The technology known as deep learning allows a chatbot to learn completely from scratch. During this phase, machine learning algorithms are used to construct the chatbot. Chatbots with deep learning capabilities learn everything from data and interactions with real people. For the modelling and training of chatbot systems, advanced ideas and techniques such as NLP approaches and deep learning techniques like deep neural networks (DNNs) and deep reinforcement learning (DRL) are being employed, in addition to the classic rule-based approach that was previously used in chatbot development and other straightforward machine learning methodology. Machine learning algorithms can make wise decisions based on what they have learned, but they need structured data to learn from. An artificial neural

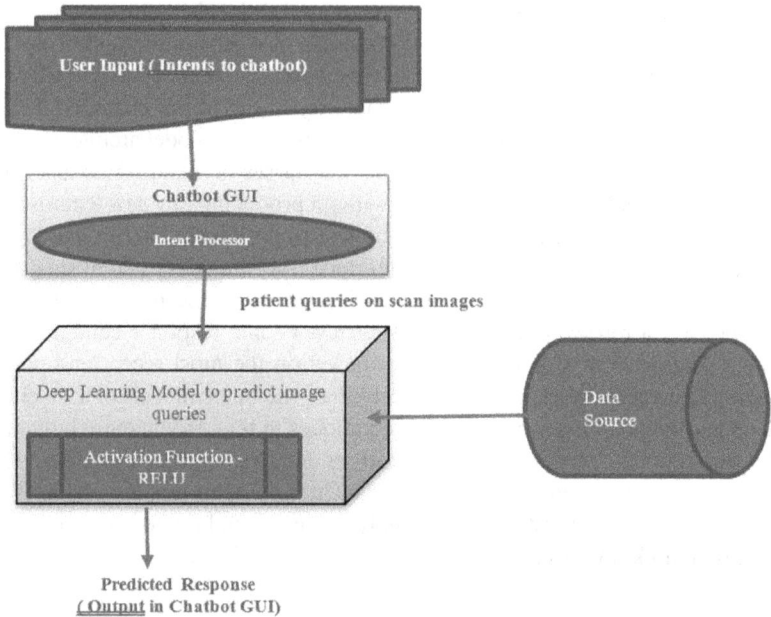

FIGURE 21.3   Chatbot architecture using deep learning techniques

network that can learn and make wise judgments on its own is created using deep learning, which builds the algorithms in layers. The architecture of a deep learning network along with chatbot architecture is shown below in Figure 21.3

21.3   NATURAL LANGUAGE PROCESSING TO ANALYZE SCAN REPORTS

Based on three characteristics – interaction, conversation, and architecture – Montenegro et al. suggested a taxonomy for chatbots in the health field. Health aims (help, diagnosis, education, etc.), health contexts (patient, physician, student), and health domains (dermatology, hospital, therapy, cardiology, mindfulness, etc.) were further separated into three groups. Three further categories are included in the dialogue attribute: communication models (multimodal, speech, text), agent types (counselling, coach), and dialogue types (dialogue generation, planner, engine, and management). Chatbots are distinguished by their architecture in terms of systems and techniques (such as reinforcement learning, convolutional neural networks, and pattern-matching)

21.3.1   NATURAL LANGUAGE UNDERSTANDING

The user utterance must be converted by the NLU unit into a specified semantic frame in accordance with the system's norms in order for the system to interpret it (Vamsi et al., 2020; Adamopoulou and Moussiades, 2020). Intent detection and slot filling are tasks included in this. Intent detection and slot filling are viewed as sequence tagging problems. The process can be implemented using long short-term memory (LSTM). The left-to-right sequences were ignored by the LSTM architecture, which only trained datasets using the right context when they were read from left to right. The network can be trained to utilize both sequences using the bidirectional LSTM (Bi-LSTM) architecture, which can then combine the two independent outputs into a single final result. Because of this, the NLU component is typically implemented as a conditional random field (CRF) layer on top of an LSTM-based recurrent neural network. The model that is being described is a sequence-to-sequence model that employs a bidirectional LSTM network that simultaneously fills the slots and predicts the intent.

To train the provided input using two different sequences: a normal sequence and a reverse sequence. Using x to represent the input and h to represent the feature vector of the sequences, which includes the current word's context and the words that came before it. Since the algorithm has both directions, the word vector can be obtained from the normal sequence $h^{\wedge}$ and another reverse sequence h^. By using the sigmoid function to activate the hidden state, we achieve the desired results. The formulas are displayed as follows.

$$h = [h^{\wedge}, h^{\wedge}]$$

$$y = \delta(h)$$

21.3.2 NATURAL LANGUAGE GENERATOR

The creation of text using natural language from a meaning representation is known as natural language generation (NLG) (Ayanouz et al., 2020). Text summarization, machine translation, and conversation systems all rely heavily on NLG systems. The system's response is mapped back to a comprehensible natural language sentence in the NLG as a semantic frame. A statistical model is used to rate the candidate utterances that trainable NLG systems can produce in a variety of ways (such as scholastically or using a rule base). Each speech is given a score by the statistical model, which is trained using textual data. The majority of these systems generate utterances using bigram and trigram language models. However, an NLG based on a semantically controlled LSTM recurrent network can learn from unaligned input by jointly optimizing its surface realization and sentence planning components using a simple cross-entropy training criterion without any heuristics, and good quality language variety is obtained simply by randomly sampling the network outputs.

21.3.2.1 Sequence-to-Sequence Models

One decoder node giving output corresponding to one encoder node is how sequence-to-sequence models are conceptualized (Bhagwat et al., 2019; Fadhi, 2019). This concept is easily used in machine translation since the decoder can produce an equivalent term for the target language by just examining one word from the input

Who   are   you

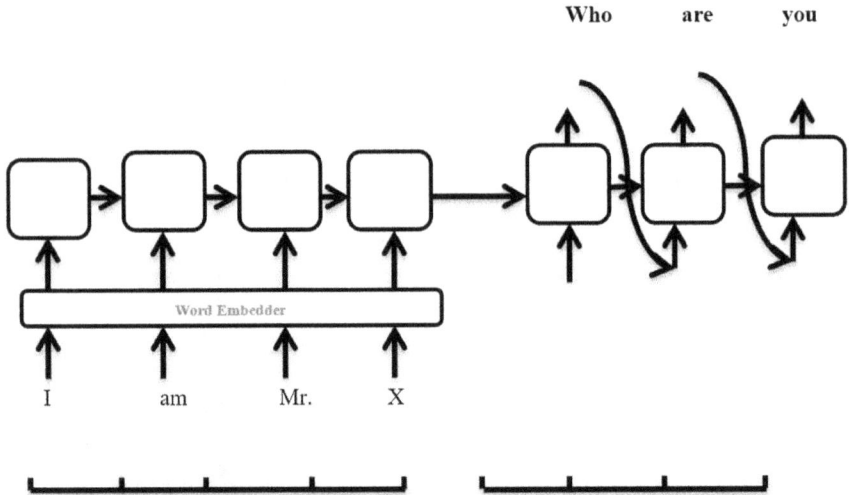

FIGURE 21.4   Encoder and decoder architecture for sequence-to-sequence model

language at a time. The architecture of a sequence-to-sequence (Seq2Seq) model is given below in Figure 21.4

The Seq2Seq model is well-suited for sequence-based problems where the input size and capacities of the sequence vary from each other. The encoder, intermediate vector, and decoder are the three components that make up the Seq2Seq model. The encoder is a stack of recurrent units where each accepts a single input sequence element and propagates information for that element forward. A collection of all the words from the question is used as the input sequence in a problem involving answering a question. A decoder is a stack of recurrent units, each of which forecasts the value y(t) of the output at time-step t. The advantage of this model is that it can map sequences of different lengths to one another.

21.3.2.2   Dialogue Management

The DM may be linked to an external knowledge base (KB) or database (DB) in order to generate more insightful responses. The dialogue state tracker (DST) and policy learning, a reinforcement learning (RL) agent, are the two parts that make up the dialogue Manager. Given the entire history up until that turn, the dialogue state tracker (DST), a sophisticated and crucial component, should accurately deduce the belief about the state of the dialogue. Policy learning is in charge of choosing the best course of action, or the system's reaction to the user's utterance, which should move the user closer to the desired outcome with the fewest possible dialogue turns.

The majority of strong retrieval systems use deep neural networks (DNNs) to learn representations (Wu and Yan 2022). DNNs are highly automated learning tools that may automatically extract underlying abstract features from data by investigating various nonlinear transformation layers. Convolution neural networks (CNNs) and recurrent neural networks (RNNs) are the dominant DNNs for modelling sentences.

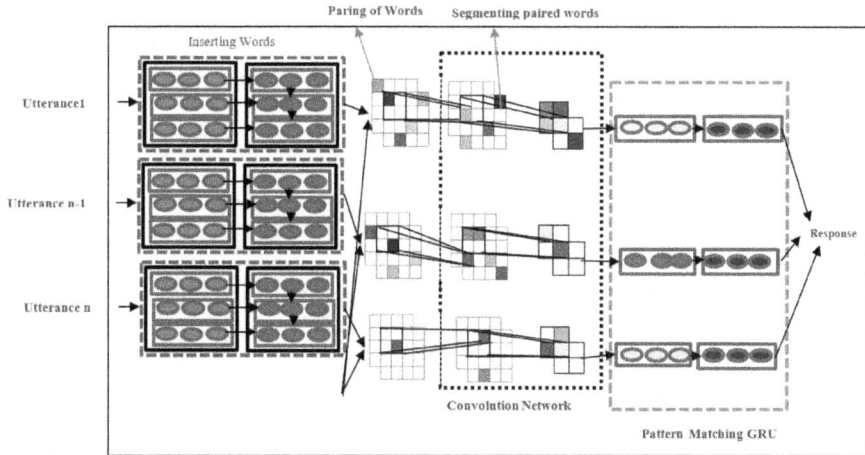

FIGURE 21.5 Architecture of response system

Short-text dialogues can be matched using a variety of techniques for retrieval-based systems. In essence, these techniques build abstractive representations by modelling utterances using convolutional or recurrent networks. The architecture of an answer retrieval system with deep learning layers is shown below in Figure 21.5.

21.4 DEEP LEARNING ALGORITHMS TO ANALYZE SCANS AND X-RAY IMAGES

Clinical techniques (Shen et al., 2017) utilized for early detection, monitoring, diagnosis, and therapy evaluation of numerous medical problems are only a few examples of how medical imaging plays a vital part in these clinical applications. Understanding medical image analysis in computer vision requires an understanding of the fundamental concepts and applications of artificial neural networks and deep learning. The need for medical image services, such as radiography, endoscopy, computed tomography (CT), mammography images (MG), ultrasound images, magnetic resonance imaging (MRI), magnetic resonance angiography (MRA), nuclear medicine imaging, positron emission tomography (PET), and pathological diagnostics has dramatically increased within the healthcare system. In addition, the lack of radiologists makes it frequently difficult and time-consuming to examine medical images. Examples of supervised DL techniques include recurrent neural networks (RNNs) and convolutional neural networks. Unsupervised learning techniques, such as deep belief networks (DBNs), restricted Boltzmann machines (RBMs), autoencoders, and generative adversarial networks (GANs), have also been researched in the context of medical picture analysis. Deep learning accelerator (DLA) is typically used to identify an anomaly and categorize a certain illness type. Convolutional neural networks are perfectly suited for classification, segmentation, object recognition, registration, and other tasks when DLA is applied to medical images.

21.4.1 STEPS TO CONSTRUCT CHATBOTS

The chatbots with deep learning techniques can be constructed using the following steps:

Create intents.

Do data preprocessing using tokenization and the stop words removal technique.

Prepare and reshape the data.

Classify intents and recognize entities. If text recognizes entities using NLP and the image is given, use deep learning techniques.

Create a bag of words or word vectors.

Train the model with a neural network.

Predict the class of input and answer user queries.

21.5 REGULATORY STANDARDS FOR HEALTHCARE CHATBOTS

Software as a medical device (SaMD) applications for healthcare that have already received regulatory approval provide a preview of what's to come (Heinz-Uwe and Dirk, 2021). The effectiveness of SaMD is being investigated in a variety of medical specialties, including dermatology, radiology, surgery, disease diagnosis, pharmacy, and even psychiatry, where chatbots are being designed to automatically identify diseases. In order to address the regulatory gap and provide the first legislative framework for AI, the European Commission (EC) proposed the Artificial Intelligence Act, which was released in April 2021. This would transform Europe into what the commission refers to as "a global centre for trustworthy artificial intelligence."

Four levels of AI danger are identified and categorized in the proposal as unacceptable risk, high risk, restricted risk, and minimum risk. The following requirements must be met for the regulatory clearance of healthcare AI applications, which typically fall into the high-risk category (Udit, 2022).

Systems for evaluating and reducing risks are adequate.

Datasets feeding the system are of high quality, reducing risks and discriminatory effects.

Activity recording to guarantee results can be tracked.

Complete documentation that gives authorities all the details they need to evaluate the system's compliance.

Information that is adequate and clear for the user.

Suitable human oversight procedures to lower risk.

High level of accuracy, security, and toughness.

Despite the fact that general data protection regulation (GDPR) (Sağlam and Nurse 2020) and its consequences have been extensively discussed in many technologies such as cloud computing, the Internet of Things, and blockchain technologies, it is interesting to note that relatively limited emphasis has been placed on potential design and implementation concerns in the chatbot environment. To begin, a lack of algorithmic transparency is a significant impediment to GDPR compliance in chatbots. There are initiatives to increase user awareness of how personal information is processed, however they are quite limited in scope. Transparency is critical for organizations in the banking and health industries that provide customized chatbots that process sensitive or personally identifiable information. Another related right, the right of access, raises significant difficulties because it is unclear how agents should or could grant access to the personal information they hold. The accuracy with which the agent processes the interactions will determine whether this condition is met. A difficulty for the data minimization principle is presented by chatbots' interactive and conversational character. A chatbot may end up processing multiple pieces of sensitive personal information that it did not expect (or request). When voluntarily or accidentally responding to an agent's questions regarding their degree of stress, a user might, for instance, opt to reveal their ethnicity. Finding the right approach for a chatbot that can still provide the user with realistic responses while also properly upholding their privacy can be challenging, especially when processing unique categories of personal data (such as ethnicity or sexual orientation). To create and develop chatbots, personal user information is necessary, but it's also crucial to take into account ethical standards, legal justifications, and legal rights under laws like the GDPR. It is obvious that further research is needed in this field as our society attempts to strike a balance between the benefits of agents and the requirement for privacy and the relevant data protection rules and regulations.

21.6   SECURITY AND ETHICAL ISSUES

A new opinion paper (Hasal et al., 2021) supporting 12 clinical, legal, and ethical problems that must be taken into account before using artificial intelligence-driven conversation agents in healthcare was published in the Journal of the American Medical Association (JAMA). The authors outlined 12 categories that practitioners should take into consideration, including patient safety, scope, trust and transparency, content decisions, data use, privacy and integration, bias and health equality, third-party engagement, cybersecurity, legal and licensing, research and development questions, governance, testing and evaluation, supporting innovation, and related topics. The algorithms used by the chatbots mainly rely on data. The data's correctness, security, privacy, and integrity are crucial. If not, people won't give the health chatbots their sensitive medical information.

Chatbots are trained to give pre-set answers to questions or, in many situations, to suggest an action based on a pattern of normal human responses that has been previously analyzed (Abhinav et al., 2021). The trustworthiness of the AI's indications and replies may need to be further established among users in these applications of AI when the human is removed from the equation in order to support its ethical use.

When designing any component, privacy and security must be taken into consideration. Threats and vulnerabilities that come with security can be viewed as a concern for businesses because there is a possibility of a system hack. It is crucial to protect user data when using chatbots, especially in the healthcare industry, since the system needs to process user data to operate. Our systematic review was influenced by two research issues. Firstly, what roles do chatbots play in the healthcare industry? And secondly, what security and privacy safeguards are currently in place for healthcare chatbots?

21.6.1 AUTHENTICATION AND AUTHORIZATION

The two key security procedures used by chatbots are authentication and authorization. Using authentication, chatbots may confirm the user's identity and authorization, so they can give the user access to data or a function. Authentication of the user's identity is not always required. When the user requests assistance with personal identification, then authentication and authorization become mandatory. Authentication can be done in two ways, either using biometric authentication or with the two-factor authentication method. Two-factor authentication ensures a user's data and communications are protected to a greater extent. For instance, the user may be requested to confirm their account credentials via email and text message. Personal data cannot be stored or shared online without additional security measures. A security layer of a biometric scan would authenticate the user's confirmation by the bots when engaging with them.

21.6.2 END-TO-END ENCRYPTION

End-to-end encryption (E2EE) was another important technology option that received significant attention. With end-to-end encryption, the message can only be accessed by the intended sender and recipient.

The message can only be viewed by legitimate personnel, which enforces encryption. The usage of an encryption algorithm similar to the RSA algorithm is suggested by Hasal et al. The user of this method will create a public key and a private key, with the public key being used for encryption and the private key for decryption. With the use of a private key that only the users are aware of, this technique guarantees that users can interact. Most chatbots that don't work with personal data don't use E2EE. Several chatbots are exclusively used on one website. HTTPS, or hypertext transfer protocol, encrypts connections and uses Secure Sockets Layer (SSL) or Transport Layer Security (TSL) to send data. In contrast to end-to-end encryption, HTTPS uses point-to-point encryption. The user's connection to a load balancer is secure when using HTTPS, but after that, the data are decrypted and returned to plain text. Because of this, all services following the load balancer can then assault the data. The secure exchange of data between such parties is only guaranteed by E2EE.

21.6.3 PRIVACY-PRESERVING CHATS

Chatbots have five privacy-related problems, as follows:

Variations in the interaction's goals.
Turn-taking fosters reciprocal connections between humans and chatbots.

Identity management activity.

Chatbots' conversational expectations.

Handling unanticipated, frequently sensitive information.

21.6.4 ENTITY-BASED PRIVACY PRESERVATION

Providing "entities" is crucial for personalizing chatbots, together with "intents" and "utterances". The entities correspond to the terminology used in a certain domain. On the client/app side, a module known as the privacy-preserving chat module (PPCM) implements the entities-based method. Understanding the original chatbot material and the underlying NLP strategies employed by the chatbot platform is necessary for the PPCM design. To solve the user's chat privacy issues, a combination of privacy-preserving approaches based on filtering and transformation are used. The text-extraction method used by PPCM is the same as that of the chatbot's NLP engine. The query is then filtered or deleted so that it is not submitted to the backend NLP engine, and the user is then given the proper notification. In order for the chatbot NLP engine to classify the user sentiment of the converted question as "neutral", the PPCM must modify the original user query to a more "neutral" response with the same semantics.

21.6.5 SEARCHABLE ENCRYPTION

Using a method known as searchable encryption (SE), sensitive data can be protected while yet allowing for server-side search (cloud) (Jayati, 2022). The server can search encrypted data using SE without disclosing any plaintext data. Searchable symmetric encryption (SSE) and public key encryption with keyword search (PEKS) are the two main subfields of SE. SE consists of the following polynomial time randomized algorithms, as shown in Figure 21.6.

The architecture of deep learning healthcare chatbots along with the security is given below, in Figure 21.7.

- $KGEN(1^k)$ outputs a public-private key pair: (A_pub, A_priv).

- $SENC(A\_pub, w, m)$ outputs a searchable encryption s_w of chat message m under entity w and public key A_pub.

- $DOOR(A\_priv, w)$ outputs a trapdoor t_w that allows to search by entity w.

- $TEST(A\_pub, s\_w, t\_w')$ outputs the message m if $w = w'$.

FIGURE 21.6 Polynomial randomized algorithm of SE

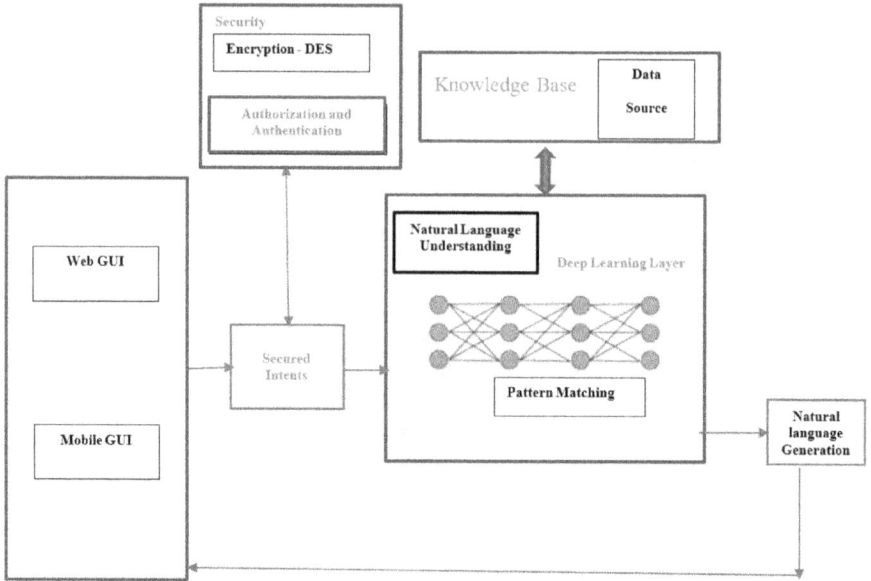

FIGURE 21.7   Framework of deep learning chatbot with security

21.7   ISSUES AND FUTURE RESEARCH TRENDS

Every technology has advantages and disadvantages. Chatbots are the same way. They do not always work perfectly. Below is a list of the dangers they pose.

21.7.1   PARTIAL INSPECTION AND EVALUATION

Numerous medical professionals think chatbots could aid in the self-diagnosis of minor illnesses. The technology has not yet advanced enough to completely replace doctor visits. They are unable to determine whether a person speaks more casually or seriously. Additionally, they struggle to keep the same tone of voice throughout every interaction.

21.7.2   UNRELIABLE INTERPRETATION

If the AI chatbot is unable to understand the precise circumstances, patients could experience severe harm or even die. The results of choosing the incorrect medication might be disastrous. Patients frequently suffer due to flaws in the healthcare system, even if the usage of AI chatbot services is less common.

21.7.3   DATA BREACHES AND USER PRIVACY

Not all end users feel safe giving bots their private information. AI also requires training, which involves obtaining fresh data as fresh scenarios arise. Such data may be hacked, resulting in privacy violations. This is one of the most important problems at hand right now.

21.7.4 LACK OF HUMAN INTERACTION

The immersive joy of human interaction will always be superior to robotic discourse, regardless of how quickly it is automated. A person can always join in on numerous informational threads to provide pertinent remarks that ultimately benefit the sufferer more.

21.7.5 LACK OF SINCERE FEELINGS AND RESPONSIBILITY

Empathy is a crucial component of communication that is frequently necessary for someone who is worried about their health. Patients feel better and are more willing to cooperate with procedures when caregivers demonstrate empathy in the healthcare system. There is now a principle-based approach to AI in healthcare, however, the absence of the trust that underpins a patient-physician connection remains.

21.8 SCOPE OF RESEARCH

Existing models of regulation are designed for locked healthcare solutions, whereas AI is flexible and evolves over time. Visionary legislation in this field will surely put more compliance pressure on legal teams, but it will also bring much-needed clarity, lower the danger of legal action for complying businesses, and give SaMD manufacturers the assurance they need to develop and fully utilize AI in the healthcare industry.

Future research can be especially helpful in three key areas: diagnostics, patient engagement outside of hospitals, and mental health. The topic of whether the technology can further engage patients to improve results is raised by chatbots that are made to not just actively capture but also captivate the patients in their care. A conversational chatbot for healthcare can be used by people seeking mental health counselling as a forum for talking about their emotions. A healthcare expert stepping in and taking over can be avoided if the patient's needs are met and can be automated.

Developing chatbots for medical insurance can have a great impact. Nobody wants to deal with insurance companies, claims, or medical costs. Thankfully, AI chatbots for healthcare can help with these chores. A chatbot for healthcare has the ability to verify current coverage, assist with the filing of claims, and monitor the progress of claims. Medical AI systems can also assist doctors with billing questions and the pre-authorization procedure.

REFERENCES

Abhinav, V., Krisstina, R., Vivek, E., & Yukti, S. (July 2021). Regulating AI in public health: Systems challenges and perspectives, ORF. *Occasional Paper*, 261.

Adamopoulou, E., & Moussiades, L. (2020a). An overview of chatbot technology. In Maglogiannis, I., Iliadis, L., Pimenidis, E. (Eds.), *Artificial Intelligence Applications and Innovations. AIAI 2020. IFIP Advances in Information and Communication Technology*, Vol. 584. Springer, Cham. doi: 10.1007/978-3-030-49186-4_31.

Adamopoulou, E., & Moussiades, L. (2020b). Chatbots: History, technology, and applications. *Machine Learning with Applications*, 2, 100006.

Ahmad, N. A., Che, M. H., Zainal, A., Abd Rauf, M. F., & Adnan, Z. (2018). Review of chatbots design techniques. *International Journal of Computer and Applications*, 181(8), 7–10.

Athota, L., Shukla, V. K., Pandey, N., & Rana, A. (2020). Chatbot for healthcare system using artificial intelligence. In *8th International Conference on Reliability, Infocom Technologies and Optimization (Trends and Future Directions) (ICRITO), 2020*, pp. 619–622. doi: 10.1109/ICRITO48877.2020.9197833.

Ayanouz, S., Abdelhakim, B. A., & Benhmed, M. (2020, March). A smart chatbot architecture based NLP and machine learning for health care assistance. In *Proceedings of the 3rd International Conference on Networking Information Systems & Security*, 756, pp. 1–6.

Bagwan, F., Phalnikar, R., & Desai, S. (2021). Artificially intelligent health chatbot using deep learning. In *2nd International Conference for Emerging Technology (INCET)*, 2021, pp. 1–5. doi: 10.1109/INCET51464.2021.9456195.

Bhagwat, S., Bhagwat, V. A., & Gaikwad, V. (2019). Deep learning for chatbots, scholar works, link: "Deep learning for chatbots" by Vyas Ajay Bhagwat (sjsu.edu).

Bhattad, H., & Atkar, M. G. (2021). Review on different types of Chatbots. *International Research Journal of Modernization in Engineering Technology and Science (IRJMETS)*, 3(5), 1347–1349.

Bhirud, N., Tataale, S., Randive, S., & Nahar, S. (2019). A literature review on chatbots in healthcare domain. *International Journal of Scientific and Technology Research*, 8(7), 225–231.

Cahn, J. (2017). Chatbot: Architecture, design and development, Senior Thesis, Department of Computer and Information Science, University of Pennsylvania.

Chopde, A., & Agrawal, M. (2022, June 19). Chatbot using deep learning. Available at SSRN: doi: 10.2139/ssrn.4140506.

Chuan, C. H., & Morgan, S. (2020). Creating and evaluating chatbots as eligibility assistants for clinical trials: An active deep learning approach towards user-centered classification. *ACM Transactions on Computing for Healthcare*, 2(1), 1–19.

Csaky, R. (2019). Deep learning based chatbot models. arXiv Preprint ArXiv:1908.08835.

Davenport, T., & Kalakota, R. (2019, June). The potential for artificial intelligence in healthcare. *Future Healthcare Journal*, 6(2), 94–98. doi: 10.7861/futurehosp.6-2-94; PMID: 31363513; PMCID: PMC6616181.

Dolianiti, F., Tsoupouroglou, I., Antoniou, P., Konstantinidis, S., Anastasiades, S., & Bamidis, P. (2020, October). Chatbots in healthcare curricula: The case of a conversational virtual patient. In *International Conference on Brain Function Assessment in Learning*. Springer, Cham, pp. 137–147.

Fadhil, A., & Schiavo, G. (2019). Designing for health chatbots. arXiv Preprint ArXiv:1902.09022.

Hasal, M., Nowaková, J., Ahmed Saghair, K., Abdulla, H., Snášel, V., & Ogiela, L. (2021). Chatbots: Security, privacy, data protection, and social aspects. *Concurrency and Computation: Practice and Experience*, 33(19), e6426.

Heinz-Uwe, D., & Dirk, T.W. (2021, November). Artificial Intelligence is forcing healthcare regulators to catch up and reimage the regulation rule book. https://www.ey.com/en_lv/law/how-the-challenge-of-regulating-ai-in-healthcare-is-escalating.

Jayati, D. (2022). Privacy-preserving conversational interfaces, thesis, University Graduate School, Indiana University.

Jiang, F., Jiang, Y., Zhi, H., et al. (2017). Artificial intelligence in healthcare: past, present and future. *Stroke and Vascular Neurology*, 2(4). doi: 10.1136/svn-2017-000101.

Karri, S. P. R., & Kumar, B. S. (2020, January). Deep learning techniques for implementation of chatbots. In *International Conference on Computer Communication and Informatics (ICCCI), 2020*. IEEE, pp. 1–5.

Khalid, H., Hussain, M., Al Ghamdi, M. A., Khalid, T., Khalid, K., Khan, M. A., Fatima, K., Masood, K., Almotiri, S. H., Farooq, M. S., Ahmed, A. (2020). A comparative systematic literature review on knee bone reports from MRI, X-rays and CT scans using deep learning and machine learning methodologies. *Diagnostics*, 10(8), 518.

Kurup, G., & Shetty, S. D. (2022). AI conversational chatbot for primary healthcare diagnosis using natural language processing and deep learning. In Das, A. K., Nayak, J., Naik, B., Dutta, S., Pelusi, D. (Eds.), *Computational Intelligence in Pattern Recognition: Advances in Intelligent Systems and Computing*, Vol. 1349. Springer, Singapore. doi: 10.1007/978-981-16-2543-5_22.

May, R., & Denecke, K. (2022). Security, privacy, and healthcare-related conversational agents: A scoping review. *Informatics for Health and Social Care*, 47(2), 194–210.

Nikhila, P., Jyothi, G. P., Mounika, K., Reddy, & M. C. (2019). Chatbots using artificial intelligence. *Journal of Applied Computer Science*, 6(2), 103–115.

Reis, L., Maier, C., Mattke, J., & Weitzel, T. (2020). Chatbots in healthcare: Status quo, application scenarios for physicians and patients and future directions. ECIS. 2020 Research Papers, 163. https://aisel.aisnet.org/ecis2020_rp/163.

Sağlam, R. B., & Nurse, J. R. (2020, July). Is your chatbot GDPR compliant? Open issues in agent design. In *Proceedings of the 2nd Conference on Conversational User Interfaces*, 1032, pp. 1–3.

Shen, D., Wu, G., & Suk, H. I. (2017, June 21). Deep learning in medical image analysis. *Annual Review of Biomedical Engineering*, 19, 221–248. doi: 10.1146/annurev-bioeng-071516-044442. Epub 2017 Mar 9. PMID: 28301734; PMCID: PMC5479722.

Siddique, S., & Chow, J. C. (2021). Machine learning in healthcare communication. *Encyclopedia*, 1(1), 220–239.

Surani, A., & Das, S. (2022). Understanding privacy and security postures of healthcare chatbots, *Chi*, 22, 1–7.

Suta, P., Lan, X., Wu, B., Mongkolnam, P., & Chan, J. H. (2020). An overview of machine learning in chatbots. *International Journal of Mechanical Engineering and Robotics*, 9(4), 502–510.

Udit, H. (2022, October). The role and risks of chatbots in healthcare industry, Cynotek, the role and risks of chatbots in healthcare industry - Cynoteck.

Vamsi, G. K., Rasool, A., & Hajela, G. (2020, July). Chatbot: A deep neural network based human to machine conversation model. In *2020 11th International Conference on Computing, Communication and Networking Technologies (ICCCNT)*. IEEE, pp. 1–7.

Wang, L., Wang, D., Tian, F., Peng, Z., Fan, X., Zhang, Z., & Wang, H. (2021). Cass: Towards building a social-support chatbot for online health community. *Proceedings of the ACM on Human-Computer Interaction*, 5(CSCW1), 1–31.

Wang, W., & Siau, K. (2018). Trust in health chatbots. In *Proceedings of the Thirty Ninth International Conference on Information Systems*, San Francisco, CA: Association for Information Systems.

Wu, W., & Yan, R. (2018). Deep chit-chat: Deep learning for ChatBots. In *Proceedings of the 2018 Conference on Empirical Methods in Natural Language Processing: Tutorial Abstracts*, Melbourne, Australia. Association for Computational Linguistics, vol. 696, pp. 354–368.

Wilson, L., & Marasoiu, M. (2022). The development and use of chatbots in public health: Scoping review. *JMIR Human Factors*, 9(4), e35882.

Wu, W., & Yan, R. (2019, July). Deep chit-chat: Deep learning for chatbots. In *Proceedings of the 42nd International ACM SIGIR Conference on Research and Development in Information Retrieval*, 753, pp. 1413–1414.

Yan, R., Li, J., & Yu, Z. (2022). Deep learning for dialogue systems: Chit-chat and beyond. *Foundations and Trends in Information Retrieval*, 15(5), 417–588. doi: 10.1561/1500000083.

Ye, W., & Li, Q. (2020). Chatbot security and privacy in the age of personal assistants. In *2020 IEEE/ACM Symposium on Edge Computing (SEC), 2020*, pp. 388–393. doi: 10.1109/SEC50012.2020.00057.

22 Autism, ADHD and Dyslexia Disorder Comorbidity

An Enhanced Study on Education for Children through Artificial Intelligence-Enabled Personalized Assistive Tools

K.N. Praveena, R. Mahalakshmi,
C. Manjunath, and Dipali K. Dakhole

22.1 INTRODUCTION

22.1.1 MENTAL DISORDERS

According to the Diagnostic and Statistical Manual of Mental Disorders (DSM-V), mental disorders with onset in infancy or teenage contain together neurodevelopmental disorders (NDDs), like knowledgeable frailty, and precise education incapacities, such as dyslexia, attention deficit hyperactivity disorder (ADHD), and autism spectrum disorder (ASD). With a rate of 10–20% worldwide, mental illnesses beginning in infancy are becoming more common. Additionally, the previously stated conduct, psychosis, stress, depression, and anxiety-related disorders may develop suicidal ideation. Furthermore, NDDs and MHDs frequently overlap. When NDDs and MHDs coexist, a complicated network of comorbidities can worsen a child's learning impairments and lower their quality of life [1]. The implications for modifying therapy for specific children due to this complex comorbidity include a worse long-term prognosis [2]. Children's mental disorder development is influenced by both genetics and the environment. A youngster's neurological ability and emotional well-being could be impacted by their family's financial status. In addition, a parent's personal health issues, psychological illness, social loneliness, or lack of housing can make

DOI: 10.1201/9781003363361-22

it harder for them to raise a child in a way that encourages growth and development and keeps mental health issues at bay [3]. Therefore, it is vital to comprehend the most effective ways to identify and treat early-onset MDs, and NDDs in particular. These disorders have a significant effect on people experiencing them, their relatives, and the world. There are two goals for this systematic study. First, in order to help kids with serious NDDs, an outline of how artificial intelligence (AI) technologies have been used is necessary. Second, we want to draw attention to the shortcomings of currently available AI tools in order to facilitate suggestions for future paths in AI development and further personalize instruction for these students.

22.1.1.1 ADHD

The frequency of the NDD ADHD, which ranges from 9% to 40% [4, 5] has many etiologies, with combinations of environmental and genetic factors contributing to the aetiology and its varied symptoms [6]. Brain damage, preterm labour, parental liquor use during pregnancy, and exposure to specific environmental factors have all been implicated as non-genetic risk factors. Children who satisfy the diagnostic measures for ADHD frequently also have other comorbid conditions and particular learning difficulties. Children with ADHD struggle to pay attention for long stretches of time, and they may also be hyperactive, restless, and unable to wait their turn [7]. Research in its early stages suggests that children with ADHD have different brain sizes from neurotypical kids, with the frontal and parietal cortex being particularly affected.

22.1.1.2 Dyslexia

A frequent form of education problem known as NDD dyslexia affects three to 15% of school children [8]. People who have dyslexia specifically struggle to develop their advanced reading abilities. Poor spelling and decoding skills, as well as a lack of word recognition, are all symptoms of dyslexia [9]. Compared to non-dyslexic individuals, those with dyslexia are demonstrated to exhibit changes in handy brain images, such as decreased neural changes to sustain motivation. Kids with dyslexia may also experience additional distinct learning disabilities [9], as well as lower self-esteem, anxiety, and sadness.

22.1.1.3 Autism Spectrum Disorder

During the first three years of life is normally when autism spectrum disorders occur in person, which have a described occurrence of about 2% in affluent nations. ASDs are characterized by difficulties interacting with others difficulties speaking, linguistic delays, avoidance of eye contact, inability to adapt to variations in the environment, presentation of repetitive behaviours, and variations in learning abilities. There is a great prevalence of anxiety and sadness in both kids and adults with ASDs. Kids with ASDs and typically developing children have different neurobiological profiles, according to research on the pathophysiology of ASDs. It is believed that the diminished "pruning"s of faulty neural connections during brain development is the primary cause of these excessive connections.

22.2 ARTIFICIAL INTELLIGENCE-BASED PERSONALIZED ASSISTIVE TOOLS FOR CHILDREN WITH NDD

According to the previous description, NDDs such as ASDs, ADHD, and dyslexia are extremely common conditions that are linked to reduced knowledge outcomes and a higher frequency of MHDs. More support techniques are needed, according to a recent study [2], to enable students with these disorders to learn in regular classrooms. It is crucial to use efficient technologies to enhance learning results. Personalized assistive educational technologies may enhance educational outcomes, aid afflicted people in reintegrating into society, and resolve stressful situations, which are known to frequently serve as triggers for suicide attempts. Therefore, Section 22.1 emphasises the three basic NDDs and the requirement for customized assistive devices. The issues faced by educational practices in schools are discussed in Section 22.3, along with the possible contribution of AI technologies to overcome those challenges. The research methodology is covered in Section 22.5, and the usefulness of the AI tools built for individualized education is covered in Section 22.5.1. The limits of current AI technologies are described in Section 22.6. The proposed AI tool for individualized learning, which overcomes the shortcomings of the current tools, is presented in Section 22.8. The review study is concluded in Section 22.9.

22.3 PRESENT MANAGEMENT WITH NDD CHILDREN

22.3.1 INDIVIDUALIZED EDUCATIONAL STRATEGIES FOR CHILDREN WITH ADHD

It is advised to use inclusive methods so that NDD students can attend typical schools whenever is necessary. Nevertheless, traditional school environments can exacerbate signs in kids with ADHD, particularly when they are required to sit motionless, silent, and maintain focus. Thus, mainstream education without supplementary help can harm children's self-esteem and have a detrimental effect on their interactions with instructors and peers. Therefore, it is advised that teachers use customized learning approaches in the schoolroom to meet the needs of these kids on an individual basis.

22.3.2 INDIVIDUALIZED EDUCATIONAL STRATEGIES FOR CHILDREN WITH DYSLEXIA

When teaching dyslexic students in schools, a multi-sensory approach is reportedly preferred [10]. This method involves displaying information simultaneously through a variety of channels.

The strategies listed in Table 22.2 are those that have been used successfully in school settings for kids who have been diagnosed with dyslexia.

22.3.3 INDIVIDUALIZED EDUCATIONAL STRATEGIES FOR CHILDREN WITH ASD

Variances in acoustic handling, motivation, simulation, and organization can hinder ASD children's learning success [11]. ASD children deliberate, study, and perform differently from neurotypical children [11]. As a result, individualized educational methods have been used to meet the various requirements of ASD kids.

22.3.4 Difficulties in Executing Individualized Learning Methodologies in School

Teachers encounter a number of difficulties in accomplishing the goal of individualized learning, despite the fact that evidence suggests that individualized courses are successful in assisting children in overcoming their learning problems [12]. The process of giving differentiated instructions, making sure the child has grasped them, and then achieving the objectives specified for each student takes a lot of time for teachers [12]. Appropriate learning resources are in low supply in many schools. Therefore, a learning aid that can be customized to fit each child's unique needs and learning obstacles would be incredibly beneficial for teachers and a tremendous aid in assisting students to achieve their unique goals. It may take some effort to master a new tool and educate kids to use it, but employing such technologies to facilitate customized education and enhance complete medical and educational results has evident advantages.

22.3.5 Utilization of AI in Therapy and Sympathetic Teaching for Children with Mental Disorders

22.3.5.1 AI with ML Models

Artificial intelligence includes ML, where the model can complete tasks without human intervention. The input data that is fed into the traditional machine learning models train them, and as a result, these models are able to predict outcomes very accurately. Large amounts of data are utilized to train these models in the branch of machine learning known as deep learning, which is likewise capable of highly accurate result prediction. Both models have a high degree of accuracy when used to diagnose some neurological illnesses. For the purpose of diagnosing neurological illnesses, the models are either fed with electroencephalogram (EEG) signals or images. Figure 22.1 illustrates the process of developing a machine learning model for diagnostic diseases.

22.3.5.2 Deep Learning Methods Using AI

As shown in Figures 22.3–22.5, the convolutional neural network (CNN), long short term memory model (LSTM) and autoencoder are a few often-used deep learning models [1]. In CNN models, the convolutional layer receives the input data. Each subsequent layer generates a new feature map, from which more reliable features are collected for forecasting. Classification of the dataset occurs in the last fully connected layer. Input, Forget, and Output Gates are the three primary blocks of memory cells that make up the LSTM, and they are responsible for managing the information that is read, written, and stored on the cell as information is received. The LSTM functions primarily by retaining crucial data from earlier states and

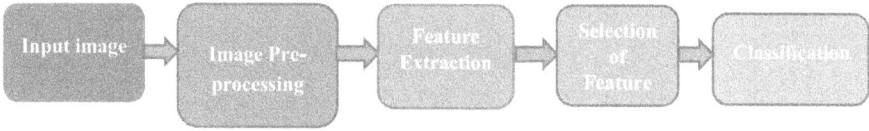

FIGURE 22.1 Steps involved in training the machine learning model

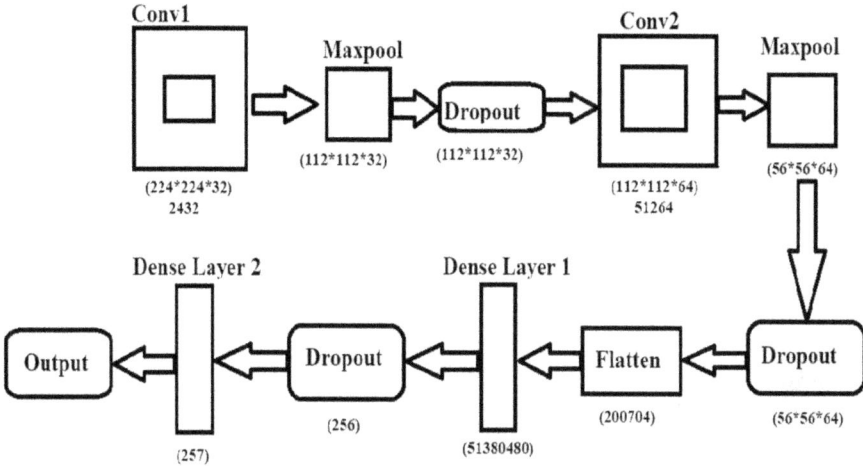

FIGURE 22.2 Sample convolution model

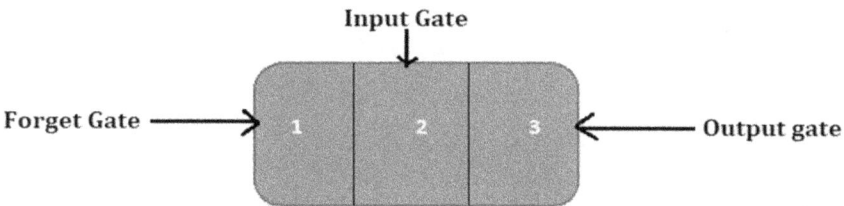

FIGURE 22.3 LSTM model

building on them. The deeper autoencoder model is formed by the arrangement of encoders. Autoencoders work by encrypting unlabelled data and then accurately reconstructing the data.

22.3.5.3 Treatments and Sympathetic Teaching: The Role of AI

Children with ASDs have been trained to recognize and respond to social cues with the help of artificial intelligence. A machine learning technique was utilized by Belpaeme et al. [6] to examine ASD manners and stages of engagement for treatment. According to the results, the model performed better than non-personalized

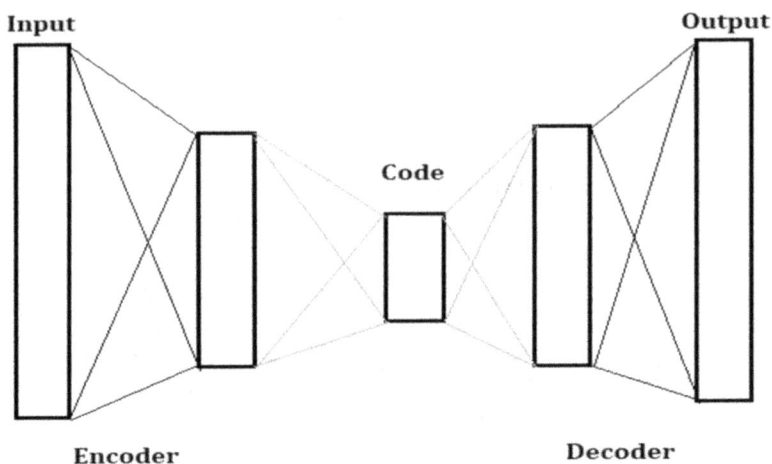

FIGURE 22.4 Autoencoder aodel

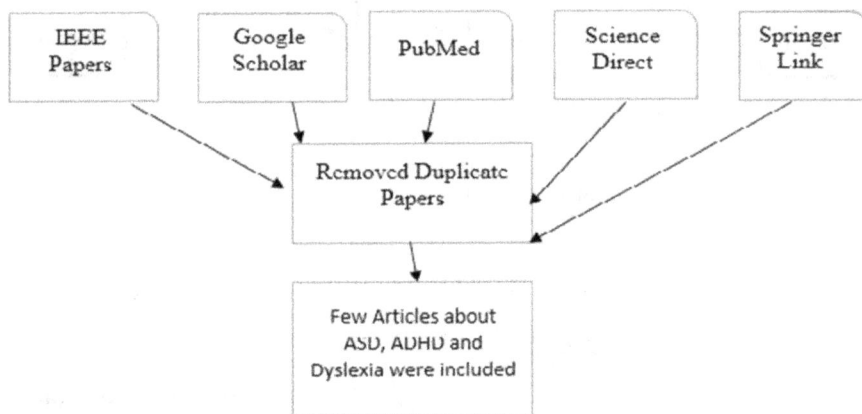

FIGURE 22.5 PRISMA flowchart for collection of related articles

machine learning solutions, in terms of how well it predicted impact and engagement in comparison to human experts, with an accuracy of roughly 60%. In other training, an amalgam teaching instrument for physical education was formed using artificial intelligence and speech recognition to create a voice-activated, interactive educational robot. According to the findings, the robot was able to respond to learners' inquiries with an accuracy of greater than 90%. The findings listed above therefore confirm that AI is a potential way to enhance social contact and sympathetic teaching for kids with psychological problems. Figure 22.2 represents a sample CNN model. Figures 22.3 and 22.4 represent the LSTM model and autoencoder model, respectively.

22.4   RELATED WORK

22.4.1   Summary of Articles Which Used AI Tools

The summaries of the papers that discuss using machine learning techniques and AI tools to teach kids with learning difficulties are depicted in Tables 22.1, 22.2, and 22.3.

22.5   MATERIALS AND METHODS

The maximum pertinent studies of assistive tools established to address educational incapacities using ML algorithms were analyzed in the organized review. The search was carried out between 2011 and 2021. The Institute of Electrical and Electronic Engineering, Google Scholar, PubMed, Science Direct, and Springer Link scientific repositories were used to search for the relevant journal articles. Based on three main methods from the PRISMA standards, the pertinent publications were selected from several databanks for this analysis. The procedure was completed with the selection of the 26 articles deemed to be the most pertinent. Figure 22.5 illustrates the flow-chart for the procedures involved in retrieving pertinent articles utilizing PRISMA criteria.

22.5.1   AI's Effectiveness in Delivering Individualized Education

The majority of AI learning technologies, as indicated in Table 22.3, have reported successful results. A student with ADHD who has trouble focusing on their work may benefit from using artificial intelligence tool. The application has also helped users become more engaged and show higher behavioural intentions towards it. FaceSay games were employed in a study to help autistic kids, and the results showed increases in social interaction, emotion detection, and face recognition in both low- and high-functioning autistic individuals. The creation of software games for kids with ADHD has positive effects in addressing their moods and can enhance the communication with others. It has been demonstrated that using robots and other communication tools can help kids with ASD learn math, social skills, and how to focus. Consequently, the aforementioned findings attest to the usefulness of AI tools for individualized learning.

22.6   LIMITATIONS OF AI TOOLS FOR PERSONALIZED EDUCATION

There are few community databanks about kids with specific NDDs since it is difficult to acquire information from kids whose disorders mean that they often struggle to remain still. There is also a scarcity of information for these disorders to collect from the parents. Numerous kids have complicated comorbidities, making building personalized AI tools for them difficult.

TABLE 22.1

Review of AI-Based Tools for Helping Students with ADHD

Year	Artificial Intelligence Tool	Training Model	Skill Used	Learning Area Addressed	Efficiency
2014	KAR Robot	-	Assistive Technology	Increases communal talents by telling stories	Enhances children's intellectual capabilities
2015	Kid action sensing and training tool	Machine learning model	Wearable technology	Helps students sustain attention	Assists kids with ADHD who lose concentration when working
2018	WatchMinder vibrating watch	Uses sensors and bespoke algorithm	Assistive Tools	Aids in reminding learners to focus on their task	The watch has been demonstrated to be a very basic memory aid for kids with ADHD when equipped with the auditory or vibrating alarm feature [65]
2018	Speech recognition software	Audio data, deep learning model	Assistive Technology	Writing is replaced with speech	It helps ADHD students to improve in writing, reading, and spelling
2018	Talking calculators	Built-in speech recognition	Assistive technology	Helps with hearing and doing math	Students are able to complete assignments faster

TABLE 22.2

Review of AI-Based Tools for Helping Students with Dyslexia.

Year	Artificial Intelligence Tool	Training Model	Skill Used	Learning Area Addressed	Efficiency
2013	Dyslexia AI system	Machine learning model	Assistive technology	Helps children obtain knowledge about letters and the alphabet	Improves reading and writing skills
2014	Adaptive reading system	Machine learning model	Assistive technology	Helps students to read Greek	Reading skills improved
2015	Learning model using computer	Machine learning model	-	Helps in the learning process using ML methods	-
2017	Dyslexia Quest	Audio data, deep learning model	Digital application	Reading and writing skills	Audiobooks, which are useful for learning
2018	DIMMAND, CapturaTalk application	Chatbots	Digital use	Used to improve literacy	-

22.7 DISCUSSION

Tables 22.1, 22.2, and 22.3 illustrate the AI tools used to help students with ASD, ADHD, and dyslexia learn. This study shows that the majority of these tools are created to aid autistic students in education, and application-based tools are the most frequently created tools to aid ADHD, dyslexia, and ASD students in education. Through this analysis, it has also become clear that, in contrast to ADHD and dyslexic children, ASD kids have received the most support from robotics and application-based technologies for their learning. Our review's findings also support the notion that some AI tools have produced beneficial effects and proven effective in specific educational contexts. Table 22.3 shows that most application-based tools are created to help children with ASD in many learning environments. Additionally, compared to other learning disorders, it is apparent that more types of technology have been utilized for ASD, leading to the development of more AI tools to assist kids with ASD. This might be an outcome of the difficulties that people with ASDs have with learning, social communication, and play abilities. Due to the highly heterogeneous character of ASDs, it is also clear from the review that AI tools can be used for ASD children in order to communicate with society (Tables 22.1, 22.2, and 22.3). These technologies have unique capabilities that enable each learner to receive individualized instruction. For the benefit of kids with ADHD, wearable technology, robots, and application-based aids have all been developed. Tables 22.1, 22.2, and 22.3 show our findings from the review that not all tools produced have unique

TABLE 22.3

Review of AI-Based Tools for Helping Students with Autism

Year	Artificial Intelligence Tool	Training Model	Skill Used	Learning Area Addressed	Efficiency
2011	LifeisGame	Facial features are captured from web cam	Digital application	It helps teach students to recognize facial emotions	-
2017 [17, 18]	ENABLE Me app	Feeling appreciation, Google smartglasses	Wearable technology	Enhances social communication between students and teachers	Students can improve their communication
2018 [20, 21]	Kasper automaton	Sensor information, reinforcement learning	Assistive technology	Enhances social communication between students and teachers	Students can improve their communication
2018	Flash cards, autism emotions, etc.	Deep learning/ machine learning	Digital application	Enhances social communication between students and teachers	Students can improve their communication
2019	Emotify game	Audio data, random forest classifier	Digital application	Assists schoolchildren with precise approaches	The app made students more engaged and participatory

features that enable personalization. Students' learning demands vary from one to the next, depending on the intensity and specifics of the condition that affects them. Therefore, we conclude that it is essential to incorporate specific characteristics that allow for personalization together with the improvement of AI-based support technologies in order to meet each student's unique learning needs. Regardless of its benefits, utilizing AI to create such tools has several limits, which are covered below.

22.7.1 DRAWBACKS OF EXISTING AI TOOLS FOR EDUCATING CHILDREN WITH ASD, ADHD, AND DYSLEXIA

Public databases are few, since it is difficult to collect information from kids with specific NDDs, as they often have trouble remaining still. There is also a dearth of information on the severity of such illnesses. Creating personalized AI solutions for such students can be difficult because many youngsters have complicated comorbidities.

22.8 PROPOSAL FOR A FUTURE AI TOOL

Deep learning techniques are used to create a special cloud-based model or application-based tool which allows for personalization and works as a support for tutors who help students study. To create the personalized model, a sizable amount of data containing input features like facial appearance, pictures, speech signals, medical information, age, sex, hereditary history, etc. are utilized. The trained deep learning model, stored on a cloud server, will receive data collected from each individual user. The model will then be capable of accurately estimating the individual's educational needs and delivering customized training to meet individual goals. Additionally, regionalization and customer confidentiality techniques will be integrated with the suggested tool. The suggested artificial intelligence tool for individualized education is displayed in Figure 22.6.

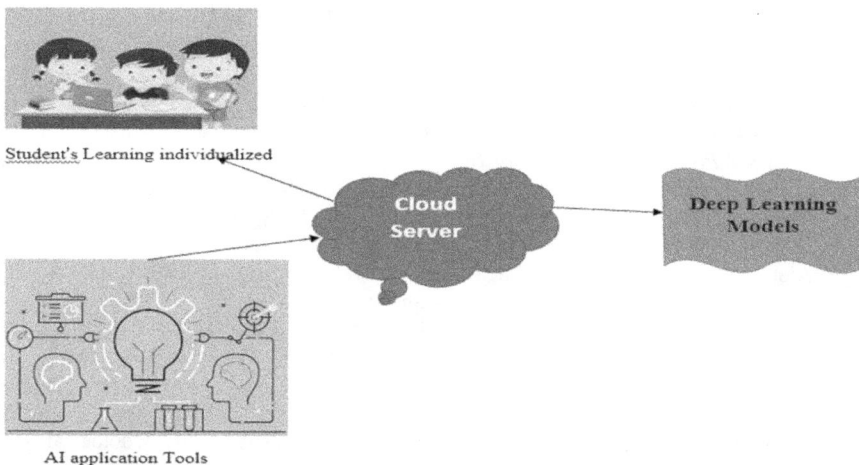

FIGURE 22.6 Proposed AI tool for individualized learning

22.9 CONCLUSION

Despite being in their infancy, supported tools have been offered to address the educational demands of the kids who are suffering from prevalent NDDs like ADHD, dyslexia, and ASDs. The popular tools discussed in previously published works about AI utilized in this context were ASD-centric. For kids with a variety of NDDs, it is obvious that an extra effort has to be made to create and evaluate assistive devices. According to research conducted so far, AI-assisted tools have a beneficial impact on students' learning, are applicable to educators, parents, special educational teachers, and psychoanalysts, and can be easily used in these settings. According to reports, AI techniques help children with learning challenges to reach their unique learning objectives with the help of AI tools. As was discussed, our review found that the current AI support tools have several limitations. For instance, the AI technologies described here are not cloud-based, which limits their capacity to offer real-time recommendations for customized learning. Digital apps with AI-based technologies could be a big leap in providing NDD-affected persons with individualized specialist instruction and learning in real time.

REFERENCES

1. Leitner, Y. (2014 April 29). The Co-Occurrence of Autism and Attention Deficit Hyperactivity Disorder in Children - What Do We Know? *Frontiers in Human Neuroscience*, 8, 268. doi: 10.3389/fnhum.2014.00268. PMID: 24808851. PMCID: PMC4010758.
2. Fucà, E., et al. (2023). Psychiatric Comorbidities in Children and Adolescents with High-Functioning Autism Spectrum Disorder: A Study on Prevalence, Distribution and Clinical Features in an Italian Sample. *Journal of Clinical Medicine*, 12(2), 677.
3. Praveena, K. N., & Mahalakshmi, R. (2022). A Survey on Early Prediction of Autism Spectrum Disorder Using Supervised Machine Learning Methods. *HWWE 2020: Technology Enabled Ergonomic Design*. Design Science and Innovation. Springer, Singapore.
4. Dinu, L. et al. (2023). The Effects of Different Exercise Approaches on Attention Deficit Hyperactivity Disorder in Adults: A Randomised Controlled Trial. *Behavioral Sciences*, 13(2), 129.
5. Nouri, A., & Tabanfar, Z. (2023). Detection of ADHD Disorder in Children Using Layer-Wise Relevance Propagation and Convolutional Neural Network: An EEG Analysis. *Frontiers in Biomedical Technologies*, 10(4).
6. Cook, J. L., & Robinson, G. E. (2023). Comparative Genomics and the Roots of Human Behavior. *Trends in Cognitive Sciences*, 27(3), 230–232 ISSN 1364-6613, https://doi.org /10.1016/j.tics.2022.12.012.
7. Alothaim, S. S. (2023) The Effectiveness of Transition to School for Children with Autism Spectrum Disorder (ASD) *A Systematic Review* 12(3).
8. Jamolovna, A. A. (2023). Development of Intellectual Algorithms and Software Tools (Artificial Intelligence) for the English Language Learners. *Nexus: Journal of Advances Studies of Engineering Science*, 2(3), 22–24.
9. Barletta, V. S., Caruso, F., Di Mascio, T., & Piccinno, A. (2023). Serious Games for Autism Based on Immersive Virtual Reality: A Lens on Methodological and Technological Challenges. In *International Conference in Methodologies and intelligent Systems for Techhnology Enhanced Learning* (pp. 181–195). Springer, Cham.

10. Mutini, L. A., & Bakar, N. A. (2023). The Role of Inclusive Schools in Developing Social Interactions of Children With Special Needs (Autism). *Jurnal Pendidikan dan Konseling (JPDK)*, 5(1), 2522–2529.
11. Quinn, A. (2023). Expanding Autism Treatment Through Social Robotics: Prospective Solutions in Clinical Therapy (Doctoral dissertation, Azusa Pacific University).
12. Zhanatkyzy, A., Telisheva, Z., Amirova, A., Rakhymbayeva, N., & Sandygulova, A. (2023, March). Multi-Purposeful Activities for Robot-Assisted Autism Therapy, What Works Best for Children's Social Outcomes? *Academic Medicine/IEEE International Conference on Human-Robot Interaction*, 2023, 34–43.

Index

For Product Safety Concerns and Information please contact our EU
representative GPSR@taylorandfrancis.com
Taylor & Francis Verlag GmbH, Kaufingerstraße 24, 80331 München, Germany

www.ingramcontent.com/pod-product-compliance
Lightning Source LLC
Chambersburg PA
CBHW060425220326
41598CB00021BA/2289